DRUG T

NATIONAL HEAI
ENGLAND AN

NOVEMBER 2000

*Compiled on behalf of the Department of Health
by the Prescription Pricing Authority*

London: The Stationery Office

Technical Specifications
are available singly from:

The Department of Health
Room 168
Richmond House
79 Whitehall
London SW1A 2NS

ISBN 0 11 782027 X
ISSN 0962 3582

TO: General Medical Practitioners, Pharmacy Contractors, Appliance Contractors (Excluding Drug Stores)

PREFACE
AMENDMENTS TO THE DRUG TARIFF
NOVEMBER 2000

1. Pursuant to Regulation 18(1) of the National Health Service (Pharmaceutical Services) Regulations 1992, the Secretary of State for Health as respects England and the National Assembly for Wales as respects Wales has amended the Drug Tariff with effect from 1 November 2000.

2. Please note that you are now being supplied each month with the Drug Tariff which incorporates all amendments to date. All entries showing a change in price are not specifically included in this preface but are indicated in the Drug Tariff by ∇ for price reduction and ∆ for price increase; changes to the t e x t relating to code, product description, or the inclusion of a new product are indicated by a vertical line in the margin.

3. While every effort is made to ensure that each monthly publication of the Drug Tariff includes all amendments made by the Secretary of State and the National Assembly for Wales to the price applicable to the relevant period, the need to observe printing deadlines sometimes defeats those efforts. Any omitted amendments will be effective from the date on which they came into force, even if publication of the details is unavoidably delayed.

4. Contractors should note the size of **Cavity Dressing Sorbalgon T** in **Part IXA - Wound Management Dressing** is **30cm/2g** not 32cm/2g as previously stated.

5. Contractors should note the **deletion** of Clindamycin Oral Suspension, Paediatric, DPF and Oxytetracycline Capsules, BP from **Part XVIIA - Dental Prescribing**. Also various entries which were formerly 'DPF' now read 'BP'.

6. **CHANGES TO NOVEMBER 2000 DRUG TARIFF**

6.1 Additions to November 2000 Drug Tariff

    6.1.1 **Part VIII - Basic Prices of Drugs**

Page 54

Chlorpromazine Tablets BP, 25mg	* 28		96p	Category C (Norton)

Page 69

Indomethacin Capsules BP, 50mg	* 28		81p	Category A

Page 85

Sodium Bicarbonate Tablets 600mg	* 56		112p	Category C (Norton)

* This pack size only (others already included)

    6.1.2 **Part IXA - Appliances**

Page 104 -Short Stretch Compresssion Bandage

Actiban	8cm x 5cm	300p
	10cm x 5cm	322p
	12cm x 5cm	392p

Page 110 - Nèlaton Catheter ('ordinary' cylindrical Catheter)

Astra Tech LoFric		Per pack of 25
(Female 15cm) (980800-981400)	8-14 gauges	3000p

Page 145 - Hypodermic Equipment
Ⓧ Resusable Pens

	Cartridge Size	Dial up unit dose	
Autopen			
(Owen Mumford)	3.0ml	1 unit (1-21 units)	1396p

Page 148 - Lubricating Jelly

Ⓧ Sutherland Lubricating Jelly (sterile)	5g sachet	18p
	42g tube	124p
	82g tube	194p

Page 154 - Saliva Stimulating Tablet

Ⓧ *SST* Saliva Stimulating Tablets	container of 100	486p

6. CHANGES TO NOVEMBER 2000 DRUG TARIFF - cont

6.1 Additions to November 2000 Drug Tariff - cont

Page 162 - Tapeless Dressing Holders

Ⓧ Breast Dressing Holder	petite	500p
	small	620p
	medium	680p
	large	800p
Ⓧ Facial Dressing Holder	small	408p
	large	468p
Ⓧ Neck Dressing Holder	one size	450p
Ⓧ T-Vest Dressing Holder	small	678p
	medium	803p
	large	873p
	extra large	950p

Tapeless IV Holders

Ⓧ Tapeless Arm IV Holder	small	230p
	medium	270p
Ⓧ Tapeless Hand IV Holder	small	220p
	medium	225p
	large	245p

Page 163 - Tracheostomy and Laryngectomy Appliances

Ⓧ Tapeless Tracheostomy Tube Holder	621	280p

6.1.3 Part IXB - Incontinence Appliances

Page 169 - Catheter Valves
L.I.N.C Medical Systems Ltd
S   CareVent Duo Catheter Valve   08.9801   5   1166p

Page 175 - Incontinence Sheaths
Manfred Sauer
⊗ K + ICS Sheath (plus 5 Sheath tip connectors) have speical removable tips which enable the sheath to be expanded over the penis with a special sheath expander tool, to allow for clean intermittent self catheterisation (see Tubing and Accessories section of this publication for Manfred Sauer Sheath Expander order no. 100.01).

18mm	103.18	30	4450p
20mm	103.20	30	4450p
22mm	103.22	30	4450p
24mm	103.24	30	4450p
26mm	103.26	30	4450p
28mm	103.28	30	4450p
30mm	103.30	30	4450p
32mm	103.32	30	4450p
35mm	103.35	30	4450p
37mm	103.37	30	4450p
40mm	103.40	30	4450p

S   These Catheter Valves are supplied sterile
⊗   Non-adhesive sheath without liner

6.   **CHANGES TO NOVEMBER 2000 DRUG TARIFF** - cont

6.1   **Additions to November 2000 Drug Tariff** - cont

Page 194 - Tubing and Accessories
Manfred Sauer

K + ICS Sheath Expander	100.01	1	6317p

(can only be used to expand Manfred Sauer K + ICS Sheaths over the penis to allow for clean intermittant self catheterisation - see Incontinence Sheaths section of this publication for Manfred Sauer K + ICS Sheaths, order no. 103.nn).

K + ICS Sheath Tips	100.05	10	1577p

(can only be used with Manfred Sauer K + ICS Sheaths - see Incontinence Sheaths section of this publication for Manfred Sauer K + ICS sheaths, order no. 103.nn).

6.1.4   **Part IXC - Stoma Appliances**

Page 229 - Bag Closures
Dansac Ltd

Opaque Longer Soft Wire Ties	095-02	50	600p

Page 262 - Colostomy Bags
Oakmed Ltd
   Option-Mini Pouch with Filter and Soft Covering to both sides
     Opaque

cut to fit 10mm - 50mm		1110k	30	5349p

   Option-Colostomy wth Filter and Soft Covering to both sides
     Opaque

starter hole	20mm	0320k	30	6048p
	25mm	0325k	30	6048p
	30mm	0330k	30	6048p
	35mm	0335k	30	6048p
	40mm	0340k	30	6048p
	45mm	0345k	30	6048p
	50mm	0350k	30	6048p
	55mm	0355k	30	6048p
	60mm	0360k	30	6048p

   Option-Colostomy Plus with Filter and Soft Covering to both sides
     Opaque

starter hole	20mm	0420k	30	6195p
	25mm	0425k	30	6195p
	30mm	0430k	30	6195p
	35mm	0435k	30	6195p
	40mm	0440k	30	6195p
	45mm	0445k	30	6195p
	50mm	0450k	30	6195p
	55mm	0455k	30	6195p
	60mm	0460k	30	6195p

6.   CHANGES TO NOVEMBER 2000 DRUG TARIFF - cont

6.1   Additions to November 2000 Drug Tariff - cont

Page 262 - Colostomy Bags
Oakmed Ltd
Option-Colostomy Maxi with Filter and Soft Covering to one side
Clear

cut to fit	20mm-100mm	0720k	30	6564p

Option-Colostomy Maxi with Filter and Soft Covering to both sides
Opaque

cut to fit	20mm-100mm	0820k	30	6698p

Page 302 - Ileostomy (Drainable) Bags
Oakmed Ltd
Option-Ileostomy Midi with Filter and Soft Covering to one side
Clear

starter hole	20mm	3220k	30	5897p
	25mm	3225k	30	5897p
	30mm	3230k	30	5897p
	35mm	3235k	30	5897p
	40mm	3240k	30	5897p
	45mm	3245k	30	5897p
	50mm	3250k	30	5897p
	55mm	3255k	30	5897p
	60mm	3260k	30	5897p

Opaque

starter hole	20mm	3320k	30	5897p
	25mm	3325k	30	5897p
	30mm	3330k	30	5897p
	35mm	3335k	30	5897p
	40mm	3340k	30	5897p
	45mm	3345k	30	5897p
	50mm	3350k	30	5897p
	55mm	3355k	30	5897p
	60mm	3360k	30	5897p

Option - Ileostomy with Filter and Soft Covering to one side
Clear

starter hole	20mm	3020k	30	6235p
	25mm	3025k	30	6235p
	30mm	3030k	30	6235p
	35mm	3035k	30	6235p
	40mm	3040k	30	6235p
	45mm	3045k	30	6235p
	50mm	3050k	30	6235p
	55mm	3055k	30	6235p
	60mm	3060k	30	6235p

6. CHANGES TO NOVEMBER 2000 DRUG TARIFF - cont

6.1 Additions to November 2000 Drug Tariff - cont

Page 302 - Ileostomy (Drainable) Bags

Oakmed Ltd

Option - Ileostomy with Filter and Soft Covering to one side

Opaque

starter hole				
	20mm	3120k	30	6235p
	25mm	3125k	30	6235p
	30mm	3130k	30	6235p
	35mm	3135k	30	6235p
	40mm	3140k	30	6235p
	45mm	3145k	30	6235p
	50mm	3150k	30	6235p
	55mm	3155k	30	6235p
	60mm	3160k	30	6235p

Page 303

Oakmed Ltd

Option-Ileostomy Midi with Filter and Soft Covering to both sides

Opaque

starter hole				
	20mm	4320k	30	6182p
	25mm	4325k	30	6182p
	30mm	4330k	30	6182p
	35mm	4335k	30	6182p
	40mm	4340k	30	6182p
	45mm	4345k	30	6182p
	50mm	4350k	30	6182p
	55mm	4355k	30	6182p
	60mm	4360k	30	6182p

Option-Ileosomy with Filter and Soft Covering to both sides

Opaque

starter hole				
	20mm	4120k	30	6512p
	25mm	4125k	30	6512p
	30mm	4130k	30	6512p
	35mm	4135k	30	6512p
	40mm	4140k	30	6512p
	45mm	4145k	30	6512p
	50mm	4150k	30	6512p
	55mm	4155k	30	6512p
	60mm	4160k	30	6512p

Page 329 - Skin Protectors (Wafers, Blankets, Foam Pads, Washers)

Dansac Ltd

Dansac Gx-tra Seals

Washers

20mm (50mm outer diameter) 725-20	30	3731p
30mm (60mm outer diameter) 725-30	30	3731p
40mm (70mm outer diameter) 725-40	30	3731p
50mm (80mm outer diameter) 725-50	30	3731p

(25 packs already available)

6.   CHANGES TO NOVEMBER 2000 DRUG TARIFF - cont

6.1   Additions to November 2000 Drug Tariff - cont

Page 333 - Stoma Caps/Dressings
Oakmed Ltd
Option Stoma Cap with Soft Covering and Filter
Opaque
cut to fit   20mm-50mm   1420k   50   5498p

Page 354 - Two Piece Ostomy Systems
Oakmed Ltd
Option Range
Option Flange
                    50mm   F500   5   1310p
                    70mm   F700   5   1310p

Colostomy with Filter and Soft Covering to one side
Clear for:-   50mm flange   CB50K   30   3256p

Colostomy with Filter and Soft Covering to both sides
Opaque for:- 50mm flange   CA50K   30   3295p

Colostomy Plus with Filter and Soft Covering to one side
Clear for:-   70mm flange   CD70K   30   3309p

Colostomy Plus with Filter and Soft Covering to both sides
Opaque for:- 70mm flange   CC70K   30   3348p

Ileostomy Midi with Filter and Soft Covering to one side
Clear for:-   50mm flange   IG50K   30   3309p
              70mm flange   IG70K   30   3309p

Ileostomy with Filter and Soft Covering to one side
Clear for:-   50mm flange   IB50K   30   3309p
              70mm flange   IB70K   30   3309p

Ileostomy Midi with Filter and Soft Covering to both sides
Opaque for:- 50mm flange   ID50K   30   3329p
              70mm flange   ID70K   30   3329p

Ileostomy with Filter and Soft Covering to both sides
Opaque for:- 50mm flange   IA50K   30   3329p
              70mm flange   IA70K   30   3329p

6. **CHANGES TO NOVEMBER 2000 DRUG TARIFF** - cont

6.2 **Other Changes to November 2000 Drug Tariff**

6.2.1 **Part VIII - Basic Prices of Drugs**

Page 78

Oxprenolol Tablets BP, 40mg		100	840p	Category A
now reads				
Oxprenolol Tablets BP, 40mg		56	259p	Category C *(Trasicor)*
Oxprenolol Tablets BP, 80mg		100	1260p	Category A
now reads				
Oxprenolol Tablets BP, 80mg		56	517p	Category C *(Trasicor)*

6.2.2 **Part IXA - Appliances**

Page 113 - Catheters, Urethral Sterile
(c) Foley Catheter - 2 Way
(ii) a For Long Term use - Adult

		Balloon Size/ml	Gauge (Ch)	Per Pack of 1
Porges Folysil all Silicone Catheter				
(male)	(AA74)	10	12-16	565p
(male)	(AA71)	10	12-18	565p
now reads				
(male) (open ended)	(AA74)	10	12-18	565p
(male)	(AA71)	10	12-24	565p

CONTENTS

11/2000

Page Commencing Cont

		Page Commencing
Preface		(i)
Definitions		2
Part I	Requirements for the Supply of Drugs, Appliances and Chemical Reagents .	3
Part II	Requirements enabling payment to be made for Drugs, Appliances and Chemical Reagents	5
Part IIIA	Professional Fees (Pharmacy Contractors)	15
IIIB	Scale of Fees (Appliance Contractors)	29
Part IV	Containers	31
Part V	Deduction Scale	33
Part VIA	Payment for additional professional services	37
Part VIB	Scale of On-cost allowances (Appliance Contractors)	39
Part VII	Drugs with Commonly Used Pack Sizes	41
Part VIII	Basic Prices of Drugs covered by Part II Clause 8A	43
Part IX	Approved list of Appliance -notes	93
	List of Technical Specifications	95
Part IXA	Approved list of Appliances	97
Part IXB	Incontinence Section including list of components and accessories	165
Part IXC	Stoma Section including lists of components and accessories	223
Part IXR	Approved List of Chemical Reagents	383
	Appendix	391
Part X	Domiciliary Oxygen Therapy Service	393
Part XI	Additional Pharmacist Access Services (formerly Rota Service)	413
Part XII	Essential Small Pharmacies Scheme	415
Part XIII	Payment in respect of Pre-Registration Trainees	419
Part XIVA	Advice to Care Homes	421
Part XIVB	Patient Medication Records	423
Part XIVC	Reward Scheme - Fraudulent Prescription Forms	425
Part XV	Borderline Substances	427
Part XVI	Prescription Charges	483
Part XVIIA	Secretary of State for Health as respects England and the National Assembly for Wales as respects Wales' List of Preparations Prescribable on FP10(D)	495
Part XVIIB	Secretary of State for Health as respects England and the National Assembly for Wales as respects Wales' List of Preparations Prescribable on FP10(CN) and FP10(PN)	497
Part XVIIIA	Drugs and other substances not to be prescribed under the NHS Pharmaceutical Services	501
Part XVIIIB	Drugs to be prescribed in certain circumstances under the NHS Pharmaceutical Services	531
Part XVIIIC	Criteria notified under the Transparency Directive	533
Index		535

a.   Except where the context otherwise requires, the terms to which a meaning is assigned by the Regulations or the Terms of Service have the same meaning in this Tariff.

b.   The term contractor has the same meaning as chemist as defined in the Regulations.

c.   A pharmacy contractor is a person with whom the Health Authority has made arrangements for the provision of pharmaceutical services in respect of the supply of drugs, appliances and chemical reagents.

d.   An appliance contractor is a person with whom the Health Authority has made arrangements for the provision of pharmaceutical services so far as it relates to the supply of appliances included within Part IXA/B/C of this Tariff.

e.   A drug store contractor is a person with whom the Health Authority has made arrangements for the provision of pharmaceutical services so far as it relates to the supply of medicinal products on a general sales list under or by virtue of the provisions of the Medicines Act.

f.   The term persons includes a body of persons corporate or unincorporate.

g.   The term Pricing Authority means, as the case may require, the Prescription Pricing Authority or the Bro Taf Health Authority.

h.   The term appliances as used in this Tariff includes dressings.

NB   In the preparation of this Tariff the Secretary of State for Health and the National Assembly for Wales have consulted the Pharmaceutical Services Negotiating Committee.

CLAUSE 1   DRUGS

Any drug included in this Tariff or in the British National Formulary including the Nurse Prescribers' Formulary, Dental Practitioner's Formulary, European Pharmacopoeia, British Pharmacopoeia or the British Pharmaceutical Codex, supplied as part of pharmaceutical services, must comply with the standard or formula specified therein unless the prescriber has indicated to the contrary. Any drug supplied which is not so included must be of a grade or quality not lower than that ordinarily used for medicinal purposes.

CLAUSE 2   APPLIANCES

The only appliances which may be supplied as part of the pharmaceutical services are those listed in Part IXA/B/C, and Part X (see Clause 4 below), of the Tariff and which comply with the specifications therein. The items within Part IXA which are **not** prescribable on Forms FP10(CN) and FP10(PN) are annotated ⊗

CLAUSE 3   CHEMICAL REAGENTS

The only chemical reagents which may be supplied as part of the pharmaceutical services are those listed in Part IXR of the Tariff. The items within Part IXR which are **not** prescribable on forms FP10(CN) and FP10(PN) are annotated ⊗

CLAUSE 4   DOMICILIARY OXYGEN THERAPY SERVICE

The requirements for the supply of domiciliary oxygen and its associated appliances together with the arrangements for reimbursement of those contractors included on the Health Authority's lists of contractors authorised to provide this service, are set out in Part X of the Tariff.

This Page Is Intentionally Blank

II

CLAUSE 5   CLAIMS FOR PAYMENT

Contractors shall endorse prescription forms as required in Clause 9 (Endorsement Requirements) of this Tariff. Contractors shall sort and despatch forms in such a manner as the Health Authority may direct. Contractors shall despatch the forms together with the appropriate claim form not later than the fifth day of the month following that in which the supply was made.

CLAUSE 6   CALCULATION OF PAYMENTS

A.   **Pharmacy Contractors**

Payment for services provided by pharmacy contractors in respect of the supply of drugs, appliances and chemical reagents supplied against prescriptions at each separate place of business shall comprise:-

(i)   (a)   The total of the prices of the drugs, appliances and chemical reagents so supplied calculated in accordance with the requirements of this Tariff.

LESS

*(b)   An amount, based on the total of the prices at (i)(a) above, calculated from the table at Part V ("Deduction Scale").

AND

(ii)   The appropriate professional fee as set out in Part IIIA

AND

(iii)   The allowance for containers and specified measuring devices as set out in Part IV.

*NOTE

No deduction will be made in respect of prescriptions for items listed on Page 10, 11 and 12 for which the contractor has not been able to obtain a discount:

CLAUSE 6 - cont

B.   **Appliance Contractors**

Payment for services provided by appliance contractors in respect of the supply of appliances so supplied against prescriptions at each separate place of business, shall comprise:-

(i)   The total of the prices of the appliances, calculated in accordance with Part IXA/B/C

PLUS

(ii)   An amount based on the number of prescriptions against which supply is made each month, calculated from the Table at Part VIB ("Oncost Allowance" scale) and applied to the total of the prices at (i) above.

PROVIDED THAT

(a)   Where prescription forms are received by the Pricing Authority from two or more contractors whose names are separately entered on the pharmaceutical list for the supply of appliances only in respect of the provision of services at the same place of business, all such prescription forms shall be aggregated for the purpose of the calculation as at (ii) above and the rate so calculated shall be applied to the total of the prices calculated in accordance with (i) above in respect of the prescriptions received from each of those persons.

(b)   A contractor's name shall not be entered on the Pharmaceutical List separately for the same place of business in respect of (1) the supply of appliances, (2) the supply of drugs and appliances, or (3) the supply of drugs, except in the case of a contractor for whom separate entries on the Pharmaceutical List relating to the same place of business were allowed prior to the first day of November 1961.

(c)   Where a contractor's name is entered on the Pharmaceutical List in respect of the provision of services at more than one place of business, the calculation as at (ii) above shall be made separately in relation to the total of the prices calculated in accordance with (i) above in respect of prescriptions received in respect of the services provided at each place of business.

AND

(iii)   The appropriate fees as set out in Part IIIB

C.   **Drug Store Contractors**

Payments to drug store contractors for pharmaceutical services relating to drugs supplied against prescriptions at each separate place of business are made on the same basis as payments to pharmacy contractors set out in Clause 6A (i)(a), plus an on-cost of 10.5% and attract the fee set out in Part IIIA(1) and the container allowances set out in Part IV.

CLAUSE 7   **PAYMENTS FOR DRUGS, APPLIANCES AND CHEMICAL REAGENTS**

A.   The price on which payment is based for a quantity of a drug, appliance or chemical reagent supplied is calculated proportionately from the basic price (see Clause 8 - Basic Price).

B.   Subject to the provisions of Clause 10 (Quantity to be supplied) payment will be calculated on the basis that the exact quantity ordered by the prescriber has been supplied.

C.   Where a prescription form has been returned to the contractor for endorsement or elucidation and it is returned to the Pricing Authority unendorsed, or incompletely endorsed, or without further explanation, then the price for the drug, appliance or chemical reagent which it orders shall be determined by the Secretary of State for Health and the National Assembly for Wales.

D.   If a contractor's overall supply of a product appears to justify payment being based on the cost of a larger size than that normally required pursuant to orders on prescription forms and notice has been given to that effect to the contractor, the basic price will be the price of that larger size, the prescription form being deemed to have been endorsed.

CLAUSE 8   **BASIC PRICE**

A.   The basic price for those drugs, appliances and chemical reagents ordered by a name, or a synonym of that name, included in Parts VIII or IX shall be the price listed in the Drug Tariff.

B.   The basic price for a drug which is not listed in part VIII of the Tariff shall be the list price, for supplying to contractors, of the pack size to be used for a prescription for that quantity, published by the manufacturer, wholesaler or supplier. In default of any such list price, the price shall be determined by the Secretary of State for Health and the National Assembly for Wales.

CLAUSE 9   **ENDORSEMENT REQUIREMENTS**

A.   Contractors shall endorse prescription forms for drugs, appliances and chemical reagents listed in this Tariff as required by this Clause and when so required by the provisions of Part II Clauses 10 (Quantity to be Supplied) and 11 (Broken Bulk), Part III (Fees) and Note 2 to Part IXA/B/C (Appliances).

B.   Every other prescription form shall be endorsed by the contractor with the pack size from which its order was supplied and, if the order is in pharmacopoeial or 'generic' form, with the brand name or the name of the manufacturer or wholesaler from whom the supply was purchased. Where additional specific endorsement is necessary contractors shall endorse prescription forms when so required by the provisions of Part II Clauses 10 (Quantity to be Supplied) and 11 (Broken Bulk), Part III (Fees).

C.   Where insufficient information is available to enable the Pricing Authority process the prescription, the form shall be returned to the contractor who shall endorse the prescription form with the information requested.

D.   Where a contractor supplies a quantity at variance with that ordered, ie under the provisions set out in Clause 10 (Quantity to be Supplied), the prescription shall be endorsed with the quantity supplied. An exception to this requirement is where a drug is supplied in a Calendar Pack and the quantity ordered differs from that pack. In such cases and in the absence of an endorsement to the contrary, the contractor will be deemed to have supplied the quantity available in the nearest number of packs or sub-packs to that ordered.

CLAUSE 10   QUANTITY TO BE SUPPLIED

A.   Subject to the requirements of the Weights and Measures (Equivalents for Dealing with Drugs)
Regulation, 1970, with regard to the supply in metric quantities of orders expressed in imperial
quantities, payment will normally be calculated on the basis that the exact quantity ordered by
the prescriber has been supplied, except only of those preparations referred to in B and C
below:

B.   **Drugs and Chemical Reagents in Special Containers.**

Where the quantity ordered by the prescriber does not coincide with that of an original pack and
the drug or chemical reagent is:

(i)   Sterile

(ii)   Effervescent or hygroscopic, or

(iii)   (a)   Liquid preparations for addition to bath water

(b)   Coal Tar preparations

(c)   Viscous external preparations

(iv)   Packed in a castor, collapsible tube, drop-bottle, pressurised aerosol, puffer pack, roll-
on-bottle, sachet, shaker, spray, squeeze pack, container with an integral means of
application, or any other container from which it is not practicable to dispense the
exact quantity:

the contractor shall supply in the special container or containers the quantity nearest to that
ordered and endorse the prescription form with the number and size of those containers.
Although payment will normally be based on the quantity nearest to that ordered, some items
are available in a larger size pack or container than that normally required pursuant to orders
on prescription forms. Where the amount ordered on a prescription form, or the frequency of
supply, justifies supply from such larger size pack or container, payment will be based on the
cost of that larger size in the absence of endorsement.

C.   **Manufacturers' Calendar Packs (including Oral Contraceptives)**

(i)   A manufacturer's calender pack is a blister or strip pack showing the days of the
week or month against each of the several units in the pack. Although payment is
normally based on the number of packs or sub-packs nearest to the quantity ordered
(see Clause 9D (Endorsement Requirements)) there may be occasions when, in the
pharmacist's professional opinion, the prescriber's intention is that an exact quantity
should be supplied. In such cases the contractor should supply accordingly and
endorse the prescription form with the quantity supplied. Payment will then be based
on the quantity shown by the endorsement.

(ii)   Payment for a Manufacturer's Calendar Pack or Original Pack will be based on the
smallest pack size available when one or a number of such packs are ordered. Some
original packs contain more than one monthly cycle and prescriptions ordering three
or more such packs will be returned to the contractor for clarification.

*   Products included in Clause 10B(iii) are listed on page 13 and 14.

CLAUSE 11   BROKEN BULK

A.   This clause applies to drugs, incontinence and stoma appliances in Part IXB and IXC and chemical reagents other than items supplied in special containers covered by Clause 10B.

B.   When the quantity ordered on a prescription form is other than the minimum quantity the manufacturer, wholesaler or supplier is prepared to supply and the contractor, having purchased such minimum quantity as may be necessary to supply the quantity ordered cannot readily dispose of the remainder, payment will be made for the whole of the quantity purchased. Subsequent prescriptions, received during the next six months, will be deemed to have been supplied from the remainder and no further payment will be made to drug costs other than fees and container allowances until that remainder has been used up. Thereafter contractors must endorse prescription forms to indicate when a claim for payment is being made.

CLAUSE 12   OUT OF POCKET EXPENSES

Where, in exceptional circumstances, out-of-pocket expenses have been incurred in obtaining a drug, appliance or chemical reagent other than those priced in Part VIII Category A, Part IXA and Part IXR of the Tariff and not required to be frequently supplied by the contractor, or where out-of-pocket expenses have been incurred in obtaining oxygen from a manufacturer, wholesaler or supplier specially for supply against a prescription, payment of the amount by which such expenses on any occasion exceed 10p may be made where the contractor sends a claim giving full particulars to the Pricing Authority with the appropriate prescription form.

CLAUSE 13   DRUG PREPARATIONS REQUIRING RECONSTITUTION FROM GRANULES OR POWDER

A.   This clause applies to a drug preparation requiring reconstitution from granules or powder by the contractor and resulting in a liquid of limited stability.

B.   When the quantity reconstituted from an original pack or packs is unavoidably greater than the quantity ordered, and it has not been possible for the contractor to use the remainder for or towards supplying against another prescription (see Clause 11 - Broken Bulk) payment, which attracts the standard professional fee (but see also Part IIIA, E), will be calculated from the Basic Price of the preparation and will be based on the nearest pack or number of packs necessary to cover the quantity ordered.

ZERO DISCOUNT LIST A

Contractors who have not received discount in respect of the following products need not endorse the prescription "ZD". The prescription price reimbursement will have no discount deduction applied.

Actinac Treatment Pack
Air Cylinders (Medical Grade)
Alexan Ampoule
Alkeran Tablets
Alternative Medicines
Ametop Gel
Amphocil I/V Infusion (Zeneca)
Ativan Injection 4mg/1ml Ampoule
Avonex Injection (dist. Caremark)
Benefix
Betaferon (Schering)
Bismuth Subnitrate and Iodoform Paste
     BPC 1954
Borderline Substance Foods*
Britaject Ampoule (Britannia Pharmaceuticals)
Britaject Pen (Britannia Pharmaceuticals)
Calciferol Injection
     300,000u/1ml and 600,000u/2ml
Calcisorb Powder Sachets
Calsynar
CAPD Fluids
Carbon Dioxide J-size Cylinders
     (L.H. Medical)
Caverject Injection 40 microgram only
Chloramphenicol Eye Drops BP, 0.5% w/v
Chloromycetin Redidrops 0.5%
Choragon Injection (Ferring Pharmaceuticals)
Clomid Tablets (Hoechst Marion Roussel)
Combivir Tablets
Controlled Drugs in schedules 1,2 and 3 of the
     Misuse of Drugs Regulations 1985
Covermark Products listed in Drug Tariff*
     (Covermark)
Cuplex Gel
Cystagon Capsules
Cytosar Injection (Pharmacia & Upjohn)
Daktacort Cream
Dalivit Drops
DaunoXome Infusion (Nexstar)
DDAVP Injection
DDAVP Intranasal
Debrisoquine Tablets (Cambridge Laboratories)
Dentomycin Gel 2%
Dermablend Products listed in Drug Tariff*
     (Brodie and Stone)
Dermacolor Products listed in Drug Tariff*
     (Charles H Fox)
Desferal Injection 500mg
Desmopressin Intranasal Solution BP,
     100 micrograms/ml
Diprivan Injection (Zeneca)
Drugs available only on a named patient basis
Eldisine Injection
Eprex (Janssen Cilag)
Fertiral (Hoechst Marion Roussel)
Fibro-Vein Injection

Fortovase Capsules
Fragmin Injection 12,500iu
Fungizone Intravenous
Fungizone Tissue Culture (Bristol-Myers Squibb)
Gammabulin (Baxter)
Genotropin
Genotropin Kabiquick
Genotropin Kabivial
Genotropin Miniquick
GlucaGen Kit
Glucagon Injection
Gonadotraphon LH Injection
     (Ferring Pharmaceuticals)
Granocyte Injection (Rhone-Poulenc Rorer)
G.T.O. Oil (S.H.S.)
Haemate
Healonid Injection (Pharmacia & Upjohn)
Helixate
Heminevrin 0.8% Infusion
Heminevrin Syrup
Histoacryl Tissue Adhesive
Homoeopathic Products
     (including Iscador Injection (Weleda))
HRF Injection (Monmouth)
Humatrope
Hydrocortisone and Miconazole Cream
Hypostop
Insulin
Insulin, Human
Intron - A Injection (Schering Plough)
Isocarboxazid Tablets
Kabiglobulin (KabiVitrum)
Keromask Products listed in Drug Tariff *
     (Innoxa)
Ketovite Liquid
Ketovite Tablets
Kogenate
Latanoprost Eye Drops
Lentaron IM Depot
Leucomax Injection
Leukeran Tablets
Lofepramine Suspension (Rosemont)
Loprazolam Tablets
Lorenzo's Oil (S.H.S.)
Lysuride Tablets (Cambridge Laboratories)
Made to measure elastic hosiery & trusses
Medihaler Ergotamine
Meronem Injection (Zeneca)
Miacalcic Injection
Minims (all preparations)
Monoclate P
Mononine
Multibionta Infusion
Muse Urethral Stick (Astra)

*Part XV

ZERO DISCOUNT LIST A

Contractors who have not received discount in respect of the following products need not endorse the prescription "ZD". The prescription price reimbursement will have no discount deduction applied.

Mustine Hydrochloride Injection 10mg
Mydrilate Solution
Myleran Tablets
Nabilone Capsules 1mg (Cambridge Laboratories)
Nardil Tablets
Natures Own Products
NeoRecormon (formerly Recormon)
NeoRecormon with Syringe
    (formerly Recormon S)
Neosporin Eye Drops
Neupogen (Roche)
Norditropin Pen Set
Norvir Capsules (Abbott)
Norvir Oral Solution (Abbott)
Noxyflex-S
Ocusert Pilo
One-Alpha Drops
One-Alpha Injection
Ophthaine Solution 0.5%
Otosporin Ear Drops
Pancrex Granules
Pancrex V Capsules
Pancrex V 125 Capsules
Pancrex V Forte Tablets
Pancrex V Powder
Pancrex V Tablets
Partobulin Injection
Pavulon Injection 4mg/2ml
Ped-El Injection
Perfan Injection
Pharmorubicin Injection
Phenelzine Tablets 15mg
Phosex Tablets
Pregnyl Injection
Pro-Epanutin Conc for Injection
Prograf Capsules 0.5mg, 1mg & 5mg (Fujisawa)
Prograf Injection 5mg/ml (Fujisawa)
Pulmozyme Ampoule (Roche)
Puregon Injections
Pyopen Injection
Recombinate
Rebif Injection (Serono)
Refacto Injections
Regranex Gel
Replenate
Replenine-VF
Restandol Capsules 40mg
Roferon - A Injection (Roche)
Sandimmun Infusion (Novartis)
Sandimmun Oral Solution (Novartis)
Sandoglobulin (Novartis)
Sandostatin Injection
Sandostatin LAR Injection
Saventrine I.V. Injection
Scoline Injection

Scopaderm TTS Patches
SDV
Simulect Injection
Sno Phenicol
Sno Pilo
Sodium Bicarbonate Intravenous Infusion BP
Somatuline LA Injection (Ipsen)
STD Injection
Synacthen Ampoule
Synacthen Depot Ampoule
Synercid Vials
Syntometrine Injection
Tacrolimus Capsules 0.5mg, 1mg & 5mg
Taxotere Injection
Tenormin Injection (Stuart)
Testosterone Enanthate 250mg/1ml Ampoule
    (Cambridge Laboratories)
Testosterone Undecanoate Capsules 40mg
Tetrabenazine Tablets
Thiotepa Wyeth Lederle Injection
Ticar Injection/Infusion (Link)
Timodine Cream
Tobi
Total Parenteral Nutrition (TPN)
Tracrium Injection
Vaccines
Varidase Combi-pack
Varidase Topical
Veil Products listed in Drug Tariff*
    (Thomas Blake)
Videx Tablets (Bristol-Myers Squibb)
Viraferon Injection (Schering-Plough)
Viramune Tablets
Voltarol Ophtha
Wellferon Injection (Glaxo Wellcome)
Xalatan Eye Drops
Xyloproct Ointment
Xyloproct Suppositories
Zenapax Infusions
Zomacton Injection (Ferring)

*Part XV

ZERO DISCOUNT LIST B

Contractors who have not received discount in respect of the following products should endorse the prescription "ZD". The prescription price reimbursement will then have no discount deduction applied.

Achromycin Ointment 3%
Amyl Nitrite Vitrellae BPC
Aramine Injection 10mg/1ml
Audicort Drops
Aureomycin Cream 3%
Aureomycin Eye Ointment 1%
Aureomycin Ointment 3%
Aveeno Bath Oil, Colloidal Sachets and Cream
Calcitare Injection 160 units
Ceredase
Chlormethiazole Oral Solution BP,
        sugar free 250mg/5ml
Clexane Injection 60mg, 80mg
Co-danthramer Capsules
Co-danthramer Capsules Strong
Co-danthramer Suspension 25/200 in 5ml
Co-danthramer Suspension Strong 75/1000 in 5ml
Co-danthrusate Capsules
Co-danthrusate Suspension
Crixivan Capsules
Cyclopentolate Eye Drops BP, 0.5% and 1% w/v
Cyclosporin Oral Solution
De-capeptyl SR
Desmopressin Nasal Spray 10micrograms
Desmospray Spray
Dysport
Eminase 30 Unit Vial
Eminase IV Injection Pack
Endobulin
Epipen
Ergometrine Injection 500 micrograms/1ml
Estracyt Capsules 140mg
Flolan
Fortum Injection
Furamide Tablets (Knoll)
Gonal-F (Serono)
Hepsal Solution 50iu/5ml
Human Normal Immunoglobulin
Humegon (Organon)
Hyoscine Injection BP,
        400 micrograms/1ml Ampoule
Innohep Injection (Leo)
Intraval Sodium
Isovorin Injection
Kabikinase Injection
Kay Cee L Syrup
Ketalar Injection
Lignocaine Antiseptic Gel
Lignocaine Gel
Magnesium Sulphate Injection 50%
Marcain Preparations
Metrodin High Purity Injection (Serono)
Metrozol
Min-I-Jet

Monoparin Injection
Naprosyn Suppositories 500mg
Naproxen Suppositories 500mg
Norditropin SimpleXx
Normax Suspension
Normegon (Organon)
Orgafol (Organon)
Oxycel Sterilised Gauze Pad
Paracetamol Suppositories 500mg
Pergonal Injection (Serono)
Phenylephrine Eye Drops BP, 10% w/v
Profasi Injection (Serono)
Proleukin Injection
Relefact LH-RH (Hoechst Marion Roussel)
Relefact LH-RH/TRH (Hoechst Marion Roussel)
Ro-A-Vit Ampoule
Saizen Injection 4iu, 10iu, 24iu vials(Serono)
Sandimmun Capsules (Novartis)
Securopen Injection 2g vial
Skin-Cap Preparations (Cheminova)
Sodium Chloride Intravenous Infusion BP,
        0.9% w/v 100ml
Solivito N Solution
Special formulations
Sulphadimidine Tablets BP, 500mg
Surgicel
Sustiva Capsules
Temopen Injection
Tetabulin Injection
Tilarin Nasal Spray
Triclofos Oral Solution BP
Trifluoperazine Syrup 5mg/5ml
Ukidan Injection
Velbe Injection
Vigam Liquid (BPL)
Vitamin A Injection (Cambridge Laboratories)
Vivotif Capsules
Water for Injection 100ml
Xylocaine 2% Adrenaline Injection Cartridge
Xylocaine Adrenaline Injection Vial
Xylotox E80 Injection Cartridge
Zerit Capsules

Products included in Clause 10B(iii) are listed below.
Liquid preparations for external use:

Sub Para	Name	Pack(s)
(c)	Alcoderm Lotion	(200ml)
(a)	Alpha Keri Bath Oil	(240ml and 480ml)
(b)	Alphosyl Lotion	(250ml)
(c)	Alphosyl Shampoo 2 in 1	(125ml and 250ml)
(c)	Ascabiol Emulsion	(100ml)
(a)	Aveeno Bath Oil	(250ml)
(a)	Balneum Bath Oil	(200ml, 500ml and 1000ml)
(a)	Balneum Plus Bath Oil 82.95%/15%	(500ml)
(c)	Betadine Shampoo	(250ml)
(b)	Capasal Therapeutic Shampoo	(250ml)
(c)	Ceanel Concentrate	(50ml, 150ml and 500ml)
(a)	Cetraben Bath Oil	(500ml)
(c)	Dentinox Cradle Cap Shampoo	(125ml)
(a)	Dermalo Bath Emollient	(500ml)
(c)	Dermol 200 Shower Emollient	(200ml)
(c)	Dermol 500 Lotion	(500ml pump)
(c)	Dermol 600 Bath Emollient	(600ml)
(a)	Diprobath Emollient	(500ml)
(a)	E45 Bath Oil	(250ml and 500ml)
(c)	E45 Lotion	(200ml and 500ml pump)
(c)	E45 Wash	(250ml)
(a)	Eurax Dermatological Bath Oil	(200ml)
(a)	Emmolate Bath Oil	(200ml)
(a)	Emulsiderm Emollient	(300ml and 1 litre)
(a)	Epaderm Emollient	(125g)
(b)	Exorex Lotion	(100ml and 250ml)
(b)	Gelcosal Gel	(50g)

(b)	Gelcotar Gel	(50g and 500g)
(b)	Gelcotar Liquid	(150ml and 350ml)
(a)	Hydromol Emollient	(150ml, 350ml and 1 litre)
(c)	Keri Therapeutic Lotion	(190ml and 380ml pump packs)
(a)	Imuderm Therapeutic Oil	(250ml)
(a)	Infaderm Therapeutic Oil	(250ml)
(c)	Lacticare Lotion	(150ml)
(c)	Meted Shampoo	(120ml)
(a)	Oilatum Bath Formula	(150ml and 300ml)
(a)	Oilatum Emollient	(250ml and 500ml)
(a)	Oilatum Emollient, Fragrance Free	(500ml)
(a)	Oilatum Junior Bath Formula	(150ml and 300ml)
(a)	Oilatum Junior Flare-Up Bath Treatment	(150ml)
(a)	Oilatum Plus Emollient	(500ml and 1 litre)
(b)	Pentrax Shampoo	(120ml)
(b)	Polytar AF Liquid	(150ml)
(b)	Polytar Emollient	(350ml and 500ml)
(b)	Polytar Liquid	(150ml and 250ml)
(b)	Polytar Plus (Scalp Cleanser)	(350ml and 500ml)
(b)	Pragmator Cream	(25g and 100g)
(b)	Psorin Ointment	(50g and 100g)
(b)	Psoriderm Bath Emulsion	(200ml)
(b)	Psoriderm Cream	(225ml)
(b)	Psoriderm Scalp Lotion Shampoo	(250ml)
(c)	Quellada-M Cream Shampoo	(40g)
(a)	Quellada-M Liquid (Aqueous)	(50ml and 200ml)
(c)	Quinoderm Lotio-Gel 5%	(30ml)
(c)	Selsun Suspension	(50ml, 100ml and 150ml)
(a)	Ster-Zac Bath Concentrate	(28.5ml)
(b)	T-Gel Shampoo	(125ml and 250ml)
(b)	T-Gel Shampoo Anti-Dandruff	(125ml and 250ml)

See Part II, Clause 6A(ii) (Page 5)

		Fee per prescription P	*Endorsements required by contractors
1.	**ALL PRESCRIPTIONS** (except the Special Fee at 3) attract a Professional Fee with a value of:	97.50 NIL	

IIIA

2.   **ADDITIONAL FEES:**

A.   PREPARATIONS WHEN EXTEMPORANEOUSLY DISPENSED *AND ENDORSED*

(a)   "Extemporaneously dispensed"

		Fee	Endorsement
(i)	Unit dosage forms, eg cachets, capsules, pills, lozenges, pastilles, pessaries, powders	256 per 10 or part thereof	"Extemporaneously dispensed"
(ii)	Liquids being 'special formula preparations'. eg mixtures, lotions, nasal drops (not including dilutions)	155	"Extemporaneously dispensed"
(iii)	Liquid preparations prepared by straight forward dilution (not including reconstitution)	85	"Extemporaneously dispensed"
(iv)	Special formula powders	155	"Extemporaneously dispensed"
(v)	Ointments, creams, pastes being 'special formula preparations' (not including dilutions)	310	"Extemporaneously dispensed"
(vi)	Ointments, creams, pastes prepared by dilution or admixture of standard or proprietary ointments, creams and pastes	155	"Extemporaneously dispensed"

(b)   "Aseptically dispensed"
Preparations when aseptically dispensed (excluding proprietary preparations)

		Fee	Endorsement
(i)	Unit dosage forms, eg injections	1277 per 10 or part thereof	"Aseptically dispensed"
(ii)	Non-unit dosage forms, eg Eye Drops	767	"Aseptically dispensed"

(c)   "Extemporaneously sterilised"
Liquids, semi-solids, solids prepared with a BP sterilization process   767   "Extemporaneously sterilised"

*   See page 17

See Part II, Clause 6A(ii) (Page 5)

		Fee per prescription P	*Endorsements required by contractors
2.	**ADDITIONAL FEES:** Cont		
B.	APPLIANCES AND DRESSINGS		
(a)	Elastic Hosiery (Compression Hosiery) requiring measurement and endorsed "measured and fitted"	128	"Measured and fitted"
(b) (i)	Trusses requiring measurement and endorsed "measured and fitted"	197	"Measured and fitted
(ii)	Repairs to Trusses	69	NIL
(c)	Stoma Appliances, Suprapubic Belts, Incontinence Appliances		
(i)	Replacement of complete appliance and/or	}	
(ii)	One or more types of spare parts and accessories	} 128	NIL
C.	BULK PRESCRIPTIONS for schools or institutions supplied in accordance with the regulations (See Note 6, Part VIII, page 46)	644	NIL
D.	Where liquid preparations extemporaneously dispensed other than at 2A(b) and 2A(c) above are ordered by the prescriber to be supplied in more than one container, each extra quantity ordered	128	NIL
E.	Where a preparation which requires the addition of a vehicle/diluent by the pharmacy contractor results in a liquid of stability of less than 14 days, and for pharmaceutical reasons necessitates supply in more than one container and the prescription form is endorsed with the number of extra quantities supplied, for each extra supply	155	Number of extra containers supplied
F.	Where the prescription is for a Controlled Drug in Schedule 2 or 3 of the Misuse of Drugs Regulations 1985 and is endorsed "CD" by the contractor		
	Schedule 2 drug	128	"CD"
	Schedule 3 drug (from 1 Jan 1997) (including Temazepam)	43	"CD"

*   See page 17

See Part II, Clause 6A(ii) (Page 5)

2.   **ADDITIONAL FEES:** Cont

G.   When the prescription has been dispensed at a time when the premises are not open for dispensing on the day or (in the case of a prescription dispensed after midnight) the day following that on which it was written and

IIIA

		FEE PER CALL-OUT Resident P	Non-Resident† P	*Endorsements required by contractors
(i)	Is endorsed "urgent" by the prescriber and dispensed between the time the premises close for dispensing and 11 pm on days other than Sundays and public holidays	713	1756	Time and date. Where appropriate "non-resident"
(ii)	Is endorsed "urgent" by the prescriber or "dispensed urgently" by the contractor and is signed by the patient (or his representative) and dispensed between 11 pm and the time the premises open for dispensing or on Sundays and public holidays	920	2118	Time and date. Where appropriate "non-resident" Where appropriate "dispensed urgently" (signature of patient or representative required)

Urgent fees are not payable for prescriptions dispensed after the normal working hours agreed between the contractor and the Health Authority before the actual closing of the pharmacy and the contractor still being present.

ALL "URGENT" PRESCRIPTIONS MUST BE ENDORSED WITH THE TIME AND DATE OF DISPENSING

In order to qualify for the non-resident rates, a contractor who normally lives elsewhere than on his business premises will need to have left those premises and to return to open them to dispense an "urgent" prescription. In the absence of an endorsement "non-resident" on "urgent" prescription forms, payments will automatically be made at the "resident" rate.

*   Abbreviated endorsements, eg "Extemp prep" are acceptable. Endorsements under this heading apply only to claims for the appropriate professional fee. Further endorsement may be necessary for other purposes eg Part II Clause 8 (Basic Price), Clause 9 (Endorsement Requirements) and Notes to Part VIII (page 43).

H.   FEE RELATED TO THRESHOLD QUANTITY

An additional fee of 40p will be paid in respect of each prescription with the exception of bulk prescriptions, for an oral solid dose preparation (as listed below, pages 18 to 27) where the quantity ordered exceeds the threshold listed against the preparation.

(See Appendix to 2H pages 18 to 27)

PROFESSIONAL FEES (Pharmacy Contractors) - cont

See Part II, Clause 6A(ii) (page 5)

2.   **ADDITIONAL FEES** : Cont

I.   **Expensive Prescription Fee**
      A fee equivalent to 2% of the net ingredient cost will be payable on all prescriptions
      over £100.
      Note - Expensive Prescription Fee is not included in calculation of ESPS payments

3.   **SPECIAL FEE** (ie not paid in addition to professional fee)

	Fee per prescription P	Endorsements required by contractors
Appliances not covered by 2B (including Elastic Hosiery and Trusses not measured and fitted) and		
Dressings	85	NIL

APPENDIX TO PARAGRAPH 2.H.

Drug	Threshold quantity	Drug	Threshold quantity
Acepril Tablets 12.5mg	102	Amiloride Tablets BP, 5mg	64
Acepril Tablets 25mg	123	Aminoglutethimide Tablets 250mg	120
Acepril Tablets 50mg	132	Aminophylline Tablets BP, 100mg	109
Acetazolamide Tablets BP, 250mg	91	Amiodarone Tablets BP, 100mg	63
Achromycin Capsules 250mg	49	Amitriptyline Tablets BP, 10mg	86
Aciclovir Tablets, Dispersible 200mg	35	Amitriptyline Tablets BP, 25mg	92
Aciclovir Tablets, Dispersible 800mg	47	Amitriptyline Tablets BP, 50mg	79
Acupan Tablets 30mg	133	Amix-250 Capsules	29
Adalat 5 Capsules	131	Amoram Capsules 250mg	27
Adalat Capsules 10mg	146	Amoxil Capsules 250mg	28
Adalat LA 30 Tablets	60	Amoxil Capsules 500mg	28
Adalat Retard 10 Tablets	105	Amoxil Tablets Disp 500mg	26
Adalat Retard Tablets 20mg	115	Amoxycillin Capsules BP, 250mg	27
Adifax Capsules 15mg	80	Amoxycillin Capsules BP, 500mg	27
Aldactide 25 Tablets	81	Ampicillin Capsules BP, 250mg	34
Aldactide 50 Tablets	68	Ampicillin Capsules BP, 500mg	33
Aldactone Tablets 25mg	98	Amytal Tablets 50mg	120
Aldactone Tablets 50mg	65	Anafranil Capsules 10mg	105
Aldactone Tablets 100mg	57	Anafranil Capsules 25mg	110
Aldomet Tablets 125mg	125	Anafranil Capsules 50mg	92
Aldomet Tablets 250mg	142	Anafranil SR Tablets 75mg	53
Aldomet Tablets 500mg	140	Androcur Tablets 50mg	127
Allegron Tablets 25mg	115	Antabuse 200 Tablets	65
Allopurinol Tablets BP, 100mg	92	Antepsin Tablets 1g	138
Allopurinol Tablets BP, 300mg	62	Anturan Tablets 100mg	135
Almodan Capsules 250mg	29	Anturan Tablets 200mg	160
Aloxiprin Tablets 600mg	165	Apisate Tablets	55
Alrheumat Capsules 50mg	120	Apresoline Tablets 25mg	133
Alu-Cap Capsules 475mg	283	Apresoline Tablets 50mg	135
Aluminium Hydroxide Tablets BP, 500mg	145	Aprinox Tablets 2.5mg	53
		Aprinox Tablets 5mg	56
Alupent Tablets 20mg	129	Apsifen Tablets 600mg	95
Ambaxin Tablets 400mg	24	Artane Tablets 2mg	122
Amfipen Capsules 250mg	33	Artane Tablets 5mg	116
Amilco Tablets	64	Arthrotec 50 Tablets	79

Asacol Tablets 400mg	197
Ascorbic Acid Tablets BP, 25mg	83
Ascorbic Acid Tablets BP, 50mg	99
Ascorbic Acid Tablets BP, 100mg	95
Ascorbic Acid Tablets BP, 200mg	88
Ascorbic Acid Tablets BP, 500mg	100
Aspirin Nuseal 300mg	67
Aspirin Nuseal 600mg	120
Aspirin Tablets BP, 75mg	79
Aspirin Tablets BP, 300mg	69
Aspirin Tablets Disp BP, 75mg	65
Aspirin Tablets Disp BP, 300mg	70
Astemizole Tablets 10mg	47
Atarax Tablets 10mg	84
Atarax Tablets 25mg	76
Atenolol Tablets BP, 25mg	62
Atenolol Tablets BP, 50mg	63
Atenolol Tablets BP, 100mg	62
Atromid-S Capsules 500mg	154
Augmentin Tablets Disp	30
Augmentin Tablets 375mg	29
Avloclor Tablets 250mg	48
Avomine Tablets 25mg	68
Axid Capsules 150mg	71
Azathioprine Tablets BP, 50mg	110
Baclofen Tablets BP, 10mg	164
Bactrim Drapsules	35
Baratol Tablets 25mg	116
Baxan Capsules 500mg	22
Baycaron Tablets 25mg	68
Bendogen Tablets 10mg	155
Bendrofluazide Tablets BP, 2.5mg	63
Bendrofluazide Tablets BP, 5mg	62
Benemid Tablets 500mg	109
Benoral Tablets 750mg	166
Benorylate Tablets 750mg	150
Benzhexol Tablets BP, 2mg	125
Benzhexol Tablets BP, 5mg	116
Beta-Adalat Capsules	77
Beta-Cardone Tablets 40mg	118
Beta-Cardone Tablets 80mg	87
Betahistine Dihydrochloride	
Tablets 8mg	138
Betaloc Tablets 50mg	103
Betaloc Tablets 100mg	105
Betaloc-SA Tablets	66
Bethanidine Sulph Tablets 10mg	155
Betim Tablets 10mg	92
Betnelan Tablets 0.5mg	71
Betnesol Tablets 0.5mg	67
Bezalip Tablets 200mg	136
Bezalip Mono Tablets 400mg	58
Bisacodyl Tablets BP, 5mg (e/c)	84
Blocadren Tablets 10mg	92
Bolvidon Tablets 10mg	87
Bolvidon Tablets 20mg	67
Bradosol Lozenges	45
Brevinor Tablets	131
Bricanyl SA Tablets	81
Bricanyl Tablets 5mg	116
Bromocriptine Tablets BP, 2.5mg	126
Brufen Tablets 200mg	122
Brufen Tablets 400mg	110
Brufen Tablets 600mg	107

Brufen Retard Tablets 800mg	73
Buccastem Tablets	39
Burinex-A Tablets	61
Burinex K Tablets	72
Burinex Tablets 1mg	81
Burinex Tablets 5mg	60
Buscopan Tablets	82
Buspar Tablets 5mg	84
Cafergot Tablets	51
Calcichew Tablets 1.2518g	124
Calciferol Tablets BP,	
250microgram (10,000 units)	92
Calciferol Tablets BP,	
1.25mg (50,000 units)	69
Calcium Gluconate Tablets BP,	
600mg	128
Calcium Lactate Tablets BP, 300mg	126
Calcium & Ergocalciferol Tablets	96
Camcolit 250 Tablets	144
Camcolit Tablets 400mg	91
Capoten Tablets 12.5mg	101
Capoten Tablets 25mg	123
Capoten Tablets 50mg	121
Capozide Tablets	71
Captopril Tablets BP, 25mg	119
Captopril Tablets BP, 50mg	132
Carace Tablets 5mg	65
Carace Tablets 10mg	64
Carbamazepine Tablets BP, 100mg	136
Carbamazepine Tablets BP, 200mg	141
Carbamazepine Tablets BP, 400mg	113
Cardene Capsules 20mg	136
Cardene Capsules 30mg	128
Cardura Tablets 1mg	68
Cardura Tablets 2mg	70
Catapres Perlongets 0.25mg	77
Catapres Tablets 0.1mg	139
Catapres Tablets 0.3mg	144
Caved S Tablets	157
Cedocard Retard Tablets 20mg	108
Cedocard Retard Tablets 40mg	100
Cedocard Tablets 5mg	127
Cedocard-10 Tablets	153
Cedocard-20 Tablets	121
Cefaclor Capsules 250mg	28
Cefaclor Capsules 500mg	28
Celectol Tablets 200mg	64
Celevac Tablets	212
Cephalexin Capsules BP, 250mg	33
Cephalexin Capsules BP, 500mg	29
Cephalexin Tablets BP, 250mg	33
Cephalexin Tablets BP, 500mg	28
Ceporex Capsules 250mg	34
Ceporex Capsules 500mg	30
Ceporex Tablets 250mg	34
Ceporex Tablets 500mg	30
Charcoal Tablets BPC34	182
Chloractil Tablets 25mg	109
Chloractil Tablets 50mg	107
Chloractil Tablets 100mg	103
Chlordiazepoxide Capsules BP, 5mg	87
Chlordiazepoxide Capsules	
BP, 10mg	105
Chlordiazepoxide Tablets 5mg	94

IIIA

Chlordiazepoxide Tablets 10mg	93
Chlordiazepoxide Tablets 25mg	97
Chlorpheniramine Tablets BP, 4mg	69
Chlorpromazine Tablets BP, 25mg	109
Chlorpromazine Tablets BP, 50mg	107
Chlorpromazine Tablets BP, 100mg	103
Chlorpropamide Tablets BP, 100mg	85
Chlorpropamide Tablets BP, 250mg	79
Choledyl Tablets 100mg	126
Choledyl Tablets 200mg	132
Cimetidine Tablets BP, 200mg	110
Cimetidine Tablets BP, 400mg	81
Cimetidine Tablets BP, 800mg	53
Cinnarizine Tablets 15mg	122
Cinobac Capsules 500mg	24
Ciproxin Tablets 250mg	27
Ciproxin Tablets 500mg	19
Clarityn Tablets 10mg	43
Clemastine Tablets BP, 1mg	64
Clinoril Tablets 100mg	124
Clinoril Tablets 200mg	93
Clobazam Capsules BP, 10mg	97
Clomid Tablets 50mg	30
Clomiphene Tablets BP, 50mg	30
Co-amilofruse Tablets BP, 2.5/20	52
Co-amilofruse Tablets BP, 5/40	64
Co-amilozideTablets BP, 2.5/25	60
Co-amilozide Tablets BP, 5/50	62
Co-Betaloc Tablets	77
Co-codamol Tablets BP, 8mg/500mg	128
Co-codamol Tablets Effer 8mg/500mg	138
Co-codaprin Tablets BP	122
Co-codaprin Tablets Disp BP	113
Codafen Continus Tablets	95
Co-danthrusate Capsules BP	79
Codeine Phosphate Tablets BP, 15mg	101
Codeine Phosphate Tablets BP, 30mg	117
Codeine Phosphate Tablets BP, 60mg	134
Co-dydramol Tablets BP	133
Cogentin Tablets 2mg	75
Colchicine Tablets BP, 500microgram	90
Colofac Tablets 135mg	115
Colpermin Capsules 0.2ml	126
Concordin Tablets 5mg	106
Concordin Tablets 10mg	124
Conova 30 Tablets	136
Co-phenotrope Tablets 2.5/0.025	72
Co-proxamol Tablets BP	144
Coracten Capsules 10mg	98
Coracten Capsules 20mg	107
Cordarone X Tablets 200mg	57
Cordilox Tablets 40mg	146
Cordilox Tablets 80mg	139
Cordilox Tablets 120mg	138
Cordilox Tablets 160mg	98
Corgard Tablets 40mg	76
Corgard Tablets 80mg	74
Corgaretic Tablets 40mg	70
Corgaretic Tablets 80mg	64
Corlan Pellets	41
Cortisone Acetate MSD Tablets 25mg	93
Cortistab Tablets 5mg	198
Cortistab Tablets 25mg	93
Cortisyl Tablets 25mg	93
Co-trimoxazole Tablets BP	40
Co-trimoxazole Tablets Disp BP	40
Co-trimoxazole Tablets BP,160/800	22
Cyclophosphamide Tablets BP, 50mg	84
Cytotec Tablets 200 microgram	106
Dalacin C Capsules 150mg	38
Daneral SA Tablets	57
Danol Capsules 100mg	86
Danol Capsules 200mg	81
Dantrium Capsules 25mg	180
Daonil Tablets 5mg	109
Dapsone Tablets BP, 50mg	102
Dapsone Tablets BP, 100mg	81
Daraprim Tablets	30
De-Nol Tablets 120mg	156
Decadron Tablets 0.5mg	133
Declinax Tablets 10mg	127
Deltacortril Tablets ec 2.5mg	108
Deltacortril Tablets ec 5mg	85
Dequadin Lozenges	48
Deseril Tablets 1mg	128
Detecto Tablets 300mg	27
Dexamethasone Tablets BP, 500 microgram	133
Dexedrine Tablets 5mg	76
Dextropropoxyphene Capsules BP, 60mg	106
DHC Continus Tablets 60mg	84
Diabinese Tablets 100mg	91
Diabinese Tablets 250mg	89
Diamicron Tablets 80mg	96
Diamorphine HCl Tablets 10mg	170
Diamox Tablets 250mg	91
Diazepam Tablets BP, 2mg	75
Diazepam Tablets BP, 5mg	69
Diazepam Tablets BP, 10mg	57
Dibenyline Capsules 10mg	90
Diclofenac Tablets BP, 25mg (e/c)	108
Diclofenac Tablets BP, 50mg (e/c)	98
Diclofenac Sodium Tablets 75mg (m/r)	68
Diclomax Retard Capsules 100mg	44
Diconal Tablets	63
Dicynene Tablets 500mg	53
Diflucan Capsules 150mg	2
Diflunisal Tablets BP, 250mg	103
Diflunisal Tablets BP, 500mg	76
Digoxin Tablets BP, 62.5microgram	65
Digoxin Tablets BP, 125microgram	60
Digoxin Tablets BP, 250microgram	61
Dihydrocodeine Tablets BP, 30mg	113
Diltiazem HCl Tablets 60mg (m/r)	141
Diltiazem HCl Tablets 90mg (m/r)	99
Dimotane LA Tablets 12mg	65
Dimotane Tablets 4mg	68
Dindevan Tablets 10mg	153

Dindevan Tablets 50mg	146
Dipyridamole Tablets BP, 25mg	195
Dipyridamole Tablets BP, 100mg	148
Disipal Tablets 50mg	127
Disopyramide Capsules BP, 100mg	142
Distaclor Capsules 250mg	28
Distaclor Capsules 500mg	28
Distaclor MR Tablets 375mg	18
Distamine Tablets 125mg	114
Distamine Tablets 250mg	98
Ditropan Tablets 2.5mg	104
Ditropan Tablets 5mg	100
Diumide-K Tablets	63
Diurexan Tablets 20mg	63
Dixarit Tablets 0.025mg	164
Dolmatil Tablets 200mg	118
Dolobid Tablets 250mg	103
Dolobid 500 Tablets	76
Domical Tablets 50mg	72
Doralese Tiltabs 20mg	84
Dothiepin Capsules BP, 25mg	90
Dothiepin Tablets BP, 75mg	57
Doxycycline Capsules BP, 100mg	15
Dramamine Tablets 50mg	94
Duphaston Tablets 10mg	96
Duromine Capsules 15mg	47
Duramine Capsules 30mg	45
Dyazide Tablets	62
Dytac Capsules 50mg	80
Dytide Capsules	70
Economycin Capsules 250mg	49
Efamast Capsules 40mg	289
Effercitrate Tablets	66
Elantan 10 Tablets	113
Elantan Tablets 20mg	111
Elantan Tablets 40mg	113
Elantan LA 50 Capsules	54
Eldepryl Tablets 5mg	83
Eltroxin Tablets 50microgram	107
Eltroxin Tablets 100microgram	80
Emflex Capsules 60mg	84
Enalapril Maleate Tablets 5mg	75
Enalapril Maleate Tablets 10mg	72
Endoxana Tablets 50mg	84
Epanutin Capsules 25mg	90
Epanutin Capsules 50mg	100
Epanutin Capsules 100mg	142
Ephedrine HCl Tablets BP, 30mg	114
Ephynal Tablets 50mg	137
Ephynal Tablets 200mg	130
Epilim Tablets Crushable 100mg	205
Epilim Tablets ec 200mg	188
Epilim Tablets ec 500mg	155
Epogam 40 Capsules 40mg	267
Equanil Tablets 200mg	102
Equanil Tablets 400mg	104
Ergometrine Tablets 500microgram	22
Erymax Capsules 250mg	41
Erythrocin Tablets 250mg	38
Erythrocin 500 Tablets	26
Erythromid Tablets 250mg	39
Erythromycin Stearate Tablets BP, 250mg	38
Erythromycin Stearate Tablets BP, 500mg	26
Erythromycin Tablets BP, 250mg (e/c)	43
Erythroped A Tablets 500mg	37
Esidrex Tablets 50mg	61
Ethinyloestradiol Tablets BP, 10microgram	91
Euglucon Tablets 2.5mg	90
Euglucon Tablets 5mg	109
Eugynon 30 Tablets	133
Exirel Capsules 15mg	125
Famotidine Tablets 40mg	52
Fansidar Tablets	18
Farlutal Tablets 100mg	134
Fectrim Tablets Forte	22
Feldene Capsules 10mg	87
Feldene Capsules 20mg	52
Feldene Tablets Disp 10mg	61
Feldene Tablets Disp 20mg	46
Femulen Tablets	154
Fenbid Capsules 300mg	117
Fenopron Tablets 300mg	128
Fenopron Tablets 600mg	105
Fentazin Tablets 2mg	107
Fentazin Tablets 4mg	122
Ferrocontin Continus Tablets	57
Ferrocontin Folic Continus Tablets	60
Ferrograd-Folic Tablets	62
Ferrograd Tablets 325mg	58
Ferrous Gluconate Tablets BP, 300mg	106
Ferrous Sulphate Tablets Compound BPC	119
Ferrous Sulphate Tablets BP, 200mg	108
Ferrous Sulphate Tablets BP, 300mg	83
Fersaday Tablets	53
Fersamal Tablets 200mg	114
Flagyl Tablets 200mg	29
Flagyl Tablets 400mg	27
Florinef Tablets 0.1mg	68
Floxapen Capsules 250mg	39
Floxapen Capsules 500mg	34
Fluanxol Tablets 0.5mg	73
Fluanxol Tablets 1mg	59
Flucloxacillin Capsules BP, 250mg	39
Flucloxacillin Capsules BP, 500mg	43
Flurbiprofen Tablets BP, 50mg	120
Flurbiprofen Tablets BP, 100mg	112
Folic Acid Tablets BP, 5mg	70
Franol Plus Tablets	135
Franol Tablets	127
Froben Tablets 50mg	120
Froben Tablets 100mg	112
Froben SR Capsules 200mg	50
Frumil LS Tablets	52
Frumil Tablets	64
Frusemide Tablets BP, 20mg	58
Frusemide Tablets BP, 40mg	75
Frusemide Tablets BP, 500mg	43
Frusene Tablets 40mg	65

IIIA

Fucidin Tablets ec 250mg	95	Imipramine Tablets BP, 10mg	104
Fulcin Tablets 125mg	155	Imipramine Tablets BP, 25mg	129
Fulcin Tablets 500mg	75	Imodium Capsules 2mg	61
Fungilin Lozenges 10mg	53	Imuran Tablets 50mg	114
Furadantin Tablets 50mg	66	Indapamide Tablets 2.5mg	62
Furadantin Tablets 100mg	45	Inderal LA Capsules 160mg	64
Galenamox Capsules 250mg	48	Inderal Tablets 10mg	142
Galpseud Tablets 60mg	27	Inderal Tablets 40mg	122
Gamanil Tablets 70mg	78	Inderal Tablets 80mg	137
Gastrocote Tablets	153	Inderetic Capsules	86
Gastrozepin Tablets 50mg	93	Inderex Capsules	66
Gaviscon Tablets	138	Indocid Capsules 25mg	118
Glibenclamide Tablets BP, 2.5mg	77	Indocid Capsules 50mg	109
Glibenclamide Tablets BP, 5mg	115	Indocid-R Capsules 75mg	71
Glibenese Tablets 5mg	118	Indolar SR Capsules	63
Gliclazide Tablets BP, 80mg	96	Indomethacin Capsules BP, 25mg	116
Glipizide Tablets BP, 5mg	143	Indomethacin Capsules BP, 50mg	102
Glucophage Tablets 500mg	124	Indomod Capsules 75mg	63
Glucophage Tablets 850mg	104	Innovace Tablets 2.5mg	69
Glurenorm Tablets 30mg	133	Innovace Tablets 5mg	71
Glyceryl Trinitrate Tablets BP,		Innovace Tablets 10mg	72
500microgram	150	Innovace Tablets 20mg	70
Glyceryl Trinitrate Tablets BP,		Ionamin Capsules 15mg	48
600microgram	150	Ionamin Capsules 30mg	47
Grisovin Tablets 125mg	155	Ipral Tablets 100mg	41
Grisovin Tablets 500mg	88	Ipral Tablets 200mg	22
Haldol Tablets 5mg	101	Ismelin Tablets 10mg	116
Haldol Tablets 10mg	124	Ismelin Tablets 25mg	91
Half-Inderal LA Capsules 80mg	54	Ismo 10 Tablets	115
Halibut Liver Oil Capsules BP	109	Ismo 20 Tablets	114
Haloperidol Capsules BP,		Isoket Retard Tablets 20mg	108
500 microgram	99	Isoket Retard Tablets 40mg	100
Haloperidol Tablets BP, 1.5mg	115	Isoniazid Tablets BP, 100mg	122
Haloperidol Tablets BP, 5mg	101	Isordil Tablets Sublingual 5mg	127
Haloperidol Tablets BP, 10mg	124	Isordil Tablets 10mg	153
Harmogen Tablets 1.5mg	103	Isordil Tablets 30mg	152
Heminevrin Capsules 192mg	71	Isordil Tembids 40mg	116
Hexopal Forte Tablets 750mg	147	Isosorbide Dinitrate Tablets BP,	
Hexopal Tablets 500mg	153	10mg	155
Hiprex Tablets 1g	79	Isosorbide Dinitrate Tablets BP,	
Hismanal Tablets 10mg	47	20mg	145
Honvan Tablets	102	Isosorbide Mononitrate Tablets	
Hydergine Tablets 1.5mg	130	10mg	119
Hydergine Tablets 4.5mg	63	Isosorbide Mononitrate Tablets	
Hydralazine Tablets BP, 25mg	141	20mg	122
Hydralazine Tablets BP, 50mg	132	Isosorbide Mononitrate Tablets	
Hydrenox Tablets 50mg	92	40mg	113
Hydromet Tablets	117	Istin Tablets 5mg	60
Hydrocortistab Tablets 20mg	93	Istin Tablets 10mg	58
Hydrocortone Tablets 10mg	142	Kalspare Tablets	56
Hydrocortone Tablets 20mg	93	Kalten Capsules	65
HydroSaluric Tablets 25mg	69	Keflex Capsules 250mg	33
HydroSaluric Tablets 50mg	61	Keflex Capsules 500mg	29
Hygroton Tablets 50mg	69	Keflex Tablets 250mg	34
Hypovase Tablets 0.5mg	128	Keflex Tablets 500mg	29
Hypovase Tablets 1mg	142	Kelfizine W Tablets 2g	7
Hypovase Tablets 2mg	143	Kemadrin Tablets 5mg	106
Hypovase Tablets 5mg	140	Kerlone Tablets 20mg	47
Ibuprofen Tablets BP, 200mg	105	Ketoprofen Capsules BP, 50mg	120
Ibuprofen Tablets BP, 400mg	99	Ketoprofen Capsules BP, 100mg	98
Ibuprofen Tablets BP, 600mg	94	Ketovite Tablets	108
Ilosone Capsules 250mg	36	Kinidin Durules	136
Imdur Durules 60mg	53	Klaricid Tablets 250mg	21
Imigran Tablets 100mg	9	Kloref Tablets	175

Labetolol Tablets BP, 100mg	125	Medrone Tablets 4mg	69
Labetolol Tablets BP, 200mg	135	Medroxyprogesterone Acetate	
Labetolol Tablets BP, 400mg	132	Tablets 100mg	134
Lamisil Tablets 250mg	45	Mefenamic Acid Capsules BP,	
Lanoxin PG Tablets	70	250mg	91
Lanoxin Tablets 0.125mg	58	Mefenamic Acid Tablets BP, 500mg	83
Lanoxin Tablets 0.25mg	55	Melleril Tablets 10mg	94
Largactil Tablets 10mg	108	Melleril Tablets 25mg	88
Largactil Tablets 25mg	100	Melleril Tablets 50mg	89
Largactil Tablets 50mg	98	Melleril Tablets 100mg	100
Largactil Tablets 100mg	104	Meprobamate Tablets BP, 200mg	91
Lasikal Tablets	73	Meprobamate Tablets BP, 400mg	95
Lasilactone Capsules	71	Meptid Tablets 200mg	109
Lasix Tablets 20mg	60	Merbentyl Tablets 10mg	92
Lasix Tablets 40mg	70	Merbentyl 20 Tablets	74
Lasma Tablets 300mg	80	Merocaine Lozenges	43
Lasoride Tablets	60	Merocet Lozenges	45
Ledercort Tablets 2mg	88	Mestinon Tablets	251
Ledercort Tablets 4mg	68	Metenix 5 Tablets	61
Lederfen Capsules 300mg	113	Metformin Tablets BP, 500mg	130
Lederfen Tablets 300mg	125	Metformin Tablets BP, 850mg	115
Lederfen 450 Tablets	86	Methotrexate Tablets BP, 2.5mg	37
Lentizol Capsules 25mg	76	Methyldopa Tablets BP, 125mg	125
Lentizol Capsules 50mg	66	Methyldopa Tablets BP, 250mg	141
Lioresal Tablets 10mg	159	Methyldopa Tablets BP, 500mg	146
Lipostat Tablets 10mg	60	Metoclopramide Tablets BP, 10mg	79
Lisinopril Tablets 5mg	65	Metoprolol Tablets BP, 50mg	102
Liskonium Tablets 450mg	95	Metoprolol Tablets BP, 100mg	109
Livial Tablets 2.5mg	103	Metronidazole Tablets BP, 200mg	25
Lodine Capsules 300mg	81	Metronidazole Tablets BP, 400mg	28
Loestrin 20 Tablets	126	Mexitil Capsules 200mg	144
Loestrin 30 Tablets	121	Mianserin Tablets BP, 10mg	87
Lofepramine Tablets 70mg	78	Mianserin Tablets BP, 20mg	67
Lomotil Tablets	72	Mianserin Tablets BP, 30mg	62
Loniten Tablets 10mg	134	Microgynon 30 Tablets	133
Loprazolam Tablets BP, 1mg	51	Micronor Tablets	152
Lopresor Tablets 50mg	103	Microval Tablets	178
Lopresor Tablets 100mg	105	Midamor Tablets 5mg	80
Lopresor SR Tablets 200mg	66	Midrid Capsules	68
Lopresoretic Tablets	79	Migraleve Tablets pink	46
Lorazepam Tablets BP, 1mg	79	Migraleve Tablets yellow	42
Lorazepam Tablets BP, 2.5mg	90	Migravess Tablets	59
Lormetazepam Tablets BP, 1mg	56	Migravess Forte Tablets	57
Losec Capsules 20mg	70	Migril Tablets	49
Ludiomil Tablets 25mg	80	Minocin Tablets 50mg	107
Ludiomil Tablets 50mg	63	Minocin Tablets 100mg	73
Ludiomil Tablets 75mg	51	Minocin MR Capsules 100mg	69
Lustral Tablets 50mg	52	Minocycline Tablets BP, 50mg	114
Macrodantin Capsules 50mg	49	Minodiab Tablets 5mg	118
Macrodantin Capsules 100mg	45	Mobiflex Tablets 20mg	46
Madopar 62.5 Capsules	152	Moditen Tablets 1mg	68
Madopar 125 Capsules	170	Moducren Tablets	70
Madopar 250 Capsules	148	Moduret 25 Tablets	60
Magnapen Capsules 500mg	37	Moduretic Tablets	66
Magnesium Trisilicate Co		Molipaxin Capsules 50mg	83
Tablets BP	155	Molipaxin Capsules 100mg	89
Malaprim Tablets	24	Monit LS Tablets 10mg	112
Marevan Tablets 1mg	114	Monit Tablets 20mg	110
Marevan Tablets 3mg	87	Mono-Cedocard 20 Tablets	111
Marevan Tablets 5mg	74	Mono-Cedocard 40 Tablets	113
Marplan Tablets 10mg	113	Monocor Tablets 5mg	59
Marvelon Tablets	126	Monocor Tablets 10mg	63
Maxolon Tablets 10mg	71	Monotrim Tablets 100mg	38
Mebeverine Tablets BP, 135mg	111	Monotrim Tablets 200mg	23

IIIA

Motilium Tablets 10mg	78	One-alpha Capsules 0.25microgram	69
Motipress Tablets	51	One-alpha Capsules 1microgram	67
Motival Tablets	90	Opilon Tablets 40mg	143
Motrin Tablets 400mg	110	Optimax WV Tablets 500mg	143
Motrin Tablets 600mg	95	Optimine Tablets 1mg	62
MST Continus Tablets 10mg	95	Orap Tablets 2mg	99
MST Continus Tablets 30mg	90	Orap Tablets 4mg	76
MST Continus Tablets 60mg	92	Orimeten Tablets 250mg	120
Myambutol Tablets 100mg	111	Orphenadrine Hydrochloride Tablets BP,	
Myambutol Tablets 400mg	101	50mg	127
Mycardol Tablets	141	Ortho-Novin Tablets 1/50	123
Mysoline Tablets	134	Orudis Capsules 50mg	120
Mysteclin Tablets	44	Orudis Capsules 100mg	98
Nacton Tablets 2mg	141	Oruvail Capsules 100mg	75
Nacton Forte Tablets 4mg	129	Oruvail 200 Capsules	49
Naftidrofuryl Capsules BP, 100mg	162	Ossopan 800 Tablets	135
Nalcrom Capsules 100mg	186	Ovran Tablets	108
Naprosyn Tablets 250mg	107	Ovran-30 Tablets	130
Naprosyn Tablets 500mg	90	Ovranette Tablets	137
Naprosyn Tablets EC 250mg	92	Ovysmen Tablets	129
Naprosyn Tablets EC 500mg	79	Oxazepam Capsules 30mg	83
Naproxen Tablets BP, 250mg	99	Oxazepam Tablets BP, 10mg	82
Naproxen Tablets BP, 500mg	81	Oxazepam Tablets BP, 15mg	100
Nardil Tablets	114	Oxazepam Tablets BP, 30mg	83
Narphen Tablets 5mg	106	Oxprenolol Tablets BP, 20mg	129
Natrilix Tablets 2.5mg	62	Oxprenolol Tablets BP, 40mg	122
Navidrex Tablets 0.5mg	69	Oxprenolol Tablets BP, 80mg	127
Navispare Tablets	70	Oxprenolol Tablets BP, 160mg	93
Negram Tablets 500mg	74	Oxybutynine Hydrochloride	
Neo Mercazole 5 Tablets	141	Tablets 5mg	100
Neo-Naclex Tablets 5mg	65	Oxytetracycline Capsules BP,	
Neo-Naclex-K Tablets	79	250mg	50
Neocon Tablets	123	Oxytetracycline Tablets BP, 250mg	86
Neogest Tablets	180	Palfium Tablets 5mg	75
Nephril Tablets 1mg	70	Palfium Tablets 10mg	90
Neulactil Tablets 2.5mg	131	Paludrine Tablets 100mg	169
Nicotinamide Tablets BP, 50mg	121	Pancrex V Capsules	356
Nicotinic Acid Tablets BP, 50mg	152	Pancrex V Tablets	417
Nifedipine Capsules BP, 5mg	129	Pancrex V Tablets Forte	514
Nifedipine Capsules BP, 10mg	142	Paracetamol Tablets BP, 500mg	136
Nifensar XL Tablets 20mg	87	Paracetamol Tablets Sol BP, 500mg	110
Nitoman Tablets 25mg	130	Paramax Tablets	66
Nitrazepam Tablets BP, 5mg	63	Parlodel Capsules 10mg	135
Nitrazepam Tablets BP, 10mg	58	Parlodel Tablets 2.5mg	126
Nitrocontin Tablets 2.6mg	95	Parnate Tablets	109
Nitrofurantoin Tablets BP, 50mg	66	Paroven Capsules 250mg	136
Nitrofurantoin Tablets BP, 100mg	45	Parstelin Tablets	101
Nivaquine Tablets 200mg	34	Penbritin Capsules 250mg	37
Nizoral Tablets 200mg	33	Penbritin Capsules 500mg	36
Noctec Capsules 500mg	60	Pendramine Tablets 125mg	114
Nolvadex Tablets 10mg	118	Pendramine Tablets 250mg	98
Nolvadex-D Tablets 20mg	69	Penicillin VK Capsules 250mg	38
Nordox Capsules 100mg	14	Penicillin VK Tablets 125mg	34
Norethisterone Tablets BP, 5mg	93	Penicillin VK Tablets 250mg	39
Norgeston Tablets	208	Pentazocine Capsules BP, 50mg	101
Noriday Tablets	156	Pentazocine Tablets BP, 25mg	118
Norimin Tablets	129	Pepcid Tablets 40mg	52
Norinyl-1 Tablets	127	Periactin Tablets 4mg	95
Norval Tablets 20mg	67	Persantin Tablets 25mg	195
Nuelin Tablets 125mg	126	Persantin Tablets 100mg	146
Nuelin SA 175 Tablets	98	Pertofran Tablets 25mg	143
Nuelin SA 250 Tablets	100	Pethidine Tablets BP, 50mg	61
Nystan Tablets oral	55	Phenergan Tablets 10mg	67
Nystan Pastilles	70	Phenergan Tablets 25mg	61

Phenobarbitone Tablets BP, 15mg	115
Phenobarbitone Tablets BP, 30mg	128
Phenobarbitone Tablets BP, 60mg	113
Phenobarbitone Tablets BP, 100mg	85
Phenytoin Capsules BP, 50mg	100
Phenytoin Capsules BP, 100mg	142
Phenytoin Tablets BP, 50mg	107
Phenytoin Tablets BP, 100mg	149
Phyllocontin Tablets paed	104
Phyllocontin Tablets 225mg	113
Phyllocontin Tablets Forte 350mg	95
Physeptone Tablets 5mg	48
Piriton Tablets 4mg	64
Piroxicam Capsules BP, 10mg	86
Piroxicam Capsules BP, 20mg	50
Plaquenil Tablets 200mg	79
Ponderax PA Capsules 60mg	57
Pondocillin Tablets 500mg	18
Ponstan Capsules 250mg	89
Ponstan Tablets Forte 500mg	81
Potassium Chloride Tablets Slow BP, 600mg	111
Potassium Tablets Effervescent BPC 1968	250
Praxilene Capsules 100mg	162
Prednesol Tablets 5mg	50
Prednisolone Tablets BP, 1mg	145
Prednisolone Tablets BP, 5mg	83
Prednisolone Enteric-coated Tablets BP, 2.5mg	98
Prednisolone Enteric-coated Tablets BP, 5mg	87
Prednisone Tablets BP, 1mg	150
Prednisone Tablets BP, 5mg	83
Pregaday Tablets	62
Premarin Tablets 625microgram	113
Premarin Tablets 1.25mg	112
Premarin Tablets 2.5mg	108
Prepulsid Tablets 10mg	125
Prestim Tablets	77
Priadel Tablets	95
Priadel 200 Tablets	98
Primalan Tablets 5mg	64
Primolut N Tablets 5mg	93
Primperan Tablets 10mg	70
Pro-Actidil Tablets 10mg	56
Pro-Banthine Tablets 15mg	119
Prochlorperazine Tablets BP,5mg	82
Procyclidine Tablets BP, 5mg	102
Progesic Tablets 200mg	103
Progynova Tablets 1mg	68
Progynova Tablets 2mg	77
Promethazine Hydrochloride Tablets BP, 25mg	61
Propranolol Tablets BP, 10mg	144
Propranolol Tablets BP, 40mg	117
Propranolol Tablets BP, 80mg	128
Propranolol Tablets BP, 160mg	127
Proscar Tablets 5mg	50
Prothiaden Capsules 25mg	90
Prothiaden Tablets 75mg	57
Provera Tablets 5mg	69
Provera Tablets 100mg	134
Pro-Viron Tablets 25mg	118
Prozac Capsules 20mg	47
Pseudoephedrine Tablets BP, 60mg	55
Pyridoxine Tablets BP, 10mg	71
Pyridoxine Tablets BP, 20mg	102
Pyridoxine Tablets BP, 50mg	112
Pyrogastrone Tablets	148
Quinidine Sulph Tablets 200mg	103
Quinine Bisulph Tablets BP, 300mg	60
Quinine Sulph Tablets BP, 200mg	57
Quinine Sulph Tablets BP, 300mg	55
Ranitidine Tablets BP, 150mg	85
Rastinon Tablets 500mg	128
Relifex Tablets 500mg	87
Rheumox Capsules 300mg	101
Rheumox 600 Tablets	84
Rifadin Capsules 300mg	68
Rifampicin Capsules BP, 300mg	68
Rifinah 300 Tablets	93
Rimactane Capsules 300mg	68
Rimactazid 300 Tablets	93
Rivotril Tablets 0.5mg	117
Rivotril Tablets 2mg	104
Robaxin -750 Tablets	102
Ronicol Tablets 25mg	134
Ronicol Timespan Tablets	89
Rythmodan Capsules 100mg	142
Rythmodan Retard Tablets	92
Sabril Tablets 500mg	177
Salazopyrin EN Tablets	199
Salazopyrin Tablets	210
Salbutamol Tablets BP, 2mg	101
Salbutamol Tablets BP, 4mg	112
Saluric Tablets 500mg	75
Sando-K Tablets	130
Sandocal 400 Tablets	130
Sandocal 1000 Eff Tablets	65
Sanomigran Tablets 500microgram	94
Sanomigran Tablets 1.5mg	57
Saventrine Tablets 30mg	148
Secadrex Tablets	66
Seconal Sodium Pulvules 100mg	92
Sectral Capsules 100mg	113
Sectral 200 Capsules	103
Sectral 400 Tablets	67
Securon Tablets 120mg	96
Securon SR Tablets 240mg	63
Semi-Daonil Tablets 2.5mg	72
Senna Tablets BP, 7.5mg	95
Septrin Tablets Disp	40
Septrin Tablets Forte	22
Septrin Tablets Paed	74
Septrin Tablets	40
Serc-8 Tablets	138
Serc-16 Tablets	112
Serenace Capsules 0.5mg	99
Serenace Tablets 1.5mg	115
Serenace Tablets 5mg	101
Serenace Tablets 10mg	124
Serophene Tablets 50mg	30
Seroxat Tablets 20mg	46
Simvastatin Tablets 20mg	67
Sinemet-Plus Tablets	172
Sinemet-110 Tablets	161
Sinemet-275 Tablets	140

IIIA

Sinequan Capsules 10mg	98	Surmontil Tablets 25mg	85
Sinequan Capsules 25mg	89	Suscard Buccal Tablets 1mg	103
Sinequan Capsules 50mg	73	Suscard Buccal Tablets 2mg	114
Sinequan Capsules 75mg	52	Suscard Buccal Tablets 5mg	140
Sinthrome Tablets 1mg	124	Sustac Tablets 2.6mg	308
Slo-Phyllin Capsules 60mg	96	Sustac Tablets 6.4mg	128
Slo-Phyllin Capsules 125mg	87	Sustac Tablets 10mg	125
Slo-Phyllin Capsules 250mg	95	Sustamycin Capsules 250mg	46
Slow-Fe Folic	57	Symmetrel Capsules 100mg	88
Slow-Fe Tablets	62	Synflex Tablets 275mg	81
Slow-K Tablets 600mg	114	Tagamet Tablets 400mg	83
Slow Trasicor Tablets 160mg	73	Tagamet Tablets 800mg	46
Sodium Amytal Pulvules 60mg	108	Tagamet Tiltabs 200mg	117
Sodium Amytal Pulvules 200mg	78	Tambocor Tablets 100mg	108
Sodium Amytal Tablets 200mg	81	Tamoxifen Tablets BP, 10mg	113
Sodium Valproate Tablets		Tamoxifen Tablets BP, 20mg	75
BP, 100mg	205	Tarivid Tablets 200mg	18
Solpadol Caplets	106	Tavegil Tablets 1mg	64
Solpadol Eff Tablets	112	Tegretol Tablets 100mg	147
Soneryl Tablets 100mg	82	Tegretol Tablets 200mg	159
Soni-Slo Capsules 40mg	116	Tegretol Tablets 400mg	113
Sorbichew Tablets 5mg	108	Tegretol Retard Tablets 200mg	144
Sorbid - 40 SA Capsules	100	Temazepam Tablets 10mg	51
Sorbitrate Tablets 10mg	151	Temazepam Tablets 20mg	49
Sorbitrate Tablets 20mg	141	Temgesic Tablets Sublingual 0.2mg	97
Sotacor Tablets 80mg	99	Tenif Capsules	75
Sotacor Tablets 160mg	65	Tenoret 50 Tablets	65
Sotazide Tablets	66	Tenoretic Tablets	64
Spasmonal Capsules 60mg	105	Tenormin 25 Tablets	60
Spiroctan Capsules 100mg	52	Tenormin LS Tablets 50mg	60
Spiroctan Tablets 25mg	77	Tenormin Tablets 100mg	60
Spiroctan Tablets 50mg	69	Tenoxicam Tablets 20mg	46
Spirolone Tablets 25mg	85	Tenuate Dospan Tablets 75mg	47
Spirolone Tablets 50mg	63	Terfenadine Tablets 60mg	74
Spirolone Tablets 100mg	61	Terfenadine Tablets 120mg	49
Spironolactone Tablets BP, 25mg	95	Terramycin Capsules 250mg	50
Spironolactone Tablets BP, 50mg	65	Terramycin Tablets 250mg	43
Spironolactone Tablets BP, 100mg	56	Tertroxin Tablets 20microgram	152
Sporanox Capsules 100mg	12	Tetrabid-Organon Capsules 250mg	28
Staril Tablets 10mg	59	Tetrachel Capsules 250mg	49
Stelazine Spansules 2mg	84	Tetracycline Capsules BP, 250mg	49
Stelazine Spansules 10mg	70	Tetracycline Tablets BP, 250mg	57
Stelazine Spansules 15mg	77	Theo-Dur Tablets 200mg	100
Stelazine Tablets 1mg	102	Theo-Dur Tablets 300mg	87
Stelazine Tablets 5mg	106	Thephorin Tablets 25mg	82
Stemetil Tablets 5mg	85	Thiamine HCl Tablets 10mg	84
Stemetil Tablets 25mg	88	Thioridazine Tablets BP, 50mg	89
Stilboestrol Tablets BP, 1mg	130	Thioridazine Tablets BP, 100mg	100
Stilboestrol Tablets BP, 5mg	105	Thyroxine Tablets BP,	
Strepsils Lozenges	44	25 microgram	95
Stromba Tablets 5mg	76	Thyroxine Tablets BP,	
Stugeron Capsules Forte 75mg	109	50 microgram	115
Stugeron Tablets 15mg	122	Thyroxine Tablets BP,	
Sucralfate Tablets 1g	138	100 microgram	85
Sudafed Tablets 60mg	55	Tildiem Tablets 60mg	152
Sudafed Plus Tablets	53	Tildiem Retard 90 Tablets	99
Sulphasalazine Tablets 500mg	198	Tildiem Retard 120 Tablets	102
Sulpiride Tablets 200mg	118	Titralac Tablets	156
Suprax Tablets 200mg	12	Tofranil Tablets 10mg	108
Surgam Tablets 200mg	117	Tofranil Tablets 25mg	119
Surgam Tablets 300mg	81	Tolbutamide Tablets BP, 500mg	128
Surgam SA Capsules 300mg	82	Topal Tablets	128
Surmontil Capsules 50mg	72	Trancopal Tablets 200mg	73
Surmontil Tablets 10mg	85	Trandate Tablets 100mg	125

Trandate Tablets 200mg	135	Warfarin Tablets 5mg WB	74
Trandate Tablets 400mg	132	Welldorm Tablets	63
Trasicor Tablets 20mg	127	Zaditen Capsules 1mg	102
Trasicor Tablets 40mg	129	Zaditen Tablets 1mg	97
Trasicor Tablets 80mg	131	Zantac Tablets 150mg	85
Trasicor Tablets 160mg	124	Zantac Tablets 300mg	61
Trasidrex Tablets	76	Zarontin Capsules 250mg	147
Trental 400 Tablets	122	Zestril Tablets 2.5mg	63
Triludan Tablets 60mg	72	Zestril Tablets 5mg	64
Triludan Forte Tablets 120mg	49	Zestril Tablets 10mg	63
Trimethoprim Tablets BP, 100mg	42	Zestril Tablets 20mg	64
Trimethoprim Tablets BP, 200mg	19	Zimovane Tablets 7.5mg	41
Trimopan Tablets 200mg	25	Zinnat Tablets 250mg	114
Triptafen Tablets	99	Zirtek Tablets 10mg	45
Triptafen-M Tablets	100	Zocor Tablets 10mg	61
Tritace Capsules 5mg	71	Zocor Tablets 20mg	67
Tryptizol 75 Capsules	57	Zopiclone Tablets 7.5mg	41
Tryptizol Tablets 10mg	100	Zovirax Tablets 200mg	35
Tryptizol Tablets 25mg	97	Zovirax Tablets 800mg	47
Tryptizol Tablets 50mg	72	Zyloric Tablets 100mg	113
Tuinal Pulvules 100mg	104	Zyloric-300 Tablets	60
Tylex Capsules	114		
Tyrozets Lozenges	48		
Uniphyllin Continus Tablets 200mg	84		
Uniphyllin Continus Tablets 300mg	78		
Uniphyllin Continus Tablets 400mg	74		
Urantoin Tablets 50mg	66		
Urantoin Tablets 100mg	45		
Urispas Tablets 100mg	160		
Utinor Tablets 400mg	14		
Utovlan Tablets 5mg	84		
Vallergan Tablets 10mg	67		
Valoid Tablets 50mg	60		
Velosef Capsules 250mg	36		
Velosef Capsules 500mg	33		
Ventolin Tablets 2mg	106		
Ventolin Tablets 4mg	117		
Verapamil Tablets BP, 40mg	152		
Verapamil Tablets BP, 80mg	144		
Verapamil Tablets BP, 120mg	131		
Vibramycin Capsules 50mg	60		
Vibramycin Capsules 100mg	14		
Vibramycin-D Tablets 100mg	18		
Viskaldix Tablets	65		
Visken Tablets 5mg	116		
Visken Tablets 15mg	88		
Vitamin A & D Capsules BPC	87		
Vitamin Capsules BPC	85		
Vitamin B Compound Tablets BPC	90		
Vitamin B Compound Tablets Strong BPC	98		
Volital Tablets 20mg	109		
Volmax Tablets 4mg	73		
Volmax Tablets 8mg	79		
Volraman Tablets 50mg	91		
Voltarol Retard Tablets 100mg	51		
Voltarol SR Tablets 75mg	68		
Voltarol Tablets 25mg	112		
Voltarol Tablets 50mg	102		
Warfarin Tablets BP, 1mg	113		
Warfarin Tablets 1mg WB	114		
Warfarin Tablets BP, 3mg	86		
Warfarin Tablets 3mg WB	87		
Warfarin Tablets BP, 5mg	76		

IIIA

This Page Is Intentionally Blank

See Part II, Clause 6B(iii)(page 6)

			Fee per prescription P
1.	APPLIANCES		
	ELASTIC HOSIERY (Compression Hosiery)		
	Anklets, Kneecaps, Leggings		13
	Below-knee, Above-knee and Thigh Stockings		18
	TRUSSES		
	Spring	Single	50
	. . . .	Double	78
	Elastic Band	Single	23
	. . . .	Double	30
	Repairs		5
2.	OTHER APPLIANCES		2

IIIB

This Page Is Intentionally Blank

See Part II Clause 6A(iii) and 6C (pages 5 and 6)

1. A Pharmacy Contractor shall supply in a *suitable container* any drug which he is required to supply under Part 1 of the Fourth Schedule to the Regulations.

    Capsules, tablets, pills, pulvules etc shall be supplied in airtight containers of glass, aluminium or rigid plastics; card containers may be used only for foil/strip packed tablets etc. For ointments, creams, pastes, card containers shall not be used

    Eye, ear and nasal drops shall be supplied in dropper bottles, or with a separate dropper where appropriate.

2. *Payment for containers* is at the average rate of **6.50p** per prescription for every prescription (except a "Bulk" or oxygen prescription) supplied by contractors whether or not a container is supplied.

    This payment includes provision for supply of a *5ml plastic measuring spoon* which shall comply with BS 3221:Part 6:1993 and shall be made with every oral liquid medicine except where the manufacturer's pack includes one. However, when the prescribed dose is not 5ml or whole multiples of 5ml, and the pack does not already contain a suitable measuring device, a 5ml plastics oral syringe measure, wrapped together with a bottle adaptor and instruction leaflet, shall be supplied. This shall comply with BS 3221: Part 7: 1993, or an equivalent European Standard.

    In very exceptional circumstances, or where specifically requested by the prescriber dilution may still take place. The prescription should be endorsed accordingly.

3. Payment for containers is payable to pharmacy contractors and drug store contractors only.

IV

(Revised with effect from 1st April 2000)
See Part II Clause 6A(i)(b) (page 5)

Monthly Total of Prices £ From	To	Deduction Rate %	Monthly Total of Prices £ From	To	Deduction Rate %	Monthly Total of Prices £ From	To	Deduction Rate %
			6751	6875	8.22	13626	13750	9.96
1	125	6.51	6876	7000	8.25	13751	13875	10.00
126	250	6.54	7001	7125	8.28	13876	14000	10.03
251	375	6.57	7126	7250	8.32	14001	14125	10.06
376	500	6.61	7251	7375	8.35	14126	14250	10.09
501	625	6.64	7376	7500	8.38	14251	14375	10.12
626	750	6.67	7501	7625	8.41	14376	14500	10.15
751	875	6.70	7626	7750	8.44	14501	14625	10.19
876	1000	6.73	7751	7875	8.48	14626	14750	10.22
1001	1125	6.76	7876	8000	8.51	14751	14875	10.25
1126	1250	6.80	8001	8125	8.54	14876	15000	10.28
1251	1375	6.83	8126	8250	8.57	15001	15125	10.31
1376	1500	6.86	8251	8375	8.60	15126	15250	10.34
1501	1625	6.89	8376	8500	8.63	15251	15375	10.38
1626	1750	6.92	8501	8625	8.67	15376	15500	10.41
1751	1875	6.95	8626	8750	8.70	15501	34000	10.44
1876	2000	6.99	8751	8875	8.73	34001	34250	10.45
2001	2125	7.02	8876	9000	8.76	34251	34750	10.46
2126	2250	7.05	9001	9125	8.79	34751	35000	10.47
2251	2375	7.08	9126	9250	8.82	35001	35250	10.48
2376	2500	7.11	9251	9375	8.86	35251	35500	10.49
2501	2625	7.14	9376	9500	8.89	35501	36000	10.50
2626	2750	7.18	9501	9625	8.92	36001	36250	10.51
2751	2875	7.21	9626	9750	8.95	36251	36500	10.52
2876	3000	7.24	9751	9875	8.98	36501	37000	10.53
3001	3125	7.27	9876	10000	9.01	37001	37250	10.54
3126	3250	7.30	10001	10125	9.05	37251	37500	10.55
3251	3375	7.33	10126	10250	9.08	37501	37750	10.56
3376	3500	7.37	10251	10375	9.11	37751	38250	10.57
3501	3625	7.40	10376	10500	9.14	38251	38500	10.58
3626	3750	7.43	10501	10625	9.17	38501	38750	10.59
3751	3875	7.46	10626	10750	9.20	38751	39000	10.60
3876	4000	7.49	10751	10875	9.24	39001	39500	10.61
4001	4125	7.52	10876	11000	9.27	39501	39750	10.62
4126	4250	7.56	11001	11125	9.30	39751	40000	10.63
4251	4375	7.59	11126	11250	9.33	40001	40250	10.64
4376	4500	7.62	11251	11375	9.36	40251	40750	10.65
4501	4625	7.65	11376	11500	9.39	40751	41000	10.66
4626	4750	7.68	11501	11625	9.43	41001	41250	10.67
4751	4875	7.71	11626	11750	9.46	41251	41500	10.68
4876	5000	7.75	11751	11875	9.49	41501	42000	10.69
5001	5125	7.78	11876	12000	9.52	42001	42250	10.70
5126	5250	7.81	12001	12125	9.55	42251	42500	10.71
5251	5375	7.84	12126	12250	9.58	42501	43000	10.72
5376	5500	7.87	12251	12375	9.62	43001	43250	10.73
5501	5625	7.90	12376	12500	9.65	43251	43500	10.74
5626	5750	7.94	12501	12625	9.68	43501	43750	10.75
5751	5875	7.97	12626	12750	9.71	43751	44250	10.76
5876	6000	8.00	12751	12875	9.74	44251	44500	10.77
6001	6125	8.03	12876	13000	9.77	44501	44750	10.78
6126	6250	8.06	13001	13125	9.81	44751	45000	10.79
6251	6375	8.09	13126	13250	9.84	45001	45500	10.80
6376	6500	8.13	13251	13375	9.87	45501	45750	10.81
6501	6625	8.16	13376	13500	9.90	45751	46000	10.82
6626	6750	8.19	13501	13625	9.93	46001	46250	10.83

V

DEDUCTION SCALE (Pharmacy Contractors)

(Revised with effect from 1st April 2000)
See Part II Clause 6A(i)(b) (page 5)

Monthly Total of Prices £		Deduction Rate %	Monthly Total of Prices £		Deduction Rate %	Monthly Total of Prices £		Deduction Rate %
From	To		From	To		From	To	
46251	46750	10.84	63501	63750	11.38	101751	102750	11.92
46751	47000	10.85	63751	64000	11.39	102751	103500	11.93
47001	47250	10.86	64001	64250	11.40	103501	104250	11.94
47251	47500	10.87	64251	64750	11.41	104251	105250	11.95
47501	48000	10.88	64751	65000	11.42	105251	106000	11.96
48001	48250	10.89	65001	65250	11.43	106001	106750	11.97
48251	48500	10.90	65251	65750	11.44	106751	107750	11.98
48501	49000	10.91	65751	66000	11.45	107751	108500	11.99
49001	49250	10.92	66001	66250	11.46	108501	109250	12.00
49251	49500	10.93	66251	66500	11.47	109251	110000	12.01
49501	49750	10.94	66501	67000	11.48	110001	111000	12.02
49751	50250	10.95	67001	67250	11.49	111001	111750	12.03
50251	50500	10.96	67251	67750	11.50	111751	112500	12.04
50501	50750	10.97	67751	68500	11.51	112501	113500	12.05
50751	51000	10.98	68501	69500	11.52	113501	114250	12.06
51001	51500	10.99	69501	70250	11.53	114251	115000	12.07
51501	51750	11.00	70251	71000	11.54	115001	116000	12.08
51751	52000	11.01	71001	72000	11.55	116001	116750	12.09
52001	52250	11.02	72001	72750	11.56	116751	117500	12.10
52251	52750	11.03	72751	73500	11.57	117501	118500	12.11
52751	53000	11.04	73501	74500	11.58	118501	119250	12.12
53001	53250	11.05	74501	75250	11.59	119251	120000	12.13
53251	53750	11.06	75251	76000	11.60	120001	121000	12.14
53751	54000	11.07	76001	77000	11.61	121001	121750	12.15
54001	54250	11.08	77001	77750	11.62	121751	122500	12.16
54251	54500	11.09	77751	78500	11.63	122501	123500	12.17
54501	55000	11.10	78501	79500	11.64	123501	124250	12.18
55001	55250	11.11	79501	80250	11.65	124251	125000	12.19
55251	55500	11.12	80251	81000	11.66	125001	126000	12.20
55501	55750	11.13	81001	82000	11.67	126001	126750	12.21
55751	56250	11.14	82001	82750	11.68	126751	127500	12.22
56251	56500	11.15	82751	83500	11.69	127501	128500	12.23
56501	56750	11.16	83501	84500	11.70	128501	129250	12.24
56751	57000	11.17	84501	85250	11.71	129251	130000	12.25
57001	57500	11.18	85251	86000	11.72	130001	130750	12.26
57501	57750	11.19	86001	87000	11.73	130751	131750	12.27
57751	58000	11.20	87001	87750	11.74	131751	132500	12.28
58001	58250	11.21	87751	88500	11.75	132501	133250	12.29
58251	58750	11.22	88501	89250	11.76	133251	134250	12.30
58751	59000	11.23	89251	90250	11.77	134251	135000	12.31
59001	59250	11.24	90251	91000	11.78	135001	135750	12.32
59251	59750	11.25	91001	91750	11.79	135751	136750	12.33
59751	60000	11.26	91751	92750	11.80	136751	137500	12.34
60001	60250	11.27	92751	93500	11.81	137501	138250	12.35
60251	60500	11.28	93501	94250	11.82	138251	139250	12.36
60501	61000	11.29	94251	95250	11.83	139251	140000	12.37
61001	61250	11.30	95251	96000	11.84	140001	140750	12.38
61251	61500	11.31	96001	96750	11.85	140751	141750	12.39
61501	61750	11.32	96751	97750	11.86	141751	142500	12.40
61751	62250	11.33	97751	98500	11.87	142501	143250	12.41
62251	62500	11.34	98501	99250	11.88	143251	144250	12.42
62501	62750	11.35	99251	100250	11.89	144251	145000	12.43
62751	63000	11.36	100251	101000	11.90	145001	145750	12.44
63001	63500	11.37	101001	101750	11.91	145751	146750	12.45

(Revised with effect from 1st April 2000)
See Part II Clause 6A(i)(b) (page 5)

Monthly Total of Prices £		Deduction Rate %	Monthly Total of Prices £		Deduction Rate %	Monthly Total of Prices £		Deduction Rate %
From	To		From	To		From	To	
146751	147500	12.46						
147501	148250	12.47						
148251	149250	12.48						
149251	150000	12.49						
150001	& Over	12.50						

V

(Revised with effect from 1st April 2000)
See Part II Clause 6A(i)(b) (page 5)

This Page Is Intentionally Blank

PAYMENT FOR ADDITIONAL PROFESSIONAL SERVICES

1. Contractors who have had passed for payment by the Pricing Authority between 1,100 and 1,600 prescriptions in the relevant month will, subject to (i) - (iii) below, receive a payment rising from £755 at 1,100 prescriptions to £1,460 (from April 1999) at 1,600 prescriptions. The rate of £1,460 (from April 1999) will apply to all contractors who have had passed for payment 1,600 or more prescriptions in the relevant month.

    The following additional conditions must be satisfied:

    1.1   the pharmacy must produce a practice leaflet;

    1.2   the pharmacy must display up to a maximum of eight health promotion leaflets. Contractors may display additional health promotion material if they wish, but are not required to do so to receive payment;

    1.3   the contractor must, subject to the provisions of Part XIVB, keep patient medication records.

2. Contractors who had passed for pricing 13,200 or more prescriptions between 1 April 1999 and 31 March 2000, but did not receive a professional allowance in each month of the relevant period may apply for top up payment.

3. Contractors will be eligible for a payment of £755 for each month in which no payment was made between April 1999 and March 2000 provided that the following conditions are met:

    3.1   the relevant number of prescriptions was passed for pricing in the period as a whole;

    3.2   the other criteria for the professional allowance has been met throughout the period (see (i) to (iii) above);

    3.3   prescriptions have been regularly submitted to the Pricing Authority each month and the Pricing Authority has made no abatement;

    3.4   the contractor has been open throughout the period for which the claim has been made.

4. Contractors should make a claim for top up payments to their Health Authority by 31 October 2000. They should submit copies of FP34 statements for the relevant period (April 1999 to March 2000) as evidence of the total number of prescriptions passed for pricing during this period.

Note: Contractors in receipt of ESPS payments are not eligible for top up professional allowance payments at the end of the year. Non-payment of the professional allowance in a particular month will have been taken into account in calculating the level of ESPS subsidy due.

These arrangements apply for 1999/2000 only. Instructions for 2000/2001 will be given in the April 2001 Drug Tariff.

VIA

This Page Is Intentionally Blank

See Part II Clause 6B(ii) (page 6)

Number of prescriptions dispensed during month		On-cost %	Number of prescriptions dispensed during month		On-cost %
From	To		From	To	
1	505	25.0	1036	1048	20.3
506	515	24.9	1049	1062	20.2
516	526	24.8	1063	1076	20.1
527	537	24.7	1077	1090	20.0
538	549	24.6	1091	1105	19.9
550	561	24.5	1106	1120	19.8
562	574	24.4	1121	1136	19.7
575	588	24.3	1137	1152	19.6
589	602	24.2	1153	1169	19.5
603	617	24.1	1170	1186	19.4
618	632	24.0	1187	1203	19.3
633	649	23.9	1204	1221	19.2
650	666	23.8	1222	1240	19.1
667	684	23.7	1241	1259	19.0
685	704	23.6	1260	1279	18.9
705	724	23.5	1280	1300	18.8
725	746	23.4	1301	1321	18.7
747	756	23.3	1322	1342	18.6
757	762	23.2	1343	1365	18.5
763	770	23.1	1366	1388	18.4
771	777	23.0	1389	1413	18.3
778	785	22.9	1414	1438	18.2
786	792	22.8	1439	1463	18.1
793	800	22.7	1464	1490	18.0
801	808	22.6	1491	1518	17.9
809	816	22.5	1519	1547	17.8
817	824	22.4	1548	1577	17.7
825	833	22.3	1578	1608	17.6
834	841	22.2	1609	1641	17.5
842	850	22.1	1642	1675	17.4
851	859	22.0	1676	1710	17.3
860	868	21.9	1711	1747	17.2
869	878	21.8	1748	1785	17.1
879	887	21.7	1786	1825	17.0
888	897	21.6	1826	1867	16.9
898	907	21.5	1868	1911	16.8
908	918	21.4	1912	1957	16.7
919	928	21.3	1958	2006	16.6
929	939	21.2	2007	2056	16.5
940	950	21.1	2057	2110	16.4
951	961	21.0	2111	2166	16.3
962	973	20.9	2167	2226	16.2
974	984	20.8	2227	2288	16.1
985	996	20.7	2289	2355	16.0
997	1009	20.6	2356	2425	15.9
1010	1022	20.5	2426	2500	15.8
1023	1035	20.4			

VIB

See Part II Clause 6B(ii) (page 6)

This Page Is Intentionally Blank

LIST OF DRUGS WITH A COMMONLY USED PACK SIZE
See Part II, Clause 7D (page 7)

If a drug specified in this list is supplied but the relative prescription form is not endorsed payment will be calculated on the basis of the price for the pack size listed

Drug	Common Pack	
Anusol Suppositories	24	
Azathioprine Tablets, 50mg	100	
Benadryl Allergy Relief Capsules 8mg	24	
Betahistine Dihydrochloride Tablets 8mg	84	
Brufen 400 Tablets	250	
Capoten Tablets, 25mg	56	
Ceporex Capsules, 250mg	100	
Ceporex Capsules, 500mg	100	
Ceporex Tablets, 250mg	100	
Ceporex Tablets, 500mg	100	
Co-amilozide Tablets BP, 2.5/25	100	
Co-codamol Tablets BP, 8/5000	500	
(Syn: Codeine Phosphate and Paracetamol Tablets 8/500)		
Co-dydramol Tablets BP, 10/500	500	
(Syn: Dihydrocodeine and Paracetamol Tablets 10/500)		
Deltacortril Enteric Tablets, 2.5mg	100	
Deltacortril Enteric Tablets, 5mg	100	
Dexamethasone Tablets BP, 2mg	500	
Dexomon SR Tablets 75mg	56	
Diclofenac Tablets BP, 25mg (e/c)	100	
Diclofenac Tablets BP, 50mg (e/c)	100	
Diclovol SR Tablets 75mg	28	
Dihydrocodeine Tablets BP, 30mg	100	
Dipyridamole Tablets BP, 25mg	100	
Diumide-K Tablets Continus	250	
Elantan 10 Tablets, 10mg	84	
Elantan 20 Tablets, 20mg	84	
Enprin Tablets, 75mg	56	
Erythrocin 250 Tablets	500	
Frusemide Tablets BP, 500mg	28	
Fybogel Orange Sachets	60	(2x30)
Galpseud Linctus	2	litre
Galpseud Tablets	100	
Gaviscon Liquid Aniseed	500	ml
Gaviscon Liquid Peppermint	500	ml
Glibenclamide Tablets BP, 2.5mg	100	
Haloperidol Tablets BP, 1.5mg	250	
Haloperidol Tablets BP, 5mg	28	
Hexopal Tablets	500	

VII

Drug	Common Pack	

Imodium Capsules	250	
Imodium Plus Tablets	18	
Keflex Pulvules, 250mg	100	
Keflex Pulvules, 500mg	100	
Keflex Tablets, 250mg	100	
Keflex Tablets, 500mg	100	
Kolanticon Gel	500	ml
Lasix Tablets 40mg	28	
Melleril Tablets, 25mg	1,000	
Melleril Tablets, 50mg	1,000	
Metformin Tablets, 850mg	300	
Metoprolol Tartrate Tablets BP, 50mg	100	
Metoprolol Tartrate Tablets BP, 100mg	100	
Minocin Tablets, 100mg	20	
Monit Tablets	100	
Natrilix Tablets, 2.5mg	60	
Nicef Capsules, 250mg	100	
Nicef Capsules, 500mg	100	
Nifedipine Capsules BP, 5mg	84	
Novonorm Tablets, 500 microgram	90	
Novonorm Tablets, 1mg	90	
Nurofen for Children Oral Suspension 100mg/5ml sugar free	150	ml
Oxybutinin Hydrochloride Tablets 5mg	56	
Penbritin Capsules, 250mg	100	
Praxilene Capsules	500	
Prednisolone Enteric-coated Tablets BP, 2.5mg	100	
(Syn: Gastro-resistant Prednisolone Tablets 2.5mg)		
Prednisolone Enteric-coated Tablets BP, 5mg	100	
(Syn: Gastro-resistant Prednisolone Tablets 5mg)		
Proflavine Cream	500ml	
(Syns: Flavine Cream, Proflavine Emulsion)		
Prothiaden Capsules	600	
Prothiaden Tablets	500	
Provera Tablets, 100mg	100	
Redoxon Slow Release Vit C Capsules	40	
Senokot Syrup	500	ml
Slo-phyllin Capsules 250mg	100	
Stugeron Tablets	100	
Sudafed Elixir	1	litre
Sudafed Tablets	100	
Theophylline Capsules, 250mg (m/r)	100	
Trandate Tablets, 100mg	250	
Trandate Tablets, 200mg	250	
Velosef Capsules, 250mg	100	
Velosef Capsules, 500mg	100	

BASIC PRICE OF DRUGS
COVERED BY PART II CLAUSE 8A

The price listed in respect of a drug specified in the following list is
the basic price (see Part II, Clause 8) on which payment will be calculated
pursuant to Part II Clause 6A for the dispensing of that drug

NOTES:

1.   All drugs listed in this Part have a pack size and price which has been determined by the Secretary of State for Health as respects England and the National Assembly for Wales as respects Wales.

2.   Categories A,B,C,D and E of the drugs (appearing in Col.4) are as under:

     2.1   Category A - Drugs which are readily available. Endorsement of pack size is required if more than one pack size is listed. Broken Bulk may be claimed if necessary.

     2.2   Category B - Drugs whose usage has declined over time. No endorsement is required other than a claim for Broken Bulk if necessary.

     2.3   Category C - Priced on the basis of a particular brand or particular manufacturer. Endorsement of pack size is required if more than one pack is listed. Broken Bulk may be claimed if necessary.

     2.4   Category D - Drugs for which there is a problem of availability at the lowest price. Endorsement of manufacturer/supplier and pack size is needed. In the absence of such an endorsement payment will default to the lowest price as listed. Broken Bulk may be claimed if necessary.

     2.5   Category E - Extemporaneously prepared items for which the fee listed under Part III A(a)(ii), (iii), (iv) or (v) will be claimed. No endorsement is required. Broken Bulk is not allowed, but may be paid on the ingredients.

3.   Methylated Spirit

     Industrial Methylated Spirit should be supplied or used and payment will be calculated accordingly, where:

     3.1   "Methylated Spirit", "Spirit", "Spt. Vini. Meth.", "SVM", "IMS", is ordered alone or as an ingredient of a preparation for external use, or

     3.2   A liniment, lotion, etc., in the preparatioin of which Methylated Spirit is permitted, is ordered and the prescriber has not indicated to the contrary.

4.   Rectified Spirit

     4.1   Where Alcohol (96%), or Rectified Spirit (Ethanol 90%), or any other of the dilute Ethanols is prescribed alone or as an ingredient in a medicament for external application, payment will be made for supply of Industrial Methylated Spirit unless the prescriber has indicated that no alternative may be used.

     4.2   Where Alcohol (96%), or Rectified Spirit (Ethanol 90%), or any other of the dilute Ethanols is prescribed as an ingredient of a medicine for internal use, the price of the duty paid to Customs and Excise will be allowed, unless the contractor endorses the prescription form "rebate claimed".

VIII

5.   Purified Water
        (Exclusive of ordinary potable water)

        Payment for Purified Water will be made:

        5.1   where it is ordered:

        5.2   where the water is included in any preparation intended for application to the eye;

        5.3   where, in the opinion of the pharmacist the use of ordinary potable water in a particular
                preparation would result in an undesirable change in the medicament prescribed and he endorses
                the prescription form accordingly;

        5.4   where the Health Authority, after consultation with the Local Medical Committee and Local
                Pharmaceutical Committee, has decided with the approval of the Secretary of State for Health
                as respects England and the National Assembly for Wales as respects Wales that the water
                ordinarily available is unsuitable for dispensing purposes, and has notified the contractor
                accordingly.

        When Purified Water is used instead of potable water, it should be freshly boiled and cooled.

6.   A "Bulk" prescription is an order for two or more patients, bearing the name of a school or institution
        in which at least 20 persons normally reside, for the treatment of at least 10 of whom a particular doctor
        is responsible. Such a prescription must be an order for a drug which is prescribable under the NHS and
        which is not designated a "Prescription Only Medicine" (POM) under Section 58(1) of the Medicines Act
        1968, or for a prescribable dressing which does not contain a product which is designated POM.

Drug	Quantity		Basic Price p	Category	
Acacia Powder BP 1993	500	g	880	B	
Acarbose Tablets 50mg	90		968	C	*(Glucobay 50)*
Acarbose Tablets 100mg	90		1251	C	*(Glucobay 100)*
Acebutolol Capsules 100mg (as hydrochloride)	84		1610	C	*(Sectral)*
Acebutolol Capsules 200mg (as hydrochloride)	56		2063	C	*(Sectral 200)*
Acebutolol Tablets 400mg (as hydrochloride)	♦ 28		2002	C	*(Sectral 400)*
Aceclofenac Tabs 100mg	60		1495	C	*(Preservex)*
Acemetacin Capsules 60mg	90		2136	C	*(Emflex)*
Acetazolamide Capsules 250mg (m/r)	♦ 28		1050	C	*(Diamox SR)*
Acetazolamide Tablets BP 250mg	112		1153	C	*(Diamox)*
Acetic Acid (33 per cent) BP (Syn: Acetic Acid)	500	ml	225	A	
Acetone BP	500	ml	177	A	
Acetylsalicylic Acid Mixture BPC 1963	200	ml	37	E	
(Asprin Mixture)					
Aciclovir Cream BP, 5% w/w	■ 2	g	290	A	
(Syn: Acyclovir Cream 5% w/w)	■ 10	g	809 ▽	A	
Aciclovir Eye Ointment BP, 3% w/w	■ 4.5	g	1067	C	*(Zovirax)*
Aciclovir Oral Suspension BP, 200mg/5ml sugar free .	125	ml	2889	C	*(Zovirax)*
(Syn: Acyclovir Oral Suspension 200mg/5ml					
sugar free)					
Aciclovir Oral Suspension BP, 400mg/5ml sugar free .	■ 50	ml	1614	C	*(Zovirax*
(Chickenpox Treatment)					*Chickenpox*
(Syn: Acyclovir Oral Suspension 400mg/5ml					*Treatment)*
sugar free)					
Aciclovir Tablets BP, 200mg	25		562 △	A	
(Syn: Acyclovir Tablets 200mg)					
Aciclovir Tablets BP, 400mg	56		1490 △	A	
(Syn: Acyclovir Tablets 400mg)					
Aciclovir Tablets, Dispersible 200mg	25		510	A	
Aciclovir Tablets, Dispersible 400mg	♦ 56		1846	A	
Aciclovir Tablets, Dispersible 800mg	35		1899	A	
Acriflavine Emulsion - (See Proflavine Cream BPC) . . .	-		-	-	
Acrivastine Capsules 8mg	84		481	C	*(Semprex)*
Adrenaline Injection BP, 0.5ml ampoules	10		486	A	
(Syn: Adrenaline Tartrate Injection 0.5ml					
ampoules)					
Adrenaline Injection BP, 1ml ampoules	10		364	A	
(Syn: Adrenaline Tartrate Injection 1ml					
ampoules)					
Alcohol 90% v/v (See Ethanol 90 per-cent BP)	-		-	-	
Alendronic Acid Tablets 10mg	♦ 28		2312	C	*(Fosamax)*
(as alendronate sodium)					
Alfacalcidol Capsules 250 nanogram	■ 30		337	C	
Alfacalcidol Capsules 500 nanogram	■ 30		674	C	*(One-Alpha)*
Alfacalcidol Capsules 1 microgram	■ 30		1006	C	

VIII

■ Special Containers
♦ Manufacturers' Calendar Packs

Drug	Quantity		Basic Price p		Category	
Alfuzosin Hydrochloride Tablets 2.5mg	60		1900		C	(Xatral)
. . . .	90		2500		C	(Xatral)
Alfuzosin Hydrochloride Tablets 5mg (m/r)	60		2380		C	(Xatral SR)
Alkaline Ipecacuanha Mixture BPC 1963	200	ml	22		E	
(Syn: Mist. Expect Alk)						
Allopurinol Tablets BP, 100mg	28		90		A	
Allopurinol Tablets BP, 300mg	28		217		A	
Almond Oil BP	500	ml	411		A	
§ Alprostadil Injection 10 microgram/ml	■ 1		735		C	
1ml vial + diluent -filled syringe						
§ Alprostadil Injection 20 microgram/ml	■ 1		950		C	
1ml vial + diluent-filled syringe						
Alum BP (Granular Powder)	100	g	30		A	
(Syns: Potash Alum,						
Aluminium Potassium Sulphate)						
Alverine Citrate Capsules 60mg	100		1092		C	(Spasmonal)
Alverine Citrate Capsules 120mg	60		1310		C	(Spasmonal Forte)
Amantadine Capsules BP, 100mg	56		1535		C	(Symmetrel)
Amantadine Oral Solution BP, 50mg/5ml	■ 150	ml	505		C	(Symmetrel Syrup)
Amaranth Solution BP 1988	500	ml	395		C	(Loveridge)
Amiloride Tablets BP, 5mg	28		164	▽	A	
Aminoglutethimide Tablets 250mg	56		2022		C	(Orimeten)
. . . .	100		3611		A	
Aminophylline Injection BP, 250mg/10ml ampoules . .	10		673	△	A	
Amiodarone Tablets BP, 100mg	♦ 28		426		A	
Amiodarone Tablets BP, 200mg	♦ 28		646		A	
Amitriptyline Tablets BP, 10mg	28		78		A	
Amitriptyline Tablets BP, 25mg	28		80		A	
Amitriptyline Tablets BP, 50mg	28		120		A	
Amitriptyline Hydrochloride Capsules 25mg (m/r) . . .	56		258		C	(Lentizol)
Amitriptyline Hydrochloride Capsules 50mg (m/r) . . .	56		479		C	(Lentizol)
Amitriptyline Hydrochloride Oral Solution						
50mg/5ml sugar free	500	ml	3550		A	
Amlodipine Besylate Tablets 5mg	♦ 28		1185		C	(Istin)
Amlodipine Besylate Tablets 10mg	♦ 28		1770		C	(Istin)
Ammonia Aromatic Solution BP	500	ml	354		A	
(Syn: Sal. Volatile Solution)						
Ammonia and Ipecacuanha Mixture BP	500	ml	170		C	(AAH)
(Syn: Ammonia and Ipecacuanha Oral Solution)						
Ammonium Acetate Solution, Strong BP	500	ml	350		A	
Ammonium Bicarbonate BP	500	g	205		C	(Thornton & Ross)
Ammonium Chloride BP	500	g	295		C	(Thornton & Ross)

§ Only allowed to be prescribed in certain circumstances, see Part XVIIIB
■ Special Containers
♦ Manufacturers' Calendar Packs

Drug	Quantity		Basic Price p	Category	
Ammonium Chloride Mixture BP	200	ml	39	E	
(Syn: Ammonium Chloride Oral Solution)					
Amorolfine Cream 0.25% w/w (as hydrochloride) . . . ■	20	g	483	C	(Loceryl)
Amorolfine Nail Lacquer 5% w/v . . . . ■	5	ml	2994	C	(Loceryl)
(as hydrochloride)					
Amoxycillin Capsules BP, 250mg	21		124	A	
Amoxycillin Capsules BP, 500mg	21		184	A	
. . . .	100		528	A	
Amoxycillin Injection BP, 250mg	10		344	C	(Amoxil)
(as sodium salt) vials					
Amoxycillin Injection BP, 500mg	10		626	C	(Amoxil)
(as sodium salt) vials					
Amoxycillin Injection BP, 1 g	10		1252	C	(Amoxil)
(as sodium salt) vials					
Amoxycillin Oral Powder DPF, 3 g	2		467	A	
(Amoxycillin Sachets 3g (as trihydrate), sugar free)	14		3194	A	
Amoxycillin Oral Suspension BP, 125mg/1.25ml (paediatric)					
●	20	ml	363	C	(Amoxil)
(Syns: Amoxycillin Mixture 125mg/1.25ml (paediatric)					
Amoxycillin Syrup 125mg/1.25ml (paediatric))					
Amoxycillin Oral Suspension BP, 125mg/5ml . . . . . . ●	100	ml	114	A	
(Syns: Amoxycillin Mixture 125mg/5ml,					
Amoxycillin Syrup 125mg/5ml)					
Amoxycillin Oral Suspension BP, ... ●	100	ml	129	A	
125mg/5ml sugar free					
(Syns: Amoxycillin Mixture 125mg/5ml sugar free					
Amoxycillin Syrup 125mg/5ml sugar free)					
Amoxycillin Oral Suspension BP, 250mg/5ml . . . . . . ●	100	ml	179	A	
(Syns: Amoxycillin Mixture 250mg/5ml					
Amoxycillin Syrup 250mg/5ml)					
Amoxycillin Oral Suspension BP, ... ●	100	ml	225	A	
250mg/5ml sugar free					
(Syns: Amoxycillin Mixture 250mg/5ml sugar free					
Amoxycillin Syrup 250mg/5ml sugar free)					
Amphotericin Lozenges BP, 10mg	60		395	C	(Fungilin)
Amphotericin Oral Suspension DPF, 100mg/ml sugar free ■	12	ml	231	C	(Fungilin)
Amphotericin Tablets 100mg	56		832	C	(Fungilin)
Ampicillin Capsules BP, 250mg	28		182 ∇	A	
. . . .	500		1559	A	
Ampicillin Capsules BP, 500mg	28		359	A	
. . . .	250		1494	A	
Ampicillin Oral Suspension BP, 125mg/5ml . . . . ●	100	ml	175	A	
(Syns: Ampicillin Mixture 125mg/5ml					
Ampicillin Syrup 125mg/5ml)					
Ampicillin Oral Suspension BP, 250mg/5ml . . . . ●	100	ml	323	A	
(Syns: Ampicillin Mixture 250mg/5ml					
Ampicillin Syrup 250mg/5ml)					
Anastrozole Tablets 1mg . . . . ♦	28		8316	C	(Arimidex)
Anise Oil BP (Syn: Aniseed Oil)	100	ml	455	A	
Anise Water, Concentrated BP	100	ml	692	A	
Aqueous Cream BP	500	g	105	A	

VIII

■ Special Containers
♦ Manufacturers' Calendar Packs
● Preparations Requiring Reconstitution

Drug	Quantity		Basic Price p	Category	
Arachis Oil BP (Syns: Ground-nut Oil; Peanut Oil) . . .	200	ml	136	A	
Arachis Oil Enema in 130ml single-dose	■ 130	ml	102	C	*(Fletchers)*
disposable packs					
Ascorbic Acid BP (Syn: Vitamin C)	100	g	345	C	(Thornton & Ross)
Ascorbic Acid Tablets BP, 100mg	100		90	A	
(Syn: Vitamin C Tablets 100mg)					
Ascorbic Acid Tablets BP, 200mg	100		112	A	
(Syn: Vitamin C Tablets 200mg)					
Ascorbic Acid Tablets BP, 500mg	28		125	A	
(Syn: Vitamin C Tablets 500mg)	100		199 ▽	A	
Aspirin BP (Syn: Acetylsalicylic Acid)	500	g	900	C	(Thornton & Ross)
Aspirin Tablets BP, 300mg	32		31	A	
(Syn: Acetylsalicylic Acid Tablets 300mg)					
Aspirin Tablets 75mg (e/c)	28		149 ▽	A	
. . . .	♦ 56		301	A	
Aspirin Tablets 300mg (e/c)	100		510	A	
Aspirin Tablets Dispersible BP, 75mg	28		32	A	
. . . .	100		56 ▽	A	
Aspirin Tablets, Dispersible BP, 300mg	32		34	A	
(Soluble Aspirin Tablets)	100		110	A	
Atenolol Oral Solution BP, sugar free 25mg/5ml	300	ml	777	C	*(Tenormin*
					Syrup)
Atenolol Tablets BP, 25mg	♦ 28		72 ▽	A	
Atenolol Tablets BP, 50mg	♦ 28		82 ▽	A	
Atenolol Tablets BP, 100mg	♦ 28		103	A	
Atorvastatin Tablets 10mg	♦ 28		1888	C	*(Lipitor)*
(as calcium trihydrate)					
Atorvastatin Tablets 20mg	♦ 28		3060	C	*(Lipitor)*
(as calcium trihydrate)					
Atorvastatin Tablets 40mg	♦ 28		4704	C	*(Lipitor)*
(as calcium trihydrate)					
Atropine Eye Drops BP, 1% w/v	■ 10	ml	83	A	
Atropine Eye Ointment BP, 1%	■ 3	g	258	A	
Atropine Injection BP, 600 microgram/1ml ampoule . .	10		461	A	
Atropine Tablets BP, 600 microgram	28		598	A	
Auranofin Tablets 3mg	60		2240	C	*(Ridaura)*
Azapropazone Capsules BP, 300mg	100		1432	C	*(Rheumox)*
Azapropazone Tablets BP, 600mg	100		2488	C	*(Rheumox 600)*
Azathioprine Tablets BP, 25mg	28		908	A	
. . . .	100		3322	A	
Azathioprine Tablets BP, 50mg	♦ 56		997	A	
. . . .	★ 100		1589	A	
Azelastine Hydrochloride Aqueous Nasal Spray					
140 microgram (0.14ml)/metered spray	■ 136	dose	1192	C	*(Rhinolast)*
Azithromycin Capsules 250mg (as dihydrate)	4		895	C	*(Zithromax)*
. . . .	6		1343	C	*(Zithromax)*
Azithromycin Oral Suspension 200mg/5ml	● 15	ml	508	C	*(Zithromax)*
(as dihydrate)	● 22.5	ml	762	C	*(Zithromax)*
. . . .	● 30	ml	1380	C	*(Zithromax)*
Azithromycin Tablets 500mg	3		1099	C	*(Zithromax)*
(as dihydrate)					

■ Special Containers
♦ Manufacturers' Calendar Packs
● Preparations Requiring Reconstitution
★ Common Pack

Drug	Quantity		Basic Price p	Category	
Baclofen Oral Solution BP, 5mg/5ml sugar free	300	ml	746	C	*(Lioresal Liquid)*
Baclofen Tablets BP, 10mg	28		102	A	
. . . .	84		305	A	
. . . .	100		284	A	
Bambuterol Hydrochloride Tablets 10mg	28		1095	C	*(Bambec)*
Bambuterol Hydrochloride Tablets 20mg	28		1314	C	*(Bambec)*
Beclomethasone Nasal Spray BP, ...	■ 200	dose	346	A	
50 micrograms/metered spray (Aqueous)					
Beclomethasone Pressurised Inhalation BP, ...	■ 200	dose	425	A	
50 microgram per actuation					
Beclomethasone Pressurised Inhalation BP, ...	■ 200	dose	824	A	
100 microgram per actuation					
Beclomethasone Pressurised Inhalation BP, ...	■ 200	dose	1961	C	*(Becotide 200)*
200 microgram per actuation					
Beclomethasone Pressurised Inhalation BP, ...	■ 200	dose	1779	A	
250 microgram per actuation					
Beclomethasone Dipropionate Dry Powder Capsules .	112		847	C	*(Becotide*
for Inhalation 100 microgram					*Rotacaps)*
Beclomethasone Dipropionate Dry Powder Capsules .	112		1607	C	*(Becotide*
for Inhalation 200 microgram					*Rotacaps)*
Beclomethasone Dipropionate Dry Powder Capsules .	112		3054	C	*(Becotide*
for Inhalation 400 microgram					*Rotacaps)*
Beeswax, White BP (Plates)	500	g	645	C	(AAH)
Beeswax, Yellow BP	500	g	1095	C	(Thornton & Ross)
Belladonna Tincture BP	500	ml	402	A	
Bendrofluazide Tablets BP, 2.5mg	28		74	A	
Bendrofluazide Tablets BP, 5mg	28		73	A	
Benorylate Oral Suspension BP sugar free	300	ml	1105	A	
(Syn: Benorylate Mixture sugar free)					
Benorylate Tablets BP, 750mg	100		867	A	
Benzhexol Tablets BP, 2mg	84		267 ∇	A	
. . . .	100		299	A	
Benzhexol Tablets BP, 5mg	100		391	A	
Benzoic Acid Ointment, Compound BP	500	g	313	A	
(Syn: Whitfield's Ointment)					
Benzoin Tincture BPC	500	ml	470	C	(Thornton & Ross)
Benzoin Tincture Compound BP (Syn: Friars' Balsam) .	500	ml	440	C	(Thornton & Ross)
Benztropine Tablets BP, 2mg	60		87	C	*(Cogentin)*
Benzydamine Cream BP, 3% w/v	■ 100	g	669	C	*(Difflam)*
Benzydamine Mouthwash BP 0.15% w/v	■ 300	ml	392	C	*(Difflam)*
(Benzydamine Hydrochloride Oral Rinse Solution 0.15% w/v)					
Benzydamine Oromucosal Spray BP, 0.15% w/v	■ 30	ml	341	C	*(Difflam)*
(Benzydamine Hydrochloride Oral Spray 0.15% w/v)					
Benzyl Benzoate BP	500	g	340	C	(Loveridge)
Benzyl Benzoate Application BP	500	ml	245	A	
Benzylpenicillin Injection BP, 600mg vials	25		1048	C	*(Crystapen)*
Benzylpenicillin Injection BP, 1200mg vials	25		2096	C	*(Crystapen)*

VIII

■ Special Containers

Drug	Quantity		Basic Price p	Category
Betahistine Dihydrochloride Tablets 8mg	★ 84		551	A
. . . .	120		725	A
Betahistine Dihydrochloride Tablets 16mg	◆ 84		1466	A
Betamethasone Eye Drops BP, 0.1% w/v	■ 10	ml	131	C *(Betnesol)*
Betamethasone Sodium Phosphate Ear Drops . . . . . 0.1% w/v	■ 10	ml	131	C *(Betnesol)*
Betamethasone Sodium Phosphate Nasal Drops 0.1% w/v	■ 10	ml	131	C *(Betnesol)*
Betamethasone Valerate Cream BP, 0.025% w/w . . .	■ 100	g	326	C *(Betnovate-RD)*
Betamethasone Valerate Cream BP, 0.1% w/w	■ 30	g	140	C *(Betnovate)*
. . . .	■ 100	g	395	C *(Betnovate)*
Betamethasone Valerate Ointment BP, 0.025% w/w .	■ 100	g	326	C *(Betnovate-RD)*
Betamethasone Valerate Ointment BP, 0.1% w/w . . .	■ 30	g	140	C *(Betnovate)*
. . . .	■ 100	g	395	C *(Betnovate)*
Betamethasone Valerate Scalp Application BP, ... 0.1% w/w	■ 100	ml	422	C *(Betacap)*
Betaxolol Hydrochloride Eye Drops . . . . 0.25% w/v	■ 5	ml	477	C *(Betoptic Suspension)*
Betaxolol Hydrochloride Eye Drops 0.5% w/v	■ 5	ml	381	C *(Betoptic Ophthalmic Solution)*
Bezafibrate Tablets 200mg	100		984	C *(Bezalip)*
Bezafibrate Tablets 400mg (m/r)	◆ 28		812	C
Bicalutamide Tablets 50mg	◆ 28		12800	C *(Casodex)*
Bisacodyl Suppositories BP, 5mg	5		89	C *(Dulcolax)*
Bisacodyl Suppositories BP, 10mg	12		76	A
Bisacodyl Tablets BP, 5mg (e/c)	1000		2950	A
Bismuth Subcarbonate BP (Syn: Bismuth Carbonate) .	250	g	1420	A
Bisoprolol Fumarate Tablets 5mg	◆ 28		856	C
Bisoprolol Fumarate Tablets 10mg	◆ 28		961	C
Black Currant Syrup BP	500	ml	375	A
Boric Acid BP	100	g	39	C (Thornton & Ross)
Bromocriptine Capsules BP, 5mg	100		3434	C *(Parlodel)*
Bromocriptine Capsules BP, 10mg	100		6353	C *(Parlodel)*
Bromocriptine Tablets BP, 1mg	100		905	C *(Parlodel)*
Bromocriptine Tablets BP, 2.5mg	30		528	C
Brompheniramine Tablets BP, 4mg	28		83	C *(Dimotane)*
Brompheniramine Maleate Elixir 2mg/5ml	200	ml	142	C *(Dimotane)*
Brompheniramine Maleate Tablets 12mg (m/r)	28		125	C *(Dimotane LA)*
Budesonide Aqueous Nasal Spray . . . . 100 microgram/metered spray	■ 100	dose	585	C *(Rhinocort Aqua)*
Budesonide Breath-actuated Dry Powder . . . . Inhaler 100 microgram/inhalation	■ 200	dose	1850	C *(Pulmicort Turbohaler 100)*
Budesonide Breath-actuated Dry Powder . . . . Inhaler 200 microgram/inhalation	■ 100	dose	1850	C *(Pulmicort Turbohaler 200)*
Budesonide Breath-actuated Dry Powder . . . . Inhaler 400 microgram/inhalation	■ 50	dose	1850	C *(Pulmicort Turbohaler 400)*

■ Special Containers
◆ Manufacturers' Calendar Packs
★ Common Pack

Drug		Quantity		Basic Price p		Category
Buffered Cream BP		500	g	264		A
Bumetanide Oral Solution BP, 1mg/5ml sugar free . . .		150	ml	317		C (Burinex Liquid)
Bumetanide Tablets BP, 1mg	♦	28		171		A
Bumetanide Tablets BP, 5mg	♦	28		1117		A
Bumetanide 1mg and Amiloride Hydrochloride . . . . . 5mg Tablets	♦	28		306		C (Burinex A)
Bumetanide and Slow Potassium Tablets BP, ... 500 microgram/7.7mmol		28		114		C (Burinex K)
Buprenorphine Tablets 200 microgram . . . . (as hydrochloride) (sublingual)		50		573		C (Temgesic)
Buprenorphine Tablets 400 microgram . . . . (as hydrochloride) (sublingual)		7		160		C (Subutex)
		50		1146		C (Temgesic)
Buspirone Hydrochloride Tablets 5mg		90		2808		C (Buspar)
. . . .		100		3115	▽	A
Buspirone Hydrochloride Tablets 10mg		90		4212		C (Buspar)
. . . .		100		3980	▽	A
Cabergoline Tablets 500 microgram	■	8		3004		C (Dostinex)
Cabergoline Tablets 1mg	■	20		7545		C (Cabaser)
Cabergoline Tablets 2mg	■	20		7545		C (Cabaser)
Cabergoline Tablets 4mg	■	16		6036		C (Cabaser)
Cade Oil BPC		100	ml	653		A
Calamine BP (Syn: Prepared Calamine)		500	g	306		A
Calamine Lotion BP		500	ml	160		B
Calamine Lotion Oily BP 1980		100	ml	53		C (Thornton & Ross)
Calamine Aqueous Cream BP		100	ml	61	▽	A
Calamine Compound Application BPC		50	g	67		C (AAH)
Calciferol Injection BP, 300,000 u/1 ml ampoules . . .		10		5924		A
Calciferol Injection BP, 600,000 u/2 ml ampoules . . .		10		7070		A
Calciferol Tablets BP, ... 250 microgram (10,000 units)		100		2199		A
Calciferol Tablets BP, ... 1.25mg (50,000 units)		100		3033		A
Calcipotriol Cream 50 micrograms/g	■	30g		778		C (Dovonex)
. . . .	■	60g		1557		C (Dovonex)
. . . .	■	120g		2808		C (Dovonex)
Calcipotriol Ointment 50 micrograms/g	■	30g		778		C (Dovonex)
. . . .	■	60g		1557		C (Dovonex)
. . . .	■	120g		2808		C (Dovonex)
Calcipotriol Scalp Solution 50 microgram/ml	■	60	ml	2128		C (Dovonex)
Calcium and Ergocalciferol Tablets 400iu . . . . (Calcium with Vitamin D Tablets)		28		68		A
Calcium Carbonate BP		1	kg	310		A
Calcium Carbonate Mixture, Compound, ... Paediatric BPC		100	ml	7		E

■ Special Containers
♦ Manufacturers' Calendar Packs

VIII

Drug	Quantity		Basic Price p		Category	
Calcium Carbonate Tablets 1.25g, Chewable . . . . . . (500mg calcium)	100		982		C	(Calcichew)
Calcium Carbonate Tablets 2.5g, Chewable . . . . (1g calcium)	100		2194		C	(Calcichew Forte)
Calcium Gluconate Tablets, Effervescent BP, 1g	28		462		A	
Calcium Lactate Tablets BP, 300mg	84		291	△	A	
Calcium Sulphate, Dried BP . . . . (Syns: Calcium Sulphate, Exsiccated, Plaster of Paris)	5	kg	495		C	(Thornton & Ross)
Camphor BP 1988	100	g	198		A	
Camphor Water Concentrated BP	100	ml	150		B	
Camphorated Opium Tincture BP (Syn: Paregoric) . . .	500	ml	568		A	
Capsicum Ointment BPC	500	g	490		A	
Capsicum Tincture BPC	500	ml	305		A	
Captopril Tablets BP, 12.5mg	56		222	▽	A	
Captopril Tablets BP, 25mg	♦ 56		295	▽	A	
Captopril Tablets BP, 50mg	♦ 56		375	▽	A	
Carbamazepine Oral Liquid 100mg/5ml sugar free . . .	300	ml	572		C	(Tegretol)
Carbamazepine Tablets BP, 100mg	♦ 28		113		A	
. . . .	84		243		C	(Tegretol)
Carbamazepine Tablets BP, 200mg	♦ 28		156	△	A	
. . . .	84		450		C	(Tegretol)
Carbamazepine Tablets 200mg (m/r)	56		482		C	
Carbamazepine Tablets BP, 400mg	28		434	△	A	
. . . .	56		590		C	(Tegretol)
Carbamazepine Tablets 400mg (m/r)	56		948		C	
Carbaryl Lotion BP, 0.5% w/v (Alcoholic)	■ 50	ml	228		C	(Carylderm)
. . . .	■ 200	ml	585		C	(Carylderm)
Carbaryl Lotion BP, 1% w/v (Aqueous)	■ 50	ml	228		C	(Carylderm Liquid)
. . . .	■ 200	ml	585		C	(Carylderm Liquid)
Carbimazole Tablets BP, 5mg	100		287		C	(Neo-Mercazole 5)
Carbimazole Tablets BP, 20mg	100		1065		C	(Neo-Mercazole 20)
§ Carbocisteine Capsules (Carbocysteine Caps) 375mg	30		448		C	(Mucodyne)
§ Carbocisteine Syrup (Carbocysteine Syrup) 125mg/5ml	300	ml	491		C	(Mucodyne)
§ Carbocisteine Syrup (Carbocysteine Syrup) 250mg/5ml	300	ml	628		C	(Mucodyne)

§ Only allowed to be prescribed in certain circumstances, see Part XVIIIB
■ Special Containers
♦ Manufacturers' Calendar Packs

Drug	Quantity		Basic Price p	Category	
Cardamom Tincture, Aromatic BP	500	ml	525	C	(AAH)
Cardamom Tincture, Compound BP	500	ml	365	C	(Thornton & Ross)
Carmellose Gelatin Paste DPF	■ 30	g	181	C	*(Orabase)*
. . . .	■ 100	g	403	C	*(Orabase)*
Carteolol Eye Drops BP, 1% w/v	■ 5	ml	460	C	*(Teoptic)*
Carteolol Eye Drops BP, 2% w/v	■ 5	ml	540	C	*(Teoptic)*
Castor Oil BP	500	ml	409	A	
Caustic Pencil (Toughened Silver Nitrate BP 1980, 95%)	■ each		166	C	*(Avoca Wart Treatment Set)*
Cefaclor Capsules 250mg	21		680	C	
Cefaclor Capsules 500mg	50		5415	C	
Cefaclor Suspension 125mg/5ml	● 100	ml	503	A	
Cefaclor Suspension 250mg/5ml	● 100	ml	890	A	
Cefaclor Tablets 375mg	14		693	C	*(Distaclor MR)*
(as monohydrate) (m/r)					
Cefadroxil Capsules 500mg (as monohydrate)	100		2819	C	*(Baxan)*
Cefadroxil Suspension 125mg/5ml (as monohydrate) .	● 60	ml	175	C	*(Baxan)*
Cefadroxil Suspension 250mg/5ml (as monohydrate) .	● 60	ml	348	C	*(Baxan)*
Cefadroxil Suspension 500mg/5ml (as monohydrate) .	● 60	ml	521	C	*(Baxan)*
Cefixime Oral Suspension 100mg/5ml	●37.5	ml	790	C	*(Suprax)*
. . . .	● 75	ml	1418	C	*(Suprax)*
Cefixime Tablets 200mg	7		1203	C	*(Suprax)*
Cefpodoxime Tablets 100mg (as 130mg Proxetil) . . .	10		926	C	*(Orelox)*
Cefuroxime Axetil Tablets BP, 125mg	14		473	C	*(Zinnat)*
Cefuroxime Axetil Tablets BP, 250mg	14		945	C	*(Zinnat)*
Celiprolol Hydrochloride Tablets 200mg	♦ 28		1719	C	
Celiprolol Hydrochloride Tablets 400mg	♦ 28		3438	C	
Cephalexin Capsules BP, 250mg	28		261	A	
	100		932	A	
Cephalexin Capsules BP, 500mg	21		397 ▽	A	
	100		1932	A	
Cephalexin Oral Suspension BP, 125mg/5ml	● 100	ml	133	A	
(Syn: Cephalexin Mixture 125mg/5ml)					
Cephalexin Oral Suspension BP, 250mg/5ml	● 100	ml	232	A	
(Syn: Cephalexin Mixture 250mg/5ml)					
Cephalexin Oral Suspension BP, 500mg/5ml	● 100	ml	619	C	*(Ceporex Syrup)*
(Syn: Cephalexin Mixture 500mg/5ml)					
Cephalexin Tablets BP, 250mg	28		265 ▽	A	
. . . .	100		952	A	
Cephalexin Tablets BP, 500mg	100		1814	A	
Cephalexin Tablets BP, 1g	14		872	C	*(Ceporex)*
Cephradine Capsules BP, 250mg	20		355	C	
	100		1708	C	
Cephradine Capsules BP, 500mg	20		700	C	
. . . .	100		3372	C	
Cephradine Oral Solution DPF, 250mg/5ml	● 100	ml	422	C	*(Velosef Syrup)*
Cetirizine Dihydrochloride Tablets 10mg	30		873	C	*(Zirtek)*
Cetomacrogol Cream BP 1988 (Formula A)	500	g	239	A	
Cetomacrogol Cream BP 1988 (Formula B)	500	g	248	A	

VIII

■ Special Containers
♦ Manufacturers' Calendar Packs
● Preparations Requiring Reconstitution

Drug	Quantity		Basic Price p	Category	
Chalk BP (Powder) (Syn: Prepared Chalk)	2	kg	398	A	
Chloral Mixture BP	200	ml	89	E	
(Syns: Chloral Oral Solution; Chloral Hydrate Mixture)					
Chloral Betaine Tablets 707mg	30		243	C	*(Welldorm)*
Chloral Hydrate BP	100	g	413	A	
Chloramphenicol Capsules BP, 250mg	60		2094	A	
Chloramphenicol Ear Drops BP, 5% w/v	■ 10	ml	140	A	
Chloramphenicol Eye Drops BP, 0.5% w/v	■ 10	ml	96	A	
Chloramphenicol Eye Ointment BP, 1% w/v	■ 4	g	105	A	
Chlordiazepoxide Capsules BP, 5mg	500		1976	A	
Chlordiazepoxide Capsules BP, 10mg	500		2811	A	
Chlordiazepoxide Hydrochloride Tablets BP, 5mg	100		393	C	*(Tropium)*
Chlordiazepoxide Hydrochloride Tablets BP, 10mg . . .	100		546	C	*(Tropium)*
Chlorhexidine Mouthwash DPF, 0.2% w/v	300	ml	193	C	*(Corsodyl)*
(Chlorhexidine Gluconate Mouthwash 0.2% w/v)					
Chlorhexidine Gluconate Gel DPF, 1% w/w	■ 50	g	121	C	*(Corsodyl)*
Chlorhexidine Gluconate Oral Spray DPF 0.2%	■ 60	ml	410	C	*(Corsodyl)*
Chlormethiazole Capsules BP, 192mg	60		434	C	*(Heminevrin)*
Chlormethiazole Oral Solution BP, 250mg/5ml sugar free	300	ml	363	C	*(Heminevrin Syrup)*
Chloroform Spirit BP	500	ml	248	A	
Chloroform Water Concentrated BPC 1959	500	ml	187	A	
Chloroform and Morphine Tincture BP	500	ml	482	A	
(Syn: Chlorodyne)					
Chloroquine Phosphate Tablets BP, 250mg	20		111	C	*(Avloclor)*
Chloroquine Sulphate Tablets BP, 200mg	28		134	C	*(Nivaquine)*
Chlorpheniramine Oral Solution BP 2mg/5ml	150	ml	216	C	*(Piriton Syrup)*
(Syn: Chlorpheniramine Elixir 2mg/5ml)					
Chlorpheniramine Tablets BP, 4mg	28		42	△ A	
Chlorpromazine Oral Solution BP, 25mg/5ml	150	ml	135	A	
(Syn: Chlorpromazine Elixir 25mg/5ml)					
Chlorpromazine Tablets BP, 10mg	56		71	C	*(Largactil)*
Chlorpromazine Tablets BP, 25mg	28		96	C	(Norton)
. . . .	1000		764	▽ A	
Chlorpromazine Tablets BP, 50mg	28		95	A	
. . . .	500		1517	▽ A	
Chlorpromazine Tablets BP, 100mg	28		115	A	
. . . .	500		1101	▽ A	
Chlorthalidone Tablets BP, 50mg	28		168	C	*(Hygroton)*
Cholestyramine (anhydrous) Powders 4g/sachet	60		2106	C	*(Questran)*
Cholestyramine (anhydrous) Powders 4g/sachet, ...	180		6616	△ A	
with aspartame					

■ Special Containers

Drug		Quantity		Basic Price p	Category	
Choline Salicylate Dental Gel BP sugar free	■	10	g	131	C	(Dinneford's Teejel)
. . . .	■	15	g	163	C	(Bonjela)
Cimetidine Oral Solution BP, 200mg/5ml		600	ml	2849	C	(Tagamet Syrup)
Cimetidine Oral Suspension BP, 200mg/5ml sugar free		600	ml	2408	C	(Dyspamet)
Cimetidine Tablets BP, 200mg		60		264	A	
Cimetidine Tablets BP, 400mg	♦	60		526	A	
Cimetidine Tablets BP, 800mg	♦	30		538	A	
Cinnarizine Tablets 15mg		84		457	A	
Ciprofibrate Tablets 100mg		28		1338	C	(Modalim)
Ciprofloxacin Tablets BP, 100mg		6		280	C	(Ciproxin)
Ciprofloxacin Tablets BP, 250mg		10		750	C	(Ciproxin)
Ciprofloxacin Tablets BP, 500mg		10		1420	C	(Ciproxin)
Ciprofloxacin Tablets BP, 750mg		10		2000	C	(Ciproxin)
Cisapride Suspension 5mg/5ml (as monohydrate) . . .		500	ml	1560	C	(Prepulsid)
Cisapride Tablets 10mg (as monohydrate)		120		2820	C	(Prepulsid)
Citalopram Tablets 10mg (as hydrobromide)	♦	28		964	C	(Cipramil)
Citalopram Tablets 20mg (as hydrobromide)	♦	28		1603	C	(Cipramil)
Citalopram Tablets 40mg (as hydrobromide)	♦	28		2710	C	(Cipramil)
Citric Acid Monohydrate BP		500	g	290	C	(Thornton & Ross)
Clarithromycin Suspension 125mg/5ml	●	70	ml	600	C	(Klaricid)
. . . .	●	100	ml	1032	C	(Klaricid)
Clarithromycin Suspension 250mg/5ml	●	70	ml	1200	C	(Klaricid)
Clarithromycin Tablets 250mg	♦	14		1124	C	(Klaricid)
Clarithromycin Tablets 500mg	♦	14		2249	C	(Klaricid)
. . . .	♦	20		3213	C	(Klaricid 500)
Clemastine Oral Solution BP, 500 microgram/5ml . . .		150	ml	92	C	(Tavegil Elixir)
sugar free						
Clemastine Tablets BP, 1mg		60		235	C	(Tavegil)
Clindamycin Capsules BP, 75mg		24		593	C	(Dalacin C)
Clindamycin Capsules BP, 150mg		24		1092	C	(Dalacin C)
Clindamycin Lotion 1% w/v (as phosphate)	■	30	ml	508	C	(Dalacin T Topical Lotion)
. . . .	■	50	ml	847	C	(Dalacin T Topical Lotion)
Clindamycin Topical Solution 1% w/v (as phosphate) .	■	30	ml	434	C	(Dalacin T)
Clindamycin Phosphate Cream 2% w/w	■	40	g	864	C	(Dalacin)
§ Clobazam Tablets 10mg		30		998	C	(Frisium)

VIII

§ Only allowed to be prescribed in certain circumstances, see Part XVIIIB
■ Special Containers
♦ Manufacturers' Calendar Packs
● Preparations Requiring Reconstitution

Drug		Quantity		Basic Price p		Category	
Clobetasol Cream BP, 0.05% w/v	■	30	g	256		C	(Dermovate)
. . . .	■	100	g	752		C	(Dermovate)
Clobetasol Ointment BP, 0.05% w/w	■	30	g	256		C	(Dermovate)
. . . .	■	100	g	752		C	(Dermovate)
Clobetasone Cream BP, 0.05% w/v	■	30	g	176		C	(Eumovate)
. . . .	■	100	g	516		C	(Eumovate)
Clobetasone Ointment BP, 0.05% w/v	■	30	g	176		C	(Eumovate)
. . . .	■	100	g	516		C	(Eumovate)
Clomiphene Tablets BP, 50mg		30		838	△	A	
Clomipramine Capsules BP, 10mg		28		121		A	
(Syn: Clomipramine Hydrochloride Capsules 10mg)							
Clomipramine Capsules BP, 25mg		28		193		A	
(Syn: Clomipramine Hydrochloride Capsules 25mg)		100		460		A	
Clomipramine Capsules BP, 50mg		28		242		A	
(Syn: Clomipramine Hydrochloride Capsules 50mg)							
Clomipramine Hydrochloride Tablets 75mg (m/r)		28		751		C	(Anafranil SR)
Clonazepam Tablets 500 microgram		100		422		C	(Rivotril)
Clonazepam Tablets 2mg		100		562		C	(Rivotril)
Clonidine Tablets BP, 25 microgram		112		711		C	(Dixarit)
(Syn: Clonidine Hydrochloride Tablets 25 microgram)							
Clonidine Tablets BP, 100 microgram		100		560		C	(Catapres)
(Syn: Clonidine Hydrochloride Tablets 100 microgram)							
Clonidine Tablets BP, 300 microgram		100		1304		C	(Catapres)
(Syn: Clonidine Hydrochloride Tablets 300 microgram)							
Clotrimazole Cream BP, 1% w/w	■	20	g	214		C	(Canesten)
. . . .	■	50	g	444		C	
Clotrimazole Cream BP, 10% w/w	■	5	g	348		C	(Canesten VC)
Clotrimazole Pessaries BP, 100mg	■	6		362		C	(Canesten)
Clotrimazole Pessaries BP, 200mg	■	3		362		C	(Canesten)
Clotrimazole Pessaries BP, 500mg	■	1		348		C	
Clotrimazole 1% and Hydrocortisone 1% Cream w/w	■	30	g	217		C	(Canesten HC)
Clove Oil BP		100	ml	378		B	
Coal Tar Solution BP		500	ml	398		A	
Coal Tar Solution Strong BP		500	ml	588		A	
Co-amilofruse Tablets BP, 2.5/20	♦	28		438		A	
(Syn: Amiloride and Frusemide Tablets 2.5/20) .	♦	56		949		C	(Frumil LS)
Co-amilofruse Tablets BP, 5/40	♦	28		258		A	
(Syn: Amiloride and Frusemide Tablets 5/40) . .	♦	56		471		A	
Co-amilofruse Tablets BP, 10/80	♦	28		754		A	
Co-amilozide Tablets BP, 2.5/25	♦	28		185		C	(Moduret 25)
(Syn: Amiloride and Hydrochlorothiazide Tablets 2.5/25)	★	100		492		A	
Co-amilozide Tablets BP, 5/50		28		199		A	
(Syn : Amiloride and Hydrochlorothiazide Tablets 5/50)							

■ Special Containers
♦ Manufacturers' Calendar Packs
★ Common Pack

Drug	Quantity	Basic Price p	Category	
Co-amoxiclav Suspension 125/31 in 5ml sugar free .. (Amoxycillin and Potassium Clavulanate Suspension 125/31 sugar free)	● 100 ml	457	C	
Co-amoxiclav Suspension 250/62 in 5ml sugar free .. (Amoxycillin and Potassium Clavulanate Suspension 250/62 sugar free)	● 100 ml	642	C	
Co-amoxiclav Suspension 400/57 in 5ml sugar free .. (Amoxycillin and Potassium Clavulanate	● 35 ml	471	C	*(Augmentin-Duo 400/57)*
Suspension 400/57 sugar free)	● 70 ml	661	C	*(Augmentin-Duo 400/57)*
Co-amoxiclav Tablets BP, 250/125	21	979	C	
(Syn: Amoxycillin and Potassium Clavulanate Tablets 250/125)	100	4720	C	
Co-amoxiclav Tablets BP, 500/125 . . . . (Syn: Amoxycillin and Potassium Clavulanate . Tablets 500/125)	21	1573	C	
Co-amoxiclav Tablets, Dispersible 250/125 . . . . (Amoxycillin and Potassium Clavulanate Tablets, Dispersible 150/125)	21	1099	C	*(Augmentin Dispersible)*
Co-beneldopa Capsules 12.5/50 . . . . (Benserazide Hydrochloride and Levodopa Capsules 12.5/50)	■ 100	667	C	*(Madopar 62.5)*
Co-beneldopa Capsules 25/100 . . . . (Benserazide Hydrochloride and Levodopa Capsules 25/100)	■ 100	929	C	*(Madopar 125)*
Co-beneldopa Capsules 50/200 . . . . (Benserazide Hydrochloride and Levodopa Capsules 50/200)	■ 100	1584	C	*(Madopar 250)*
Co-beneldopa Tablets, Dispersible 12.5/50 . . . . (Benserazide Hydrochloride and Levodopa Tablets, Dispersible 12.5/50)	■ 100	792	C	*(Madopar 62.5 Dispersible)*
Co-beneldopa Tablets, Dispersible, 25/100 . . . . (Benserazide Hydrochloride and Levodopa Tablets, Dispersible 25/100)	■ 100	1404	C	*(Madopar 125 Dispersible)*
Cocaine Hydrochloride BP	5 g	5497	A	
Co-careldopa Tablets BP, 10/100 . . . . (Syn: Levodopa 100mg and Carbidopa 10mg Tablets)	100	760 Δ	A	
Co-careldopa Tablets BP, 12.5/50 . . . . (Syn: Levodopa 50mg and Carbidopa 12.5mg Tablets)	90	703	C	*(Sinemet 62.5)*
Co-careldopa Tablets BP, 25/100 . . . . (Syn: Levodopa 100mg and Carbidopa 25mg Tablets)	100	1066 Δ	A	
Co-careldopa Tablets BP, 25/250 . . . . (Syn: Levodopa 250mg and Carbidopa 25mg Tablets)	100	1416 Δ	A	

■ Special Containers
● Preparations Requiring Reconstitution

Drug	Quantity		Basic Price p		Category	
Co-codamol Capsules 30/500	100		821	△	C	*(Tylex)*
(Codeine Phosphate and Paracetamol Capsules 30/500)						
Co-codamol Tablets BP, 8/500	30		72	▽	A	
(Syn: Codeine Phosphate and Paracetamol ...	32		72		A	
Tablets, 8/500)	100		167	▽	A	
....	★ 500		570		A	
Co-codamol Tablets BP, 30/500	100		749	▽	A	
(Syn: Codeine Phosphate and Paracetamol Tablets)						
Co-codamol Tablets, Effervescent 8/500	100		463		A	
(Codeine Phosphate and Paracetamol Tablets Dispersible 8/500)						
Co-codaprin Tablets, Dispersible BP	100		367		A	
(Syn: Aspirin and Codeine Tablets, Dispersible)	500		1834		A	
Coconut Oil BP	500	g	310		C	(Thornton & Ross)
Coconut Oil, Fractionated BP	250	ml	665		B	
Co-danthramer Capsules NPF, 25/200	60		1286		A	
Co-danthramer Capsules Strong NPF, 37.5/500	60		1555		A	
Co-danthramer Oral Suspension NPF, 25/200 in 5ml .	300	ml	1127		A	
sugar free						
(Danthron and Poloxamer 188 Suspension, 25/200 sugar free)						
Co-danthramer Oral Suspension Strong NPF, ...	300	ml	3013		A	
75/1000 in 5ml sugar free						
(Danthron and Poloxamer 188 Suspension, Strong 75/1000 sugar free)						
Co-danthrusate Capsules BP, 50/60	63		1346		C	
(Syn: Danthron and Docusate Sodium Capsules 50/60)						
Co-danthrusate Oral Suspension NPF sugar free	200	ml	875		C	*(Normax)*
Codeine Linctus BP	2	litre	797		A	
Codeine Linctus BP, sugar free	2	litre	601		A	
Codeine Linctus Diabetic BP	500	ml	363	▽	C	(Thornton & Ross)
Codeine Linctus Paediatric BP	100	ml	21		E	
Codeine Phosphate BP	25	g	3795		C	(Thornton & Ross)
Codeine Phosphate Oral Solution BP	500	ml	447	▽	A	
(Syn: Codeine Phosphate Syrup)						
Codeine Phosphate Tablets BP, 15mg	28		101		A	
....	30		111	△	A	
Codeine Phosphate Tablets BP, 30mg	28		145		A	
....	30		155	△	A	
Codeine Phosphate Tablets BP, 60mg	28		258		A	
....	30		277	△	A	
Co-dergocrine Tablets BP, 1.5mg	100		1078		C	*(Hydergine)*
Co-dergocrine Tablets BP, 4.5mg	◆ 28		1078		C	*(Hydergine)*
Co-dydramol Tablets BP, 10/500	30		81	▽	A	
(Syn: Dihydrocodeine and Paracetamol	100		205	▽	A	
Tablets 10/500)	★ 500		684		A	

◆ Manufacturers' Calendar Packs
★ Common Pack

Drug	Quantity		Basic Price p	Category	
Co-fluampicil Capsules BP, 250/250	28		878	A	
(Syn: Flucloxacillin Sodium and	100		2326	A	
Ampicillin Capsules 250/250)					
Co-fluampicil Syrup 125/125 in 5ml	● 100	ml	499	C	*(Magnapen)*
(Flucloxacillin Magnesium and Ampicillin					
Syrup 125/125)					
Co-flumactone Tablets 25/25	100		1686	C	*(Aldactide 25)*
(Hydroflumethiazide and Spironolactone Tablets 25/25)					
Co-flumactone Tablets 50/50	100		3186	C	*(Aldactide 50)*
(Hydroflumethazide and Spironolactone Tablets 50/50)					
Colchicine Tablets BP, 500 microgram	100		1662	A	
Copper Sulphate Pentahydrate BP	500	g	250	A	
(Syn: Copper Sulphate)					
Co-prenozide Tablets 160/0.25	♦ 28		740	C	*(Trasidrex)*
(Oxprenolol Hydrochloride 160mg (m/r) and					
Cyclopenthiazide 250 microgram Tablets)					
Co-proxamol Tablets BP, 32.5/325	100		120	A	
(Syn: Dextroproxyphene Hydrochloride 32.5mg					
and Paracetamol 325 mg Tablets)					
Cortisone Tablets BP, 25mg	56		324	C	*(Cortisyl)*
Co-simalcite Suspension 125/500 in 5ml sugar free .	500	ml	196	C	*(Altacite Plus)*
(Activated Dimethicone and Hydrotalcite					
sugar free Suspension 125/500)					
Co-tenidone Tablets BP, 50/12.5	♦ 28		272	A	
(Syn: Atenolol and Chlorthalidone Tablets 50/12.5)					
Co-tenidone Tablets BP, 100/25	♦ 28		384	A	
(Syn: Atenolol and Chlorthalidone Tablets 100/25)					
Co-triamterzide Tablets BP, 50/25	30		169	C	*(Triam-Co)*
(Syn: Triamterene and					
Hydrochlorothiazide Tablets)					
Crotamiton Cream BP, 10% w/w	■ 30	g	223	C	*(Eurax)*
. . . .	■ 100	g	382	C	*(Eurax)*
Cyanocobalamin Injection BP, 1mg/1ml ampoules . . .	5		833	C	*(Cytamen)*
§ Cyanocobalamin Tablets BP, 50 microgram	50		277	C	*(Cytacon)*
(§ Syn: Vitamin B12 Tablets 50 microgram)					
Cyclizine Injection BP, 50mg/ml, 1ml ampoules	5		271	C	*(Valoid)*
(Syn: Cyclizine Lactate Injection 50mg/ml)					
Cyclizine Tablets BP, 50mg	100		475	C	*(Valoid)*
Cyclopenthiazide Tablets BP, 500 microgram	28		127	C	*(Navidrex)*
Cyclopenthiazide 250 microgram and	♦ 28		206	C	*(Navispare)*
Amiloride Hydrochloride 2.5mg Tablets					

VIII

§   Only allowed to be prescribed in certain circumstances, see Part XVIIIB
■   Special Containers
♦   Manufacturers' Calendar Packs
●   Preparations Requiring Reconstitution

Drug		Quantity		Basic Price p	Category	
Cyclopentolate Eye Drops BP, 0.5% w/v	■	5	ml	73	C	*(Mydrilate)*
Cyclopentolate Eye Drops BP, 1% w/v	■	5	ml	98	C	*(Mydrilate)*
Cyclophosphamide Tablets BP, 50mg		100		1058	A	
Cyclosporin Capsules 10mg		30		822	C	*(Neoral)*
Cyclosporin Capsules 25mg		30		2054	C	
Cyclosporin Capsules 50mg		30		4022	C	
Cyclosporin Capsules 100mg		30		7633	C	
Cyclosporin Oral Solution 100mg/ml sugar free	■	50	ml	11438	C	
Cyproterone Acetate Tablets 100mg		84		9670	C	
Danazol Capsules 100mg	♦	60		1484	A	
....		100		2452	A	
Danazol Capsules 200mg		60		2850	A	
....		100		4670	A	
Dantrolene Sodium Capsules 25mg		100		1266	C	*(Dantrium)*
Dantrolene Sodium Capsules 100mg		100		4427	C	*(Dantrium)*
Dapsone Tablets BP, 50mg		28		203	A	
Dapsone Tablets BP, 100mg		28		294	A	
Desmopressin Intranasal Solution BP, ...	■	2.5	ml	950	C	*(DDAVP Nasal*
100 micrograms/ml						*Solution)*
Desmopressin Nasal Spray	■	60	dose	2800	C	*(Desmospray)*
10 micrograms/metered spray						
Dexamethasone Tablets BP, 500 microgram		30		96	C	*(Decadron)*
....		50		160	A	
....		100		320	A	
....		500		1594	A	
Dexamethasone Tablets BP, 2mg		50		550	A	
....		100		1095	A	
....	★	500		4333	A	
Dexamethasone 0.1% w/v and	■	5	ml	149	C	*(Maxidex)*
Hypromellose 0.5% w/v Eye Drops	■	10	ml	295	C	*(Maxidex)*
Dexamphetamine Sulphate Tablets 5mg		28		96	C	*(Dexedrine)*
Dextropropoxyphene Capsules BP, 60mg		100		820	C	*(Doloxene)*
Dextrose, Strong Injection	-			-	-	
(See Glucose Intravenous Infusion BP)						
Diamorphine Injection BP, 5mg ampoules		5		591	A	
Diamorphine Injection BP, 10mg ampoules		5		679	A	
Diamorphine Injection BP, 30mg ampoules		5		811	A	
Diamorphine Injection BP, 100mg ampoules		5		2249	A	
Diamorphine Injection BP, 500mg ampoules		5		10342	A	
Diamorphine Hydrochloride BP		2	g	1296	A	
Diamorphine Hydrochloride Tablets 10mg		100		1230	A	

■ Special Containers
★ Common Pack
♦ Manufacturers' Calendar Packs

Drug	Quantity		Basic Price p		Category	
Diazepam Solution 2mg/ml, 2.5ml	5		670		A	
Rectal Tube						
Diazepam Solution 4mg/ml, 2.5ml	5		864		A	
Rectal Tube						
Diazepam Syrup 2mg/5ml	100	ml	160	▽	A	
Diazepam Tablets BP, 2mg	28		53		A	
Diazepam Tablets BP, 5mg	28		58		A	
Diazepam Tablets BP, 10mg	28		84		A	
Diclofenac Diethylammonium Salt Gel 1.16%	■ 100	g	700		C	(Voltarol
(equivalent to Diclofenac Sodium 1%)						Emulgel)
Diclofenac Tablets BP, 25mg (e/c)	84		237	▽	A	
	★ 100		338	△	A	
Diclofenac Tablets BP, 50mg (e/c)	84		356	▽	A	
	★ 100		499	▽	A	
Diclofenac Sodium Capsules 75mg (m/r)	♦ 56		1301		C	(Diclomax SR)
Diclofenac Sodium Capsules 100mg (m/r)	♦ 28		936		C	(Diclomax
						Retard)
Diclofenac Sodium Capsules	56		1499		C	(Motifene
dual-release 25mg (e/c)/50mg (m/r)						75mg)
Diclofenac Sodium Suppositories 25mg	10		115		C	(Voltarol)
Diclofenac Sodium Suppositories 50mg	10		189		C	(Voltarol)
Diclofenac Sodium Suppositories 100mg	10		338		C	(Voltarol)
Diclofenac Sodium Suppositories, Paediatric 12.5mg	10		65		C	(Voltarol)
Diclofenac Sodium Dispersible Tablets 50mg	21		515		C	(Voltarol
						Dispersible)
Diclofenac Sodium 50mg (e/c) and	60		1331		C	(Arthrotec 50)
Misoprostol Tablets 200 microgram						
Diclofenac Sodium 75mg (e/c) and	60		1759		C	(Arthrotec 75)
Misoprostol Tablets 200 microgram						
Dicyclomine Oral Solution BP, 10mg/5ml	120	ml	198		C	(Merbentyl
(Syn: Dicyclomine Elixir 10mg/5ml)						Syrup)
Dicyclomine Tablets BP, 10mg	100		542		C	(Merbentyl)
Dicyclomine Tablets BP, 20mg	84		911		C	(Merbentyl 20)
Dienoestrol Cream 0.01% w/w (with applicator)	■ 78	g	261		C	(Ortho-
						Dienoestrol)
Diethylamine Salicylate Cream 10% w/w	■ 50	g	75		C	(Algesal)
Diflunisal Tablets BP, 250mg	60		541		C	(Dolobid)
Diflunisal Tablets BP, 500mg	60		1082		C	(Dolobid 500)
Digitoxin Tablets BP, 100 microgram	28		399		A	
Digoxin Oral Solution, Paediatric BP	■ 60	ml	523		C	(Lanoxin-
(Syn: Paediatric Digoxin Elixir)						PG Elixir)
Digoxin Tablets BP, 62.5 microgram	28		72		A	
Digoxin Tablets BP, 125 microgram	28		56		A	
Digoxin Tablets BP, 250 microgram	28		56		A	
Dihydrocodeine Injection BP, 50mg/1ml ampoules	5		970	△	A	
Dihydrocodeine Oral Solution BP, 10mg/5ml	150	ml	320		A	
(Syn: Dihydrocodeine Elixir 10mg/5ml)						
Dihydrocodeine Tablets BP, 30mg	28		161	▽	A	
	30		153	▽	A	
	★ 100		402	▽	A	
	500		1827		A	
Dihydrocodeine Tartrate Tablets 60mg (m/r)	56		628		C	(DHC Continus)
Dihydrocodeine Tartrate Tablets 90mg (m/r)	56		989		C	(DHC Continus)
Dihydrocodeine Tartrate Tablets 120mg (m/r)	56		1321		C	(DHC Continus)

VIII

■ Special Containers
♦ Manufacturers' Calendar Packs
★ Common Pack

Drug		Quantity		Basic Price p		Category
Dill Water Concentrated BPC		100	ml	485		C	(AAH)
Diltiazem Hydrochloride Capsules 60mg (m/r)		56		832		C	(Dilzem SR 60)
Diltiazem Hydrochloride Capsules 200mg (m/r)	♦	28		1161		C	(Tildiem LA 200)
Diltiazem Hydrochloride Tablets 60mg (m/r)		84		498	∇	A	
		100		523		A	
Dimethicone Cream BPC		500	g	365		A	
Dipivefrine Hydrochloride Eye Drops 0.1% w/v	▪	5	ml	381		C	(Propine)
	▪	10	ml	477		C	(Propine)
Dipyridamole Tablets BP, 25mg		84		170		C	(Persantin)
	★	100		201		A	
Dipyridamole Tablets BP, 100mg		84		473		C	(Persantin)
Disodium Etidronate Tablets 200mg		60		4388		C	(Didronel)
Disopyramide Capsules BP, 100mg		84		1582		C	(Rythmodan)
Disopyramide Capsules BP, 150mg		84		2099		C	(Rythmodan)
		100		1277	∆	A	
Disopyramide Tablets 150mg		100		1235		C	(Dirythmin SA)
(as phosphate) (m/r)							
Disopyramide Tablets 250mg		56		3102		C	(Rythmodan Retard)
(as phosphate) (m/r)							
Disulfiram Tablets BP, 200mg		50		1925		C	(Antabuse)
Dithranol BP		25	g	3100		C	(AAH)
Docusate Capsules NPF, 100mg		30		167		C	(Dioctyl)
		100		444		C	(Dioctyl)
Docusate Oral Solution NPF, 50mg/5ml		300	ml	248		C	(Docusol)
(1%) sugar free							
Docusate Oral Solution, Paediatric NPF,		300	ml	163		C	(Docusol)
(0.25%) sugar free							
Domperidone Suppositories 30mg		10		265		C	(Motilium)
Domperidone Suspension 5mg/5ml sugar free		200	ml	180		C	(Motilium)
Domperidone Tablets 10mg (as maleate)		30		250		A	
		100		833		A	
Dorzolamide Ophthalmic Solution	▪	5	ml	931		C	(Trusopt)
2% (as hydrochloride)							
Dothiepin Capsules BP, 25mg		28		146		A	
		100		362		A	
Dothiepin Tablets BP, 75mg	♦	28		279		A	
Doxazosin Tablets 1mg (as mesylate)	♦	28		1056		C	(Cardura)
Doxazosin Tablets 2mg (as mesylate)	♦	28		1408		C	(Cardura)
Doxazosin Tablets 4mg (as mesylate)	♦	28		1760		C	(Cardura)
Doxepin Capsules BP, 10mg		56		121		C	(Sinequan)
Doxepin Capsules BP, 25mg		28		87		C	(Sinequan)
Doxepin Capsules BP, 50mg		28		143		C	(Sinequan)
Doxepin Capsules BP, 75mg		28		226		C	(Sinequan)
Doxycycline Capsules BP, 50mg	♦	28		677		A	
Doxycycline Capsules BP, 100mg		8		247		A	
		50		1022		A	
Droperidol Tablets 10mg		50		1230		C	(Droleptan)
Dydrogesterone Tablets BP, 10mg		60		449		C	(Duphaston)

▪ Special Containers
♦ Manufacturers' Calendar Packs
★ Common Pack

Drug		Quantity		Basic Price p	Category	
Emulsifying Ointment BP		500	g	149	A	
Emulsifying Wax BP (Syn: Anionic Emulsifying Wax) .		500	g	390	C	(Thornton & Ross)
Enalapril Maleate Tablets 2.5mg	♦	28		253	A	
Enalapril Maleate Tablets 5mg	♦	28		390	A	
Enalapril Maleate Tablets 10mg	♦	28		509	A	
Enalapril Maleate Tablets 20mg	♦	28		634	A	
Ephedrine Elixir BP, 15mg/5ml		500	ml	430	A	
(Syn: Ephedrine Oral Solution 15mg/5ml)						
Ephedrine Nasal Drops BP, 0.5% w/v	■	10	ml	108	A	
Ephedrine Nasal Drops BP, 1% w/v	■	10	ml	115	A	
Ephedrine Hydrochloride Tablets BP, 15mg		28		156	∇ A	
Ephedrine Hydrochloride Tablets BP, 30mg		28		163	∇ A	
Erythromycin Capsules 250mg (e/c)		30		608	C	(Tiloryth)
Erythromycin Tablets BP, 250mg (e/c)		28		308	A	
. . . .		100		1100	C	(Abbott)
. . . .		500		5500	C	(Abbott)
Erythromycin Topical Solution 2%	■	50	ml	860	C	(Stiemycin)
Erythromycin Ethyl Succinate Oral Suspension BP, . . Paediatric, 125mg/5ml	●	100	ml	112	A	
Erythromycin Ethyl Succinate Oral Suspension BP, . . Paediatric, 125mg/5ml sugar free	●	100	ml	104	A	
Erythromycin Ethyl Succinate Oral Suspension BP, . . 250mg/5ml	●	100	ml	178	A	
Erythromycin Ethyl Succinate Oral Suspension BP, . . 250mg/5ml sugar free	●	100	ml	176	∇ A	
Erythromycin Ethyl Succinate Oral Suspension BP, . . 500mg/5ml	●	100	ml	282	A	
Erythromycin Ethyl Succinate Oral Suspension BP, . . 500mg/5ml sugar free	●	100	ml	317	∇ A	
Erythromycin Ethyl Succinate Tablets BP, 500mg . . .	♦	28		926	C	(Erythroped A)
Erythromycin Stearate Tablets BP, 250mg		100		1359	C	(Erythrocin)
. . . .		500		6620	C	(Erythrocin)
Erythromycin Stearate Tablets BP, 500mg		100		2730	C	(Erythrocin 500)
Erythromycin 40mg/ml and Zinc Acetate	■	30	ml	709	C	(Zineryt)
12mg/ml Lotion	■	90	ml	2062	C	(Zineryt)
Estropipate Tablets BP, 1.5mg		28		300	C	(Harmogen)
Ethamsylate Tablets 500mg		100		2113	C	(Dicynene)
Ethanol 90 per cent BP						
(Syns: Alcohol 90 per cent; Rectified Spirit)						
(Excluding rebate)		100	ml	560	A	
(Including Duty) (See Note 4, page 45)		100	ml	736	A	
Ethanolamine Oleate Injection BP, 5% 2ml ampoules .		10		2466	A	
Ethanolamine Oleate Injection BP, 5% 5ml ampoules .		10		2099	A	
Ether Solvent BP		500	ml	632	A	
Ethinyloestradiol Tablets BP, 10 microgram		21		1299	A	
Ethinyloestradiol Tablets BP, 50 microgram		21		1549	A	
Ethinyloestradiol Tablets BP, 1mg		28		2885	A	
Ethosuximide Capsules BP, 250mg		56		451	C	(Zarontin)
Ethosuximide Oral Solution BP		200	ml	373	C	(Zarontin)
(Syn: Ethosuximide Elixir)						
Eucalyptus Oil BP		500	ml	783	A	

VIII

■ Special Containers
♦ Manufacturers' Calendar Packs
● Preparations Requiring Reconstitution

Drug		Quantity		Basic Price p	Category	
Famciclovir Tablets 125mg		10		2812	C	(Famvir Tiltab)
Famciclovir Tablets 250mg		15		8435	C	(Famvir Tiltab)
		21		11808	C	(Famvir Tiltab)
		56		31490	C	(Famvir Tiltab)
Famciclovir Tablets 500mg		14		15747	C	(Famvir Tiltab)
		30		33734	C	(Famvir Tiltab)
		56		62989	C	(Famvir Tiltab)
Famciclovir Tablets 750mg	♦	7		11272	C	(Famvir Tiltab)
Famotidine Tablets 20mg	♦	28		1337	C	
Famotidine Tablets 40mg	♦	28		2540	C	
Felbinac Foam Aerosol 3.17% w/w	■	100	g	700	C	(Traxam)
Felbinac Gel 3% w/w	■	30	g	226	C	(Traxam Pain Relief Gel)
	■	100	g	700	C	(Traxam)
Felodipine Tablets 2.5mg (m/r)	♦	28		609	C	(Plendil)
Felodipine Tablets 5mg (m/r)	♦	28		812	C	(Plendil)
Felodipine Tablets 10mg (m/r)	♦	28		1092	C	(Plendil)
Fenbufen Capsules BP, 300mg	♦	84		1521 ▽	A	
Fenbufen Tablets BP, 300mg	♦	84		1413	A	
Fenbufen Tablets BP, 450mg	♦	56		1318	A	
Fenofibrate Capsules 200mg (micronised)	♦	28		2175	C	(Lipantil Micro)
Fenoterol Hydrobromide Aerosol Inhalation 100 microgram per actuation	■	200	dose	236	C	(Berotec 100)
Fenoterol Hydrobromide Aerosol Inhalation 200 microgram per actuation	■	200	dose	278	C	(Berotec 200)
Fenoterol Hydrobromide 100 microgram and Ipratropium Bromide 40 microgram Aerosol Inhalation	■	200	dose	538	C	(Duovent)
Ferric Chloride Solution BPC		500	ml	330	C	(Loveridge)
Ferrous Fumarate Oral Solution 140mg (45mg iron)/5ml		200	ml	235	C	(Fersamal Syrup)
Ferrous Fumarate Oral Solution 140mg (45mg iron)/5ml sugar free		300	ml	486	C	(Galfer Syrup)
Ferrous Fumarate Tablets BP, 210mg		100		120	C	(Fersamal)
Ferrous Gluconate Tablets BP, 300mg		1000		3405	A	
Ferrous Sulphate Tablets BP, 200mg	♦	28		90	A	
Flavoxate Tablets BP, 200mg		90		1187	C	(Urispas 200)
Flecainide Acetate Tablets 50mg		60		1555	C	
Flecainide Acetate Tablets 100mg		60		2221	C	
Flexible Collodion BP (Methylated)		500	ml	984	A	
Flucloxacillin Capsules BP, 250mg		28		291	A	
Flucloxacillin Capsules BP, 500mg		28		474	A	
Flucloxacillin Oral Solution BP, 125mg/5ml (Syns: Flucloxacillin Elixir 125mg/5ml Flucloxacillin Syrup 125mg/5ml)	●	100	ml	322	A	
Flucloxacillin Oral Suspension BP, 125mg/5ml (Syn: Flucloxacillin Mixture 125mg/5ml)	●	100	ml	349	C	(Floxapen)
Flucloxacillin Oral Suspension BP, 250mg/5ml (Syn: Flucloxacillin Mixture 250mg/5ml)	●	100	ml	697	C	(Floxapen)

■ Special Containers
♦ Manufacturers' Calendar Packs
● Preparations Requiring Reconstitution

Drug		Quantity		Basic Price p	Category
Fluconazole Capsules DPF, 50mg	♦	7		1661	C	(Diflucan)
Fluconazole Capsules 150mg	■	1		712	C	(Diflucan)
Fluconazole Capsules 200mg	♦	7		6642	C	(Diflucan)
Fluconazole Oral Suspension DPF, 50mg/5ml	●	35	ml	1661	C	(Diflucan)
Fluconazole Oral Suspension 200mg/5ml	●	35	ml	6642	C	(Diflucan)
Fludrocortisone Tablets BP, 100 microgram		56		269	C	(Florinef)
Flunisolide Nasal Spray 25 microgram/0.1ml	■	24	ml	525	C	(Syntaris)
Fluoxetine Liquid 20mg/5ml (as hydrochloride)	■	70	ml	1852	C	(Prozac)
Fluoxetine Hydrochloride Capsules 20mg	♦	30		685	A	
Fluoxetine Hydrochloride Capsules 60mg		30		5951	C	(Prozac 60)
Flupenthixol Tablets 500 microgram		60		310	C	(Fluanxol)
(as dihydrochloride)						
Flupenthixol Tablets 1mg (as dihydrochloride)		60		523	C	(Fluanxol)
Flupenthixol Tablets 3mg (as dihydrochloride)		100		1497	C	(Depixol)
Flurbiprofen Capsules 200mg (m/r)		30		1088	C	(Froben SR)
Flurbiprofen Tablets BP, 50mg		100		908	C	
Flurbiprofen Tablets BP, 100mg		100		1722	C	
Flutamide Tablets 250mg	♦	84		6547	A	
Fluticasone Cream BP, 0.05%	■	15	g	235	C	(Cutivate)
	■	50	g	695	C	(Cutivate)
Fluticasone Propionate Aerosol	■	120	dose	686	C	(Flixotide
Inhalation 25 microgram						Inhaler)
Fluticasone Propionate Aerosol	■	120	dose	585	C	(Flixotide
Inhalation 50 microgram						Inhaler)
Fluticasone Propionate Aerosol	■	120	dose	2286	C	(Flixotide
Inhalation 125 microgram						(Inhaler)
Fluticasone Propionate Aerosol	■	120	dose	3886	C	(Flixotide
Inhalation 250 microgram						Inhaler)
Fluticasone Propionate Aqueous Nasal Spray	■	150	dose	1143	C	(Flixonase)
50 microgram/metered spray						
Fluvastatin Capsules 20mg (as sodium salt)	♦	28		1272	C	(Lescol)
Fluvastatin Capsules 40mg (as sodium salt)	♦	28		1272	C	(Lescol)
Fluvoxamine Tablets BP, 50mg		60		1900	C	(Faverin 50)
Fluvoxamine Tablets BP, 100mg		30		1900	C	(Faverin 100)
Folic Acid Syrup 2.5mg/5ml sugar free		150	ml	974	C	(Lexpec)
Folic Acid Tablets BP, 400 microgram		90		219	C	(Preconceive)
Folic Acid Tablets BP, 5mg		28		44	A	
Formaldehyde Solution BP (Syn: Formalin)		500	ml	215	C	(Loveridge)
		2	litre	427	A	
Fosinopril Sodium Tablets 10mg	♦	28		1204	C	(Staril)
Fosinopril Sodium Tablets 20mg	♦	28		1300	C	(Staril)
Frusemide Tablets BP, 20mg		28		64	A	
		250		437	A	
Frusemide Tablets BP, 40mg	♦	28		78	A	
Frusemide Tablets BP, 500mg	★	28		901	A	
		100		3221 ∇	A	

VIII

■ Special Containers
♦ Manufacturers' Calendar Packs
● Preparations Requiring Reconstitution
★ Common Pack

Drug		Quantity	Basic Price p	Category
Fusidic Acid Cream 2% w/w	■	15 g	274	C *(Fucidin)*
	■	30 g	462	C *(Fucidin)*
Fusidic Acid Gel 2% w/w	■	15 g	237	C *(Fucidin)*
	■	30 g	410	C *(Fucidin)*
Fusidic Acid Viscous Eye Drops 1%	■	5 g	209	C *(Fucithalmic Viscous Drops)*
Fusidic Acid 2% and Betamethasone	■	15 g	357	C *(Fucibet)*
Valerate 0.1% Cream	■	30 g	604	C *(Fucibet)*
	■	60 g	1207	C *(Fucibet)*
Fusidic Acid 2% and Hydrocortisone	■	15 g	308	C *(Fucidin H)*
Acetate 1% Cream	■	30 g	530	C *(Fucidin H)*
Gabapentin Capsules 100mg		100	2286	C *(Neurontin)*
Gabapentin Capsules 300mg		100	5300	C *(Neurontin)*
Gabapentin Capsules 400mg		100	6133	C *(Neurontin)*
Gemfibrozil Capsules BP, 300mg		112	2390 ▽	A
Gemfibrozil Tablets BP, 600mg		30	1548	A
	♦	56	2964	C *(Lopid 600)*
Gentamicin Ear Drops 0.3% w/v	■	10 ml	179	C *(Garamycin)*
Gentamicin Eye Drops BP, 0.3% w/v	■	10 ml	179	C *(Garamycin)*
Gentamicin 0.3% (as sulphate) and	■	10 ml	397	C *(Gentisone HC)*
Hydrocortisone Acetate 1% Ear Drops				
Gentian Infusion, Compound Concentrated BP		500 ml	626	A
Gentian Acid Mixture BP		200 ml	37	E
(Syn: Gentian Acid Oral Solution)				
Gentian Alkaline Mixture BP		2 litre	626	A
(Syn: Gentian Alkaline Oral Solution)				
Gentian Alkaline with Phenobarbitone Mixture BPC		200 ml	66	E
Ginger Syrup BPC		500 ml	119	E
Ginger Tincture, Strong BP (Syn: Ginger Essence)		500 ml	845	A
Glibenclamide Tablets BP, 2.5mg	♦	28	96	A
Glibenclamide Tablets BP, 5mg		28	121	A
Gliclazide Tablets BP, 80mg		28	250	A
		60	619	A
Glipizide Tablets BP, 2.5mg		28	148	C *(Minodiab 2.5)*
Glipizide Tablets BP, 5mg		56	429	A
Glucose for Oral Use BP 1980		500 g	80	A
Glucose Intravenous Infusion BP, 50% w/v 25ml ampoules		10	3106	A
Glucose Intravenous Infusion BP, 50% w/v 50ml vials	■	1	163	A
Glucose Liquid BPC 1963		140 g	62	A
Glycerol BP (Syn: Glycerin)		100 ml	64	A

■ Special Containers
♦ Manufacturers' Calendar Packs

Drug	Quantity	Basic Price p	Category
Glycerol Suppositories BP, (Syn: Glycerin Suppositories) Infants size, mould size, 1g wrapped	12	81	A
Glycerol Suppositories BP, (Syn: Glycerin Suppositories) Child's size, mould size, 2g wrapped	12	83	A
Glycerol Suppositories BP, (Syn: Glycerin Suppositories) Adult's size, mould size, 4g wrapped	12	71	A
Glyceryl Trinitrate Spray 400 microgram/dose	■ 200 dose	313	C
Glyceryl Trinitrate Tablets BP, 300 microgram (Syns: Trinitrin Tablets, 300 microgram Nitroglycerin Tablets, 300 microgram)	■ 100	291	C (GTN)
Glyceryl Trinitrate Tablets BP, 500 microgram (Syns: Trinitrin Tablets, 500 microgram Nitroglycerin Tablets, 500 microgram)	■ 100	105	A
Glyceryl Trinitrate Tablets BP, 600 microgram (Syns: Trinitrin Tablets, 600 microgram Nitroglycerin Tablets, 600 microgram)	■ 100	231	A
Goserelin Implant 3.6mg (as acetate) in Syringe Applicator	■ 1	12227	C (Zoladex)
Goserelin Implant 10.8mg (as acetate) in Syringe Applicator	■ 1	36681	C (Zoladex LA)
Griseofulvin Tablets BP, 125mg	100	233	C (Grisovin)
Griseofulvin Tablets BP, 500mg	100	875	C (Grisovin)
Halibut-Liver Oil Capsules BP (4000 units of vitamin A activity)	100	105	C (AAH)
Haloperidol Capsules BP, 500 microgram	30	98	C (Serenace)
Haloperidol Oral Solution BP, 0.2% w/v (2mg/1ml) sugar free (Syns: Haloperidol Oral Drops 0.2% w/v sugar free Haloperidol Solution 0.2% w/v sugar free)	500 ml	4383	A
Haloperidol Tablets BP, 1.5mg	28	159	A
	100	521 Δ	A
	★ 250	1004	A
Haloperidol Tablets BP, 5mg	★ 28	456	A
	100	1222 ▽	A
	250	2995	A
Haloperidol Tablets BP, 10mg	50	1197 ▽	A
Haloperidol Tablets BP, 20mg	50	2081 Δ	A
Hamamelis Water BPC	500 ml	205	A
Homatropine Eye Drops BP, 1% w/v	■ 10 ml	195	A
Homatropine Eye Drops BP, 2% w/v	■ 10 ml	206	A
Hydralazine Tablets BP, 25mg	56	150	A
Hydralazine Tablets BP, 50mg	56	296	A
Hydrochloric Acid, Dilute BP	500 ml	285	A
Hydrochlorothiazide Tablets BP, 25mg	30	44	C (Hydrosaluric)
Hydrochlorothiazide Tablets BP, 50mg	30	81	C (Hydrosaluric)

■ Special Containers
★ Common Pack

Drug	Quantity		Basic Price p		Category	
Hydrocortisone BP	1	g	450		C	(Thornton & Ross)
	5	g	1573		A	
Hydrocortisone Cream BP, 0.1% w/w	■ 15	g	151		C	(Dermacort)
	■ 30	g	269		C	(Dioderm)
Hydrocortisone Cream BP, 0.5% w/w	■ 15	g	36		A	
	■ 30	g	60		C	(Efcortelan)
Hydrocortisone Cream BP, 1% w/w	■ 15	g	39		A	
	■ 30	g	80		A	
Hydrocortisone Cream BP, 2.5% w/w	■ 15	g	86		A	
	■ 30	g	166		C	(Efcortelan)
Hydrocortisone Eye Ointment BPC, 2.5% w/w	■ 3	g	222		C	(AAH)
Hydrocortisone Ointment BP, 0.5% w/w	■ 15	g	37		A	
	■ 30	g	60		C	(Efcortelan)
Hydrocortisone Ointment BP, 1% w/w	■ 15	g	37	▽	A	
	■ 30	g	69	▽	A	
Hydrocortisone Ointment BP, 2.5% w/w	■ 15	g	102		A	
	■ 30	g	166		C	(Efcortelan)
Hydrocortisone Tablets 10mg	30		70		C	(Hydrocortone)
Hydrocortisone Tablets 20mg	30		107		C	(Hydrocortone)
Hydrocortisone and Miconazole Cream DPF	■ 30	g	224		C	(Daktacort)
Hydrocortisone and Miconazole Ointment DPF	■ 30	g	225		C	(Daktacort)
Hydrocortisone Butyrate Cream 0.1% w/w	■ 30	g	204		C	(Locoid)
	■ 100	g	626		C	(Locoid)
Hydrocortisone Butyrate Ointment 0.1% w/w	■ 30	g	204		C	(Locoid)
	■ 100	g	626		C	(Locoid)
Hydrocortisone Sodium Succinate Injection BP, 100mg vial	■ 1		97		C	(Solu-Cortef)
Hydrogen Peroxide Ear Drops BP 1980	10	ml	1		E	
Hydrogen Peroxide Solution BP (6 per cent) (Syn: Hydrogen Peroxide Solution)	2	litre	310		A	
Hydrotalcite Suspension 500mg/5ml	500	ml	196		C	(Peckforton Pharmaceuticals Ltd
Hydrous Ointment BP (Syn: Oily Cream)	500	g	207		A	
Hydrous Wool Fat Ointment BPC	500	g	358		A	
Hydroxocobalamin Injection BP, 1mg/1ml ampoules	5		1249	▽	C	
Hydroxychloroquine Tablets BP, 200mg	60		455		C	(Plaquenil)
Hydroxyurea Capsules BP, 500mg	100		1195		C	(Hydrea)
Hydroxyzine Hydrochloride Tablets 10mg	84		152		C	(Atarax)
Hydroxyzine Hydrochloride Tablets 25mg	28		102		C	(Atarax)
Hyoscine Injection BP, 400 microgram/1ml ampoules (Syn: Hyoscine Hydrobromide Injection 400 microgram/1ml ampoules	10		2712		A	
Hyoscine Butylbromide Tablets BP, 10mg	56		259		C	(Buscopan)
Hyoscyamus Tincture BP 1980	500	ml	474		C	(AAH)

■ Special Containers

Drug		Quantity		Basic Price p	Category	
Hypromellose Eye Drops BP, 0.3% w/v	■	10	ml	74	A	
(Syns: Alkaline Eye Drops 0.3% w/v						
Artificial Tears 0.3% w/v)						
Hypromellose Eye Drops BP, 0.5% w/v	■	10	ml	85	C	*(Isopto Plain)*
(Syns: Alkaline Eye Drops 0.5% w/v						
Artificial Tears 0.5% w/v)						
Hypromellose Eye Drops BP, 1% w/v	■	10	ml	99	C	*(Isopto Alkaline)*
(Syns: Alkaline Eye Drops 1% w/v						
Artificial Tears 1% w/v)						
Ibuprofen Cream BP, 5% w/w	■	30	g	259	C	*(Proflex Pain Relief Cream)*
....	■	100	g	650	C	*(Proflex)*
Ibuprofen Gel BP, 5% w/w	■	30	g	242	C	*(Ibuleve)*
....	■	50	g	258	A	
....	■	100	g	595	C	*(Ibugel)*
Ibuprofen Granules Effervescent 600mg/sachet		20		567	C	*(Brufen)*
Ibuprofen Oral Suspension BP, 100mg/5ml sugar free		100	ml	194	C	*(Nurofen)*
....		150	ml	291	C	*(Nurofen)*
Ibuprofen Syrup 100mg/5ml		500	ml	807	C	*(Brufen)*
Ibuprofen Tablets BP, 200mg		84		165	A	
Ibuprofen Tablets BP, 400mg		84		244	A	
Ibuprofen Tablets BP, 600mg		84		366	▽ A	
....		100		460	A	
Ibuprofen Tablets BP, 800mg		90		1052	C	*(Motrin)*
Ibuprofen Tablets 800mg (m/r)	♦	56		965	C	*(Brufen Retard)*
Ichthammol BP (Syn: Ammonium Ichthosulphonate) .		100	g	395	A	
Ichthammol Glycerin BPC		500	ml	587	A	
Imipramine Tablets BP, 10mg		28		85	A	
....		250		318	▽ A	
Imipramine Tablets BP, 25mg		28		101	A	
....		1000		795	A	
Imipramine Hydrochloride Syrup 25mg/5ml		150	ml	311	C	*(Tofranil)*
Indapamide Tablets 2.5mg (as hemihydrate)		28		275	A	
....		56		510	A	
Indomethacin Capsules BP, 25mg		28		72	A	
Indomethacin Capsules BP, 50mg		28		81	A	
....		100		215	A	
Indomethacin Suppositories BP, 100mg		10		128	A	
Indoramin Tablets BP, 20mg		60		1230	C	*(Doralese Tiltab)*
Indoramin Tablets BP, 25mg		84		900	C	*(Baratol)*
Indoramin Tablets BP, 50mg		84		1700	C	*(Baratol)*
Industrial Methylated Spirit BP		500	ml	135	C	(Thornton & Ross)
(Syns: Industrial Methylated Spirits; IMS)						
Iodine BP		100	g	625	C	(AAH)
Iodine Solution, Strong BP 1958		500	ml	640	C	(AAH)
Iodine Aqueous Oral Solution BP		100	ml	170	C	(Thornton & Ross)
(Syns: Iodine Aqueous Solution, Lugol's Solution)						
....		500	ml	545	A	

■ Special Containers
♦ Manufacturers' Calendar Packs

Drug	Quantity		Basic Price p	Category
Ipecacuanha Mixture (See Alk. Ipecac Mixture)	-		-	-
Ipecacuanha Mixture, Paediatric BPC	100	ml	12	E
Ipecacuanha Tincture BP	500	ml	847	A
Ipecacuanha and Ammonia Mixture Paediatric BPC . .	100	ml	10	E
Ipecacuanha Opiate Mixture, Paediatric BPC	100	ml	16	E
Ipratropium Bromide Aerosol Inhalation . . . . ■	200	dose	421	C _(Atrovent)_
20 microgram per actuation				
Ipratropium Bromide Aerosol Inhalation . . . . ■	200	dose	622	C _(Atrovent Forte)_
40 microgram per actuation				
Ipratropium Bromide Aqueous Nasal Spray . . . . ■	15	ml	455	C _(Rinatec_
21 microgram/ pump spray 180 dose				_Aqueous)_
Isoniazid Tablets BP, 50mg	56		578	C (Penn Pharm)
Isoniazid Tablets BP, 100mg	28		577	C (Penn Pharm)
Isosorbide Dinitrate Tablets BP, 5mg	100		143	C _(Isordil)_
(Syn: Sorbide Nitrate Tablets 5mg)				
Isosorbide Dinitrate Tablets BP, 10mg	56		100	A
(Syn: Sorbide Nitrate Tablets 10mg)	100		140	A
Isosorbide Dinitrate Tablets BP, 20mg	56		173	A
(Syn: Sorbide Nitrate Tablets 20mg)	100		220	A
Isosorbide Dinitrate Tablets BP, 30mg	112		386	C _(Isordil)_
(Syn: Sorbide Nitrate Tablets 30mg)				
Isosorbide Mononitrate Capsules 25mg (m/r) . . . . . . ♦	28		669	C _(Elantan LA 25)_
Isosorbide Mononitrate Tablets 10mg	56		112	A
Isosorbide Mononitrate Tablets 20mg	56		179	A
Isosorbide Mononitrate Tablets 40mg	56		373	A
Ispaghula Husk Granules, Effervescent BP, ...	265	g	643	C _(Fybozest)_
sugar and gluten-free	(Bulk Pack)			
Ispaghula Husk Granules, Effervescent BP, ...	60		424	C _(Fybogel)_
3.5g/sachet sugar and gluten-free	(2x30)			
Ispaghula Husk Powder, BP, ...	30		157	C _(Regulan)_
3.4g/5.85g sachet sugar and gluten-free				
Itraconazole Capsules 100mg	4		572	C _(Sporanox)_
. . . .	15		2145	C _(Sporanox)_
. . . .	60		8580	C _(Sporanox)_
Kaolin Light BP	1	kg	320	A
Kaolin Mixture BP (Syn: Kaolin Oral Suspension)	200	ml	51	C (AAH)
. . . .	2	litre	421	A
Kaolin Mixture, Paediatric BP 1980	500	ml	186	A
Kaolin Poultice BP . . . . ■	200	g	191	A
(To be supplied in lever-lidded tins, ... ■	500	g	335	A
or approved polypropylene jars)				
Kaolin and Morphine Mixture BP	2	litre	387	A
(Syn: Kaolin and Morphine Oral Suspension)				

■ Special Containers
♦ Manufacturers' Calendar Packs

Drug		Quantity		Basic Price p	Category	
Ketoconazole Cream 2% w/w	■	30	g	381	C	(Nizoral)
Ketoconazole Shampoo 2% w/v	■	120	ml	584	C	(Nizoral)
Ketoprofen Capsules BP, 50mg		28		447	A	
....		100		1595	A	
Ketoprofen Gel 2.5% w/w	■	30	g	262	C	(Oruvail)
....		50	g	325	C	(Powergel)
....	■	100	g	678	C	(Oruvail)
Ketotifen Elixir 1mg		300	ml	964	C	(Zaditen)
(as hydrogen fumarate)/5ml sugar free						

Drug		Quantity		Basic Price p	Category	
Labetalol Tablets BP, 50mg	♦	56		505	C	(Trandate)
(Syn: Labetalol Hydrochloride Tablets 50mg)						
Labetalol Tablets BP, 100mg		56		477	A	
(Syn: Labetalol Hydrochloride Tablets 100mg)						
Labetalol Tablets BP, 200mg		56		646	A	
(Syn: Labetalol Hydrochloride Tablets 200mg) ..						
Labetalol Tablets BP, 400mg		56		1112	A	
(Syn: Labetalol Hydrochloride Tablets 400mg)						
Lacidipine Tablets 2mg	♦	28		1023	C	(Motens)
Lacidipine Tablets 4mg	♦	28		1530	C	(Motens)
Lactic Acid BP		500	ml	585	C	(AAH)
Lactitol Powder NPF, 10g per sachet		10		100	C	(Importal)
Lactose BP		500	g	258	A	
(Syn: Lactose Monohydrate)						
Lactulose Solution BP, 3.1-3.7g/5ml.		500	ml	244	A	
....		1	litre	491	A	
Lamotrigine Dispersible Tablets 5mg		28		796	C	(Lamictal Dispersible)
Lamotrigine Dispersible Tablets 25mg		56		1997	C	(Lamictal Dispersible)
Lamotrigine Dispersible Tablets 100mg		56		5857	C	(Lamictal Dispersible)
Lamotrigine Tablets 25mg		21		749	C	(Lamictal)
....		42		1497	C	(Lamictal)
....		56		1997	C	(Lamictal)
Lamotrigine Tablets 50mg		56		3395	C	(Lamictal)
Lamotrigine Tablets 100mg		56		5857	C	(Lamictal)
Lamotrigine Tablets 200mg	♦	56		9956	C	(Lamictal)
Lansoprazole Capsules 15mg (e/c granules)	♦	28		1298	C	(Zoton)
....	♦	56		2596	C	(Zoton)
Lansoprazole Capsules 30mg (e/c granules)	♦	14		1188	C	(Zoton)
....	♦	28		2375	C	(Zoton)
Lansoprazole Granules 30mg		28		3414	C	(Zoton)
(Lansoprazole Sachets 30mg)						
Latanoprost Eye Drops	■	2.5	ml	1528	C	(Xalatan)
50 microgram/ml w/v						

VIII

■ Special Containers
♦ Manufacturers' Calendar Packs

Drug		Quantity		Basic Price p	Category	
Lemon Spirit BP		100	ml	590	A	
Levobunolol Eye Drops BP, 0.5% w/v	■	5	ml	466	C	*(Betagan)*
Levodopa Tablets BP, 500 mg		200		6000	A	
(Syn: L-Dopa Tablets 500mg)						
Levodopa and Carbidopa Tablets - see Co-careldopa Tablets						
Lignocaine Gel BP, 2% w/v	■	20	g	76	C	*(Xylocaine)*
(Syn: Lignocaine Hydrochloride Gel 2% w/v)						
Lignocaine Injection BP, 1% 2ml ampoules		10		217	A	
(Syn: Lignocaine Hydrochloride Injection 1% 2ml ampoules)						
Lignocaine Injection BP, 1% 5ml ampoules		10		209	A	
(Syn: Lignocaine Hydrochloride Injection 1% 5ml ampoules)						
Lignocaine Injection BP, 1% 10ml ampoules		10		339	A	
(Syn: Lignocaine Hydrochloride Injection 1% 10ml ampoules)						
Lignocaine Injection BP, 1% 20ml ampoules		10		521	A	
(Syn: Lignocaine Hydrochloride Injection 1% 20ml ampoules)						
Lignocaine Injection BP, 2% 2ml ampoules		10		273	A	
(Syn: Lignocaine Hydrochloride Injection 2% 2ml ampoules)						
Lignocaine Injection BP, 2% 5ml ampoules		10		227	A	
(Syn: Lignocaine Hydrochloride Injection 2% 5ml ampoules)						
Lignocaine Injection BP, 2% 20ml ampoules		10		606	A	
(Syn: Lignocaine Hydrochloride Injection 2% 20ml ampoules)						
Lignocaine Ointment DPF, NPF, 5%	■	15	g	80	C	*(Xylocaine)*
Linseed Oil BP		500	ml	215	A	
Liothyronine Tablets BP, 20 microgram		100		1492	C	*(Tertroxin)*
(Syn: L-Tri-iodothyronine Sodium Tablets 20 microgram)						
Liquefied Phenol BP		200	ml	425	E	
Liquid Paraffin Oral Emulsion BP		500	ml	200	C	(Loveridge)
(Syn: Liquid Paraffin Emulsion)						
Liquid Paraffin and Magnesium Hydroxide		2	litre	660	A	
Oral Emulsion BP						
(Syn: Liquid Paraffin and Magnesium Hydroxide Emulsion)						
Liquorice Liquid Extract BP		500	ml	512	A	
Lisinopril Tablets 2.5mg (as dihydrate)	♦	28		626	C	*(Zestril)*
Lisinopril Tablets 5mg (as dihydrate)	♦	28		786	C	*(Zestril)*
Lisinopril Tablets 10mg (as dihydrate)	♦	28		970	C	*(Zestril)*
Lisinopril Tablets 20mg (as dihydrate)	♦	28		1097	C	*(Zestril)*

■ Special Containers
♦ Manufacturers' Calendar Packs

Drug	Quantity		Basic Price p	Category	
Lithium Carbonate Tablets BP, 250mg	100		288	C	(Camcolit 250)
Lithium Carbonate Tablets Slow BP, 200mg	100		250	C	(Priadel 200)
Lithium Carbonate Tablets Slow BP, 450mg	60		282	C	(Liskonum)
Lodoxamide Eye Drops 0.1% w/v ■	10	ml	548	C	(Alomide Ophthalmic Solution)
(as trometamol)					
Lofepramine Tablets 70mg (as hydrochloride) ♦	56		1002	A	
Loperamide Hydrochloride Capsules 2mg	30		180	A	
Loperamide Hydrochloride Syrup	100	ml	105	C	(Imodium)
1mg/5ml sugar free					
Loprazolam Tablets BP, 1mg	28		446	C	(Aventis Pharma)
Loratadine Syrup 5mg/5ml	100	ml	757	C	(Clarityn)
Loratadine Tablets 10mg	30		757	C	(Clarityn)
Lorazepam Tablets BP, 1mg	28		108	A	
	100		175	A	
Lorazepam Tablets BP, 2.5mg	28		157	A	
	100		235	A	
Lormetazepam Tablets BP, 500 microgram	28		105	A	
	30		268	A	
Lormetazepam Tablets BP, 1mg	28		154	A	
	30		320	A	
Losartan Potassium Tablets 25mg	7		431	C	(Cozaar Half Strength)
Losartan Potassium Tablets 50mg ♦	28		1723	C	(Cozaar)
Magnesium Carbonate, Heavy BP	500	g	415	A	
Magnesium Carbonate, Light BP	500	g	360	A	
Magnesium Carbonate, Mixture BPC	2	litre	544	A	
Magnesium Carbonate Aromatic Mixture BP	2	litre	612	A	
(Syn: Magnesium Carbonate Aromatic Oral Suspension)					
Magnesium Hydroxide Mixture BP	500	ml	212	A	
(Syn: Magnesium Hydroxide Oral Suspension, Cream of Magnesia)					
Magnesium Sulphate BP (Syn: Epsom Salts)	1.5	kg	308	A	
Magnesium Sulphate, Dried BP (Powder)	500	g	315	B	
(Syn: Epsom Salts, Dried)					
Magnesium Sulphate Injection BP, 50% w/v 2ml ampoules	10		3062	A	
Magnesium Sulphate Mixture BP	200	ml	30	E	
(Syn: Magnesium Sulphate Oral Suspension)					
Magnesium Sulphate Paste BP (Syn: Morison's Paste)	25	g	52	A	
	50	g	60	A	
	500	g	400	C	(Thornton & Ross)
Magnesium Trisilicate BP					
(Syns: Magnesium Trisilicate Powder) Magnesium Trisilicate Oral Powder)					
Magnesium Trisilicate Mixture BP	2	litre	461	A	
(Syns: Magnesium Trisilicate Oral Suspension Compound Magnesium Trisilicate Mixture)					

■ Special Containers
♦ Manufacturers' Calendar Packs

Drug		Quantity		Basic Price p		Category	
Magnesium Trisilicate Oral Powder Compound BP . . .		500	g	250		E	
(Syn: Magnesium Trisilicate Powder Compound)							
Magnesium Trisilicate and Belladonna Mixture BPC . .		200	ml	52		E	
Maize Starch - See Starch Maize BP (Powder)							
Malathion Alcoholic Lotion 0.5% w/v	■	50	ml	216		C	*(Suleo M)*
. . . .	■	200	ml	528		C	*(Suleo M)*
Malathion Aqueous Lotion 0.5% w/v	■	50	ml	216		C	*(Derbac-M)*
. . . .	■	200	ml	528		C	*(Derbac-M)*
Malathion Shampoo 1% w/w	■	40	g	259		C	*(Prioderm)*
Mebendazole Oral Suspension NPF, 100mg/5ml	■	30	ml	177		C	*(Vermox)*
sugar free							
Mebendazole Tablets NPF, 100mg (Chewable)		6		153		C	*(Vermox)*
Mebeverine Tablets BP, 135mg		100		767		A	
Medroxyprogesterone Acetate Injection							
(Aqueous Suspension) 150mg/ml							
1ml pre-filled syringe	■	1		455		C	*(Depo-Provera)*
3.3ml vials	■	1		1249		C	*(Depo-Provera)*
Medroxyprogesterone Acetate Tablets 2.5mg		30		184		C	*(Provera)*
Medroxyprogesterone Acetate Tablets 5mg		10		123		C	*(Provera)*
Medroxyprogesterone Acetate Tablets 10mg		10		247		C	*(Provera)*
. . . .		90		2216		C	*(Provera)*
Medroxyprogesterone Acetate Tablets 100mg		100		3975		C	*(Provera)*
Medroxyprogesterone Acetate Tablets 200mg		30		2360		C	*(Provera)*
Medroxyprogesterone Acetate Tablets 250mg		50		4845		C	*(Farlutal 250)*
Medroxyprogesterone Acetate Tablets 400mg		30		4669		C	*(Provera)*
Medroxyprogesterone Acetate Tablets 500mg	♦	56		10852		C	*(Farlutal 500)*
Mefenamic Acid Capsules BP, 250mg		100		250		A	
. . . .		500		1248		A	
Mefenamic Acid Tablets 500mg		28		254		A	
. . . .		100		726		A	
Megestrol Tablets BP, 40mg		120		3048		C	*(Megace)*
Megestrol Tablets BP, 160mg		30		2930		C	*(Megace)*
Meloxicam Suppositories 7.5mg		12		400		C	*(Mobic)*
Meloxicam Suppositories 15mg		12		600		C	*(Mobic)*
Meloxicam Tablets 7.5mg		30		1000		C	*(Mobic)*
Meloxicam Tablets 15mg		30		1390		C	*(Mobic)*
Menthol BP		5	g	86		C	(AAH)
Menthol and Eucalyptus Inhalation BP 1980		100	ml	59		A	
Meptazinol Tablets BP, 200mg		112		2457		C	*(Meptid)*
Mesalazine Tablets 400mg (e/c)		90		3269		C	*(Asacol)*
. . . .		120		4358		C	*(Asacol)*
Metformin Tablets BP, 500mg		28		78	Δ	A	
Metformin Tablets BP, 850mg		56		229	∇	A	
. . . .	★	300		1001	Δ	A	
Methadone Injection BP, 10mg/ml, 1ml ampoules . . .		10		859		A	
Methadone Injection BP, 10mg/ml, 2ml ampoules . . .		10		1450		A	
Methadone Injection BP, 10mg/ml, 3.5ml ampoules . .		10		1783		A	
Methadone Injection BP, 10mg/ml, 5ml ampoules . . .		10		1923		A	
Methadone Linctus BP		500	ml	520		A	

■ Special Containers
♦ Manufacturers' Calendar Packs
★ Common Pack

Drug	Quantity		Basic Price p		Category	
Methadone Mixture 1mg/1ml	30	ml	44		C	*(Physeptone)*
(Methadone Oral Solution 1mg/1ml)	50	ml	73		C	*(Physeptone)*
. . . .	100	ml	145		C	*(Physeptone)*
. . . .	500	ml	759		A	
Methadone Mixture 1mg/1ml sugar free	30	ml	44		C	*(Physeptone)*
(Methadone Oral Solution 1mg/1ml sugar free) .	50	ml	73		C	*(Physeptone)*
. . . .	100	ml	145		C	*(Physeptone)*
. . . . , . . .	500	ml	725		C	*(Physeptone)*
Methadone Tablets BP, 5mg	50		297		C	*(Physeptone)*
Methadone Hydrochloride BP	2	g	984		A	
Methionine Tablets 250mg	250		8212		A	
Methocarbamol Tablets 750mg	100		1265		C	*(Robaxin - 750)*
Methotrexate Tablets BP, 2.5mg	100		1138		A	
Methotrexate Tablets BP, 10mg	100		5507		A	
Methylcellulose '20' BP	500	g	1795		A	
Methylcellulose Tablets BP	112		269		C	*(Celevac)*
Methyldopa Tablets BP, 125mg	56		131		A	
Methyldopa Tablets BP, 250mg	56		169	Δ	A	
Methyldopa Tablets BP, 500mg	56		345		A	
Methylphenidate Hydrochloride Tablets 10mg	30		557		C	*(Ritalin)*
Methyl Salicylate BP	500	ml	542		A	
Methyl Salicylate Liniment BP	500	ml	300		A	
Methyl Salicylate Ointment BP	500	g	483		A	
(Syn: Strong Methyl Salicylate Ointment)						
Metoclopramide Tablets BP, 5mg	84		469		C	*(Maxolon)*
Metoclopramide Tablets BP, 10mg	28		86		A	
Metolazone Tablets 5mg	100		2037		C	*(Metenix 5)*
Metoprolol Tartrate Tablets BP, 50mg	28		117	∇	A	
. . . .	♦ 56		228		A	
. . . .	★ 100		313		A	
Metoprolol Tartrate Tablets BP, 100mg	28		183	∇	A	
. . . .	♦ 56		381		A	
. . . .	★ 100		594		A	
Metronidazole Oral Suspension DPF	100	ml	768		A	
(Metronidazole Oral Suspension 200mg						
(as benzoate)/5ml)						
Metronidazole Tablets BP, 200mg	21		133		A	
. . . .	250		496		A	
Metronidazole Tablets BP, 400mg	21		154		A	
. . . .	100		415		A	
Metronidazole Tablets BP, 500mg	21		352		A	
Mianserin Tablets BP, 10mg	28		271		A	
Mianserin Tablets BP, 20mg	28		416		A	
. . . .	♦ 56		760	∇	A	
Mianserin Tablets BP, 30mg	♦ 28		540		A	
. . . .	100		1832		A	
Miconazole Cream BP, 2% w/w	■ 30	g	207		C	*(Daktarin)*
(Syn: Miconazole Nitrate Cream 2% w/w)						
Miconazole Oral Gel DPF, NPF, 24mg/ml sugar free . .	■ 15	g	227		C	*(Daktarin)*
. . . .	■ 80	g	500		C	*(Daktarin)*
Miconazole and Hydrocortisone Cream						
(See Hydrocortisone and Miconazole Cream DPF)	-		-		-	
Miconazole and Hydrocortisone Ointment						
(See Hydrocortisone and Miconazole Ointment DPF)	-		-		-	

■ Special Containers
♦ Manufacturers' Calendar Packs
★ Common Pack

VIII

Drug	Quantity		Basic Price p		Category	
Minocycline Tablets BP, 50mg	28		765		A	
Minocycline Tablets BP, 100mg	28		1145		A	
Minocycline Hydrochloride Capsules 100mg (m/r)	♦ 56		3523		C	(Minocin MR)
Misoprostol Tablets 200 microgram	60		1114		C	(Cytotec)
Moclobemide Tablets 150mg	30		1003		C	(Manerix)
Moclobemide Tablets 300mg	30		1504		C	(Manerix)
Mometasone Furoate Cream 0.1%	■ 30	g	488		C	(Elocon)
	■ 100	g	1405		C	(Elocon)
Mometasone Furoate Ointment 0.1%	■ 30	g	488		C	(Elocon)
	■ 100	g	1405		C	(Elocon)
Morphine and Cocaine Elixir BPC	200	ml	541	△	E	
Morphine Hydrochloride BP	2	g	1274		A	
Morphine Sulphate BP	2	g	1042		A	
Morphine Sulphate Injection BP, 10mg/1ml ampoules	5		329		A	
Morphine Sulphate Injection BP, 15mg/1ml ampoules	5		381		A	
Morphine Sulphate Injection BP, 30mg/1ml ampoules	5		495		A	
Morphine Sulphate Suppositories BP, 15mg	12		586		A	
Morphine Sulphate Suppositories BP, 30mg	12		988		A	
Morphine Sulphate Tablets 5mg (m/r)	60		430		C	(MST Continus)
Morphine Sulphate Tablets 15mg (m/r)	60		1257		C	(MST Continus)
Morphine Sulphate Tablets 200mg (m/r)	60		10634		C	(MST Continus)
Mouthwash Solution Tablets DPF, NPF	■ 100		214		A	
Mupirocin Nasal Ointment 2% w/w	■ 3g		624		C	(Bactroban Nasal)
Mupirocin Ointment 2% w/w	■ 15	g	471		C	(Bactroban)
Myrrh Tincture BPC	100	ml	255		B	
Nabumetone Oral Suspension BP, 500mg/5ml sugar free	300	ml	2522		C	(Relifex)
Nabumetone Tablets BP, 500mg	56		1811		C	
Naftidrofuryl Capsules BP, 100mg	84		781		A	
	100		1023		C	(Praxilene)
	500		4975		C	(Praxilene)
Naproxen Suppositories BP, 500mg	10		228		C	(Naprosyn)
Naproxen Tablets BP, 250mg	28		157		A	
	60		333		A	
	250		1328		A	
Naproxen Tablets BP, 500mg	28		348	▽	A	
	60		593		A	
	100		1249		A	
Naproxen Sodium Tablets 275mg	60		811		C	(Synflex)
Naproxen Tablets 250mg (e/c)	56		446		A	
Naproxen Tablets 500mg (e/c)	56		816		A	
Naratriptan Tablets 2.5mg (as hydrochloride)	6		2400		C	(Naramig)
Nedocromil Sodium Aqueous Eye Drops 2% w/v	■ 5	ml	975		C	(Rapitil)
Nefazodone Hydrochloride Tablets 100mg	♦ 56		1680		C	(Dutonin)
Nefazodone Hydrochloride Tablets 200mg	♦ 56		1680		C	(Dutonin)
Nefopam Hydrochloride Tablets 30mg	90		1093		C	(Acupan)

■ Special Containers
♦ Manufacturers' Calendar Packs

Drug	Quantity		Basic Price p	Category	
Neomycin Cream BPC	■ 15	g	109	C	(AAH)
Neomycin Eye Ointment BP, 0.5%	■ 3	g	232	A	
(Syn: Neomycin Sulphate Eye Ointment 0.5%)					
Nicardipine Hydrochloride Capsules 20mg	56		838	C	(Cardene)
Nicardipine Hydrochloride Capsules 30mg	56		973	C	(Cardene)
Nicardipine Hydrochloride Capsules 30mg (m/r)	56		968	C	(Cardene SR)
Nicardipine Hydrochloride Capsules 45mg (m/r)	56		1344	C	(Cardene SR)
Nicorandil Tablets 10mg	60		779	C	(Ikorel)
. . . .	(6x■10)				
Nicorandil Tablets 20mg	60		1480	C	(Ikorel)
. . . .	(6x■10)				
Nifedipine Capsules BP, 5mg	★ 84		372	A	
. . . .	100		410	A	
Nifedipine Capsules BP, 10mg	84		440	▽ A	
. . . .	100		489	A	
Nifedipine Capsules 10mg (m/r)	60		625	C	(Coracten SR)
Nifedipine Capsules 20mg (m/r)	60		867	C	(Coracten SR)
Nifedipine Tablets 60mg (m/r)	♦ 28		1540	C	(Adalat LA 60)
Nitrazepam Oral Suspension BP, 2.5mg/5ml	150	ml	530	C	(Somnite)
(Syn: Nitrazepam Mixture 2.5mg/5ml)					
Nitrazepam Tablets BP, 5mg	28		82	A	
Nitrofurantoin Capsules 50mg	30		305	C	(Macrodantin)
Nitrofurantoin Capsules 100mg	30		576	C	(Macrodantin)
Nitrofurantoin Capsules 100mg (m/r)	14		489	C	(Macrobid)
Nitrofurantoin Tablets BP, 50mg	100		881	A	
Nitrofurantoin Tablets BP, 100mg	100		1630	A	
Nizatidine Capsules 150mg	♦ 30		827	C	(Axid)
Nizatidine Capsules 300mg	♦ 30		1640	C	(Axid)
Norethisterone Tablets BP, 1mg	36		375	C	(Micronor HRT)
. . . .	(3x■12)				
Norethisterone Tablets BP, 5mg	30		216	C	
Norfloxacin Tablets 400mg	6		219	C	(Utinor)
. . . .	14		511	C	(Utinor)
Nortriptyline Tablets BP, 10mg	100		1139	C	(Allegron)
Nortriptyline Tablets BP, 25mg	100		2317	C	(Allegron)
Nystatin Cream 100,000 units/g	■ 30	g	218	C	(Nystan)
Nystatin Ointment BP, 100,000 units/g	■ 30	g	175	C	(Nystan)
Nystatin Oral Suspension BP, 100,000 u/ml	■ 30	ml	220	A	
(Syns: Nystatin Mixture 100,000u/ml,					
Nystatin Oral Drops 100,000u/ml,					
Nystatin Suspension 100,000u/ml)					
Nystatin Oral Suspension BP, 100,000u/ml sugar free	■ 30	ml	196	C	(Nystamont)
(Syns: Nystatin Mixture 100,000u/ml sugar free,					
Nystatin Oral Drops 100,000u/ml sugar free					
Nystatin Suspension 100,000u/ml sugar free)					
Nystatin Pastilles DPF, NPF, 100,000 units	■ 28		324	C	(Nystan)
Nystatin Pessaries BP, 100,000 units	■ 28		196	C	(Nystan)
Nystatin Tablets BP, 500,000 units	56		470	C	(Nystan)
Nystatin Vaginal Cream 100,000 units/4g application	■ 60	g	277	C	(Nystan)

VIII

■ Special Containers
♦ Manufacturers' Calendar Packs
★ Common Pack

Drug		Quantity		Basic Price p	Category	
Oestradiol Implant 25mg	■	1		959	A	
Oestradiol Implant 50mg	■	1		1916	A	
Oestradiol Implant 100mg	■	1		3340	A	
Oestrogens, Conjugated Tablets 625 microgram	♦	84 (3x28)		810	C	*(Premarin)*
Oestrogens, Conjugated Tablets 1.25mg	♦	84 (3x28)		1099	C	*(Premarin)*
Oestrogens, Conjugated Tablets 2.5mg	♦	84 (3x28)		1170	C	*(Premarin)*
Ofloxacin Tablets 200mg		10		1026	C	*(Tarivid)*
		20		2050	C	*(Tarivid)*
		100		10251	C	*(Tarivid)*
Ofloxacin Tablets 400mg		5		1024	C	*(Tarivid 400)*
		10		2043	C	*(Tarivid 400)*
		50		10208	C	*(Tarivid 400)*
Oily Cream (See Hydrous Ointment BP)		-		-	-	
Olanzapine Tablets 2.5mg		28		3170	C	*(Zyprexa)*
Olanzapine Tablets 5mg		28		4878	C	*(Zyprexa)*
Olanzapine Tablets 7.5mg		56		14634	C	*(Zyprexa)*
Olanzapine Tablets 10mg		28		9756	C	*(Zyprexa)*
		56		19511	C	*(Zyprexa)*
Oleic Acid BP		500	ml	300	C	(Thornton & Ross)
Olive Oil BP		2	litre	1450	C	(Thornton & Ross)
Olsalazine Sodium Capsules 250mg		112		2742	C	*(Dipentum)*
Omeprazole Capsules 10mg (e/c)		28		1891	C	*(Losec)*
Omeprazole Capsules 20mg (e/c)		28		2856	C	*(Losec)*
Omeprazole Capsules 40mg (e/c)		7		1428	C	*(Losec)*
Omeprazole Tablets, Dispersible 10mg	♦	28		1891	C	*(Losec MUPS)*
Omeprazole Tablets, Dispersible 20mg	♦	28		2856	C	*(Losec MUPS)*
Omeprazole Tablets, Dispersible 40mg	♦	7		1428	C	*(Losec MUPS)*
Opium Tincture BP		100	ml	465	C	(Unichem)
Orange Syrup BP		500	ml	330	C	(Thornton & Ross)
Orange Tincture BP		100	ml	595	A	
Orciprenaline Oral Solution BP, 10mg/5ml sugar free (Syn: Orciprenaline Elixir 10mg/5ml sugar free)		300	ml	226	C	*(Alupent Syrup)*
Orphenadrine Hydrochloride Tablets BP, 50mg		250		859	C	*(Disipal)*
Oxazepam Tablets BP, 10mg		28		91	A	
		100		120	A	
Oxazepam Tablets BP, 15mg		28		110	A	
		100		116	A	
Oxerutins Capsules 250mg		120		1305	C	*(Paroven)*
Oxitropium Bromide Inhaler 100 microgram	■	200	dose	669	C	*(Oxivent)*
Oxpentifylline Tablets 400mg (m/r)		90		2381	C	*(Trental 400)*
Oxprenolol Tablets BP, 20mg		56		129	C	*(Trasicor)*
Oxprenolol Tablets BP, 40mg		56		259 ▽	C	*(Trasicor)*
Oxprenolol Tablets BP, 80mg		56		517 ▽	C	*(Trasicor)*
Oxybutynin Hydrochloride Oral Solution 2.5mg/5ml		150	ml	478	C	*(Ditropan)*
Oxybutynin Hydrochloride Tablets 2.5mg		56		408 ▽	A	
Oxybutynin Hydrochloride Tablets 3mg		56		818	A	
Oxybutynin Hydrochloride Tablets 5mg	★	56		1066 △	A	
		84		1741	A	
Oxytetracycline Tablets BP, 250mg		28		81	A	

■ Special Containers
♦ Manufacturers' Calendar Packs
★ Common Pack

Drug	Quantity		Basic Price p	Category	
Pantoprazole Tablets 20mg (e/c)	28		1288	C	(Protium)
(as sodium sequihydrat¬)					
Pantoprazole Tablets 40mg (e/c)	28		2365	C	(Protium)
(as sodium sequihydrate)					
Paracetamol Oral Solution, Paediatric BP	2	litre	580	A	
(Syn: Paracetamol Elixir, Paediatric)					
Paracetamol Oral Solution, Paediatric BP, sugar free .	2	litre	618	▽ A	
(Syn: Paracetamol Elixir, Paediatric sugar free)					
Paracetamol Oral Suspension BP, 120mg/5ml (Paediatric)	500	ml	206	C	(Paldesic)
Paracetamol Oral Suspension BP, 120mg/5ml (Paediatric)	150	ml	65	C	(Medinol)
sugar free	200	ml	86	C	(Medinol)
....	500	ml	216	C	(Disprol Paediatric)
....	1	litre	345	C	(Calpol)
Paracetamol Oral Suspension BP, 250mg/5ml	500	ml	369	A	
Paracetamol Soluble Tablets BP, 500mg	60		279	A	
Paracetamol Suppositories 60mg	10		951	C	(Alvedon)
Paracetamol Suppositories 120mg	10		925	A	
Paracetamol Suppositories, Paediatric 125mg	10		1098	C	(Alvedon)
Paracetamol Suppositories 240mg	10		950	A	
Paracetamol Suppositories 250mg	10		2197	C	(Alvedon)
Paracetamol Suppositories 500mg	10		970	▽ A	
Paracetamol Tablets BP, 500mg	32		45	△ A	
....	100		74	△ A	
Paracetamol 500mg and Metoclopramide	42		669	C	(Paramax)
Hydrochloride 5mg Tablets					
Paraffin, Hard BP	500	g	218	A	
Paraffin, Hard BP (MP 43-46°C)	450	g	215	A	
Paraffin, Liquid BP	2	litre	492	A	
Paraffin Liquid Light BP	500	ml	205	A	
Paraffin Soft, White BP (Syn: White Petroleum Jelly) .	500	g	161	A	
Paraffin Soft, Yellow BP (Syn: Yellow Petroleum Jelly)	500	g	163	A	
Paroxetine Tablets 20mg (as hydrochloride) ...... ♦	30		1776	C	(Seroxat)
Paroxetine Tablets 30mg (as hydrochloride) ...... ♦	30		3116	C	(Seroxat)
Penciclovir Cream DPF, 1% w/w .... ▣	2g		420	C	(Vectavir Cold Sore Cream)
....					
Penicillamine Tablets BP, 125mg	56		548	A	
Penicillamine Tablets BP, 250mg	56		954	A	
Pentazocine Capsules BP, 50mg	100		1868	A	
Pentazocine Injection BP, 30mg/1ml ampoules	10		1671	C	(Sterwin)
(Syn: Pentazocine Lactate Injection, 30mg/1ml ampoules)					
Pentazocine Injection BP, 60mg/2ml ampoules	10		3214	C	(Sterwin)
(Syn: Pentazocine Lactate Injection 60mg/2ml ampoules)					
Pentazocine Suppositories BP, 50mg	20		1993	C	(Sterwin)
Pentazocine Tablets BP, 25mg	28		227	A	
....	100		788	A	
Peppermint Emulsion, Concentrated BP	500	ml	265	C	(AAH)
Peppermint Oil BP	100	ml	695	A	
Peppermint Oil Capsules 0.2ml (m/r) (e/c)	20		275	C	(Colpermin)
....	100		1096	C	(Colpermin)
Peppermint Oil Capsules 0.2ml (e/c)	12		123	C	(Mintec)
....	25		240	C	(Mintec)
....	84		704	C	(Mintec)
Peppermint Water Concentrated BP 1973	100	ml	448	A	

VIII

▣ Special Containers
♦ Manufacturers' Calendar Packs

Drug		Quantity		Basic Price p		Category	
Pergolide Tablets 50 microgram (as mesylate)		100		2703		C	(Celance)
Pergolide Tablets 250 microgram (as mesylate)		100		4C77		C	(Celance)
Pergolide Tablets 1mg (as mesylate)		100		14715		C	(Celance)
Perindopril Tert-butylamine (Erbumine) Tablets 2mg ..		30		883		C	(Coversyl)
Perindopril Tert-butylamine (Erbumine) Tablets 4mg ..		30		1304		C	(Coversyl)
Permethrin Cream 5% w/w	■	30	g	552		C	(Lyclear Dermal)
Permethrin Cream Rinse 1% w/v	■	59	ml	226		C	(Lyclear)
....	■	118	ml	417		C	(Lyclear)
Pethidine Injection BP, 50mg/1ml		10		513		A	
Pethidine Injection BP, 100mg/2ml		10		534		A	
Pethidine Tablets BP, 50mg		50		492		A	
Phenelzine Tablets BP, 15mg		100		1995		C	(Nardil)
Phenobarbitone Elixir BP		500	ml	386		A	
(Syn: Phenobarbitone Oral Solution)							
Phenobarbitone Tablets BP, 30mg		28		66		A	
Phenobarbitone Tablets BP, 60mg		28		73		A	
Phenobarbitone Sodium BP		25	g	294		A	
Phenol BP (Crystals)		100	g	260		B	
Phenothrin Alcoholic Lotion NPF, 0.2% w/v	■	50	ml	216		C	(Full Marks)
Phenoxymethylpenicillin Oral Solution BP, 125mg/5ml	●	100	ml	164		A	
Phenoxymethylpenicillin Oral Solution BP, 250mg/5ml	●	100	ml	226		A	
Phenoxymethylpenicillin Tablets BP, 250mg		28		176	▽	A	
(Syn: Penicillin VK Tablets, 250mg)							
Phenylephrine Eye Drops BP, 10% w/v	■	10	ml	304		A	
Phenytoin Capsules BP, 25mg		28		55		C	(Epanutin)
Phenytoin Capsules BP, 50mg		28		56		C	(Epanutin)
Phenytoin Capsules BP, 100mg		84		236		C	(Epanutin)
Phenytoin Capsules BP, 300mg		28		236		C	(Epanutin)
Phenytoin Oral Suspension BP, 30mg/5ml		500	ml	356		C	(Epanutin)
Phenytoin Tablets BP, 50mg	♦	28		125	△	A	
Phenytoin Tablets BP, 100mg	♦	28		170	△	A	
Pholcodine Linctus, 2mg/5ml sugar free	■	90	ml	111		C	(Galenphol Paediatric)
(Pholcodine Linctus Paediatric sugar free)							
....		2	litre	352		C	(Galenphol Paediatric)
Pholcodine Linctus BP, 5mg/5ml		2	litre	493		A	
Pholcodine Linctus BP, 5mg/5ml sugar free		2	litre	487		A	
Pholcodine Linctus, Strong BP, 10mg/5ml		2	litre	669		A	
Pholcodine Linctus, Strong BP, 10mg/5ml sugar free .		2	litre	710		A	
Phosphates Enema BP, (Formula B) Standard Tube ..	▥	1	bottle	44		C	(Fletcher's)
(Syn: Sodium Phosphate Enema, Standard Tube)							
Phosphates Enema BP, (Formula B) Long Tube	▥	1		61		C	(Fletcher's)
(Syn: Sodium Phosphate Enema, Long Tube)							
Phytomenadione Injection BP, 1mg/0.5 ml ampoules .		10		230		C	(Konakion)
(Syn: Vitamin K1 Injection 1mg/0.5ml ampoules)							
Phytomenadione Injection BP, 10mg/1ml ampoules ..		10		431		C	(Konakion MM)
(Syn: Vitamin K1 Injection 10mg/1ml ampoules)							
Phytomenadione Tablets BP, 10mg		10		177		C	(Konakion)
(Syn: Vitamin K1 Tablets 10mg)							

■ Special Containers
● Preparations Requiring Reconstitution

Drug		Quantity	Basic Price p	Category
Pilocarpine Hydrochloride Eye Drops BP, 0.5% w/v . .	■	10 ml	136	A
(Syn: Pilocarpine Eye Drops 0.5% w/v)				
Pilocarpine Hydrochloride Eye Drops BP, 1% w/v . . .	■	10 ml	105	A
(Syn: Pilocarpine Eye Drops 1% w/v)				
Pilocarpine Hydrochloride Eye Drops BP, 2% w/v . . .	■	10 ml	119	A
(Syn: Pilocarpine Eye Drops 2% w/v				
Pilocarpine Hydrochloride Eye Drops BP, 3% w/v . . .	■	10 ml	141	A
(Syn: Pilocarpine Eye Drops 3% w/v)				
Pilocarpine Hydrochloride Eye Drops BP, 4% w/v . . .	■	10 ml	157	A
(Syn: Pilocarpine Eye Drops 4% w/v)				
Pimozide Tablets 2mg		100	1585	C	*(Orap)*
Pimozide Tablets 4mg		100	3067	C	*(Orap)*
Pimozide Tablets 10mg		100	5881	C	*(Orap)*
Piperazine and Senna Powder NPF (2 dose dual pack)	■	1	125	C	*(Pripsen)*
Piroxicam Capsules BP, 10mg		56	283	A
. . . .		60	316	A
Piroxicam Capsules BP, 20mg		28	313	A
. . . .		30	352	A
Piroxicam Gel BP, 0.5% w/w	■	60 g	500	C	*(Feldene)*
. . . .	■	112 g	784	C	*(Feldene)*
Piroxicam Tablets, Dispersible 20mg		28	934	A
Pizotifen Elixir 250 microgram		300 ml	412	C	*(Sanomigran)*
(as hydrogen malate)/5ml sugar free				
Pizotifen Tablets BP, 500 microgram		60	257	C	*(Sanomigran)*
Pizotifen Tablets BP, 1.5mg	♦	28	428	C
Podophyllin Paint BPC 1954		10 ml	47	E
Podophyllin Paint, Compound BP		100 ml	483	A
Podophyllum Resin BP (Syn: Podophyllin)		25 g	450	A
Potassium Effervescent Tablets BPC 1968	■	56	382	A
. . . .	■	100	429	A
Potassium Bromide BP		500 g	480	A
Potassium Bromide Mixture BPC 1963		200 ml	43	E
Potassium Chlorate BPC		500 g	695	C	(Loveridge)
Potassium Chloride BP		500 g	290	C	(Thornton & Ross)
Potassium Chloride Tablets, Slow BP, 600mg		100	275	C	*(Slow-K)*
Potassium Chloride Effervescent Tablets BP, ...		100	765	C	*(Sando K)*
470mg (potassium ions) (Formula A)	(5x■20)			
Potassium Citrate BP		500 g	280	A
Potassium Citrate Mixture BP Concentrated (5 in 4) . .		2 litre	505	A
Potassium Citrate Mixture BP		200 ml	76	A
(Syn: Potassium Citrate Oral Solution)				
Potassium Citrate and Hyoscyamus Mixture BPC . . .		200 ml	78	E
Potassium Iodide BP		250 g	950	A
Potassium Iodide Mixture Ammoniated BPC		200 ml	39	E
(Syn: Potassium Iodide and Ammonia Mixture)				
Potassium Nitrate BP		500 g	640	A
Potassium Permanganate BP		500 g	365	A
Potassium Permanganate Solution BNF, 0.1%		100 ml	1	E

VIII

■ Special Containers
♦ Manufacturers' Calendar Packs

Drug		Quantity		Basic Price p	Category
Povidone-Iodine Dry Powder Spray 1.14% w/w	■	50	ml	216	C	*(Savlon Dry)*
Povidone Iodine Mouthwash BP, 1%		250	ml	112	C	*(Betadine Gargle*
....						*& Mouthwash)*
Pravastatin Sodium Tablets 10mg	♦	28		1618	C	*(Lipostat)*
Pravastatin Sodium Tablets 20mg	♦	28		2969	C	*(Lipostat)*
Pravastatin Sodium Tablets 40mg	♦	28		2969	C	*(Lipostat)*
Prazosin Tablets BP, 500 microgram		56		229	▽ A
Prazosin Tablets BP, 1mg		56		282	A
Prazosin Tablets BP, 2mg		56		406	▽ A
Prazosin Tablets BP, 5mg		56		879	A
Prednisolone Tablets BP, 1mg		28		52	A
Prednisolone Tablets BP, 5mg		28		67	A
Prednisolone Tablets BP, 25mg		56		426	C	*(Precortisyl*
						Forte)
Prednisolone Enteric-coated Tablets BP, 2.5mg		30		26	C	*(Deltacortril)*
(Syn: Gastro-resistant Prednisolone Tablets 2.5mg) ★		100		57	C	*(Deltacortril)*
Prednisolone Enteric-coated Tablets BP, 5mg		30		43	C	*(Deltacortril)*
(Syn: Gastro-resistant Prednisolone Tablets 5mg) ★		100		102	C	*(Deltacortril)*
Prednisolone Acetate Eye Drops 1% w/v	■	5	ml	152	C	*(Pred Forte)*
....	■	10	ml	305	C	*(Pred Forte)*
Prednisolone Sodium Phosphate Ear Drops 0.5% w/v .	■	10	ml	131	C	*(Predsol Ear/*
						Eye Drops)
....						
Prednisolone Sodium Phosphate Eye Drops BP, 0.5% w/v	■	10	ml	131	C	*(Predsol Ear/*
						Eye Drops)
....						
Prednisolone Sodium Phosphate Tablets 5mg		100		576	C	*(Prednesol)*
Primidone Tablets BP, 250mg		100		177	C	*(Mysoline)*
Prochlorperazine Oral Solution BP, 5mg/5ml		100	ml	374	C	*(Stemetil*
						Syrup
Prochlorperazine Tablets BP, 5mg		28		167	A
Prochlorperazine Maleate Buccal Tablets, 3mg		50		575	C	*(Buccastem)*
Prochlorperazine Maleate Suppositories 5mg		10		940	C	*(Stemetil)*
(as prochlorperazine)						
Prochlorperazine Maleate Suppositories 25mg		10		1232	C	*(Stemetil)*
(as prochlorperazine)						
Prochlorperazine Mesylate Granules		21		695	C	*(Stemetil*
effervescent 5mg/sachet						*Effervescent)*
(as prochlorperazine) sugar free						
Procyclidine Tablets BP, 5mg		28		151	A
Procyclidine Hydrochloride Syrup 2.5mg/5ml sugar free		150	ml	449	C	*(Arpicolin)*
Procyclidine Hydrochloride Syrup 5mg/5ml sugar free		150	ml	802	C	*(Arpicolin)*
Proflavine Cream BPC (Syns: Flavine Cream, ...		50	ml	46	A
Proflavine Emulsion) ★		500	ml	250	A
Proflavine Solution BPC 1949		100	ml	10	E
Proflavine Hemisulphate BPC		5	g	305	B

■ Special Containers
♦ Manufacturers' Calendar Packs
★ Common Pack

Drug		Quantity		Basic Price p		Category
Proguanil Tablets BP, 100mg	◆	98		743		C	*(Paludrine)*
Promazine Tablets BP, 25mg		250		550		A
Promazine Tablets BP, 50mg		250		999		A
Promazine Hydrochloride Suspension		150	ml	176	△	A
50mg (as embonate)/5ml						
Promethazine Oral Solution BP, 5mg/5ml sugar free		100	ml	135		C	*(Phenergan Elixir)*
(Syn: Promethazine Elixir 5mg/5ml sugar free)						
Promethazine Hydrochloride Tablets BP, 10mg		56		143		C	*(Phenergan)*
Promethazine Hydrochloride Tablets BP, 25mg		56		213		C	*(Phenergan)*
Propafenone Hydrochloride Tablets 150mg		90		2143		C	*(Arythmol)*
Propafenone Hydrochloride Tablets 300mg		60		2143		C	*(Arythmol)*
Propranolol Tablets BP, 10mg		28		59		A
Propranolol Tablets BP, 40mg		28		64		A
Propranolol Tablets BP, 80mg		56		96		A
Propranolol Tablets BP, 160mg		56		236		A
Propylene Glycol BP		500	ml	255		A
Propylthiouracil Tablets BP, 50mg		100		4361		A
Pseudoephedrine Tablets BP, 60mg		100		480		C	*(Sudafed)*
Pseudoephedrine Hydrochloride Elixir 30mg/5ml		1	litre	767		C	*(Sudafed)*
Pseudoephedrine Hydrochloride Linctus 30mg/5ml		140	ml	170		C	*(Galpseud)*
sugar free		2	litre	1375		C	*(Galpseud)*
Purified Talc BP (Sterile)		500	g	225		C	(Thornton & Ross)
Purified Talc BP		500	g	225		A
Purified Water BP		5	litre	219		A
Pyridostigmine Tablets BP, 60mg		200		5015		C	*(Mestinon)*
Pyridoxine Tablets BP, 50mg		28		52		A
(Syn: Vitamin B6 Tablets 50mg)						
Quinapril Tablets 5mg	◆	28		717		C	*(Accupro)*
Quinapril Tablets 10mg	◆	28		717		C	*(Accupro)*
Quinapril Tablets 20mg	◆	28		899		C	*(Accupro)*
Quinapril Tablets 40mg	◆	28		975		C	*(Accupro)*
Quinine Bisulphate Tablets BP, 300mg		28		145		A
(Syn: Quinine Acid Sulphate Tablets, 300mg)		500		2031	△	A
Quinine Sulphate Tablets BP, 200mg		28		141		A
Quinine Sulphate Tablets BP, 300mg		28		136		A
		500		1995	▽	A

◆ Manufacturers' Calendar Packs

Drug		Quantity	Basic Price p	Category	
Ramipril Capsules 1.25mg	♦	28	530	C	*(Tritace)*
Ramipril Capsules 2.5mg	♦	28	751	C	*(Tritace)*
Ramipril Capsules 5mg	♦	28	955	C	*(Tritace)*
Ramipril Capsules 10mg	♦	28	1300	C	*(Tritace)*
Ranitidine Oral Solution BP,75mg/5ml		300 ml	2232	C	*(Zantac Syrup)*
sugar free					
Ranitidine Tablets BP, 150mg	♦	60	731	A	
Ranitidine Tablets BP, 300mg	♦	30	731	A	
Ranitidine Effervescent Tablets 150mg		60	2789	C	*(Zantac)*
(as hydrochloride)		(4x■15)			
Ranitidine Effervescent Tablets 300mg		30	2743	C	*(Zantac)*
(as hydrochloride)		(2x■15)			
Raspberry Syrup BP 1988		500 ml	380	C	(AAH)
Rectified Spirit BP (See Ethanol 90 per cent)		-	-	-	
Rifampicin Capsules BP, 150mg		56	1139	C	*(Rimactane)*
. . . .		100	1825	A	
Rifampicin Capsules BP, 300mg		56	2277	C	*(Rimactane)*
. . . .		100	3618	A	
Risperidone Tablets 1mg		20	1345	C	*(Risperdal)*
Risperidone Tablets 2mg		60	7956	C	*(Risperdal)*
Risperidone Tablets 3mg		60	11700	C	*(Risperdal)*
Risperidone Tablets 4mg		60	15444	C	*(Risperdal)*
Saccharin Sodium BP (Syn: Soluble Saccharin)		100 g	205	C	(Thornton & Ross)
Salbutamol Dry Powder Capsules for Inhalation		112	533	C	*(Ventolin Rotacaps)*
200 microgram (as sulphate)					
Salbutamol Dry Powder Capsules for Inhalation		112	901	C	*(Ventolin Rotacaps)*
400 microgram (as sulphate)					
Salbutamol Nebuliser Solution 1mg/1ml (as sulphate) 2.5ml		20	274	C	*(Salamol)*
Salbutamol Nebuliser Solution 2mg/1ml (as sulphate) 2.5ml		20	547	C	*(Salamol)*
Salbutamol Pressurised Inhalation BP	■	200 dose	172	A	
100 microgram per actuation					
(Syn: Salbutamol Aerosol Inhalation)					
Salbutamol Pressurised Inhalation BP, ...	■	200 dose	197	C	
100 microgram per actuation, CFC-free					
(Syn: Salbutamol Aerosol Inhalation, CFC-free)					
Salbutamol Syrup 2mg/5ml (as sulphate) sugar free . .		150 ml	72	A	
Salbutamol Tablets BP, 2mg		28	82	A	
Salbutamol Tablets BP, 4mg		28	151	A	
Salbutamol Tablets 4mg (as sulphate) (m/r)	♦	56	1055	C	*(Volmax)*
Salbutamol Tablets 8mg (as sulphate) (m/r)	♦	56	1266	C	*(Volmax)*

■ Special Containers
♦ Manufacturers' Calendar Packs

Drug	Quantity		Basic Price p		Category
Salicylic Acid BP (Powder)	500	g	530		A
Salicylic Acid Lotion BP 1993	500	ml	148		E
Salicylic Acid Ointment BP	450	g	330		A
Salicylic Acid and Sulphur Ointment BPC	500	g	218		E
Salmeterol Aerosol Inhalation 25 microgram	■ 120	dose	2860		C	*(Serevent)*
(as xinafoate) per actuation						
Salmeterol Dry Powder for Inhalation	■ 60	dose	2860		C	*(Serevent*
50 microgram (as xinafoate) per actuation						*Accuhaler)*
Selegiline Hydrochloride Tablets 5mg	56		1075	▽	A
Selegiline Hydrochloride Tablets 10mg	♦ 28		1075	▽	A
	30		1126		A
Senna Granules, Standardised BP, 15mg/5ml	100	g	292		C	*(Senokot)*
Senna Oral Solution NPF, 7.5mg/5ml	100	ml	214		C	*(Senokot Syrup)*
	500	ml	269		C	*(Senokot Syrup)*
Senna Tablets BP, 7.5mg	500		738		C	*(Senokot)*
Sertraline Tablets 50mg (as hydrochloride)	♦ 28		1620		C	*(Lustral)*
Sertraline Tablets 100mg (as hydrochloride)	♦ 28		2651		C	*(Lustral)*
Simple Eye Ointment BP (Syn: Eye Ointment Basis)	■ 4	g	255		A
Simple Linctus BP	2	litre	330		A
Simple Linctus , Paediatric BP	2	litre	319		A
Simple Ointment BP (White)	500	g	243		A
Simvastatin Tablets 10mg	♦ 28		1803		C	*(Zocor)*
Simvastatin Tablets 20mg	♦ 28		2969		C	*(Zocor)*
Simvastatin Tablets 40mg	♦ 28		2969		C	*(Zocor)*
Soap Liniment BPC (Methylated)	500	ml	254		A
Soap Spirit BP (Methylated)	500	ml	200		A
Sodium Benzoate BP	500	g	395		B
Sodium Bicarbonate BP (Powder)	1.5	kg	260		A
Sodium Bicarbonate Capsules 500mg	100		3054		A
Sodium Bicarbonate Ear Drops BP	■ 10	ml	118		A
Sodium Bicarbonate Intravenous Infusion BP, 8.4% w/v	10		1903		A
(Syn: Sodium Bicarbonate Injection)						
10ml ampoules						
Sodium Bicarbonate Mixture, Paediatric BPC	100	ml	20		E
Sodium Bicarbonate Tablets 600mg	56		112		C	(Norton)
	500		1240		A
Sodium Bicarbonate Tablets, Compound BP	100		78		C	(AAH)
(Syn: Soda Mint Tablets)						
Sodium Chloride BP	500	g	183		A
Sodium Chloride Eye Drops BP, 0.9% w/v	■ 10	ml	229		A
Sodium Chloride Intravenous Infusion BP, 0.9% w/v .	10		230		A
2ml ampoules						
(Syn: Sodium Chloride Injection 0.9% w/v)						
Sodium Chloride Intravenous Infusion BP, 0.9% w/v .	10		303		A
5ml ampoules						
(Syn: Sodium Chloride Injection 0.9% w/v)						
Sodium Chloride Intravenous Infusion BP, 0.9% w/v .	10		319		A
10ml ampoules						
(Syn: Sodium Chloride Injection 0.9% w/v)						
Sodium Chloride Intravenous Infusion BP, 0.9% w/v .	10		968		A
20ml ampoules						
(Syn: Sodium Chloride Injection 0.9% w/v)						

VIII

■ Special Containers
♦ Manufacturers' Calendar Packs

Drug	Quantity		Basic Price p	Category	
Sodium Chloride Intravenous Infusion BP, 0.9% w/v .	10		2009	C	(Martindale)
50ml ampoules					
(Syn: Sodium Chloride Injection 0.9% w/v)					
Sodium Chloride Intravenous Infusion BP, 0.9% w/v .	■ 1		176	A	
50ml vials					
(Syn: Sodium 'Chloride Injection 0.9% w/v)					
Sodium Chloride Intravenous Infusion BP, 0.9% w/v .	■ 1		190	A	
100ml vials					
(Syn: Sodium Chloride Injection 0.9% w/v)					
Sodium Chloride Mixture, Compound BPC	200	ml	9	E	
Sodium Chloride Mouthwash, Compound BP	200	ml	10	E	
Sodium Chloride Solution BP	100	ml	5	E	
Sodium Citrate BP (Syn: Trisodium Citrate)	500	g	330	A	
Sodium Cromoglycate Aerosol Inhalation 5mg	■ 112	dose	1530	C	(Cromogen)
per actuation					
Sodium Cromoglycate Aqueous Eye Drops 2% w/v . .	■ 13.5	ml	196	A	
Sodium Cromoglycate Aqueous Nasal Spray 2% w/v .	■ 15	ml	815	C	(Vividrin)
Sodium Cromoglycate Aqueous Nasal Spray	■ 22	ml	1910	C	(Rynacrom)
4% w/v (5.2mg/squeeze)					
Sodium Dihydrogen Phosphate Dihydrate BP	500	g	445	C	(Thornton &
(Syn: Sodium Acid Phosphate)					Ross)
Sodium Fluoride Oral Drops DPF, 0.37% w/v	■ 60	ml	162	C	(En-De-Kay
(Sodium Fluoride Paediatric Drops 80 microgram/drop,					Fluodrops)
sugar free)					
Sodium Fluoride Tablets BP, 1.1mg	200		183	C	(En-De-Kay
. . . .					Fluotabs
. . . .					500 microgram)
Sodium Fluoride Tablets BP, 2.2mg	200		183	C	(En-De-Kay
. . . .					Fluotabs 1mg
Sodium Fluoride Tablets BP, 1.1mg (Chewable)	200		191	C	(Fluorigard
. . . .					500 microgram)
. . . .					Fluotabs)
Sodium Fluoride Tablets BP, 2.2mg (Chewable)	200		191	C	(Fluorigard 1mg)
Sodium Fusidate Ointment BP, 2% w/w	■ 15	g	234	C	(Fucidin)
. . . .	■ 30	g	397	C	(Fucidin)
Sodium Ironedetate Elixir 190mg	500	ml	471	C	(Sytron)
(equivalent to 27.5mg of iron)/5ml sugar free					
Sodium Metabisulphite BP	500	g	215	A	
(Syns: Sodium Disulphite,					
Sodium Pyrosulphite)					
Sodium Perborate BP	500	g	310	B	
Sodium Perborate Mouthwash DPF (Sachets)	20		177	C	(Bocasan)
Sodium Picosulphate Elixir 5mg/5ml sugar free	100	ml	185	C	(Laxoberal)
. . . .	300	ml	440	C	(Laxoberal)
Sodium Salicylate BP	500	g	625	C	(Thornton &
					Ross)

■ Special Containers

Drug	Quantity		Basic Price p		Category	
Sodium Valproate Oral Solution BP, 200mg/5ml sugar free	300	ml	542	▽	A	
Sodium Valproate Syrup 200mg/5ml	300	ml	589		C	*(Epilim Syrup)*
Sodium Valproate Tablets BP, 100mg (Crushable) . . .	100		428		A	
Sodium Valproate Enteric-coated Tablets BP, 200mg .	100		556		A	
Sodium Valproate Enteric-coated Tablets BP, 500mg .	100		1467		A	
Sorbitol Solution (70 per cent) (Non-Crystallising) BP .	1	litre	440		A	
Sotalol Tablets BP, 40mg	100		396		C	*(Beta-Cardone)*
Sotalol Tablets BP, 80mg	100		587		C	*(Beta-Cardone)*
Sotalol Tablets BP, 160mg . . . . ♦	28		616		A	
Sotalol Tablets BP, 200mg	30		415		C	*(Beta-Cardone)*
Spironolactone Tablets BP, 25mg	28		209		A	
Spironolactone Tablets BP, 50mg	28		445		A	
. . . .	30		375	▽	A	
Spironolactone Tablets BP, 100mg	28		464		A	
Squill Oxymel BP	2	litre	979		A	
Squill Tincture BP 1980	500	ml	385		B	
Starch Maize BP (Powder)	500	g	208		A	
Stearic Acid BP	500	g	370		C	(AAH)
Stilboestrol Tablets BP, 5mg	28		3960	△	A	
Sucralfate Tablets 1g	112		1067		A	
Sucrose BP (Syn: Refined Sugar)	1	kg	58		C	
Sulindac Tablets BP, 100mg	56		731		A	
Sulindac Tablets BP, 200mg	56		1303		A	
Sulphasalazine Tablets 500mg	112		774		C	*(Salazopyrin)*
. . . .	500		3371	▽	A	
Sulphasalazine Tablets 500mg (e/c)	100		959		A	
. . . .	112		969		C	
Sulphur Precipitated BP 1980	500	g	243		A	
Sulphur Sublimed BPC	500	g	228		A	
Sulphuric Acid Dilute BP	500	ml	300		C	(Thornton & Ross)
Sulpiride Tablets 200mg	30		480	▽	A	
	100		1573	▽	A	
Sulpiride Tablets 400mg	100		3629		C	*(Dolmatil)*
Sumatriptan Tablets 50mg	6		2970		C	*(Imigran 50)*
(as succinate)	12		5643		C	*(Imigran 50)*
Sumatriptan Tablets 100mg (as succinate)	6		4800		C	*(Imigran)*
Surgical Spirit BP	2	litre	398		A	
Syrup BP	2	litre	324	△	A	
Syrup BP (unpreserved)	2	litre	388		A	
Tacrolimus Capsules 1mg . . . . ▨	50		9293		C	*(Prograf)*
Tacrolimus Capsules 5mg . . . . ▨	50		37185		C	*(Prograf)*
Tamoxifen Tablets BP, 10mg	30		197		A	
Tamoxifen Tablets BP, 20mg	30		222		A	
Tamoxifen Tablets BP, 40mg	30		831		A	
Tamsulosin Hydrochloride Capsules 400microgram (m/r)	30		2390		C	*(Flomax MR)*
Tartaric Acid BP	500	g	675		A	

▨ Special Containers
♦ Manufacturers' Calendar Packs

Drug	Quantity		Basic Price p	Category	
Temazepam Oral Solution BP, 10mg/5ml sugar free .	300	ml	994	A	
(formerly Temazepam Elixir 10mg/5ml sugar free)					
Temazepam Tablets BP, 10mg	28		95 ▽	A	
. . . .	500		1676	A	
Temazepam Tablets BP, 20mg	28		163 ▽	A	
. . . .	250		1422	A	
Tenoxicam Tablets 20mg	28		1347	C	(Mobiflex)
Terbinafine Tablets 250mg (as hydrochloride)	♦ 14		2316	C	(Lamisil)
. . . .	♦ 28		4466	C	(Lamisil)
Terbinafine Hydrochloride Cream 1% w/w	■ 15	g	486	C	(Lamisil)
. . . .	■ 30	g	876	C	(Lamisil)
Terbutaline Tablets BP, 5mg	100		372	C	(Bricanyl)
Terbutaline Sulphate Aerosol Inhalation	■ 400	dose	531	C	(Bricanyl)
250 microgram per actuation					
Terbutaline Sulphate Breath Activated Powder for . . .	■ 100	dose	630	C	(Bricanyl
Inhalation 500 microgram/dose					Turbohaler)
Terfenadine Tablets 60mg	60		286	A	
Testosterone Undecanoate Capsules 40mg	28		830	C	(Restandol)
. . . .	56		1660	C	(Restandol)
Tetrabenazine Tablets 25mg	112		10000	A	
Tetracycline Capsules BP, 250mg	28		134	C	(Achromycin)
Tetracycline Tablets BP, 250mg	28		96	A	
Theophylline Capsules 60mg (m/r)	56		192	C	(Slo-Phylline)
Theophylline Capsules 125mg (m/r)	56		242	C	(Slo-Phylline)
Theophylline Capsules 250mg (m/r)	56		302	C	(Slo-Phylline)
. . . .	★ 100		539	C	(Slo-Phylline)
Theophylline Tablets 175mg (m/r)	60		343	C	(Nuelin SA)
Theophylline Tablets 250mg (m/r)	60		480	C	(Nuelin
					SA - 250)
Theophylline Tablets 400mg (m/r)	56		699	C	(Uniphyllin
					Continus)
Thiamine Tablets BP, 50mg	100		176	C	(Benerva)
(Syn: Vitamin B1 Tablets 50mg)					
Thiamine Tablets, Compound BPC	-		-	-	
(See Vitamin B Tablets Compound BPC)					
Thiamine Tablets, Compound, Strong BP	-		-	-	
(See Vitamin B Tablets, Compound, Strong)					
Thioridazine Oral Solution BP, 25mg/5ml	500	ml	267	A	
Thioridazine Oral Suspension BP, 25mg/5ml	300	ml	179	C	(Melleril)
Thioridazine Oral Suspension BP, 100mg/5ml	300	ml	653	C	(Melleril)
Thioridazine Tablets BP, 25mg	28		72	A	
. . . .	100		174	A	
Thioridazine Tablets BP, 50mg	28		142	A	
Thioridazine Tablets BP, 100mg	28		212	A	
Thymol BP	100	g	395	B	
Thymol Glycerin, Compound BP 1988 (Methylated) . .	2	litre	475	A	

■ Special Containers
♦ Manufacturers' Calendar Packs
★ Common Pack

Drug	Quantity		Basic Price p		Category	
Thyroxine Tablets BP, 25 microgram	28		84		A	
(Syn: L-Thyroxine Sodium Tablets 25 microgram)	500		1004		A	
Thyroxine Tablets BP, 50 microgram	28		56		A	
(Syn:L-Thyroxine Sodium Tablets 50 microgram)	1000		2004	Δ	A	
Thyroxine Tablets BP, 100 microgram	28		86	Δ	A	
(Syn: L-Thyroxine Sodium Tablets 100 microgram)	1000		2990		A	
Tiaprofenic Acid Capsules 300mg (m/r)	♦ 56		2048		C	*(Surgam SA)*
Tibolone Tablets 2.5mg	♦ 28		1305		C	*(Livial)*
Timolol Eye Drops BP, 0.25% w/v	■ 5	ml	375		A	
(Syn: Timolol Maleate Eye Drops, 0.25% w/v)						
Timolol Eye Drops BP, 0.5% w/v	■ 5	ml	401		A	
(Syn: Timolol Maleate Eye Drops 0.5% w/v)						
Timolol Tablets BP, 10mg	30		245		C	*(Betim)*
(Syn: Timolol Maleate Tablets 10mg)						
Tinidazole Tablets 500mg	20		1150		C	*(Fasigyn)*
Tioconazole Nail Solution 28% w/v	■ 12	ml	2738		C	*(Trosyl)*
Tocopheryl Acetate Tablets 50mg	100		369		C	*(Ephynal)*
(Vitamin E Tablets 50mg)						
Tocopheryl Acetate Tablets 200mg	50		524		C	*(Ephynal)*
(Vitamin E Tablets 200mg)						
Tolbutamide Tablets BP, 500mg	28		110		A	
Tragacanth Mucilage BPC	500	g	290		C	(Thornton & Ross)
Tragacanth Powdered BP 1993	100	g	1055		C	(Thornton & Ross)
Tragacanth Powder, Compound BP 1980	100	g	335		A	
Tramadol Hydrochloride Capsules 50mg	30		279	▽	A	
. . . .	100		1150	▽	A	
Tramadol Hydrochloride Tablets 100mg (m/r)	60		1826		C	*(Zydol SR 100)*
Tramadol Hydrochloride Tablets 150mg (m/r)	60		2739		C	*(Zydol SR 150)*
Tramadol Hydrochloride Tablets 200mg (m/r)	60		3652		C	*(Zydol SR 200)*
Tranexamic Acid Tablets BP, 500mg	60		1430		C	*(Cyklokapron)*
Tranylcypromine Tablets BP, 10mg	28		127		C	*(Parnate)*
Trazodone Hydrochloride Capsules 50mg	84		1731		C	*(Molipaxin)*
Trazodone Hydrochloride Capsules 100mg	56		2038		C	*(Molipaxin)*
Trazodone Hydrochloride Tablets 150mg	28		1162		C	*(Molipaxin)*
Triamcinolone Dental Paste BP, 0.1% w/w	■ 10	g	127		C	*(Adcortyl in Orabase)*
Triamterene Capsules BP, 50mg	30		1690		C	*(Dytac)*
Triamterene 50mg and Frusemide 40mg Tablets	♦ 56		567		C	*(Frusene)*
. . . .	100		1012		C	*(Frusene)*
Triclofos Oral Solution BP	300	ml	2823		A	
(Syn: Triclofos Elixir)						
Trifluoperazine Capsules 2mg (as hydrochloride) (m/r)	60		436		C	*(Stelazine)*
Trifluoperazine Capsules 10mg (as hydrochloride) (m/r)	30		283		C	*(Stelazine)*
Trifluoperazine Capsules 15mg (as hydrochloride) (m/r)	30		427		C	*(Stelazine)*
Trifluoperazine Tablets BP, 1mg	100		287		A	
Trifluoperazine Tablets BP, 5mg	100		370		A	

VI

■ Special Containers
♦ Manufacturers' Calendar Packs

Drug	Quantity		Basic Price p		Category
Trimeprazine Oral Solution, Paediatric BP, 7.5mg/5ml	100	ml	370		C	*(Vallergan*
(Syn: Trimeprazine Elixir, Paediatric 7.5mg/5ml)						*Syrup)*
Trimeprazine Oral Solution, Paediatric, ...	100	ml	572		C	*(Vallergan Forte*
Strong BP, 30mg/5ml						*Syrup)*
(Syn: Trimeprazine Elixir, Paediatric, Strong 30mg/5ml)						
Trimeprazine Tablets BP, 10mg	28		324		C	*(Vallergan)*
Trimethoprim Suspension 50mg/5ml sugar free	100	ml	177		C	*(Monotrim)*
Trimethoprim Tablets BP, 100mg	28		67		A	
Trimethoprim Tablets BP, 200mg	14		67		A	
. . . .	100		242	▽	A	
Trimipramine Capsules 50mg (as maleate)	28		851		C	*(Surmontil)*
Trimipramine Tablets BP, 10mg	84		1149		C	*(Surmontil)*
Trimipramine Tablets BP, 25mg	84		1516		C	*(Surmontil)*
Turpentine Liniment BP 1993	500	ml	368		A	
Turpentine Oil BP	500	ml	325		A	
Ursodeoxycholic Acid Capsules 250mg	60		3480	▽	A	
Ursodeoxycholic Acid Tablets 150mg	60		1836		A	
Valaciclovir Tablets 500mg (as hydrochloride)	10		2350		C	*(Valtrex)*
. . . .	42		9850		C	*(Valtrex)*
Valerian Tincture, Simple BPC 1949	500	ml	735		B	
Venlafaxine Tablets 37.5mg (as hydrochloride)	♦ 56		2397		C	*(Efexor)*
Venlafaxine Tablets 50mg (as hydrochloride)	42		2397		C	*(Efexor)*
Venlafaxine Tablets 75mg (as hydrochloride)	♦ 56		3997		C	*(Efexor)*
Verapamil Tablets BP, 40mg	84		163		A	
Verapamil Tablets BP, 80mg	84		211		A	
Verapamil Tablets BP, 120mg	28		133		A	
. . . .	100		363	▽	A	
Verapamil Tablets BP, 160mg	56		563		A	
Verapamil Hydrochloride Capsules 120mg (m/r)	♦ 28		751		C	*(Univer)*
Verapamil Hydrochloride Capsules 180mg (m/r)	♦ 56		1815		C	*(Univer)*
Verapamil Hydrochloride Capsules 240mg (m/r)	♦ 28		1224		C	*(Univer)*
Verapamil Hydrochloride Tablets 120mg (m/r)	♦ 28		682		C	*(Half-Securon*
						SR)
Verapamil Hydrochloride Tablets 240mg (m/r)	♦ 28		1064		C	*(Securon SR)*

♦ Manufacturers' Calendar Packs

Drug	Quantity		Basic Price p		Category	
Vigabatrin Oral Powder BP, 500mg/sachet sugar free .	50		2433		C	(Sabril)
Vigabatrin Tablets BP, 500mg	100		4485		C	(Sabril)
Vitamins Capsules BPC	1000		1062		A	
Vitamin A and D Capsules BPC	84		249	▽	A	
Vitamin B Tablets, Compound BPC	1000		372		A	
(Syns: Compound Aneurine Tablets, Compound Thiamine Tablets)						
Vitamin B Tablets, Compound, Strong BPC	1000		819		A	
(Syns: Strong Compound Aneurine Tablets, Strong Compound Thiamine Tablets)						
Vitamins B and C Injection BP, ...	10	Pairs	1855		C	(Pabrinex)
IM Strong/5ml + 2ml ampoules						
Vitamins B and C Injection BP, ...	10	Pairs	1657		C	(Pabrinex)
IV Strong/5ml + 5ml ampoules						
Vitamin B12 Injection (See Hydroxocobalamin	-		-		-	
Injection BP)						
Warfarin Tablets BP, 1mg	28		140		A	
Warfarin Tablets BP, 3mg	28		159		A	
Warfarin Tablets BP, 5mg	28		171		A	
Water for Injections BP, 1ml ampoules	10		177		A	
Water for Injections BP, 2ml ampoules	10		134		A	
Water for Injections BP, 5ml ampoules	10		214		A	
Water for Injections BP, 10ml ampoules	10		248		A	
Water for Injections BP, 20ml ampoules	10		527		A	
Water for Injections BP, 50ml ampoules	10		1906		A	
Water for Injections BP, 100ml vials	■ 1		195		A	
White Liniment BP (Syn: White Embrocation)	500	ml	180		C	(AAH)
. . . .	2	litre	547		A	
Wild Cherry Syrup BP 1980	2	litre	1360		C	(AAH)
Wool Alcohols Ointment BP	450	g	385		C	(Thornton & Ross)
Wool Fat BP (Syn: Anhydrous Lanolin)	500	g	348		A	
Wool Fat, Hydrous BP (Syn: Lanolin)	500	g	344		A	
Xipamide Tablets 20mg	◆ 140		2092		C	(Diurexan)
Xylometazoline Nasal Drops BP, 0.05% w/v	■ 10	ml	153		C	(Otrivine)
Xylometazoline Nasal Drops BP, 0.1% w/v	■ 10	ml	165		C	(Otrivine)
Xylometazoline Nasal Spray 0.1% w/v (as hydrochloride)	■ 10	ml	176		C	(Otrivine)

■ Special Containers
◆ Manufacturers' Calendar Packs

Drug	Quantity		Basic Price p	Category	
Zinc Ointment BP	500	g	278	A	
Zinc Paste, Compound BP	500	g	290	A	
Zinc and Castor Oil Ointment BP	500	g	285	A	
(Syn: Zinc and Caster Oil Cream)					
Zinc and Ichthammol Cream BP	500	g	380	A	
Zinc and Salicylic Acid Paste BP, (Syn: Lassar's Paste)	500	g	313	A	
Zinc Oxide BP	500	g	270	A	
Zinc Oxide and Dimethicone Spray NPF	■ 115	g	354	C	*(Sprilon)*
Zinc Sulphate BP	500	g	250	C	(Loveridge)
Zinc Sulphate Eye Drops BP	■ 10	ml	284	A	
Zinc Sulphate Lotion BP	200	ml	3	E	
Zinc Sulphate Mouthwash DPF	200	ml	3	E	
Zolpidem Tartrate Tablets 5mg	28		308	C	*(Stilnoct)*
Zolpidem Tartrate Tablets 10mg	28		448	C	*(Stilnoct)*
Zopiclone Tablets 3.75mg	28		306	A	
Zopiclone Tablets 7.5mg	28		443	A	
Zuclopenthixol Tablets BP, 2mg	100		321	C	*(Clopixol)*
Zuclopenthixol Tablets BP, 10mg	100		867	C	*(Clopixol)*
Zuclopenthixol Tablets BP, 25mg	100		1733	C	*(Clopixol)*
Zuclopenthixol Acetate Injection BP, ...	5		2602	C	*(Clopixol*
50mg/1ml ampoule					*Acuphase)*
Zuclopenthixol Acetate Injection BP, ...	5		5014	C	*(Clopixol*
100mg/2ml ampoule					*Acuphase)*
Zuclopenthixol Decanoate Injection BP, ...	10		3388	C	*(Clopixol)*
200mg/ml 1ml ampoule					
Zuclopenthixol Decanoate Injection BP, ...	5		3998	C	*(Clopixol-Conc)*
500mg/ml 1ml ampoules					

■ Special Containers

APPROVED LIST OF APPLIANCES
See Part II, Clause 8A (Page 7)

The price listed in respect of an appliance specified in the following list is
the basic price (see Part II, Clause 8 on which payment will be calculated
pursuant to Part II, Clause 6 in respect of the dispensing of appliances

NOTES

1. **Definition** - The appliances that may be supplied against orders on Forms FP10 are listed below and
must conform with the specifications shown. See Part 1, Clause 2 (page 3). These specifications
include published official standards ie BP, BPC or relevant British, European or International Standards
or the Drug Tariff Technical Specification. It should be emphasized that any appliance must conform
with the entry in this part of the Tariff as well as the official standard or technical specification quoted
therein. Other dressings and appliances which may be necessary will normally be provided through
the Hospital Services.

2. **Sealed Packets** - These are those which are "tamper-evident" - sealed with an easily detachable device
that prevents removal of the contents without the seal being broken. Additionally in the case of sterile
products: once a sealed package has been opened it should not be possible to re-seal it easily. Where
an appliance, other than a bandage, required by the Tariff to be supplied in a sealed packet is ordered
of a quantity or weight not listed in the Tariff, the quantity ordered should be made up as nearly as
possible with the smallest numbers of sealed packets available for the purpose. Where the quantity
ordered is less than the smallest quantity/weight, supply the smallest pack. The quantity of material
in each packet supplied should be recorded on the prescription form.

3. **Quality Systems** - Non CE marked sterile products shall be manufactured in accordance with the
requirements and guidance given in the Department of Health "Quality Systems for Sterile Medical
Devices and Surgical Products - Good Manufacturing Practice" (HMSO, ISBN0-11-321341-7), which
is the basis of the DH Manufacturer Registration Scheme (MRS) for such products.
Details of this scheme may be obtained from the MRS Registration Officer, Medical Devices Agency,
Hannibal House, Elephant & Castle, London SE1 6TQ.

   Manufacturers who have received approval to CE mark their sterile products have demonstrated that
these meet the essential requirements of the Medical Devices Regulations 1994, which incorporate
quality system requirements.

4. **Weights** - All weights specified in the Tariff in respect of appliances are exclusive of wrappings and
packing material.

5. **Invoice price** - This is the price chargeable for the appliance to the contractor by the manufacturer,
wholesaler or supplier.

6. **Technical Specifications** - Numbered Technical Specifications for the items in Part IXA/B/C were
published separately in 1981 in loose leaf volume and a revised list was published in 1983. The
Specifications will not be reprinted annually but individual specifications will be introduced, amended
and reprinted, or withdrawn, as necessary. A list of Technical Specifications is given on pages 95/96.
CE marked Devices have shown that they meet the essential requirements of the Medical Devices
Regulations 1994 and there is no further need for them to demonstrate compliance with other
specifications, such as those referred to above.

7. **Nurse Prescribing** - The items within Part IXA and Part IXR which are **not** prescribable by nurses on
form FP10(CN) or FP10(PN) are annotated Ⓝ See Part XVIIB for details of Nurse Prescribing.

APPROVED LIST OF APPLIANCES
See Part II, Clause 8A (Page 7)

The price listed in respect of an appliance specified in the following list is
the basic price (see Part II, Clause 8 on which payment will be calculated
pursuant to Part II, Clause 6 in respect of the dispensing of appliances

NOTES

Transitional Arrangements Arising from CE Marking.

1. After 14 June 1998 all products in Part IX which fall within the definition of a Medical Device (as defined in the Medical Devices Regulation 1994) will have to carry a CE marking.

2. Until this date products listed may conform **either** to a specification **or** will meet the requirements of the Medical Devices Regulations.

3. Companies are progressively CE marking their ranges of products already listed in Part IX. For practical reasons we do not intend to identify products individually as they gain their CE marking.

LIST OF TECHNICAL SPECIFICATIONS

		Spec. No.	Date of last revision
These Specifications are available from: **The Department of Health** **Room 168** **Richmond House** **79 Whitehall** **London SW1A 2NS**			
Absorbent Cotton, Hospital Quality		1	1981
Bandages			
Elastic Web with Foot Loop		2a	1983
Elastic Web without Foot Loop		2b	1983
High Compression (Extensible)		52	5/1992
Zinc Paste and Calamine		5	12/1990
Catheters			
Nelaton		38A	10/1996
Scott Female		38B	10/1992
Foley		38A	10/1996
Chemical Reagents			
Blood Glucose Testing Strips (BGTS)	Colorimetric	44	11/1994
	Biosensor	48	5/1994
Contraceptive Devices			
Intrauterine Contraceptive Devices		7	5/1990
Vaginal Contraceptive Caps (Pessaries)		8	1981
Dressings			
Hydrogel		50	4/1995
Perforated Film Absorbent		9	5/1993
Polyurethane Foam Film		47	9/1994
Povidone Iodine Fabric		43	1988
Sterile Dressing Pack		10	1981
Sterile Dressing Pack with NW Pads		35	1/1991
Elastic Hosiery			
Graduated Compression		40	1988
Suspended Belt		13	1981
Gauze Tissues			
Gauze and Cotton Tissue		14	1983

IX

LIST OF TECHNICAL SPECIFICATIONS (CONT)

	Spec. No.	Date of last revision
Hypodermic Equipment		
Non-Sterile		
Hypodermic Needles (Luer Fitting)	15	1981
Hypodermic Syringes (Luer Fitting)	16	12/1990
Pre-set Insulin Syringe 1ml.U100	36a	1983
Latex Foam Adhesive	19	1981
Peak Flow Meters	51	7/1995
Pessaries	20	1981
Protectives		
EMA Film Gloves, Disposable	21	1981
Rectal Dilators	22	10/1990
Stockinette		
Elasticated Surgical Tubular, Foam Padded	25	1983
Elasticated Viscose	46	1989
Elastic Net Surgical Tubular	26	1983
Swabs		
Non-Woven Fabric	28	3/1993
Non-Woven Fabric, Filmated	29	1981
Trusses		
Spring	31a	1981
Elastic Band	31b	1981

Appliance	Size or Weight	Basic Price p

ABSORBENT COTTONS

To be supplied in suitable sealed tamper evident packaging
as received from the manufacturer or wholesaler.
(See Note 2 Page 93)

		each
Absorbent Cotton BP 1988	25g	60
	100g	137
Where no quantity is stated on the prescription	500g	461
the 25g pack is to be supplied.		
Absorbent Cotton, Hospital Quality	100g	95
Specification 1	500g	300
To be supplied only where specifically ordered.		

APPLICATORS - VAGINAL

Plastics syringe-type applicator with transparent or
translucent barrel and opaque or translucent plunger.
The end of the barrel has an internal screw thread.
(Length not less than 11cm and capacity not less
than 5ml).

Ⓧ   **Type 1.** (*Ortho*)   75

Ⓧ   **Type 2.** (*Durex*)   75

N.B.

1. *To be supplied suitably wrapped as received from the manufacturer or wholesaler.*
2. *Where an Ortho pack ordered by the prescriber does not include an applicator, and the contractor considers that one is required, an Ortho Vaginal Applicator should be supplied and the prescription form endorsed accordingly.*
3. *Where Duracreme or Duragel Spermicide Jelly is ordered by the prescriber without an applicator and the contractor considers that one is required, a Durex Vaginal Applicator should be supplied and the prescription form endorsed accordingly.*
4. *For details of prescription charges payable, See Part XVI, page 493.*

ARM SLINGS

Web, Adjustable   160

IXA

Appliance	Size or Weight	Basic Price p

ATOMIZERS, HAND OPERATED   each

Nebulizers

Ⓧ (a) Inhalers
All-glass, plastics or plastics and glass with a rubber or plastics bulb, for use with any liquid intended for administration by inhalation and capable of producing an extremely fine mist.

(i)Type specified by the prescriber:	
Brovon Midget Inhaler	596
Riddell Minor	530
Pocket Riddopag Inhaler (without mask)	967
Rybar Standard Inhaler No. 1 (without mask)	929
Rybar Standard Inhaler No. 2 (without mask)	929

Other inhalers conforming to this specification may be supplied if specifically ordered and endorsed providing the *invoice price does not exceed   967

(ii) Type not specified by the prescriber:
The invoice price must not exceed   530

Where an atomizer or spray is ordered by the prescriber without specification and where the contractor considers an appliance for the administration of a liquid medicament by inhalation is required, a nebulizer should be supplied and the prescription form endorsed with the net cost and type or brand supplied. The basic price must not exceed that given for (ii) above.

Spare Parts for above   *Invoice Price

Ⓧ (b) Devices for use with Pressurised Aerosols.
Pressurised aerosols are generally regarded as drugs for prescribing purposes, even when supplied in a plastic container incorporating a spring mechanism operated by intake of breath, or with a collapsible 'spacer' device. However other devices are regarded as appliances.

Spacer/Holding Chamber Devices
incorporating one-way valve and mouthpiece. The device is reusable and should last for an extended period.   each

(★)   Plastic cone-shaped 750mL capacity.
(■)   Plastic cylindrical body and mouthpiece; rubber MDI adaptor. 145mL capacity.
(♦)   Plastic cone-shaped body and mouth piece; rubber MDI adaptor.   135mL capacity.

Type 1 - One piece, to take aerosol canister without actuator
(★ Astra)   428

Type 1 - with Mask - as above with Paediatric face mask
(★ Astra)   428

Type 2 - In two detachable parts, to take aerosol with actuator
(★ Allen and Hanbury)   ⎫
(★ Fisons - (Not available separately) ⎬ Not interchangeable   275

Type 2 - with Mask - as above with Paediatric face mask
(★ Allen and Hanbury only)   275

Type 3 - One piece, for use with all types of pressurised MDI aerosols   428
(■ 3M Healthcare Ltd)
(♦ Clement Clark Ltd)   420

Type 3 - with Mask - as above with Adult, child or infant face mask   714
(■ 3M Healthcare Ltd only)

*   For invoice price see Note 5 (Page 93)

Appliance	Size or Weight	Basic Price p

BANDAGES

1. The term "bandage" used in a prescription form without qualification is to be interpreted to mean an Open-Wove Bandage, Type 1 BP 5cm x 5m. All bandages supplied are to be of the lengths and widths specified in the Tariff. Where a bandage longer than those specified in the Tariff is ordered, the number of bandages which will, in total, provide the length nearest to that ordered should be supplied. Where a bandage in a width other than those specified is ordered, the next wider specified width should be supplied.

2. Except for Elastic Web, all bandages to be supplied completely wrapped as received from the manufacturer or wholesaler. Elastic Adhesive Bandages and Plaster of Paris Bandages to be supplied sealed in containers as received from the manufacturer or wholesaler. Except where otherwise stated all bandages possessing elasticity to be not less than 4.5m in length when fully stretched.

		each
Cotton Conforming Bandage BP 1988		
Type A		
Crinx	5cm x 3.5m	61
	7.5cm x 3.5m	76
	10cm x 3.5m	93
	15cm x 3.5m	127
Type B		
Kling	5cm x 3.5m	61
	7.5cm x 3.5m	79
	10cm x 3.5m	95
	15cm x 3.5m	125
Cotton Elastic Heavy Bandage - See Heavy Cotton and Rubber Elastic Bandage BP.		
Cotton Crêpe Bandage		
Hospicrepe 239	5cm	48
	7.5cm	67
	*10cm	87
	15cm	127
Cotton Crêpe Bandage BP 1988	7.5cm	269
	10cm	346
Cotton, Polyamide and Elastane Bandage		
Setocrepe	*10cm	112
Soffcrepe	5cm	63
	7.5cm	90
	*10cm	116
	15cm	169
Cotton Stretch Bandage BP 1988		
Hospicrepe 233	5cm	56
	7.5cm	78
	10cm	104
	15cm	148
Crêpe Bandage BP 1988	5cm	86
	7.5cm	120
	10cm	158
	15cm	229

IXA

* see also Multi-layer Compression Bandaging

Appliance	Size or Weight	Basic Price p
BANDAGES - cont		each
Elastic Adhesive Bandage BP	5cm	318
(Syn: Zinc Oxide Elastic Adhesive Bandage)	7.5cm	459
Where no size is stated by the prescriber	10cm	611
7.5cm size should be supplied.		
⊗ **Elastic Diachylon Bandage, Ventilated BPC**	7.5cm	354
Lestreflex, Ventilated		
		per metre
Elastic Web Bandage BP Blue Line	7.5cm	74
	10cm	106
		each
Elastic Web Bandage with Foot Loop Blue Line	7.5cm	425
Specification 2a		
Elastic Web Bandage Without Foot Loop	7.5cm x 2.75m	336
Red Line (Scott Curwen)	2.5m approx	
Specification 2b	unstretched length	
	7.5cm x 3.75m	406
To be supplied wrapped with instruction	3.5m approx	
folder and bandage fastener	unstretched length	
Elasticated Tubular Bandage - see		
Stockinettes page 154-157		
Elastomer and Viscose Bandage, Knitted		
BS compression type 2, for light support		
K-Lite	5cm	48
	7cm	68
	*10cm	89
	15cm	128
Litetex	5cm	38
	7cm	54
	10cm	71
	15cm	102
BS compression type 3a, for light compression		
Elset		
6m stretched	*10cm x 6m	246
	15cm x 6m	267
8m stretched	*10cm x 8m	310
Elset S		
12m stretched	15cm x 12m	529
K-Plus		
6m stretched	10cm x 6m	140
8.7m stretched	*10cm x 8.7m	198
Litetex +		
6m stretched	10cm x 6m	112
8.7m stretched	*10cm x 8.7m	158
Heavy Cotton and Rubber Elastic Bandage BP	7.5cm	1139

* see also Multi-layer Compression Bandaging

Appliance	Size or Weight	Basic Price p

BANDAGES - cont   each

HIGH COMPRESSION BANDAGES (Extensible)
Specification No. 52

P.E.C. High Compression Bandage

Syns: Polyamide, Elastane, and Cotton Compression (High) Extensible Bandage;
"PECCHE" Bandage

Setopress	7.5cm x 3.5m unstretched	254
	10cm x 3.5m unstretched	329

V.E.C. High Compression Bandage

Syns: Viscose, Elastane, and Cotton Compression (High) Extensible Bandage;
"VECCHE" Bandage

Tensopress	7.5cm x 3m unstretched	248
	*10cm x 3m unstretched	318

PERFORMANCE

IXA

The table below gives approximate sub-bandage pressures at the ankle according to the size of its circumference, including any sub-bandage dressings or padding. These are obtained when applied at the constant extension shown and in accordance with the technique indicated by the manufacturer:

Application Technique: Wound Spirally with 50% overlap						
	BANDAGE	EXTENSION ± 10%	Ankle Circumference			
			Less than 18cm	18-26cm	27-35cm	36-50cm
Approximate sub-bandage pressure	P.E.C.	70%	Not Applicable	38-27 mmHg	26-20 mmHg	-
		100%	Not Applicable	50-35 mmHg	34-27 mmHg	26-19 mmHg
	V.E.C.	50%	Not Applicable	36-25 mmHg	24-18 mmHg	-
		75%	Not Applicable	50-37 mmHg	37-28 mmHg	28-19 mmHg

LABELLING
1. The Drug Tariff title.
2. The label on the package states the nominal lay flat width.
3. Washing instructions in accordance with method for handwashing at 40° as defined in BS 2747.

HIGH COMPRESSION BANDAGE (Extensible)

SurePress	10cm x 3m unstretched	313

Knitted Polyamide and Cellulose Contour Bandage - See Polyamide and Cellulose Contour
Bandage, Knitted

* see also Multi-layer Compression Bandaging

Appliance	Size or Weight	Basic Price p

BANDAGES - cont
Multi-layer Compression Bandaging

A number of products are marketed as suitable for inclusion as components in a multi-layer bandaging system. Some such components are gathered together into multi-layer bandaging "kits".

The following is a list of products which have been identified by their manufacturers as suitable for inclusion in multi-layer bandaging systems, and which may be prescribed for this purpose or otherwise.

Prescribers should note that multi-layer bandaging "kits" are not prescribable as such. However, if prescribers wish to prescribe the individual components they are free to do so; and pharmacists are free to meet a prescription with a "kit" if the content of the kit exactly matches the components prescribed. Reimbursement will be as specified for the individual components.

3M Health Care Ltd | | each
Coban Self-Adherent Bandage | 10cm x 6m (stretched) | 275

ConvaTec Limited
SurePress Absorbent Padding - listed on page 104 | 10cm x 3m | 48

Johnson & Johnson Medical
Velband Absorbent Padding Bandage - listed on page 104 | 10cm x 4.5m | 72

Millpledge Healthcare
Hospi Four #1 *(Ortho-Band Plus* - listed on page 104) 10cm x 3.5m (unstretched) | | 40
Hospi Four #2 *(Hospicrepe 239* - listed on page 99) 10cm x 4.5m (stretched) | | 87
Hospi Four #3 *(Litetex +* - Boston Hospital Products - listed on page 100)
| 10cm x 8.7m (stretched) | 158
Hospi Four #4 *(AAA-Flex)* | 10cm x 6.3m (stretched) | 193

Parema Limited
K-Four Wound Dressing *(Paratex* - listed on page 122) | 9.5cm x 9.5cm | 25
K-Four # 1 *(K-Soft* - listed on page 104) | 10cm x 3.5m (unstretched) | 40
K-Four # 2 *(K-Lite* - listed on page 100) | 10cm x 4.5m (stretched) | 89
K-Four # 3 *(K-Plus* - listed on page 100) | 10cm x 8.7m (stretched) | 198
K-Four # 4 *(Ko-Flex)* | 10cm x 6m (stretched) | 270

Robinson Healthcare
Ultra Four # 1
(Sohfast Soft Absorbent Bandage
- listed on page 104) | 10cm x 3.5m (unstretched) | 42
Ultra Four # 2
(K-Lite - Parema Ltd - listed on page 100) | 10cm x 4.5m (stretched) | 89
Ultra Four # 3
(K-Plus - Parema Ltd - listed on page 100) | 10cm x 8.7m (stretched) | 198
Ultra Four # 4
(Cohfast Non Latex Cohesive Bandage) | 10cm x 6.3m (stretched) | 282

Seton Scholl Healthcare Plc
(Setoprime - listed on page 122) | 9.5cm x 9.5cm | 26
System 4 Wound Dressing
(Softexe - listed on page 104) | 10cm x 3.5m (unstretched) | 59
System 4 - #1
(Setocrepe - listed on page 99) | 10cm x 4.5m (stretched) | 112
System 4 - #2
(Elset - listed on page 100) | 10cm x 6m (stretched) | 246
System 4 - #3 | 10cm x 8m (stretched) | 310
(Coban Self-Adherent Bandage - 3M Health Care Ltd) | 10cm x 6m (stretched) | 275
System 4 - #4

Appliance	Size or Weight	Basic Price p

BANDAGES - cont

Multi-layer Compression Bandaging - cont
Smith & Nephew Healthcare Ltd
  Profore Wound Contact Layer

	Size or Weight	Basic Price p
Profore	14cm x 20cm	27
Profore #1 (*Soffban Natural* - listed on page 104)	10cm x 3.5m (unstretched)	60
Profore #2		
(*Soffcrepe* - listed on page 99)	10cm x 4.5m (stretched)	116
Profore #3 (*Litepress*)	10cm x 8.7m (stretched)	338
Profore #4 (*Co-plus*)	10cm x 2.5m (unstretched)	280
Profore + (*Tensopress* - listed on page 101)	10cm x 3m (unstretched)	318

	Size or Weight	Basic Price p
Vernon-Carus Ltd		
Cellona Undercast Padding - listed on page 104	7.5cm x 2.75m	37
	10cm x 2.75m	46
	15cm x 2.75m	59

	Size or Weight	Basic Price p
Open-Wove Bandage, Type 1 BP 1988	2.5cm x 5m	30
(Syn: White open-wove bandage)	5cm x 5m	49
	7.5cm x 5m	69
	10cm x 5m	90

	Size or Weight	Basic Price p
➀ **Plaster of Paris Bandage BP 1988**	7.5cm x 2.7m	155
Gypsona	10cm x 2.7m	205

Polyamide and Cellulose Contour Bandage, BP 1988	each	each	each
(Nylon & Viscose Stretch Bandage)	*Easifix*	*Slinky*	*Stayform*
Length 4m stretched 5cm	33	39	31
7.5cm	40	56	39
10cm	47	67	44
15cm	80	96	74

Polyamide and Cellulose Contour Bandage, Knitted BP 1988
K-Band

For dressing retention - Length 4m stretched		Basic Price p
	5cm	18
	7cm	23
	10cm	25
	15cm	44

Texband

For dressing retention - Length 4m stretched		Basic Price p
	5cm	15
	7cm	20
	10cm	21
	15cm	37

Appliance	Size or Weight	Basic Price p

BANDAGES - cont

Short Stretch Compression Bandage
Indications: Venous leg ulcers and lymphoedema

Actiban	8cm x 5m	300
	10cm x 5m	322
	12cm x 5m	392
Actico (Cohesive)	10cm x 6m	299
Comprilan	8cm x 5m	308
	10cm x 5m	350
	12cm x 5m	408
Rosidal K	8cm x 5m	308
	10cm x 5m	336
	12cm x 5m	408
Tensolan K	8cm x 5m	310
	10cm x 5m	356
	12cm x 5m	392
Varex Short Stretch	10cm x 5m	322

Sub-compression Wadding Bandage

Cellona Undercast Padding 2.75m unstretched	*7.5cm x 2.75m	37
	* 10cm x 2.75m	46
	* 15cm x 2.75m	59
Flexi-Ban 3.5m unstretched	10cm x 3.5m	45
K-Soft 3.5m unstretched	* 10cm x 3.5m	40
Ortho-Band Plus 3.5m unstretched	* 10cm x 3.5m	40
Soffban Natural (100% Natural Fleece) 3.5m unstretched	* 10cm x 3.5m	60
Softexe 3.5m unstretched	* 10cm x 3.5m	59
Sohfast Soft Absorbent Bandage 3.5m unstretched	* 10cm x 3.5m	42
SurePress Absorbent Padding	* 10cm x 3m	48
Velband Absorbent Padding Bandage 4.5m unstretched	* 10cm x 4.5m	72

* see also Multi-layer Compression Bandaging

Appliance	Size or Weight	Basic Price p

BANDAGES - cont

Suspensory Bandage, Cotton

Type 1. Cotton net bag with draw tapes and webbing waistband (Each in a carton or envelope)	Small	149
	Medium	149
	Large	149
	Ex-large	158
Type 2. Cotton net bag with elastic edge and webbing waistband (Each in a carton or envelope)	Small	165
	Medium	170
	Large	176
	Ex-large	183
Type 3. Cotton net bag with elastic edge and webbing waistband with insertion of elastic centre-front (Each in a carton or envelope).	Small	178
	Medium	178
	Large	178
	Ex-large	184

Note: Type supplied to be endorsed.

Triangular Calico Bandage BP 1980 (Individually wrapped)	Sides - 90cm Base - 127cm	108

IXA

Tubular Bandage - See Stockinettes, Pages 154-157

White Open-Wove Bandage - See Open-Wove Bandage, Type 1

Zinc Paste Bandages   each
To be supplied in sealed packages,
which prevent the passage of moisture, as
received from the manufacturer or wholesaler.

Zinc Paste Bandage BP		
Steripaste (15%)	7.5cm x 6m	317
Viscopaste PB7 (10%)	7.5cm x 6m	314
Zincaband (15%)	7.5cm x 6m	312
Zinc Paste and Coal Tar Bandage BP	7.5cm x 6m	313
Zinc Paste and Ichthammol Bandage BP		
Ichthopaste (6/2%)	7.5cm x 6m	317
Icthaband (15/2%)	7.5cm x 6m	313
Zinc Paste, Calamine and Clioquinol Bandage BP		
Quinaband	7.5cm x 6m	322
Zinc Paste and Calamine Bandage		
Calaband	7.5cm x 6m	322
Specification 5		

Appliance	Size or Weight	Basic Price p

Ⓧ **BREAST RELIEVER** — 60ml approx. — 387
Plasticised PVC polymer bulb with glass or
polycarbonate receiver

Ⓧ **BREAST SHIELDS** — — per pair

Plastic circular - each shield made in two — 363
sections with an opening in the concave
section (one pair in box). (Not to be
confused with Nipple Shields page 148)

BRUSHES — — each

Ⓧ **Iodine Brush** - Goose Quill — 23
(Camel Hair)

Ⓧ **Tracheostomy Brush** - See page 163.

CATHETERS, ACCESSORIES — — Pack of 5

Bard Comfasure Catheter Retainer Strap	Small	1250
	Adult	1250
	Abdominal	1300

CATHETER MAINTENANCE SOLUTIONS

OptiFlo G	(CSG50)	50ml	312
	(CSG100)	100ml	312
OptiFlo R	(CSR50)	50ml	312
	(CSR100)	100ml	312
OptiFlo S	(CSS50)	50ml	294
	(CSS100)	100ml	294

Appliance	Gauge (Ch) (See Note 1 - page 107)	Basic Price p

CATHETERS, URETHRAL STERILE

1. Catheter sizes are designated by the Charrière (Ch) gauge system - even numbers only. (The equivalent metric sizes for Charrière gauges 6-30 are 2.0mm-10.0mm, rising in 0.66mm). Where size is not stated by the prescriber, size 14 or 16 should be supplied.

2. If a balloon size is not stated by the prescriber when ordering a Foley catheter, a 10ml balloon catheter should be supplied - a 5ml balloon in the case of a paediatric catheter. (These are the minimum sizes available).

    N.B. BS 1695:1990 defines the balloon size as that amount of fluid required to fully inflate the balloon, including the volume of the lumen. Care should be taken to distinguish between an adult Catheter formerly labelled as "5ml" but requiring 10ml for full inflation, and a paediatric catheter labelled "5ml" in accordance with the BS.

3. Each sealed unit pack (i.e. one, five, ten or twenty-five units for Nélaton packs as appropriate; five units only for Scott packs; one unit only for Foley packs) to be supplied in an outer protective pack as received from the manufacturer or wholesaler.

IXA

4. The average period that a Foley Catheter is kept in place is given as a guide and may vary considerably with individual patients. All patients should be assessed on an individual basis and their optimum time for catheter change established.

5. Where the brand is not stated by the prescriber, the basic price of each listed catheter supplied must not exceed:

Nélaton (Male)	38
Nélaton (Female)	35
Nélaton (Paediatric)	35
Foley (Male)	199
Foley (Female)	208
Foley (Paediatric)	369

(A)(i) Nélaton Catheter ('ordinary' cylindrical Catheter)   Per Pack of 5*
Specification 38A and/or CE

Bard Reliacath PTFE Coated Latex			
	(DO159C)	14	703
			(=141 each)
Bard Reliacath Plastic (Male)	(D5030)	12-18	648
			(=130 each)
(Female)	(D5031)	12-18	648
			(=130 each)
(Paediatric)	(D5032)	8-10	648
			(=130 each)

DePuy Healthcare - see Simpla Continence Care

EMS - see Simpla Continence Care

---

*   5-units of plastic catheters, for example, represents on average one month's supply for patients practising intermittent catheterisation.
     See pages 220-222 for names and addresses of suppliers.

Appliance	Gauge (Ch) (See Note 1 - page 107)	Basic Price p

CATHETERS, URETHRAL STERILE - cont

(A)(i) Nélaton Catheter ('ordinary' cylindrical Catheter) - cont

			Per Pack of 5*
Maersk Medical Ltd			
UnoPlast (Male)	(ZT01008012-ZT01017012)	12-20	529
			(≈106 each)
UnoPlast (Male paediatric)	(ZT01001012-ZT01007012)	6-10	529
			(≈106 each)
UnoPlast (Female)	(ZT02016012-ZT02017012)	12-14	529
			(≈106 each)
UnoPlast (Female paediatric)			
	(ZT02014012-ZT02015012)	8-10	529
			(≈106 each)
Mentor Medical Systems Ltd			
Mentor Self-Cath			
(Male)	(408-418)	8-18	509
			(≈102 each)
(Female)	(208-214)	8-14	509
			(≈102 each)
(Paediatric)	(305-310)	8-10	509
			(≈102 each)

			Per Pack of 10
Pennine (Male)	(NC-1212/FP-1216/FP)	12-16	384 △
			(≈39 each) △
(Female)	(FC-1410/FP-1414/FP)	10-14	350 △
			(≈36 each) △
(Paediatric)	(NC-1206/FP/25-1210/FP/25)	6-10	350 △
			(≈36 each) △

			Per Pack of 1	Per Pack of 5*
Rüsch UK Ltd PVC Riplex Jaques				
(Male)	(DT6115-5)	8-18		690
				(≈138 each)
(Female)	(DT6114-5)	8-18		629
				(≈125 each)
Rüsch UK Ltd PVC Riplex Extra Long (76cm)				
(Male/Female)	(DT6116)	8-18		700
				(≈140 each)
Rüsch UK Ltd Soft Rubber Jaques				
	(DT5143-1/5)	8-18	142	600
				(≈120 each)

---

* 5-units of plastic catheters, for example, represents on average one month's supply for patients practising intermittent catheterisation.
See pages 220-222 for names and addresses of suppliers.

Appliance	Gauge (Ch) (See Note 1 - page 107)	Basic Price p	
		Per Pack of 1	Per Pack of 5*

CATHETERS, URETHRAL STERILE - cont

(A)(i)Nélaton Catheter ('ordinary' cylindrical Catheter) - cont

Simpla Continence Care EMS PVC			
(Male)	(T1010-T1018)	10-18	518 (=104 each)
(Female)	(T2012-T2018)	12-18	551 (=110 each)
(Paediatric)	(T3006-T3010)	6-10	551 (=110 each)
Simpla PVC Nélaton			
(Male)	(369612/14)	12-14	528 (= 106 each)
(Female)	(369912/14)	12-14	528 (=106 each)
(Paediatric)	(369908/10)	8-10	528 (=106 each)
SIMS Portex Ltd PVC (Male)	(300/111)	8-14	741 (=148 each)
(Female)	(300/113)	8-14	710 (=142 each)
PVC (Male)	(WS 850/8-14)	8-14	757 (=151 each)
(Female)	(WS 854/8-14)	8-14	731 (=146 each)

IXA

UnoPlast - see Maersk Medical Ltd

(A)(ii)Nélaton Catheter ('ordinary' cylindrical Catheter)
Single Use: *The rate of use is approximately between 6 and 45 times greater than reusable Nélaton catheters for patients practising intermittant catheterisation.*

Indications: High infection risk patients with neurogenic bladder disorders; particularly, patients with multiple sclerosis, spina bifida, diabetes and spinal cord injury.

			Per Pack of 25
Astra Tech LoFric Plus (non PVC)			
(Male)	(903800-905400)	8-24	3000 (=120 each)
(Female)	(943800-944800)	8-18	3000 (=120 each)
(Female 15cm)	(983800-984800)	8-18	3000 (=120 each)
(Paediatric)	(923600-924000)	6-10	3000 (=120 each)
(Paediatric 30cm)	(993600-994000)	6-10	3000 (=120 each)

*   5-units of plastic catheters, for example, represents on average one month's supply for patients practising intermittent catheterisation.
See pages 220-222 for names and addresses of suppliers.

Appliance	Gauge (Ch) (See Note 1 page 107)	Basic Price p

CATHETERS, URETHRAL STERILE - cont

Per Pack
of 25

(A)(ii) Nélaton Catheter ('ordinary' cylindrical Catheter) - cont

Single Use: *The rate of use is approximately between 6 and 45 times greater than reusable Nélaton catheters for patients practising intermittant catheterisation.*

Astra Tech LoFric (Male)	(900800-902400)	8-24	3000
			(=120 each)
(Female)	(940800-941800)	8-18	3000
			(=120 each)
(Female 15cm)	(980800-981400)	8-14	3000
			(= 120 each)
(Paediatric)	(920600)	6	3000
			(=120 each)
	(990800-991000)	8-10	3000
			(= 120 each)
(Tiemann Tip)	(961000-962000)	10-20	3000
			(=120 each)
Bard Interglide Coated Intermittent Catheter			
(Male)	D6030	8-18	3056
			(=122 each)
(Female)	D6031	8-18	3056
			(=122 each)
(Paediatric)	D6032	8-10	3056
			(=122 each)
Conveen EasiCath (Male Nélaton)	(5348-5362)	8-22	2640
			(= 106 each)
(Female)	(5368-5376)	8-16	2640
			(= 106 each)
(Paediatric)	(5006-5010)	6-10	2640
			(= 106 each)
(EasiCath 30cm)	(5086-5092)	6-12	2640
			(= 106 each)
(Tiemann Tip)	(5380-5388)	10-18	2640
			(= 106 each)
Hollister Incare Instant Cath			
(Male)	(9670-9673)	10-16	2899 △
			(=116 each) △
(Female)	(9674-9676)	10-14	2899 △
			(=116 each) △
(Paediatric)	(9677-9678)	6-8	2899 △
			(=116 each) △

LoFric PVC - see Astra Tech LoFric

Simcare - see SIMS Portex Ltd

Simpla Continence Care			
Aquacath (Male)	(G1008-G1018)	8-18	2636
			(= 105 each)
(Female)	(G2008-G2018)	8-18	2636
			(= 105 each)
(Paediatric)	(G3006-G3010)	6-10	2636
			(= 105 each)

See pages 220-222 for names and addresses of suppliers.

Appliance	Gauge (Ch) (See Note 1 page 107)	Basic Price p

CATHETERS, URETHRAL STERILE - cont

Per Pack of 25

(A)(ii)**Nélaton Catheter ('ordinary' cylindrical Catheter)** - cont
Single Use: *The rate of use is approximately between 6 and 45 times greater than reusable Nélaton catheters for patients practising intermittant catheterisation.*

SIMS Portex Ltd

Uro Flo Silky (Male)	(USCC8M-USCC16M)	8-16	3056 (= 122 each)
(Female)	(USCC8F-USCC16F)	8-16	3056 (= 122 each)

(A)(iii) **Nélaton Catheter (with handle) female use**

Per Pack of 5*

Simpla Continence Care Intex	(T/100/8-14)	8-14	527 (= 105 each)

(a PVC Nélaton style catheter with handle to assist those with impaired manual dexterity in inserting an intermittent catheter)

(A)(iv) **Dilatation Catheter without drainage eyes**   IXA

Single Use: *The average rate of use is between 5-30 catheters per month.*
Indications: for intermittent urethal dilatation to prevent stricture recurrence
Not indicated for bladder emptying

Per Pack of 25

Astra Tech Lofric Dila-Cath	(891600/800)	16/18	3000 (=120 each)

(B) **Scott Catheter** (short curved tubular catheter for women and girls)
Specification 38B and/or CE

Per pack of 5

Simcare - see SIMS Portex Ltd

SIMS Portex Ltd Polythene	(WS852/8-14)	8-14	1186 (=237 each)

(C) **Foley Catheter - 2 Way** (indwelling Nélaton catheter with balloon)
Specification 38A and/or CE

(i) a For Short/Medium Term Use - Adult:

Note: Average period of use is 1 to 3 weeks - See Note 4 (page 107)

Per Pack of 1

Bard PTFE Coated Latex	(Male)	(D1265LV)	10	12-26	235
		(D1266LV)	30	16-26	235
	(Female)	(D0169LV)	10	12-22	351
# Bard PTFE Coated Latex		(D1265AL)	10	12-22	268

Pre-filled with sterile water
* 5-units, of plastic catheters, for example, represents on average one month's supply for patients practising intermittent catheterisation.
See pages 220-222 for names and addresses of suppliers.

Appliance			Balloon Size (ml) (See note 2 - page 107)	Gauge (Ch) (See Note 1 - page 107)	Basic Price p

CATHETERS, URETHRAL STERILE - cont   Per Pack of 1

(C)   **Foley Catheter - 2 Way** (indwelling Nélaton catheter with balloon) - cont

    (i) a <u>For Short/Medium Term Use - Adult:</u>- cont

Rüsch UK Ltd Soft	(Male)	(DT4412)	10	12-26	468
Simplastic PVC		(DT4416)	30	16-26	468
	(Female)	(DT5442)	10	12-22	468
		(DT5446)	30	16-22	468
Rüsch UK Ltd PTFE	(Male)	(DT71002-1)	10	12-26	202
Coated Latex		(DT73002-1)	30	16-26	202
	(Female)	(DT81002-1)	10	12-22	257
		(DT83002-1)	30	16-22	257
Sims Portex Ltd Eschmann	(Male)	(41-515/41-517)	10	12-28	212
Folatex Latex		(41-525/41-527)	30	12-28	212
	(Female)	(41-915/41-917)	10	12-28	212
		(41-925/41-927)	30	12-28	212

    <u>(i) b.   For Short/Medium Term Use - Paediatric:</u>
    Note: Average period of use is 1 to 3 weeks - See Note 4 (page 107)

Bard PTFE Coated Latex	(DO165PV)	5	8-10	650

Eschmann - see Sims Portex Ltd

Rüsch UK Ltd PTFE				
Coated Latex	(DT 70502-1)	5	8-10	431
Sims Portex Ltd Eschmann	(41-585)	5	8-10	375
Folatex Latex				

    <u>(ii) a. For Long Term Use - Adult</u>
    Note: Average period of use is 3 to 12 weeks - See Note 4 (page 107)

Bard Biocath Hydrogel Coated					
	(Male)	(D2265)	10	12-26	726
		(D2266)	30	12-26	736
	(Female)	(D2269)	10	12-22	736
# Bard Biocath Hydrogel Coated					
	(Male)	(D2264)	10	12-22	747
	(Female)	(D2268)	10	12-22	751
Bard Silicone Elastomer Coated Latex					
	(Male)	(D1657)	10	12-22	799
		(D1667)	30	16-22	799
	(Female)	(D1647)	30	16-22	799

\#   Pre-filled with sterile water.

    See pages 220-222 for names and addresses of suppliers.

Appliance	Balloon Size (ml) (See note 2 - page 107)	Gauge (Ch) (See Note 1 - page 107)	Basic Price p

CATHETERS, URETHRAL STERILE - cont   Per Pack of 1

(C) **Foley Catheter - 2 Way** - cont.

(ii) a. <u>For Long Term Use - Adult</u> - cont
Note: Average period of use is 3 to 12 weeks - *See Note 4 (page 107)*

# Bard Silicone Elastomer Coated Latex				
(Male)	(D1657AL)	10	12-22	863
(Female)	(D1637AL)	10	12-22	863
Bard All Silicone				
(Male/Standard)	(D1658)	10	12-22	824
(Male/Standard)	(D1668)	30	16-22	824
(Female)	(D1661)	10	12-16	791
Bard Silastic Silicone Coated	(336)	10	12-24	753
	(334)	30	16-28	801
Kendall - see The Kendall Company (UK) Ltd				
Medasil (Surgical) Ltd				
All Silicone (Male)	(84M)	10	12-26	462
	(85M)	30	16-26	462
(Female)	(86F)	10	12-26	462
	(87F)	30	16-26	462
Porges Folysil All Silicone Catheter				
(Male) (open ended)	(AA74)	10	12-18	565
(Male)	(AA71)	10	12-24	565
(Female)	(AA75)	10	12-16	565
Rüsch UK Ltd				
Silikon 100 (Male)	(DT4292)	10	12-26	674
	(DT4293)	20	18-20	674
	(DT4293)	30	22-26	674
(Female)	(DT4294)	10	12-22	674
	(DT4295)	20	18-20	674
	(DT4295)	30	22	674
Sympacath Hydrogel Coated				
(Male)	18050599	10	12-30	647
	18053099	30	12-30	656
(Female)	18020599	10	12-26	656
	18023099	30	12-26	656
(3 way)	18313099	30	16-24	700
Rüsch UK Ltd Ultrasil Silicone Elastomer				
(Male)	(DT3111)	10	12-26	562
	(DT3113)	30	16-26	562

IXA

Pre-filled with sterile water
See pages 220-222 for names and addresses of suppliers.

Appliance		Balloon Size (ml) (See note 2 - page 107)	Gauge (Ch) (See Note 1 - page 107)	Basic Price p

CATHETERS, URETHRAL STERILE - cont   Per Pack of 1

(C) **Foley Catheter - 2 Way** - cont.

(ii) a. <u>For Long Term Use</u> - <u>Adult</u> - cont.
Note: Average period of use is 3 to 12 weeks - See Note 4 (page 107)

Simpla Continence Care All Silicone				
(Male)	367312-367314	10	12-14	821
	367516-367520	10	16-20	821
	367216-367218	20	16-18	821
	367220	30	20	821
(Female)	366312-366314	10	12-14	813
	366516-366518	10	16-18	813
	366220	30	20	813
SIMS Portex Ltd				
Transcath Clear Standard Silicone Catheter				
(Male/Female)	TC2125, TC2145, TC2165, TC2185, TC2205, TC2225, TC2245	5&10	12-24	700
	TC21630, TC21830, TC22030, TC22230, TC22430, TC22630	30	16-26	700
3 Way	TC3165, TC3185, TC3205, TC3225, TC3245, TC3265	5&10	16-26	750
	TC31630, TC31830. TC32030, TC32230, TC32430, TC32630	30	16-26	750
The Kendall Company (UK) Ltd				
Argyle All Silicone				
(Male)	(8887-805128-805227)	10	12-22	583
	(8887-830167)	20	16	583
	(8887-830183-830266)	30	18-26	583
(Female)	(8887-815127-815184)	10	12-18	583
Ultramer				
(Male)	(1612-1M/1626-1M)	5	12-26	625
(Female)	(1712-1F/1722-1F)	5	12-22	625
(Male)	(1416-1M/1426-1M)	30	16-26	625
(Female)	(1216-1F/1222-1F)	30	16-22	625

See pages 220-222 for names and addresses of suppliers

Appliance	Balloon Size (ml) (See note 2 - page 107)	Gauge (Ch) (See Note 1 - page 107)	Basic Price p

CATHETERS, URETHRAL STERILE - cont

                                                                         Per Pack of 1

(C) **Foley Catheter** - **2 Way** - cont.

(ii) b. For Long Term Use - Paediatric:
Note: Average period of use is 3 to 12 weeks - See Note 4 (page 107)

Bard Biocath Hydrogel Coated	(D2263) 5	8-10	736
Medasil (Surgical) Ltd			
All Silicone	(83P) 5	8-10	462
Rüsch UK Ltd			
Silikon 100	(DT4292) 5	8-10	674
Sympacath Hydrogel Coated	18010399 5	8-10	656
Simpla Continence Care All Silicone	5	8-10	820
Sherwood - see The Kendall Company (UK) Ltd			
SIMS Portex Ltd			
Transcath Clear Standard Silicone Catheter			
TC2061, TC2083, TC2103	1.5&3	6-10	700
The Kendall Company (UK) Ltd			
Argyle All Silicone (8887-803081-803107)	5	8-10	629

IXA

See pages 220-222 for names and addresses of suppliers

Appliance	Size or Weight	Basic Price p
		each
CELLULOSE WADDING BP 1988	500 g	234

May be supplied in stout polythene bag with clip closure as received from the manufacturer or wholesaler

---

CHIROPODY APPLIANCES

Ⓝ   **Adhesive Felt**   10.5cm x 8.3cm x 5mm thick   82

Zinc oxide or acrylic adhesive, spread on semi-compressed surgical wool felt (each in envelope)

Ⓝ   **Animal Wool BP 1988**   25 g   78

(Syn: Animal Wool for Chiropody)
(Long Strand Lamb's Wool for Chiropody)

Ⓝ   **Bunion Rings**   per box   80

Self-adhesive, semi-compressed felt (in box of 4 pieces)

Ⓝ •**Corn Plasters**

Salicylic Acid Adhesive Plaster BP 1980
(Syn. Salicylic Acid Self-Adhesive Plaster;
Salicylic Acid Plaster)   each

Plaster containing 20% w/w salicylic acid in the plaster mass (each in envelope)   7.5cm x 4.5cm   88

Plaster containing 40% w/w salicylic acid in the plaster mass (each in envelope)   7.5cm x 4.5cm   88

When the strength of the plaster is not specified by the prescriber a plaster containing 20% w/w salicylic acid in the plaster mass should be supplied

per box

Ⓝ   **Corn Rings**   5 mm thick   80
Self-adhesive, semi-compressed felt in a box of 9 pieces

per pair

Ⓝ   **Metatarsal Arch Supports** (previously Metatarsal Pads)   650
(Price of single article is half that of a pair)

each

Ⓝ   **Wool Felt BP 1988**   10.5 cm x 8.3 cm x 7 mm thick   97
(Syn: Wool Felt, Surgical)
Semi-compressed (each in envelope)

•   Temporarily Unavailable

Appliance	Size or Weight	Basic Price p

CONTRACEPTIVE DEVICES

                                                                    each
Fertility (Ovulation) Thermometer   168

A mercury-in-glass thermometer, conforming to BS691-1987 and BS 6834 - 1991 -
"Clinical maximum thermometers, section three, Ovulation thermometers". Range
35° to 39° Celsius subdivided in 0.1°C with a minimum scale length of 32 mm and an
accuracy of ± 0.1°C. Figured at each degree. Each thermometer shall bear the
BSI certification mark indicating approval under the BSI certification mark scheme,
or be supplied with an individual certificate of examination by the BSI.

To be supplied in a re-usable screw capped plastics protective case.

*NB: TEMPERATURE CHARTS (Form FP 1004) and advice on their use are given by the prescribing doctor;
they are also available from pharmacists.*

Ⓝ   **Intrauterine Contraceptive Device**

   Flexi T-300 Specification 7   865
   Each unit to be supplied in the individual carton
   containing the sealed and sterilised pack as received
   from the manufacturer or wholesaler.

                                                                    IXA

   **GyneFixIN* implant and insertion system*   2475
   Each unit to be supplied in the individual carton
   containing the sealed and sterilised pack as
   received from the manufacturer or wholesaler.

   **GyneFixPT* implant and insertion system*   2475
   Each unit to be supplied in the individual carton
   containing the sealed and sterilised pack as
   received from the manufacturer or wholesaler.

   *The Gynefix fitting technique differs in important respects from the technique
   for framed devices. The Faculty of Family Planning and Reproductive Health Care
   advises that those fitting GyneFix **must** have additional specific training.

   The manufacturers of GyneFix include the following notice on their packaging: "The
   fitting technique for GyneFix is not the same as other intrauterine devices. Before
   prescribing and fitting GyneFix a doctor **must** complete a GyneFix training course and
   be in receipt of a GyneFix training certificate of satisfactory completion of the course.
   Failure to follow correct insertion procedures may render GyneFix ineffective and could
   result in pain, expulsion or injury to the patient. For this reason the manufacturers do
   not recommend prescription and fitting of GyneFix by any doctor who has not received
   the GyneFix training certificate following satisfactory completion of an authorised
   training course.".

   Gyne-T380S Specification 7   993
   To be supplied in the individual sealed carton
   containing the sealed and sterilised pack as
   received from the manufacturer or wholesaler.

   Multiload CU 250 Specification 7   713
   To be supplied in the individual sealed carton
   containing the sealed and sterilised pack as
   received from the manufacturer or wholesaler.

Appliance	Size or Weight	Basic Price p

CONTRACEPTIVE DEVICES - cont   each

Ⓧ   **Intrauterine Contraceptive Device** - cont

     <u>Multiload CU 250/Short Specification 7</u>   713
     To be supplied in the individual sealed carton
     containing the sealed and sterilised pack as
     received from the manufacturer or wholesaler.

     <u>Multiload CU 375 Specification 7</u>   924
     To be supplied in the individual sealed carton
     containing the sealed and sterilised pack as
     received from the manufacturer or wholesaler.

     (Note: Prescribers have been advised that pain
     during and after insertion of Multiload CU 250,
     Multiload CU 250 Short or Multiload CU 375 is
     more likely to occur in nulliparous than in
     parous women).

     <u>Nova - T Specification 7</u>   1045
     To be supplied in the individual sealed carton
     containing the sealed and sterilised pack as
     received from the manufacturer or wholesaler.

     This type of the device and the size (where more
     than one is listed above) must be specified by
     the prescriber.

Ⓧ   **Vaginal Contraceptive Caps (Pessaries)**
     Specification 8

     <u>Type A (*Dumas* Vault Cap)</u>   No.1 ⎫
     Translucent rubber pessary   No.2 ⎪
     The size designation is moulded onto the rim   No.3 ⎬   607
          No.4 ⎪
          No.5 ⎭
     To be supplied in the individual pack as
     received from the manufacturer or wholesaler
     (plus postage 65p)

     <u>Type B (*Prentif* Cavity Rim Cervical Cap)</u>   22mm ⎫
     Opaque rubber pessary   25mm ⎪
     The normal internal diameter of the rim is   28mm ⎬   718
     moulded onto the rim   31mm ⎭
     To be supplied in the individual pack as
     received from the manufacturer or wholesaler
     (plus postage 65p)

     <u>Type C (*Vimule* Cap)</u>   No.1 ⎫
     Translucent rubber pessary   No.2 ⎬   607
     The size designation is moulded onto the rim   No.3 ⎭
     To be supplied in the individual pack as
     received from the manufacturer or wholesaler
     (plus postage 65p)

     The size of the pessary and the type must be specified by the prescriber.

Appliance	Size or Weight	Basic Price p

CONTRACEPTIVE DEVICES - cont   each

Ⓧ   **Vaginal Contraceptive Diaphragm**
Complies with British Standard 4028:1989
A dome-shaped occlusive reusable diaphragm
made of good quality natural or synthetic
rubber. The periphery is reinforced by an
enclosed metal spring.

Reflexions Flat Spring Diaphragm		
Diaphragm with a flat spring	55-95mm	559
The diaphragm is marked with the size.	(rising in 5 mm)	
Type B (BS 4028, Type 1)		
Diaphragm with a coil spring.		
The diaphragm is marked with the size.	60-100 mm	584
	(rising in 5 mm)	
Type C (BS 4028, Type 3)		
Diaphragm with an arcing spring (flat and		
coiled steel combination spring). The	60-95 mm	664
diaphragm is marked with the size.	(rising in 5 mm)	

IXA

Each diaphragm is enclosed in a robust
plastic case, and cardboard box. A booklet
of instruction to the patient regarding
care and use shall be included.

The size of the diaphragm, and the type
must be specified by the prescriber.

COTTON WOOLS - See Absorbent Cottons - page 97.

DOUCHES
Ⓧ   **With Rectal and Vaginal fittings**

Plastic Douche - Rigid plastics container,	1 litre	554
with 2m approx. flexible plastics tubing,	approx.	
a tap and vulcanite or rigid plastics rectal		
pipe and plastics vaginal pipe.		
Spare Plastics Tubing	2m approx.	90
Where type not specified by the prescriber,		
plastics tubing to be supplied		

Appliance	Size or Weight	Basic Price p

DRESSINGS

Absorbent, Perforated Dressing

Absorbent Cellulose Dressing with Fluid Repellent Backing
CE

Indications: Primary or secondary dressing for medium to heavily exuding wounds.

each

Mesorb	10cm x 10cm	51
	10cm x 15cm	66
	10cm x 20cm	81
	15cm x 20cm	116
	20cm x 25cm	183
	20cm x 30cm	208

Packed in outer container not exceeding 10 units.

Note: The exact number of pieces, ie packs, ordered by the prescriber is to be dispensed.

Absorbent, Perforated Plastic Film Faced, Dressing
Specification 9 and/or BP, CE

each

Cutilin	5cm x 5cm	12
	10cm x 10cm	20
	10cm x 20cm	38
Melolin	5cm x 5cm	13
	10cm x 10cm	22
	20cm x 10cm	42
Release	5cm x 5cm	12
	10cm x 10cm	20
	20cm x 10cm	38
Skintact	5cm x 5cm	10
	10cm x 10cm	17
	20cm x 10cm	34
Solvaline N	5cm x 5cm	9
	10cm x 10cm	16
	10cm x 20cm	32

Where not specified by the prescriber, the 5cm size to be supplied.

Where the brand or type is not specified by the prescriber, for the sizes listed below, the Basic Price must not exceed:

	5cm x 5cm	9
	10cm x 10cm	16
	20cm x 10cm	32

Appliance	Size or Weight	Basic Price p

DRESSINGS - cont

per pack

Absorbent, Perforated Dressing with Adhesive Border
BP and/or CE

Cosmopor E
5cm x 7.2cm (wound contact pad 2.7cm x 4cm + border 1.15 - 1.6cm)	7
6cm x 10cm (wound contact pad 2.7cm x 6.5cm + border 1.65 - 1.75cm)	13
8cm x 10cm (wound contact pad 4cm x 6.5cm + border 1.75 - 2.0cm)	15
6cm x 15cm (wound contact pad 2.7cm x 11cm + border 1.65cm - 2.0cm)	17
8cm x 15cm (wound contact pad 4cm x 11cm + border 2.0cm)	24
8cm x 20cm (wound contact pad 4cm x 16cm + border 2.0cm)	32
10cm x 20cm (wound contact pad 5.5cm x 16cm + border 2.0cm - 2.25cm)	39
10cm x 25cm (wound contact pad 5.5cm x 20cm + border 2.25cm - 2.5cm)	48
10cm x 35cm (woubd contact pad 5.5cm x 30cm + border 2.25cm - 2.5cm)	67

Mepore
6cm x 7cm (wound contact pad 3cm x 4cm + border 1.5cm)	8
9cm x 10cm (wound contact pad 5cm x 6cm + border 2cm)	18
9cm x 15cm (wound contact pad 5cm x 10cm + border 2.0 - 2.5cm)	30
9cm x 20cm (wound contact pad 5cm x 15cm + border 2.0 - 2.5cm)	36
9cm x 25cm (wound contact pad 5cm x 20cm + border 2.0 - 2.5cm)	50
9cm x 30cm (wound contact pad 5cm x 25cm + border 2.0 - 2.5cm)	57
9cm x 35cm (wound contact pad 5cm x 30cm + border 2.0 - 2.5cm)	62

Primapore
6cm x 8.3cm (wound contact pad 3.4cm x 5.7cm + border 1.3cm)	14
8cm x 10cm (wound contact pad 4.5cm x 5cm + border 1.75 - 2.5cm)	15
8cm x 15cm (wound contact pad 4.5cm x 10cm + border 1.75 - 2.5cm)	26
10cm x 20cm (wound contact pad 5cm x 14cm + border 2.5 - 3cm)	35
10cm x 25cm (wound contact pad 5cm x 18cm + border 2.5 - 3.5cm)	40
10cm x 30cm (wound contact pad 5cm x 23cm + border 2.5 - 3.5cm)	50
12cm x 35cm (wound contact pad 6.6cm x 29cm + border 2.7 - 2.95cm)	83

Sterifix (with two adhesive strips)
5cm x 7cm (wound contact pad 5cm x 5cm + border 1.0cm)	17
7cm x 10cm (wound contact pad 5cm x 10cm + border 1.0cm)	28
10cm x 14cm (wound contact pad 8cm x 14cm + border 1.0cm)	50

Note: The exact number of pieces, ie packs, ordered by the prescriber is to be dispensed.

Ⓧ   **Boil Dressing Pack**   69
The pack comprises:
Two boil dressings   38 mm x 38 mm
(Each complies with BP requirements for an
Elastic Adhesive Dressing - Wound Dressing.
There is a 2.5 mm hole punched through the
centre of the dressing. The pad may be
impregnated with a BP permitted antiseptic).

One Elastic Adhesive Dressing BP -
Wound Dressing   38 mm x 38 mm
(The dressing is impregnated with a BP
permitted antiseptic).

The dressings are contained within a suitable
protective package labelled with the contents,
instructions for use and storage conditions.

Note: The exact number of pieces, ie packs, ordered by the prescriber is to be dispensed.

IXA

Appliance	Size or Weight	Basic Price p

DRESSINGS - cont

each

Knitted Viscose Primary Dressing BP Type 1
(Sterile Knitted Viscose Dressing)
To be supplied in the individual pack, sealed and sterilised as received from the manufacturer or wholesaler.

N-A Dressing	9.5cm x 9.5cm	31
	19cm x 9.5cm	58
N-A Ultra	9.5cm x 9.5cm	29
	19cm x 9.5cm	55
Paratex	* 9.5cm x 9.5cm	25
	† 12.5cm x 14.5cm	50
Setoprime	* 9.5cm x 9.5cm	26
Tricotex	9.5cm x 9.5cm	27

Multiple Pack Dressing No. 1   341
To be supplied in sealed cartons as received
from the manufacturer or wholesaler.
Carton containing:

Absorbent Cotton BP 1988 (interleaved)	25g	
Absorbent Cotton Gauze. Type 13 Light BP,		
sterile	90 cm x 1 m	
Open-Wove Bandages BP 1988 (banded)	3 x 5 cm x 5 m	

Perforated Film Absorbent Dressing BP - See Absorbent, Perforated Plastic Film Faced, Dressing (P.F.A. Dressing).

Povidone–Iodine Fabric Dressing, Sterile
Specification 43

(*Inadine*)	5cm x 5cm	28
	9.5cm x 9.5cm	41
(*Poviderm*)	5cm x 5cm	25
	9.5cm x 9.5cm	36

Knitted Viscose Primary Dressing BP impregnated with a polyethyleneglycol/water-based ointment complying with Povidone Iodine Ointment USP 10% w/w.

Sterile one piece pack consisting of a sealed impermeable peelable pouch containing a single piece of the impregnated fabric between two protective layers.

The labelling of each pack shall include:
    The Title.
    "Contents sterile if pack is undamaged or unopened" - or similar.

Note: The exact number of packs, ie pieces, ordered by the prescriber are to be dispensed. Where not specified by the prescriber, the 5cm size is to be supplied.

Standard Dressings
To be supplied in sealed packets as received from
the manufacturer or wholesaler.

Ⓧ **No. 4 Medium Elastic Adhesive Wound Dressing**   per packet
    BPC 1963   packet of 3   57

                                                           each
Ⓧ **No. 16 Eye Pad with Bandage BPC,** sterile   54

---

* see also Multi-layer Compression Bandaging
† to be deleted 1 February 2001

Appliance	Size or Weight	Basic Price p

DRESSINGS - cont

STERILE DRESSING PACKS

These packs contain a selection of sterile dressing required in special nursing procedures (usually for post-operative re-dressing of wounds) when performed in the home. A pack is to be used for each sterile dressing operation. Prescribers have been advised to order this dressing only for an individual patient for whom such a sterile dressing operation is essential and to restrict their orders to the number of packs considered to be required for that patient. *The exact number of packs ordered by the prescriber is to be dispensed.*

Sterile Dressing Pack		each
Specification 10		73

Sterile Pack containing:
Gauze and Cotton Tissue Pad	8.5cm x 20cm	
Gauze Swabs 12 ply	4 x 10 x 10cm	
Absorbent Cotton Balls, large	4 x 0.9g approx	
Absorbent Paper Towel	45cm x 50cm	
Water Repellent Inner Wrapper opens out	50cm x 50cm	
as a sterile working field		
To be supplied in the individual pack, sealed and		
sterilised as received from the manufacturer or		
wholesaler.		

IXA

Sterile Dressing Pack with Non-Woven Pads		
Specification 35		

(Vernaid)		73
Sterile Pack containing:		
Non-woven Fabric Covered Dressing Pad	10cm x 20cm	
Non-woven Fabric Swabs	4 x 10cm x 10cm	
4 Absorbent Cotton Wool Balls		
Absorbent Paper Towel	50cm x 45cm	
Water Repellent inner Wrapper opens out	50cm x 50cm	
as a sterile working field.		

Vapour-permeable Adhesive Film Dressing		each
(Syn: Semipermeable Adhesive Dressing)		

Askina Derm	6cm x 7cm	36
	10cm x 12cm	100
	15cm x 20cm	229

Bioclusive	10.2cm x 12.7cm	134
To be supplied in the individual pack, sealed		
and sterilised as received from the manufacturer		
for wholesaler		

Cutifilm	5cm x 7.5cm	40
To be supplied in the individual pack, sealed	7.5cm x 10cm	66
and sterilised as received from the manufacturer	10cm x 14cm	113
or wholesaler		

Appliance	Size or Weight	Basic Price p

DRESSINGS - cont

Vapour-permeable Adhesive Film Dressing - cont   each
(Syn: Semipermeable Adhesive Dressing)

EpiVIEW	6cm x 7cm	41
	10cm x 12cm	109
Hydrofilm	6cm x 9cm	47
	10cm x 15cm	125
	12cm x 25cm	225
Mefilm		
To be supplied in the individual pack, sealed	6cm x 7cm	38
and sterilised as received from the	10cm x 12.7cm	102
manufacturer or wholesaler	10cm x 25cm	200
	15cm x 21.5cm	254
OpSite Flexigrid (formerly *OpSite*)	6cm x 7cm	45
To be supplied in the individual pack, sealed	12cm x 12cm	121
and sterilised as received from the manufacturer	15cm x 20cm	301
or wholesaler.		
Tegaderm	6cm x 7cm	37
To be supplied in the individual pack, sealed	12cm x 12cm	123
and sterilised as received from the manufacturer	15cm x 20cm	234
or wholesaler		

Note:
The exact number of pieces, ie packs, ordered by the prescriber is to be dispensed.

Vapour-permeable Adhesive Film Dressing - with absorbent pad
(Syn: Semipermeable Adhesive Dressing)

Mepore Ultra	6cm x 7cm	25
	9cm x 10cm	54
	9cm x 15cm	81
	9cm x 25cm	135
OpSite Plus	10cm x 12cm	95
	15cm x 15cm	220
OpSite Post-Op	5cm x 5cm	25
	9.5cm x 8.5cm	70
	23.5cm x 8.5cm	160
	35cm x 10cm	265

Note:
The exact number of pieces, ie packs, ordered by the prescriber is to be dispensed

Appliance	Size or Weight	Basic Price p

DRESSINGS - cont

Vapour-permeable Waterproof Plastic Wound Dressing BP, Sterile   8.5cm x 6cm   32

(Syn: Semipermeable Waterproof Plastic Wound Dressing) (*Elastoplast Airstrip* in which the pad consists of Perforated Film Absorbent Dressing Type 1)

To be supplied in the individual pack, sealed and sterilised as received from the manufacturer or wholesaler.

Note:
The exact number of pieces, ie packs, ordered by the prescriber is to be dispensed.

WOUND MANAGEMENT DRESSINGS

<u>Activated Charcoal Absorbent Dressing</u>

Carboflex	10cm x 10cm	255
	8cm x 15cm (Oval)	306
	15cm x 20cm	580
Lyofoam C	10cm x 10cm	255
	10cm x 25cm	521
	15cm x 20cm	580

<u>Activated Charcoal Non-Absorbent Dressing</u>

Carbopad VC	10cm x 10cm	159
	10cm x 20cm	215
CliniSorb	10cm x 10cm	154
	10cm x 20cm	205
	15cm x 25cm	330

IXA

Appliance	Size or Weight	Basic Price p

DRESSINGS - cont   each
WOUND MANAGEMENT DRESSINGS - cont

Activated Charcoal Cloth with Silver

Actisorb Silver 220 (formerly *Actisorb Plus*)	10.5cm x 10.5cm	224
	10.5cm x 19cm	407

Alginate Dressing - Sterile.
   BP and/or CE

Indications: Medium to heavily exuding wounds.
Precautions: Not the dressing of choice for infected wounds; not suitable for those which are very dry or covered with hard necrotic tissue.

each

Algisite M	5cm x 5cm	75
	10cm x 10cm	154
	15cm x 20cm	414
Algosteril	5cm x 5cm	75
	10cm x 10cm	172
	10cm x 20cm	286
SeaSorb	6cm x 4cm	75
	10cm x 10cm	155
	15cm x 15cm	321
Kaltogel	5cm x 5cm	74
	10cm x 10cm	153
Kaltostat	5cm x 5cm	76
	7.5cm x 12cm	165
	10cm x 20cm	326
	15cm x 25cm	560
Melgisorb	5cm x 5cm	74
	10cm x 10cm	153
	10cm x 20cm	288
Sorbalgon	5cm x 5cm	70
	10cm x 10cm	147
Sorbsan	5cm x 5cm	70
	10cm x 10cm	147
Tegagen (formerly *Tegagel*)	5cm x 5cm	71
	10cm x 10cm	150

Alginate Dressing with Absorbent Backing - Sterile

Sorbsan Plus	7.5cm x 10cm	149
	10cm x 15cm	263
	10cm x 20cm	335
	15cm x 20cm	465

The labelling of each pack shall include:
   The Title
   (1) The Category of the dressing, and
   (2) "Contents guaranteed sterile if pack is undamaged or unopened" - or similar.

Note: The exact number of sachets, each containing one dressing, ie packs ordered by the prescriber is to be dispensed.

Appliance	Size or Weight	Basic Price p

DRESSINGS - cont   each
WOUND MANAGEMENT DRESSINGS - cont

Cavity Dressing
Indications: Medium/heavily exuding cavity wounds

Algisite M-Rope		2cm x 30cm	275
Algosteril Rope		30cm/2g	305
Allevyn Cavity	circular	5cm diameter	334
		10cm diameter	796
	tubular	9cm x 2.5cm	324
		12cm x 4cm	570
Aquacel Ribbon		2cm x 45cm	224
Cutinova Cavity		5cm x 6cm	153
		10cm x 10cm	254
		15cm x 20cm	509
Kaltostat		2g	305
Melgisorb Cavity		2.2cm x 32cm (x3 pieces)	285
Seasorb Filler		40cm /2g	305
Sorbalgon T		30cm/2g	300
Sorbsan Packing		2g	305
Sorbsan Ribbon (with probe)		40cm	178
Tegagen		2cm x 30cm	250

Conforming Foam Cavity Wound Dressing

Cavi-Care	20g	1575

IXA

Hydrocolloid Dressing - Semi-permeable - Sterile
BP and/or CE
Indications: Light to medium exudating wounds.
Precautions: Not suitable for infected wounds. Heavy exudate leads to too frequent changes of dressing.
Dressing should seal round the borders of a wound.

Sterile one-piece pack:
With Adhesive Border

Comfeel Plus Contour Dressing
These dressings are contoured to facilitate application to difficult areas, such as elbows and heels.

6cm x 8cm	(wound contact pad 6cm x 8cm + irregular border)	176
9cm x 11cm	(wound contact pad 9cm x 11cm + irregular border)	306

Granuflex, Bordered
Square

6cm x 6cm	(wound contact pad 6cm x 6cm + border 2cm)	140
10cm x 10cm	(wound contact pad 10cm x 10cm + border 2.0 - 2.5cm)	264
15cm x 15cm	(wound contact pad 15cm x 15cm + border 2.5cm)	508

Triangular

10cm x 13cm	(wound contact pad 10cm x 13cm + border 2.0 - 2.5cm)	312
15cm x 18cm	(wound contact pad 15cm x 18cm + border 2.0 - 2.5cm)	486

Hydrocoll Border (Bevelled Edge)
Square

5cm x 5cm	(wound contact pad 3.5cm x 3.5cm + border 0.75cm)	85
7.5cm x 7.5cm	(wound contact pad 4.5cm x 4.5cm + border 1.5cm)	140
10cm x 10cm	(wound contact pad 7.75cm x 7.75cm + border 1.25cm)	205
15cm x 15cm	(wound contact pad 12.5cm x 12.5cm + border 1.5cm)	385

Contoured
These dressings are contoured to facilitate application to difficult areas such as elbows
and heels.

6cm x 14cm	(wound contact pad 10cm x 5cm + irregular border)	180

Sacral

15cm x 18cm	(wound contact pad 14cm x 11cm + irregular border)	306

Appliance	Size or Weight	Basic Price p

DRESSINGS - cont
WOUND MANAGEMENT DRESSINGS - cont

<u>Hydrocolloid Dressing - Semi-permeable - Sterile</u> - cont
     BP and/or CE

Sterile one-piece pack:
<u>With Adhesive Border</u>

		each
Tegasorb (formerly *Tegasorb Advanced Formulation*)		
<u>Oval</u>		
10cm x 12cm	(wound contact pad 7cm x 9cm + border 1.5cm)	209
13cm x 15cm	(wound contact pad 10cm x 12cm + border 1.5cm)	390

Sterile one-piece pack:
<u>Without Adhesive Border</u>

Comfeel (Bevelled Edge)		
<u>Square</u>		
10cm x 10cm		221
15cm x 15cm		443
20cm x 20cm		677
Comfeel Plus Ulcer Dressing		
<u>Square</u>		
10cm x 10cm		227
15cm x 15cm		452
20cm x 20cm		678
<u>Triangular</u>		
18cm x 20cm		456
Cutinova Foam		
<u>Square</u>		
10cm x 10cm		217
<u>Rectangular</u>		
5cm x 6cm		101
15cm x 20cm		395
Cutinova Hydro		
<u>Square</u>		
10cm x 10cm		205
<u>Rectangular</u>		
5cm x 6cm		102
15cm x 20cm		434
Granuflex (modified)		
<u>Square</u>		
10cm x 10cm		222
15cm x 15cm		420
20cm x 20cm		633
<u>Rectangular</u>		
15cm x 20cm		456
Hydrocoll Basic		
<u>Square</u>		
10cm x 10cm		208
20cm x 20cm		608
<u>Rectangular</u>		
15cm x 20cm		442

Appliance	Size or Weight	Basic Price p

DRESSINGS - cont
WOUND MANAGEMENT DRESSINGS - cont

Hydrocolloid Dressing - Semi-permeable - Sterile - cont
BP and/or CE

Indications: Light to medium exudating wounds.
Precautions: Not suitable for infected wounds. Heavy exudate leads to too frequent changes of dressing.
Dressing should seal round the borders of a wound.

Sterile one-piece pack: each
Without Adhesive Border

Replicare Ultra
  Square
  10cm x 10cm   210
  15cm x 15cm   417
  20cm x 20cm   616

  Anatomically Shaped Sacral Dressing
  15cm x 18cm   395

Tegasorb (formerly *Tegasorb Advanced Formulation*)
  Square
  10cm x 10cm   213
  15cm x 15cm   412

Hydrocolloid Dressing, Thin - Semi-permeable - Sterile
BP and/or CE

With Adhesive Border

Tegasorb Thin
  Oval
  10cm x 12cm (wound contact pad 7cm x 9cm + border 1.5cm)   139
  13cm x 15cm (wound contact pad 10cm x 12cm + border 1.5cm)   260

Without Adhesive Border

Askina Biofilm Transparent
  Square
  10cm x 10cm   95
  15cm x 15cm   215
  20cm x 20cm   281

DuoDERM Extra Thin
  Rectangular
  5cm x 10cm   60
  Square
  7.5cm x 7.5cm   63
  10cm x 10cm   105
  15cm x 15cm   226

Hydrocoll Thin Film
  Square
  7.5cm x 7.5cm   59
  10cm x 10cm   98
  15cm x 15cm   220

Appliance	Size or Weight	Basic Price p

DRESSINGS - cont
WOUND MANAGEMENT DRESSINGS - cont

Hydrocolloid Dressing, Thin - Semi-permeable - Sterile - cont
BP and/or CE

Without Adhesive Border- cont

Tegasorb Thin
Square
10cm x 10cm   142
15cm x 15cm   275

Note: The exact number of packs, ie pieces, ordered by the prescriber is to be dispensed.

Hydrocolloid Dressing - Semi-permeable - Sterile   each
BP and/or CE

Indications: Chronic and acute exudating wounds.

With Adhesive Border

CombiDERM
Square
10cm x 10cm (wound contact pad 5cm x 5cm + border 2.5cm)   132
14cm x 14cm (wound contact pad 7.5cm x 7.5cm + border 3.5cm)   183
20cm x 20cm (wound contact pad 13cm x 13cm + border 3.5cm)   352   Δ
Triangular
15cm x 18cm (wound contact pad 8cm x 11cm + border 3cm)   316
20cm x 23cm (wound contact pad 12cm x 15cm + border 4cm)   424   Δ

With Non-adhesive Border

CombiDERM-N

Square
7.5cm x 7.5cm (wound contact pad 5.5cm x 5.5cm + border 1cm)   103
14cm x 14cm (wound contact pad 11cm x 11cm + border 1.5cm)   184

Rectangular
15cm x 25cm (wound contact pad 13cm x 23cm + border 1cm)   375

Note: The exact number of packs, ie pieces, ordered by the prescriber is to be dispensed.

Hydrocolloid Dressing - Fibrous - Sterile
BP and/or CE

Indications: Medium to heavily exudating wounds.
Should be covered with a moisture retentive dressing.

Without Adhesive Border

Aquacel
Square
5cm x 5cm   92
10cm x 10cm   219
15cm x 15cm   413

Note: The exact number of packs, ie. pieces, ordered by the prescriber is to be dispensed.

Appliance	Size or Weight	Basic Price p

DRESSINGS - cont
WOUND MANAGEMENT DRESSINGS - cont   each

Hydrogel Dressing - Sterile
Specification 50 and/or CE

Indications: Dry "sloughy" or necrotic wounds; lightly exudating wounds; granulating wounds.
Precautions: Not suitable for infected or heavily-exudating wounds. Care should be taken to choose the appropriate secondary dressing.

AquaForm Hydrogel	15g	174
Granugel Hydrocolloid Gel	15g	184
IntraSite Conformable	10cm x 10cm (7.5g)	143
	10cm x 20cm (15g)	193
	10cm x 40cm (30g)	345
IntraSite Gel	8g	143
	15g	192
Nu-Gel	15g	181
Purilon Gel	8g	140
	15g	185
Sterigel	8g	140
	15g	185

IXA

Hydrogel Sheet

Novogel	Square	10cm x 10cm	275
		30cm x 30cm (0.15cm thickness)	1100
		30cm x 30cm (0.30cm thickness)	1165
	Rectangular	5cm x 7.5cm	175
		15cm x 20cm	525
		20cm x 40cm	1000
	Circular	7.5cm Diameter	250

Note: The exact number of packs ordered by the prescriber is to be dispensed.

Polyurethane Foam Dressing BP - Sterile

Indications: Light to medium exudating wounds.
Precautions: Not recommended for dry superficial wounds. Dressings should be secured at the edge by adhesive tape. Dressing should not be covered by occlusive tape or film. Secondary absorbent dressing is not required.

Lyofoam	7.5cm x 7.5cm	92
	10cm x 10cm	109
	17.5cm x 10cm	169
	20cm x 15cm	228

Sterile one piece pack consisting of:

A sealed peelable unit container or pouch containing a single piece of flatdressing which may be enclosed between two pieces of film or paper packed in an outer container not exceeding 10 units.

Note: The exact number of pieces, ie packs, ordered by the prescriber is to be dispensed.

Appliance	Size or Weight	Basic Price p

DRESSINGS - cont
WOUND MANAGEMENT DRESSINGS - cont

Polyurethane Foam Film Dressing - Sterile
Specification 47 and/or CE
Indications: Light to medium exudating wounds.
Precautions: Not recommended for dry superficial wounds.

                                                                              each

With Adhesive Border

Allevyn Adhesive (Adhesive faced pad)
Square
7.5cm x 7.5cm   (wound contact pad 5cm x 5cm + border 1.25cm)   121
12.5cm x 12.5cm   (wound contact pad 10cm x 10cm + border 1.25cm)   217
17.5cm x 17.5cm   (wound contact pad 15cm x 15cm + border 1.25cm)   429
22.5cm x 22.5cm   (wound contact pad 20cm x 20cm + border 1.25cm)   624
Anatomically Shaped Sacral Dressing
22cm x 22cm   (wound contact pad 15cm x 15cm + border 2cm)   468

Biatain Adhesive
Square
12cm x 12cm   (wound contact pad 8cm x 8cm + border 2cm)   210
18cm x 18cm   (wound contact pad 13cm x 13cm + border 2.5cm)   419

Lyofoam Extra Adhesive
Square
9cm x 9cm   (wound contact pad 5cm x 5cm + border 2cm)   114
15cm x 15cm   (wound contact pad 10cm x 10cm + border 2.5cm)   214
22cm x 22cm   (wound contact pad 15cm x 15cm + border 3.5cm)   421
30cm x 30cm   (wound contact pad 20cm x 20cm + border 5cm)   613
Sacral
15cm x 13cm   (wound contact pad 10cm x 8cm + border 2.5cm)   175
22cm x 26cm   (wound contact pad 15cm x 19cm + border 3.5cm)   332

Tielle
Square
11cm x 11cm   (wound contact pad 7cm x 7cm + border 2cm)   206
15cm x 15cm   (wound contact pad 11cm x 11cm + border 2cm)   337
18cm x 18cm   (wound contact pad 14cm x 14cm + border 2cm)   429
Rectangular
7cm x 9cm   (wound contact pad 3cm x 5cm + border 2cm)   111
15cm x 20cm   (wound contact pad 11cm x 16cm + border 2cm)   422

Tielle Sacrum
Square
18cm x 18cm   (wound contact pad 12cm x 10cm + border 3 - 5cm)   312

Packed in outer container not exceeding 10 units
Note: The exact number of pieces, ie packs, ordered by the prescriber is to be dispensed.

Appliance	Size or Weight	Basic Price p

DRESSINGS - cont
WOUND MANAGEMENT DRESSINGS - cont   each

<u>Polyurethane Foam Film Dressing - Sterile</u> - cont

<u>Without Adhesive Border</u>

Allevyn (non adhesive)
<u>Square</u>
5cm x 5cm 102
10cm x 10cm 203
20cm x 20cm 545
<u>Rectangular</u>
10cm x 20cm 326
<u>Heel (Cupped Shape)</u>
10.5cm x 13.5cm 407

Allevyn LM (non adhesive)
<u>Square</u>
5cm x 5cm 91
10cm x 10cm 165
<u>Rectangular</u>
10cm x 20cm 283
15cm x 20cm 353

Askina Transorbent (adhesive)
<u>Square</u>
10cm x 10cm 172
15cm x 15cm 316
20cm x 20cm 505
<u>Rectangular</u>
5cm x 7cm 91

Biatain Non-Adhesive
<u>Circular</u>
5cm diameter 100
8cm diameter 140
<u>Square</u>
10cm x 10cm .... 193 Δ
15cm x 15cm .... 356 Δ

Flexipore (adhesive)
<u>Square</u>
10cm x 10cm 173
20cm x 20cm 506
<u>Rectangular</u>
6cm x 7cm 93
10cm x 30cm 360
15cm x 20cm 370

Lyofoam Extra (non adhesive)
<u>Square</u>
10cm x 10cm 181
<u>Rectangular</u>
10cm x 17.5cm 307
10cm x 25cm 371
15cm x 20cm 398

Packed in outer container not exceeding 10 units.
Note: The exact number of pieces, ie packs, ordered by the prescriber is to be dispensed.

Appliance	Size or Weight	Basic Price p

DRESSINGS - cont
WOUND MANAGEMENT DRESSINGS - cont

Polyurethane Foam Film Dressing-Sterile -cont
    Without Adhesive Norder - cont
        Spyrosorb (adhesive)
            <u>Square</u>

10cm x 10cm		205
20cm x 20cm		586

Polyurethane Foam Film Dressing - Sterile
    <u>Indications</u>: Lightly to non-exuding wounds
    With Adhesive Border
        Tielle Lite
            <u>Square</u>

11cm x 11cm	(wound contact pad 7cm x 7cm + border 2cm)	201

            <u>Rectangular</u>

7cm x 9cm	(wound contact pad 3cm x 5cm + border 2cm)	107
8cm x 15cm	(wound contact pad 4cm x 11cm + border 2cm)	248
8cm x 20cm	(wound contact pad 4cm x 16cm + border 2cm)	262

Polyurethane Foam Film Dressing - Sterile
    <u>Indications</u>: Moderate to heavily exuding wounds.
    With Adhesive Border
        Tielle Plus
            <u>Square</u>

11cm x 11cm (wound contact pad 7cm x 7cm + border 2cm)		232
15cm x 15cm (wound contact pad 11cm x 11cm + border 2cm)		379

            <u>Rectangular</u>

15cm x 20cm (wound contact pad 11cm x 16cm + border 2cm)		475

    Without Adhesive Border
        Tielle Plus Borderless
            <u>Square</u>

11cm x 11cm		279

Packed in outer container not exceeding 10 units.
Note: The exact number of pieces, ie packs, ordered by the prescriber is to be dispensed.

    Silicone Gel Sheet
    <u>Indications:</u> For prevention treatment - Keloid and Hypertrophic scars.
        Cica-Care

6cm x 12cm		1180
15cm x 12cm		2300

        Silgel
            <u>Square</u>

10cm x 10cm		1350
20cm x 20cm		4000
40cm x 40cm		14400

            <u>Rectangular</u>

10cm x 5cm		750
15cm x 10cm		1950
30cm x 5cm		1950
10cm x 30cm		3150

            <u>Shaped</u>

5cm Diameter		400
25cm x 15cm		2112
44cm x 14cm		3946

Appliance	Size or Weight	Basic Price p

DRESSINGS - cont
WOUND MANAGEMENT DRESSINGS - cont

<u>Silicone Topical Cream</u>

    Indications: For prevention treatment - Keloid and Hypertrophic scars.

    Silgel
        10ml tube   1000

<u>Soft Silicone Wound Contact Dressing - Sterile</u>
    CE

    Indications: Non-exuding to heavily exuding wounds.
    Should be covered with a simple absorbent secondary dressing.
    Precautions: Dressing should be used with care in heavily bleeding wounds.

    Mepitel

5cm x 7.5cm		147
7.5cm x 10cm		256
10cm x 18cm		553
20cm x 30cm		1397

IXA

Packed in outer container not exceeding 10 units.
Note: The exact number of pieces, ie packs, ordered by the prescriber is to be dispensed.

<u>Soft Silicone Wound Contact Dressing with Polyurethane Foam Film Backing - Sterile</u>
    CE

    Precautions: Dressing should be used with care in heavily bleeding wounds.

    Mepilex

10cm x 10cm		214
10cm x 20cm		353
15cm x 15cm		398
20cm x 20cm		589

Packed in outer container not exceeding 10 units.
Note: The exact number of pieces, ie packs, ordered by the prescriber is to be dispensed.

DROPPERS 27
ⓧ   Glass, with bull-nose or curved flat end fitted (each in box) with good quality rubber teat.
    Where appropriate, a dropper should be supplied with eye, ear and nasal drops
    (See Part IV, containers, (Page 31) and Part XVI (Page 486) for details of prescription charges payable).

ELASTIC HOSIERY

Graduated Compression Hosiery
Specification 40

Explanation of Garments

N.B. The "Class" can be expressed either with roman or arabic numerals.

Class I
Light (Mild) Support
Compression at ankle 14mm Hg - 17mm Hg
Indications   - Superficial or early Varices. Varicosis during pregnancy.
Styles   - Thigh length or below knee with knitted in heel (reciprocated).

Class II
Medium (Moderate) Support
Compression at ankle 18mm Hg - 24mm Hg
Indications   - Varices of medium severity
    - Ulcer Treatment and prevention of recurrence. Mild oedema
    - Varicosis during pregnancy
    - Anklets and kneecaps: for soft tissue support
Styles   - Thigh length or below knee with knitted in heel (reciprocated)

Class III
Strong support
Compression at ankle 25mm Hg - 35mm Hg
Indications   - Gross varices
    - Post Thrombotic Venous Insufficiency
    - Gross Oedema
    - Ulcer Treatment and prevention of recurrence
    - Anklets and kneecaps: for soft tissue support
Styles   - Thigh length or below knee open or knitted in heel (reciprocated)

General Notes

Prescribing

Before the prescription can be dispensed the following details must be given by the prescriber.

1. Quantity - single or pair
2. Article including any accessories (see pages 137-139 for knit, style and price)
3. Compression Class I, II or III

Constructional Specification

The complete structural specification, as well as performance requirements are contained in Drug Tariff Specification No. 40.

Specially Made Garments

1. In cases where stock sizes are not suitable for patients owing to irregular limb dimensions, surgical stockings in the prescribed compression class, to be made to the patient's individual measurements, should be specified.
2. All such garments are specially shaped during manufacture and may have a knitted-in or open heel and open or knitted in toe.

ELASTIC HOSIERY - cont

Diagrams of the Hosiery Available

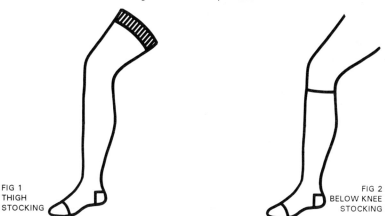

FIG 1
THIGH
STOCKING

FIG 2
BELOW KNEE
STOCKING

Figs. 1 and 2 are available in a range of stock sizes or may be made to measure.

IXA

Accessories

Any thigh length garment for men may be supplied with suspenders which are also available separately. **Suspender belts are also available.**

FIG 3   FIG 4

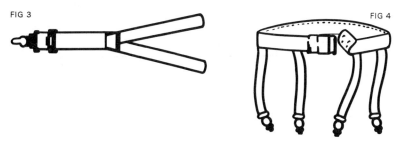

Sizing

All articles must conform to BS 6612:1985 with regard to size designation.

Labelling

All articles must state clearly on the packaging that they conform with Drug Tariff Technical Specification No 40. The packaging should also provide clear washing instructions in conformity with handwashing at 40°C as defined in BS 2747 and washing instructions should be durably and clearly marked on each garment. The packaging should clearly define the garments percentage and fibre content.

<u>Anklets and Kneecaps</u> (see page 139)

ELASTIC HOSIERY - cont

DESCRIPTION OF ARTICLES AVAILABLE			Price per pair in pence	
Compression Class (See Page 136)	Type of Garment		Standard Stock Sized Garments Supplied	* Made-to-Measure Garments Supplied
	Knit	**Style**		
1	Circular	Thigh	645	
		B. Knee	589	
	Lt. Wt Elas.Net	Thigh		1728
		B. Knee		1349
II	Circular	Thigh	959	3204
		B. Knee	862	2004
	Net	Thigh		1728
		B. Knee		1349
	Flat Bed	Thigh		3204
		B. Knee		2004
III	Circular	Thigh	1136	3204
		B. Knee	977	2004
	Flat Bed (formerly One Way Stretch)	Thigh B. Knee		3204 2004

Accessories	Price per item in pence
Additional Price for Fitted Suspender	56
Spare Suspender for thigh stockings (Fig.3)	56
Suspender Belt Drug Tariff Specification No. 13 (Fig 4)	430

NB: *The reimbursable price for one item is half the price of a pair.*

More than one prescription charge is payable where: more than one piece of elastic hosiery is supplied (see page 486).

*   All such garments are specially shaped during manufacture and many have a knitted in or open heel and open or knitted in toe with the following exceptions:

Class II/III - Flat Bed Knit can only be supplied with closed heel and open toe.

Note: Prescriptions should be endorsed with the style, ie, fabric or knit supplied.

For Above Knee Stockings - see Thigh Length.

ELASTIC HOSIERY - cont

Anklets and Kneecaps

Fig 5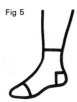

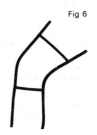 Fig 6

IXA

COMPRESSION CLASS	DESCRIPTION OF ARTICLES AVAILABLE		Price per pair in pence	
	Knit	Type of Garment	Standard Stock Sized Garments	Made to Measure Garments
CLASS II	Circular Knit	Anklet Kneecap	565 565	565 565
	Flat Bed	Anklet Kneecap	1173 1173	1173 1173
	Net	Anklet Kneecap		1110 922
CLASS III	Circular	Anklet Kneecap	788 753	788 753
(formerly One Way Stretch)	Flat Bed	Anklet Kneecap	788 753	1173 1173

NB: The reimbursable price for one item is half the price of a pair.

More than one prescription charge is payable when more than one piece of elastic hosiery is supplied. (see page 486)

Appliance	Size or Weight	Basic Price p

Ⓧ **EYE BATHS**
Squat shape, with finger grips, rigid plastics
smooth inner surface and base, rounded rim

each
20

EYE DROPS DISPENSERS

Opticare	(for 2.5, 5, 10, 15 & 20ml bottles)	475
Opticare Arthro 5	(for 2.5 & 5ml bottles)	475
Opticare Arthro 10	(for 10, 15, 20ml bottles)	475

Ⓧ **EYE SHADES**   25
Plastics, semi-rigid, non flam., perforation along
top for ventilation, to fit either eye (each individually packed in suitable container)

Ⓧ **FINGER COTS** Seamless latex   box of 10

per box
27

Ⓧ **FINGER STALLS**   per pkt

Polythene, Disposable - with apron	packet of 25	214
	packet of 50	333

To be supplied in a sealed polythene envelope
as received from the manufacturer or wholesaler   each

Simulated Leather   Small⎫
On a knitted fabric base, with adjustable elastic   Medium, Large⎬   36
wrist band   Extra-Large⎭

GAUZES
To be supplied in sealed packets* as received from
the manufacturer or wholesaler

Absorbent Cotton Gauze, Type 13 Light BP 1988,
sterile   90 cm x 1 m   90
(Syn: Absorbent Gauze)   90 cm x 3 m   188
                                         90 cm x 5 m   293
                                         90 cm x 10 m   561
(*ie. an inner sealed paper wrapper, in a film
wrapped carton)
Where no quantity is stated by the prescriber the
1 m packet should be supplied.

Absorbent Cotton Gauze, Type 13 Light BP 1988   25 m roll   1285
not sterilised
(Syn. Absorbent Gauze)
(*ie. sealed paper wrapper)

Absorbent Cotton and Viscose Ribbon Gauze
BP 1988 Sterile   1.25 cm x 5 m   68
                                         2.5 cm x 5 m   75
(*ie. an inner sealed paper wrapper, in an outer
paper wrapper).

Appliance	Size or Weight	Basic Price p

GAUZE DRESSINGS (IMPREGNATED)
To be supplied in a sealed packet or double sealed
box as received from the manufacturer or wholesaler

per pack

Ⓧ **Chlorhexidine Gauze Dressing BP**
(Syn: Chlorhexidine Tulle Gras)

Sterile one-piece pack consisting of	5cm x 5cm	23
A sealed peelable pouch containing a single piece	10cm x 10cm	49

of impregnated gauze between 2 leaves of paper or
plastics film of the size

The labelling of each pack shall include:
   "Sterile" and the size of its contents, "5cm x 5cm" or "10cm x 10cm"
   "The dressing shall not be issued nor the contents used if the wrapper or seal is broken".
Note:
   The exact number of pieces (ie packs) ordered by the prescriber are to be dispensed.
   Where not specified by the prescriber, the 5cm size to be supplied.

Ⓧ **Framycetin Gauze Dressing BP**
(Syn: Framycetin Tulle Gras)
(*Sofra Tulle*)   each
Sterile one-piece pack consisting of:
A sealed peelable foil laminate wrap containing a
single piece of impregnated gauze between two

layers of parchment	10cm x 10cm	24

The labelling of each pack shall include:
   "Sterile" "10cm x 10cm"
   "This package shall not be issued nor the contents used if the wrapper is broken".
   Each pack bears instructions for cutting to smaller sizes.

Note:
The exact number of pieces (ie packs) ordered by the prescriber are to be dispensed.

Paraffin Gauze Dressing BP Sterile
(Syn: Tulle Gras)

Sterile one-piece pack consisting of:
A peelable outer wrap containing a single piece of
impregnated gauze each piece separately enclosed
between two pieces of film or paper.

Light Loading - 90-130g/m²

Paranet	10cm x 10cm	25
Paratulle	10cm x 10cm	25

Normal Loading - 175-220g/m²

Jelonet	10cm x 10cm	33

The exact number of pieces (ie packs) ordered by the prescriber to be dispensed.

The labelling of each pack shall include:
   "Sterile" "10cm x 10cm"
   "This package shall not be issued nor the contents used if the wrapper is broken".

Appliance	Size or Weight	Basic Price p

GAUZE DRESSING (IMPREGNATED) - cont   each

Povidone Iodine "Gauze" Dressing - see Page 122

Ⓝ **Sodium Fusidate Gauze Dressing Sterile, BP**
(Fucidin Intertulle)
Cotton gauze of leno weave impregnated with
Sodium Fusidate Ointment BP 2% w/w

Sterile one-piece pack consisting of:
A sealed peelable foil laminate wrap containing
a single piece of impregnated gauze between two
layers of paper.   10cm x 10cm   23

The labelling of each pack shall include:
    "Sterile" "10cm x 10cm"
    "This package shall not be issued nor the contents used if the wrapper is broken".

Note:
The exact number of pieces (ie packs) ordered by the prescriber to be dispensed.

Gauze Pads - See SWABS page 159
Gauze Swabs - See SWABS page 159

GAUZE TISSUES
To be supplied in sealed packets* as received
from the manufacturer or wholesaler. (See
Note 2 page 93).

Gauze and Cotton Tissue BP 1988   500g   584
(Absorbent Gauze Tissue; Gauze Tissue)
(*ie sealed paper wrapper or heat-sealed stout
plastics bag)

Gauze and Cotton Tissue (Drug Tariff)   500g   427
Specification 14
(*ie sealed paper wrapper or heat-sealed stout
plastics bag)
To be supplied only where specifically ordered.

Appliance	Size or Weight	Basic Price p

each

HYPODERMIC EQUIPMENT

(N) A. **Hypodermic Needles**   30
    Specification 15
    British Standard 3522 Luer mount needles

NB:
The appropriate British Standard Needles
must be supplied if the old "Hypo" sizes
are ordered.
  B. **Hypodermic Syringes**
    Glass barrels with Luer taper conical fittings.

    (i) <u>Syringes for use with U100 Insulin</u>
        Both 0.5 and 1mL syringes are marked in units
        and are numbered every 10 units. Each
        graduation between the numbered calibrations
        represents one unit of insulin on the 0.5mL
        syringe and two units of insulin on the 1mL
        syringe.

        (a) **U100 Insulin Syringe**   0.5mL   1395
            British Standard 1619/2 1982 Luer mount 1mL   1395
            syringe bearing the BSI Certification Mark
            supplied with a dosage chart in a strong
            box.
            Where the size is not specified by the
            prescriber the 0.5mL syringe should normally
            be supplied unless the patient is known to
            take more than 50 units of insulin per
            injection.

        (b) **Pre-Set U100 Insulin Syringe** 1mL   2124
            Specification 36
            For use by blind patients.
            Supplied with a dosage chart in a strong
            box.

(N) (ii) <u>Syringes for use with drugs other than insulin</u>
        Ordinary Purpose Syringe   1mL   781
        Specification 16   2mL   781
        British Standard 1263 Luer mount syringe.
        Supplied in a strong box.

IXA

Appliance	Size or Weight	Basic Price p

HYPODERMIC EQUIPMENT - cont

C. **Single Patient-Use Products**

(i)   **U100 Insulin Syringes with Needle - Sterile, Single-use or Single Patient-use**
Shall comply with the requirements of BS 7548:1992

Sterile: intended for single use, or single patient-use, for the injection of U100 Insulin by diabetics in the community.

NB:
Intended for use immediately after filling, and not for containing insulin over extended periods of time.

The syringe may have permanently fixed needles, or detachable needles fitted ready for use.
Alternatively, syringes with a separate needle may be supplied.
The sterility of the fluid pathway and functional surfaces shall be protected by either end caps or suitable unit containers. These shall be tamper-evident.

COLOUR CODING: The colour orange is used to distinguish U100 insulin syringes.

Note:
Each scale graduation represents one unit on the 0.3mL and 0.5mL syringes and two units on the 1.0mL syringe. The graduations on the syringes are clearly numbered at every 5 units on the 0.3mL and 0.5mL syringes and at every 10 units on the 1.0mL syringe.
When the size is not specified by the prescriber the 0.5mL syringe with needle should be supplied.
If the patient is known to inject more than 50 units of insulin per injection the 1.0mL syringe shall be supplied.

Needles 8mm long shall have a needle diameter as follows: 0.3mm (30G)

Size	per 10
0.3mL syringe and needle	119
0.5mL syringe and needle	115

Needles 12mm long shall have a range of needle diameters as follows:
0.45mm (26G), 0.4mm (27G), 0.36mm (28G) and 0.33mm (29G)

Size	per 10
0.3mL syringe and needle	126
0.5mL syringe and needle	121
1.0mL syringe and needle	122

(ii)   **Hypodermic Needles-Sterile, Single-use**
Shall comply with the requirements of BS 5081: Part 2: 1987:
0.4mm size needles shall comply with the requirements of the above BS and the needle tube shall have the properties given in Annex D of BS 7548: 1992.

For use with the re-usable glass syringes listed in this Tariff on page 143. The sterility of the fluid pathway and functional surfaces shall be protected by a suitable unit container, which shall be tamper-evident.

The needles shall be of a length not less than 12mm and the following diameters may be supplied:

Size		each
0.5 mm (25G)	100	232
0.45 mm (26G)	100	232
0.4 mm (27G)	100	232

Appliance	Size or Weight	⁎Basic Price p

HYPODERMIC EQUIPMENT - cont

D. ⊗ **Reusable Pens**

	Cartridge Size	Dial up unit dose	
Autopen	3.0ml	1 unit (1-21 units)	1396
(Owen Mumford)	3.0ml	2 unit (2-42 units)	1396
	1.5ml	1 unit (1-16 units)	1396
	1.5ml	2 unit (2-32 units)	1396
BD Ultra Pen	3.0ml	1 unit	1996
(Becton Dickinson)	1.5ml	1 unit	1996
NovoPen 3 Classic	3.0ml	1 unit (2-70 units)	2200
Demi	3.0ml	0.5 unit (1-35 units)	2200
Fun	3.0ml	1 unit (2-70 units)	2200
(Novo Nordisk)			

E. ⊗ **Needles for Pre-filled and Reusable Pen Injectors**

per 100 pack

Needle length less than or equal to 6.1mm	1111
Needle length between 6.2mm and 9.9mm	787
Needle length equal to or greater than 10mm	787

IXA

The approved manufacturers of these products are Novo Nordisk, Becton Dickinson and Owen Mumford.

F. **Lancets - Sterile, Single-Use**

		Size	Price
ⒷAmes (Bayer Diagnostics)	0.5mm/25gauge	100 / 200	331 / 631
ⒶBaylet Lancet (Bayer Diagnostics)	0.5mm/25 gauge	100 / 200	331 / 631
ⒶCleanlet 25 (Gainor Medical)	0.5mm/25gauge	100 / 200	319 / 608
ⒷCleanlet 25 XL (Gainor Medical)	0.5mm/25gauge	100 / 200	319 / 608
ⒶCleanlet Fine (formerly Cleanlet 28) (Gainor Medical)	0.36mm/28gauge	100 / 200	319 / 613
ⒶFinePoint (LifeScan UK)	0.5mm/25 gauge	100	325
ⒶGlucoTip (Fine) (A. Menarani Diagnostics)	0.45mm/26 gauge	100	317
ⒶMicro-Fine + (Becton Dickinson)	0.30mm/30 gauge	200	613
ⒶMilward Steri-Let (Entaco)	0.66mm/23 gauge	100 / 200	300 / 570

Ⓐ Type A - mount fluted longitudinally
Ⓑ Type B - mount with concentric ribs

Appliance	Size or Weight		Basic Price p

HYPODERMIC EQUIPMENT - cont
F.   **Lancets - Sterile, Single-Use** - cont

Appliance	Size or Weight		Basic Price p
(A) Milward Steri-Let (Entaco)	0.36mm/28 gauge	100 / 200	300 / 570
(A) Monolet (Sherwood Medical)	0.8 mm/21gauge	100 / 200	328 / 624
(A) Monolet Extra (Sherwood Medical)	0.8 mm/21gauge	100	328
(C) Softclix II (Roche Diagnostics Ltd)	0.4mm/28 gauge	200	634
(B) Unilet Superlite (Owen Mumford Ltd)	0.66mm/23gauge	100 / 200	323 / 612
(A) Unilet G Superlite (Owen Mumford Ltd)	0.66mm/23gauge	100 / 200	323 / 612
(A) Unilet GP (Owen Mumford Ltd)	0.81mm/21gauge	100 / 200	324 / 616
(A) (B) Unilet Universal ComforTouch (Owen Mumford Ltd)	0.45mm/26gauge	100 / 200	323 / 612
(A) Vitrex Soft (Vitrex Medical Ltd)	0.65mm/23gauge	100 / 200	300 / 570
	0.36mm/28gauge	100 / 200	319 / 613

(A)   Type A - mount fluted longitudinally

(B)   Type B - mount with concentric ribs

(C)   Type C - device specific

G.   **Accessories**   each
    Needle Clipping (Chopping) Device   114

Consisting of a clipper to remove the needle from its hub, and
incorporating a suitable receptacle from which the cut-off needles cannot
be retrieved. Sufficiently robust to accommodate needles of diameter
0.45mm (26G) or finer; length: 16mm or shorter. Not generally
suitable for use with lancets. Designed to hold approximately 1,200 such needles.

INHALERS

(N) Spare Tops - mouthpiece and cork   186
    See also Nebulizers page 98

Appliance	Size or Weight	Basic Price p

INSUFFLATORS
Plastics - for inhalation of fine powders.

Ⓧ **Type 2** *(Intal Spinhaler)*. For inspiratory operation; plastics body
with detachable mouthpiece, containing a propeller, with integral
capsule piercing device of stainless steel; to hold unit dose capsules
of microfine powdered medicament. — 192

Ⓧ **Type 4** *(Becotide Rotahaler, Ventolin Rotahaler, Ventide Rotahaler)*.
For inspiratory operation; plastics body with detachable mouthpiece,
containing capsule opening device; to hold unit dose capsules of
microfine powder medicament. — 78

IRRIGATION FLUIDS
  Saline

Appliance	Container	Size or Weight	Basic Price p
Normasol Twist (Seton)	Tube	25 x 25ml	658
Askina Spray Buffered (B. Braun Medical Ltd)	Aerosol	1 x 120ml	245
		1 x 250ml	275
		1 x 350ml	320
Irriclens (ConvaTec)	Aerosol	1 x 240ml	280
Normasol (Seton)	Sachet	25 x 25ml	585
		10 x 100ml	716
Askina Jet Saline (B. Braun Medical Ltd)	Ampoules	24 x 10ml	562
		24 x 20ml	624
		24 x 30ml	720
Steripod (Seton)	Pod	25 x 20ml	683

IXA

To be supplied in sealed containers* as received from the manufacturer or wholesaler.
(*ie aerosols, ampoules, pods, sachets or tubes))

Note: *The exact number of containers (ie aerosols, ampoules, pods, sachets or tubes) ordered by the
prescriber is to be dispensed.*

Appliance	Size or Weight	Basic Price p

LARYNGECTOMY PROTECTORS - see Tracheostomy and Laryngectomy Protectors, page 164

		per piece
LATEX FOAM, ADHESIVE, raised cotton backed	22.5cm x 45cm	399
Ⓝ Specification 19	7mm thick	
	Box of 4	
Adhesive, Latex Foam, is for use with Cervical Collars		

LINT

To be supplied in sealed packets (film wrapped cartons)
as received from the manufacturer or wholesaler.

		each
Absorbent Lint BPC	25g	75
(Syn: Absorbent Cotton Lint; Cotton Lint; Plain Lint; White Lint)	100g	228
Where no quantity is stated on the prescription form	500g	960
the 25g pack is to be supplied.		
Ⓝ **Boric Acid Lint BPC 1963**	100g	259
(Syn: Boric Lint; Boracic Acid Lint)		

Ⓝ **LUBRICATING JELLY**		
Sutherland Lubricating Jelly (sterile)	5g sachet	18
	42g tube	124
	82g tube	194

NIPPLE SHIELDS, PLASTICS   53

Ⓝ Semi -rigid polypropylene base with latex teat
(each in carton). (Not to be confused with Breast Shields page 106)

Appliance	Order No.	Basic Price p

Ⓧ **PEAK FLOW METERS**
syn: P.F.M.
(Non-powered; hand-held)

Portable meters intended for single-patient use.
The standard range is suitable for use by both adults and children.
The low range model is for adults or children with severely restricted airflow.

Manufacturer   each

Standard Range
Clement Clarke	Specification	3103XXX series	686
Ferraris	51	208	653
Vitalograph		43-2XX series	665
Medic-Aid Personal Best		755EU	750

Low Range
Clement Clarke	Specification	3104XXX series (supersedes 3105XXX series)	690
Ferraris	51	209	653
Vitalograph		43-1XX series	665
Medic-Aid Personal Best		756EU	750

IXA

Each to be supplied in an individual protective pack designed to exclude dust and debris during use together with the plastics mouthpiece(s) appropriate for adults and children, instructions and chart for recording readings. The meter and its unit packaging shall carry the batch number and whether standard or low range.

The labelling of each unit package shall include:
The Title.
"Standard" or "Low Range".
"Drug Tariff Specification 51". (as appropriate)
"For single patient use".

N.B:
1. *"Low range" to be supplied only where specifically ordered.*
2. *Where the brand or manufacturer is not stated by the prescriber and has not been endorsed, the basic price must not exceed 653p.*
3. *Replacement recording charts (FP1010) are given by the prescribing doctor; they are also available from pharmacists.*

Replacement Mouthpiece (Plastics)
(Not interchangeable between brands or manufacturers)

     each

Replacement mouthpiece - suitable for both standard
and low range models for use by adults or children
(Clement Clarke)	38
(Vitalograph)	40
(Ferraris)	38

Each individually wrapped and labelled.

Appendix : see overleaf

This Page Is Intentionally Blank

APPENDIX

NOTES ON PEAK FLOW METERS

1. Peak flow meters (PFM's), for patients with reversible obstructive airways disease, enable regular home monitoring of peak expiratory flow rate (PEFR). They are primarily intended to assist in the management of asthma through regular objective measurement of peak flow rate. Such measurements are of value in the long term monitoring of treatment and compliance, and provide warning of a deteriorating function and the onset of an acute attack. Meters for short term purposes should normally be provided on loan through the hospital clinic or GP's surgery.

2. The prescribable equipment consists of non-powered, hand-held meters for single patient use. There are two ranges: standard range for use by adults and children; low range for adults or children with severely resticted peak flow. The meters are provided with detachable mouthpiece(s) of durable plastic suitable for both sizes. Replacement mouthpieces are separately prescribable. Detailed user instructions and a purpose-designed record chart are provided with each meter. Replacement charts (Form FP1010) are available to patients from GPs, also pharmacists, via Family Health Services Authorities.

3. Prescribers should ensure that patients have received adequate training when a meter is supplied. This should include advice on recording and interpretation of results, adjustment of personally administered medication and when to seek urgent medical advice in the event of abnormal readings. Instructions in the use of peak flow meters may be given by GPs or other healthcare professionals trained in PEFR monitoring techniques.

4. With careful use the prescribable meters would be expected to last at least three years. Patients should be advised to pay due regard to the manufacturer's user instructions (including maintenance and cleaning of the meter and plastic mouthpieces), and to seek professional advice on the need to replace meters over three years old or where damage is suspected.

5. The prescribable meters are designed to provide for PEF measurement within the following ranges:

    Standard Range (for adults or children)

    　　　Lower Limit - not greater than 150 litres per minute
    　　　Upper Limit - not less than 700 but not greater than 850 litres per minute

    Low Range (for use by adults or children with severely restricted peak flow)

    　　　Lower Limit - not greater than 50 litres per minute
    　　　Upper Limit - not less than 275 but not greater than 400 litres per minute

6. At present the following manufacturers and models are listed:

    Standard Range

Clement Clarke	Model No. 3103XXX series
Ferraris	Model No. 208
Medic-Aid Personal Best	Model No. 755EU
Vitalograph	Model No. 43-2XX series

    Low Range

Clement Clarke	Model No. 3105XXX series superseded by: 3104XXX series
Ferraris	Model No. 209
Medic-Aid Personal Best	Model No. 756EU
Vitalograph	Model No. 43-1XX series

Appliance		Size or Weight	Basic Price p

PESSARIES   each

Ⓧ **Hodges**
Perspex
Specification 20(i)

		8 mm thick	Diameter
		sizes	
Perspex Hodges Pessaries to be supplied against	1	60mm	375
any orders for Vulcanite and Celluloid Hodges	2	65mm	384
Pessaries. Shaped pessaries (eg. Hodges) may	3	68mm	393
revert to a circular shape if boiled.	4	73mm	403
	5	78mm	413
	6	80mm	422
	7	82mm	431
	8	85mm	441
	9	88mm	451
	10	90mm	460
	11	95mm	468
	12	100mm	480

Ring
<u>Fluid Ring</u>
Filled with combination fluid

15mm thick	
1 - 12	554
other sizes	Invoice Price
	(See note 5 Page 93)

<u>Polythene</u>
Specification 20(ii)

7.5mm thick⎫	
50-80mm ⎪	
(rising in 3mm)⎪	164
85-100mm ⎪	
(rising in 5mm)⎪	
110mm ⎭	

<u>PVC</u>
Specification 20(iii)

1.25cm thick⎫	
50-80mm ⎪	
(rising in 3mm)⎪	177
85-100mm ⎪	
(rising in 5mm)⎪	
110mm ⎭	

<u>Watch Spring</u>	Thin	1.25cm thick	
Covered with india-rubber		Sizes 1-12	404
	Medium	1.4cm thick	
		Sizes 1-12	383
		All other sizes	Invoice Price
			(See Note 5 Page 93)

<u>With Perforated Rubber Diaphragm</u>	1.3cm thick	
(Diaphragm Pessary)	Sizes 1-12	299
	51mm to 86mm	
	All other sizes	Invoice price
		(See Note 5 Page 93)

Note: Antiseptics containing phenols or cresols should be avoided as these may be absorbed causing severe irritation in use. The rings may be washed in soapy water or boiled.

Appliance	Size or Weight	Basic Price p

PLASTERS

		each
Ⓧ **Belladonna Adhesive Plaster BP 1980** (Syn: Belladonna Self-Adhesive Plaster; Belladonna Plaster)	Medium 19cm x 12.5cm Large 28cm x 17.5cm	74 126

Ⓧ **Salicylic Acid Adhesive Plaster BP 1980**

See Chiropody Appliances pages 116

Spool Plasters

See Surgical Adhesive Tapes; pages 158-159

PROTECTIVES

		per pkt
EMA Film Gloves-Disposable *(Dispos-A-Gloves)* Specification 21	Small Medium Large (packet of 30)	208
Ⓧ **Polythene Occlusives, Disposable** For use as occlusives with medicated creams.		
Ⓧ **Gloves - Polythene, 100 gauge**	packet of 25	48

			per pkt of 10
Ⓧ **Arm Sleeve - Polythene, 150 gauge**	Small Large	20cm x 30cm 20cm x 60cm	84 84
Ⓧ **Leg Sleeve - Polythene, 150 gauge**	Small Medium Large	25cm x 45cm 32.5cm x 45cm 32.5cm x 75cm	106 106 127
Ⓧ **Foot Bag - Polythene, 150 gauge**		32.5cm x 50cm	84
Ⓧ **Torso Vest - Polythene, 150 gauge**		60cm x 60cm	549
Ⓧ **Trousers - Polythene, 150 gauge**	Large		1584

To be supplied in sealed packets as received from the manufacturer or wholesaler. "The sizes given are lay-flat width x length."

Note: Packets of 10 articles containing the number nearest to the number ordered by the prescriber are to be supplied.
ie. for:

Up to 15 articles,	*1 packet of 10,*
16-25 articles,	*2 packets of 10*

IX/

Appliance	Size or Weight	Basic Price p

RECTAL DILATORS

Specification 22

Ⓧ **Perspex boilable**   each
   (a)   Cone 19mm diam. tapering to 12.5mm   Small   486
        Base 2.5cm diam. - Length 8.6cm

   (b)   Cone 19mm diam. tapering to 15mm   Large   486

The dilators may be washed in hot soapy water.

Ⓧ **SALIVA STIMULATING TABELTS**

SST Saliva Stimulating Tablets   container
                                              of 100   486

STOCKINETTE

To be supplied in sealed packets as received from the
manufacturer or wholesaler.

When Elasticated Stockinette is ordered or prescribed
without qualification, the term is to be interpreted as
Elasticated Tubular Bandage.

Cotton Stockinette, Bleached BP 1988	2.5cm x 1m	29
Heavyweight	5cm x 1m	45
(Syn: Cotton Stockinette)	7.5cm x 1m	54
	10cm x 6m	366

NB:
1m in length for use as a basic for Plaster of Paris or other bandages.
6m length for use as a compression bandage.

Appliance	Size or Weight	Basic Price p

STOCKINETTE - cont

Elasticated Tubular Bandage BP
(Elasticated Surgical Tubular Stockinette; ESTS; Elasticated Stockinette)

Size	Ref	Quantity	(easiGRIP) (P)	(Rediform) (P)	(Sigma ETB) (P)	(Textube) (P)	(Tubigrip) (P)
6.25cm	B	0.5m	61	58	61	57	82
		1.0m	110	105	110	104	149
6.75cm	C	0.5m	65	62	65	60	90
		1.0m	117	112	117	109	157
7.5cm	D	0.5m	65	63	66	60	90
		1.0m	117	114	119	109	157
8.75cm	E	0.5m	74	70	74	68	99
		1.0m	126	120	126	114	170
10.0cm	F	0.5m	74	71	74	68	99
		1.0m	126	120	126	114	170
12.0cm	G	0.5m	77	72	77	73	103
		1.0m	147	138	147	140	196

IXA

1. Where the quantity is not stated by the prescriber the 0.5 metre length should be supplied.
2. Where the size is not stated by the prescriber, the size supplied should be endorsed.
3. Where the brand is not stated by the prescriber the basic price of this stockinette must not exceed:

Size and Quantity	each (p)		each (p)		each (p)
6.25cm x 0.5m	57	7.5cm x 0.5m	60	10.00cm x 0.5m	68
6.25cm x 1.0m	104	7.5cm x 1.0m	109	10.00cm x 1.0m	114
6.75cm x 0.5m	60	8.75cm x 0.5m	68	12.00cm x 0.5m	73
6.75cm x 1.0m	109	8.75cm x 1.0m	114	12.00cm x 1.0m	140

Appliance	Size or Weight	Basic Price p

STOCKINETTE - cont

each

Elasticated Surgical Tubular Stockinette Foam Padded
(Tubipad)
Specification 25

Heel, Elbow,Knee	small 'P4'	6.5cm x 60cm	250
	medium 'P4X'	7.5cm x 60cm	269
	large 'P5'	10cm x 60cm	288
Sacral	small 'P9'	22cm x 27cm	}
	medium 'P9'	28cm x 27cm	} 1287
	large 'P9'	35cm x 27cm	}

Elasticated Viscose Stockinette
(Lightweight Elasticated Viscose Tubular Bandage)
(Tubifast)
Specification 46 and/or CE
A lightweight plain-knitted elasticated tubular fabric
for dressing retention; washable for reuse.

		Length		
		1m	3m	5m
Small Limb	3.5cm (Red Line)	76	-	-
Medium Limb	5.0cm (Green Line)	82	235	402
Large Limb	7.5cm (Blue Line)	110	309	539
Trunks (Child)	10.75cm (Yellow Line)	176	504	865
Trunks (Adult)	17.5cm (Beige Line)	222	-	-

Elastic Net Surgical Tubular Stockinette
Specification 26

A lightweight, elastic, openwork net tubular fabric for
retaining dressings, particularly on awkward sites; for
long-term re-use.

Type A *(Netelast)*

Arm/leg	1.8cm (Size C) x 40cm	36
Thigh/head	2.5cm (Size E) x 60cm	65
Trunk (adult)	4.5cm (Size F) x 60cm	95
Trunk (OS adult)	5.4cm (Size G) x 60cm	128

Type B *(Setonet)* - Now withdrawn
Type C *(Macrofix)* - Now withdrawn

NB:
The size must be specified by the prescriber.

Appliance	Size or Weight	Basic Price p

STOCKINETTE - cont

each

Ribbed Cotton and Viscose Surgical Tubular Stockinette BP1988
(Syn: Ribbed Cotton and Viscose Stockinette)
For use as protective dressings with tar-based and other non-steroid ointments

Type A Lightweight *(Seton)*		
Arm/leg (child); arm (adult)	5cm x 5m	208
Arm (OS adult); leg (adult)	7.5cm x 5m	273
Leg (OS adult)	10cm x 5m	362
Trunk (child)	15cm x 5m	522
Trunk (adult)	20cm x 5m	603
Trunk (OS adult)	25cm x 5m	721
Type B Heavyweight *(Eesiban)*		
Arm/leg (child); arm (adult)	5cm x 5m	208
Arm (OS adult); leg (adult)	7.5cm x 5m	273
Leg (OS adult)	10cm x 5m	362
Trunk (child)	15cm x 5m	522
Trunk (adult)	20cm x 5m	603
Trunk (OS adult)	25cm x 5m	721

N.B.

One 5m length of the relevant width is sufficient to provide two sets of dressing for a pair of limbs or a trunk.
Two full suits for an OS adult are provided from one pack each of the 7.5cm, 10cm and 25cm widths.
Two full suits for a standard sized adult are provided from one pack each of the 5cm, 7.5cm and 20cm widths.
Two full suits for a young child are provided from one pack each of the 5cm and 15cm widths.

SUPRAPUBIC BELTS: Replacements Only   List Price
                                             (See Clause 8B(ii))

N.B.
1. Original Belts are supplied by the Hospital Service.
2. Prescription ordering replacement of a complete Belt or Outfit may only be accepted by a pharmacy or appliance contractor who will carry out the actual measurement, fitting and supply of the belt.
3. Orders for replacement of "a belt" are to be taken as being for the belt alone and the prescription referred back to the prescriber to specify orders for a Complete Belt or Outfit where such appears to be required.

Parts may include the following:

Rubber Flaps
Rubber Shields
Rubber Understraps
Rubber Urinal, single or double-chambered (See Incontinence Appliances - Page 167)
Belt Webbing
Night Drainage Bag, Plastics (See Incontinence Appliances - Page 167)
Night Tube and Glass or Plastics Connector

Appliance	Size or Weight	Basic Price p

each

SUPRAPUBIC CATHETERS

Ⓝ **Catheters, Suprapubic, Self-retaining**
eg. de Pezzer, Malecot's, Dowse's

Invoice Price
(see note 5)
(page 93)

NB:
For prescribable Urethral Catheters including 2 way Foley Catheters see under Catheters, Urethral

Introducers ordered for use with self-retaining catheters.

SURGICAL ADHESIVE TAPES

To be supplied on spools, suitably protected, or in tins
or cartons as received from the manufacturer or
wholesaler.

each

Elastic Adhesive Tape BP 1988	2.5cm x 1.5m	76
(Syn: Elastic Surgical Adhesive Tape)	stretched	
	2.5cm x 4.5m	143
	stretched	
	5cm x 4.5m	
	(See Elastic Adhesive Bandage Page 100).	

Impermeable Plastic Adhesive Tape BP1988	2.5cm x 3m	113
(Syn: Impermeable Plastic Surgical Adhesive Tape)	2.5cm x 5m	169
	5cm x 5m	214
	7.5cm x 5m	312

Impermeable Plastic Synthetic Adhesive Tape BP 1988		
(Syn: Impermeable Plastic Surgical Synthetic Adhesive Tape)	2.5cm x 5m	161
(Blenderm)	5cm x 5m	306

Permeable Woven Synthetic Adhesive Tape BP 1988	1.25cm x 5m	67
(Syn: Permeable Woven Surgical Synthetic Adhesive	2.5cm x 5m	97
Tape)	5cm x 5m	169
(Leukosilk)		

Appliance	Size or Weight	Basic Price p

SURGICAL ADHESIVE TAPES - cont

Permeable Non-Woven Synthetic Adhesive Tape BP 1988
(Syn: Permeable Non-Woven Surgical Synthetic
Adhesive Tape)

Size or Weight	Basic Price (p) each				
	Albufilm	*Albupore*	*Leukopor*	*Micropore*	*Scanpor*
1.25cm x 5m	60	45	45	58	39
2.5 cm x 5m	92	70	70	86	63
5.0 cm x 5m	170	122	123	152	109

		each
Where no brand is stated by the prescriber, the basic	1.25cm x 5m	39
price of the tape supplied must not exceed.	2.5cm x 5m	63
	5cm x 5m	109

Permeable, Apertured Non-Woven Synthetic Adhesive Tape BP 1988
(Syn: Permeable Non-Woven Surgical Synthetic Adhesive Tape)

Mefix	2.5cm x 5m	82
	5cm x 5m	145
	10cm x 5m	232
	15cm x 5m	316
	20cm x 5m	405
	30cm x 5m	581

Zinc Oxide Adhesive Tape BP 1988
(Syn: Zinc Oxide Surgical Adhesive Tape)

	1.25cm x 5m	81
	2.5cm x 5m	117
	5cm x 5m	198
	7.5cm x 5m	297

Appliance	Basic Price p

SURGICAL SUTURES

Ethicon Code No.	Metric Gauge	Length	Needle	per pack of 12

Ⓧ **Absorbable Sutures**
Sterile Catgut Chromic BP

W480	2	75cm	16mm Curved cutting	1816
W548	2	75cm	16mm Curved Round Bodied	1816
W565	3.5	75cm	25mm Tapercut Half Circle Heavy	2356
	(Extra Chromic)			
W488	3.5	75cm	35mm Tapercut Half Circle	2082
W492	3.5	75cm	45mm Tapercut Half Circle Heavy	2177

Ⓧ **Non Absorbable Sutures**
Sterile Polyamide 6 Suture, Monofilament BP

W507	0.7	45cm(black	15mm slim blade curved cutting	1792
W319	1.5	45cm (blue)	19mm curved reverse cutting	1214
W539	1.5	45cm (blue)	25mm slim blade curved cutting	2115
W320	2.0	45cm (blue)	26mm curved reverse	1254

Sterile Polyamide 66 Suture, Braided BP

W5414	3.5	1m (black)	50mm tapercut half circle heavy	1736

Sterile Braided Silk Suture BP

W501	1.5	75cm (black)	16mm curved cutting	1214
W533	2	45cm (black)	25mm super cutting curve	1560
W321	3	45cm (black)	26mm curved reverse cutting	1178

Ⓧ **ADHESIVE, STERILE**

	pack size	
Dermabond	0.5ml	1000
Indermil	0.5g	639

Note:These items are specifically for personal administration by the prescriber.

SKIN CLOSURE STRIPS, STERILE

			per pack of 10 envelopes
Leukostrip Code No. 2952	6.4mm x 76mm	3 strips per env.	518
			12 envelopes
Steri-strip Code No.GP 41	6mm x 75mm	3 strips per env.	837

Note:These items are specifically for personal administration by the prescriber.

Appliance	Size or Weight	Basic Price p

SWABS (see note * below on sterile swabs)
N.B.
The exact number of single swabs ordered by the prescriber is to be dispensed.
(see also Note (ii) below)

<u>Gauze Swabs</u>   per pkt

Gauze Swab Type 13 Light BP 1988, Sterile* Sterile swabs of folded 8-ply undyed gauze	7.5cm sq 5 pads per pkt	33
Gauze Swab Type 13 Light BP 1988, Non Sterile Swabs of folded 8-ply undyed gauze	10cm sq 100 pads per pkt	527
Filmated Gauze Swab BP 1988 Non Sterile A thin layer of absorbent cotton enclosed within Absorbent Cotton Gauze Type 13 Light BP 1988 8-ply	10cm sq 100 pads per pkt	724

<u>Non-Woven Fabric Swabs</u>
The labelling of each pack shall include:
The Title
"Drug Tariff Specification" and number

Non-Woven Fabric Swab, Sterile* Specification 28 Sterile swabs of folded 4-ply non-woven fabric. These swabs are an alternative to gauze swabs, Type 13 Light BP 1988 sterile.	7.5cm sq 5 pads per pkt	21
Non-Woven Fabric Swab, Non Sterile Specification 28 Swabs of folded 4-ply non-woven fabric. These swabs are an alternative to gauze swabs, Type 13 Light BP 1988, for general and cleansing purposes.	10cm sq 100 pads per pkt	247
Filmated Non-Woven Fabric Swab Non-Sterile *(Regal)* Specification 29 Swabs of folded 8-ply non-woven viscose fabric containing a film of viscose fibres to increase absorbency. These swabs are an alternative to Filmated Gauze Swabs BP 1988 for general swabbing and cleansing purposes.	10cm sq 100 pads per pkt	535

*Notes: Sterile Swabs
(i) These sterile dressings are to be supplied in packs of 5 swabs 7.5cm square in a sealed packs as received from the manufacturer, supplier or wholesaler. They should not be confused with the non-sterile 10cm size in packets of 100 swabs used for general swabbing purposes.

(ii) The exact number of sterile swabs ordered are to be supplied except for orders not in multiples of 5 (See Note 2 Page 93). A packet to be used for each sterile dressing operation; unused swabs to be discarded as unsterile.

Appliance	Size or Weight	Basic Price p

⊗ SYNOVIAL FLUID — each
Fermathron — Box containing 1 pre-filled 20mg/2ml syringe — 3900

Orthovisc — Box containing 3 pre-filled 2ml syringes (1 treatment) — 19500

Box containing 1 pre-filled 2ml syringe — 6500

Supartz — Box containing 5 pre-filled 25mg/2.5ml syringes (1 treatment) — 20500

Synvisc (Hylan G-F20) — Box containing 3 pre-filled 2ml syringes (1 treatment) — 20500

⊗ SYRINGES

Bladder/Irrigating Polypropylene with catheter nozzle graduated from 0 to 100mL in 5mL graduation marks, clearly numbered in multiples of 10 — 100mL — 361

Ear Plastics-plasticised PVC polymer, moulded in one piece, fine pointed — 60mL approx — 164

Enema Higginson's: — 528
Plastics - plasticised PVC polymer or rubber bulb, with inverted flutter valve moulded in the tube, or with metal valve, (duralumin or pewter), inserted in the tube; full length tubes; polypropylene rectal pipe; PVC polymer or rubber vaginal pipe; PVC polymer shield.

Spare Vaginal Pipes Plastics or rubber, straight — 15cm — 42

⊗ TAPELESS DRESSING HOLDERS
Breast Dressing Holder — petite — 500
— small — 620
— medium — 680
— large — 800

Facial Dressing Holder — small — 408
— large — 468

Neck Dressing Holder — one size — 450

T-Vest Dressing Holder — small — 678
— medium — 803
— large — 873
— extra large — 950

⊗ TAPELESS IV HOLDERS
Tapeless Arm IV Holder — small — 230
— medium — 270

Tapeless Hand IV Holder — small — 220
— medium — 225
— large — 245

Appliance	Order No.	Basic Price p

Ⓧ TEST TUBES	12.5cm x 16mm	11

TRACHEOSTOMY AND LARYNGECTOMY APPLIANCES

Ⓧ **Tracheostomy Breathing Aids**

each

Provox Stomafilter
A filter and heat and moisture exchanger consisting of an adhesive and a filter cassette for laryngectomies.

Flexiderm adhesive round	(Transparent with	7253	271
Flexiderm adhesive oval	strong adhesive)	7254	271
Optiderm adhesive round	(Skin coloured, hydrocolloid	7255	446
Optiderm adhesive oval	for sensitive skin)	7256	446
Regular adhesive round	(Transparent, normal	7251	175
Regular adhesive oval	adhesive)	7252	175
Normal filter cassette	(Normal resistance)	7240	164
Hiflow filter cassette	(Low resistance for sport and first time users)	7241	175

IXA

Trachi-Naze Nasal Restoration System (formerly *Neo-Naze Filter System)*
A breathing aid, which helps to heat, moisten and filter, inspired air where appropriate, artificial airway resistance may improve lung function and oxygenation in patients with tracheosotomies

Blue Filter (Night filter)	resistance level	- 2 to - 3k Pas 1-[1]	LANNZ 0001A	142
Green Filter (Day filter)	resistance level	- 1 to 2k Pas 1-[2]	LANNZ 0002A	142
Orange Filter (Active filter)	resistance level less than - 1k Pas 1-[1]		LANNZ 0003A	142

Baseplate			
Hydrocolloid	(standard)	LANNZ 0004A	224
Hydrocolloid	(large)	LANNZ 0005	239
Non-Woven Adhesive (large)		LANNZ 0006	239

Ⓧ **Tracheostomy Brushes**

Tracheo Cleaning Brush (*Kapitex*)	8mm	311
	10mm	311
	12mm	311
	14mm	311

Ⓧ **Tracheostomy Dressings - Sterile**

Metalline		8cm x 9cm	49
Trachi-Dress	TR DRE 0001 Small	60mm x 82mm	60
	TR DRE 0002 Large	80mm x 100mm	60

Ⓧ **Tracheostomy Tube Holders**

Tapeless Tracheostomy Tube Holder	621	280 |

Appliance	Size or Weight	Basic Price p

TRACHEOSTOMY AND LARYNGECTOMY APPLIANCES- cont

Tracheostomy and Laryngectomy Protectors

		per pack of 10
Ⓧ *Buchanan Protector* (Laryngectomy - Permanent tracheostomy) width 21cm x mid-point height 19cm	Small Standard	2933 3182

A bib of plastics foam, covered with knitted
fabric of honeycomb pattern, bound together at
the edges by tape, which is extended for tying around
the neck.

Ⓧ *Buchanan DeltaNex Protector* (Laryngectomy - Permanent tracheostomy)	Small	2964

A bib of plastics foam, covered with knitted
fabric of honeycomb pattern, bound together
at the edges by tape. A Velcro strip is sewn
onto the top edge for attachment to the DeltaNex
neckband.
The DeltaNex neckband incorporates Velcro strips
for 'touch to close' fastening onto the strip of
Velcro on the bib and for fastening around the
neck.
Two neckbands are supplied with each pack of 10 bibs.

Ⓧ *Hirst Protector*		2689

A bib comprising two layers of a knitted,
net material bound together at the edges with
an attached neckband which fastens at the
rear of the neck with a Velcro type fastener.

		each
Ⓧ *Laryngofoam* flesh or white	5.1cm x 6.2cm 4mm thick	35 per pack of 30
An individually wrapped piece of plastics foam with an adhesive strip along the top edge.		1050

Appliance	Size or Weight	Basic Price p

TRUSSES

The price listed in respect of a truss specified in the following list is the basic price (see Part II, Clause 8) on which payment will be calculated pursuant to Part II, Clause 6A and B for the supply of such a truss. PROVIDED it is so supplied on an order by the prescriber and complies fully with the specification, included in this Part (see Note 5) and in the Drug Tariff Technical Specifications.

Before the prescription can be dispensed three details must be given by the prescriber:
(i)   Single, or double, and the side, if single
(ii)   Position, eg. Inguinal; Scrotal
(iii)   Type, eg. Spring truss; Elastic band truss

In the event of a dispute between the patient and the pharmacy or the appliance contractor about whether the truss supplied is satisfactory, the doctor's decision shall be binding.

TRUSSES
(See Part 1, Clause 2 Page 3)

Ⓧ   **Spring Truss**
Specification 31(a)
Spring Trusses shall conform to the British Standard   each
2930 : 1970 for Surgical Spring Trusses

Inguinal	Single	2681
	Double	3742
Inguinal Rat-tail	Single	3302
	Double	4934
Femoral	Single	2962
	Double	4582
Scrotal	Single	3302
	Double	4934
Double Inguinal/Scrotal		4745
Back Pad, fixed or sliding (if ordered)	extra	761
Slotted, polished Spring Ends (if ordered)	Single Extra	387
	Double Extra	779
"Special" Trusses	Single Extra	854
- conforming to the requirements in	Double Extra	1687
Specification 31b		

NB:
Requirement for a "Special" Truss should normally be confirmed by the prescriber.

Replacements and repairs:-
Understrap for Inguinal or Femoral Trusses   235

IXA

Appliance	Size or Weight	Basic Price p

TRUSSES - cont

Ⓧ   **Elastic Band Truss**
Specification 31b
Elastic Band Trusses shall conform to the British
Standard 3271: 1970 for Surgical Elastic Band Trusses   each

Inguinal	Single	1821
	Double	3033
Scrotal	Single	1896
	Double	3087
Umbilical, Single Belt		2068
Double Belt where specified by prescriber		2815
"Special" Trusses	Single Extra	535
- conforming to the requirements in	Double Extra	775
Specification 31b		

NB:
Requirement for a "Special" Truss should normally be confirmed by the prescriber

---

URINALS, PORTABLE - see Incontinence Appliances - page 167

---

                            each

URINE SUGAR ANALYSIS SET (Clinitest)   382
(For detection of glycosuria)
Test tube, dropper, colour chart, instruction sheet
and analysis record, with one bottle of 36 Diagnostic
Solution-Tablets of Copper, in a suitable container.

Replacement Test Tubes, hard glass   35

Replacement Droppers, glass with fine pointed Rubber teat   35

Replacement Diagnostic Solution Tablets of Copper (See page 383)

INCONTINENCE APPLIANCES

1.   Prescribers and suppliers should note that products not included in the list are not prescribable (See Part 1 Clause 2). Attention is drawn particularly to the information on the average life-in-use of each type of product which, together with the pack size, should enable prescribers to calculate their patients' requirements with reasonable accuracy.

2.   Only basic information on each product has been provided and prescribers may on occasions wish to seek further information about certain products eg when assessing a patient for the first time. If so, this is always available from the manufacturers (addresses and telephone numbers are given at the end of the entry). Information may also be sought from community nurses and community pharmacists. Where possible manufacturers'/suppliers' order code numbers have been shown but prescribers should note that the order numbers shown are not necessarily the full codes for the appliances they wish to order. This is particularly true of urinal systems where additional code numbers are usually necessary to denote variations from the basic design and individual sizes.

3.   Prescribers are reminded that incontinence pads (including products not necessarily described as such but using the absorption principle), incontinence garments, skin wipes and occlusive devices such as female vaginal devices and male penile clamps are not prescribable under the Drug Tariff provisions.

List of components and accessories	Page
Anal Plugs	168
Catheter Valves	169
Drainable Dribbling Appliances	170
Faecal Collectors	170
Incontinence Belts	171
Incontinence Sheaths	172
Incontinence Sheath Fixing Strips and Adhesives	180
Leg Bags	182
Night Drainage Bags	189
Suspensory Systems	192
Tubing and Accessories	193
Urinal Systems	197

IXB

Cross Reference Index of Product Ranges and Manufacturers (page 218)
Manufacturers' Addresses and Telephone Numbers (page 220)

ANAL PLUGS

Warning: This product should not be used without assessment by an appropriate medical professional.

Manufacturer	Appliance	Order No.	Quantity	List Price p
Coloplast Ltd	Conveen Anal Plug			
	Small	1450	20	3934
	Large	1451	20	3934

CATHETER VALVES

Warning: This product should not be used without assessment of bladder function by an appropriate medical professional.

Indications: For use with an indwelling urethral catheter.

Contraindications:
Reduced bladder capacity
No bladder sensation
Cognitive impairment
Insufficient manual dexterity to operate the Catheter Valve

Note: *It is recommended that the Catheter Valve is changed every 5 - 7 days.*

Manufacturer	Appliance	Order No.	Quantity	List Price p
Bard Ltd	Flip-Flo catheter valve	BFF5	5	1166
EMS Medical Ltd - see Simpla Continence Care				
Jade- Euro-Med Ltd S Euro Catheter Valve		JECV	5	1100
L.I.N.C. Medical Systems Ltd				
S CareVent Duo Catheter Valve		08.9801	5	1166
Simpla Continence Care	Simpla Catheter Valve	T180	5	1160
SIMS Portex Ltd	Uro-Flo Catheter Valve	WS856-01-A	5	1119

Catheter Valve with Integral Bag

Manufacturer	Appliance	Order No.	Quantity	List Price p
Jade-Euro-Med Ltd S Euro Bag with duel tap		JEDT	10	2650

IXB

S   These Catheter Valves are supplied sterile

DRAINABLE DRIBBLING APPLIANCES

Bags or pouches which use absorptive material to soak up urine are not prescribable.

Note: The appliances listed below may be re-used, on average, for at least a month.

Manufacturer	Appliance	Order No.	Quantity	List Price p
Body's Surgical Company - see Jade-Euro-Med Ltd				
CS Bullen Ltd	Dribblet bag	LU-15	10	2257
	Dribblet sheath bag	LU-20	10	5066
DePuy Healthcare - see Simpla Continence Care				
Jade-Euro-Med Ltd	Dribbling bag with loops and tapes	Fig 18	1	1703
	Drip Male Urinal with tap	M 100	1	4576
	Replacement belt for M100	JB 100	1	1128
Leyland Medical Ltd, (Peoplecare) - see Rüsch UK Ltd				
Rüsch UK Ltd	Peoplecare drip male urinal	755300	1	5025
Simpla Continence Care	Aquadry drip type urinal	571016	1	5329
Ward Surgical Appliance Co.	Male Dribbling bag with diaphragm and belt	WM60	1	2792

FAECAL COLLECTORS

Manufacturer	Appliance	Order No.	Quantity	List Price p
Hollister Ltd	Incare Faecal Collector			
	500ml	9822	10	3960
	1000ml	9821	10	3960

INCONTINENCE BELTS

Note: Average Life-in-Use - 6 Months

Manufacturer	Appliance	Order No.	Quantity	List Price p
Body's Surgical Company - see Jade-Euro-Med Ltd				
Downs Surgical Ltd - see SIMS Portex Ltd				
GU Manufacturing Ltd - see S G & P Payne				
Jade-Euro-Med Ltd	Waist belt for Kipper bags	KBWB	1	554
	37mm webbing/elastic waistbelt for use with Jade-Euro-Med appliances	WB	1	564
Leyland Medical Ltd (Peoplecare) - see Rüsch Ltd				
Rüsch UK Ltd	Waist and support for Kipper bag	886103	1	651
Simcare - see SIMS Portex Ltd				
SIMS Portex Ltd	Rubber belt	WS101-61-A	1	551
	Web Belt	WS105-91-C	1	1101
		WS106-01-C	1	1101
		WS107-01-G	1	1101
Ward Surgical Appliance Co	Waist belt for black kipper bag	WM62	1	513
	Rubber belt for PP Urinal	WM63	1	444

IXB

INCONTINENCE SHEATHS

The incontinence sheaths (also known as penile sheaths and external catheters) listed below, are, except where indicated, of the soft, flexible, latex type. Sheaths are available with and without fixing devices which may be applied externally (around the outside of the sheath) or internally (around the penis between the skin and the sheath). A list of fixing devices and other adhesion products is included at page 177

Note: Each Sheath may be left in place for 1 to 3 days between changes.

Manufacturer	Appliance	Order No.	Quantity	List Price p
Aldington Laboratores Ltd - See Rüsch UK Ltd				
Bard Ltd	⊙ Integrity encompass			
	Self-adhesive penile sheath on applicator			
	25mm	BUIS 25	30	4174
	30mm	BUIS 30	30	4174
	35mm	BUIS 35	30	4174
	Reliasheath Penile sheath			
	(including adhesive strip)	D52	30	3827
	20mm, 25mm, 30mm,			
	35mm, 40mm			
	⊗ Penile Sheath 20mm, 25mm,	U52	30	2564
	30mm, 35mm, 40mm			
	⊗ Uro sheath (washable - may be	1502	1	535
	re-used many times)			
	small (28.5mm),			
	medium (38mm),			
	large (44.5mm)			
CliniMed Ltd	≐ CliniFlex Medimates incontinence sheath with			
	single sided adhesive strip			
	(Straight)			
	20mm	S20S	30	2935
	25mm	S25S	30	2935
	30mm	S30S	30	2935
	35mm	S35S	30	2935
	40mm	S40S	30	2935
	(Bulb) 25mm	B25S	30	2935
	30mm	B30S	30	2935
	35mm	B35S	30	2935
	double sided adhesive strip			
	(Straight)			
	20mm	S20D	30	3131
	25mm	S25D	30	3131
	30mm	S30D	30	3131
	35mm	S35D	30	3131
	40mm	S40D	30	3131
	(Bulb) 25mm	B25D	30	3131
	30mm	B30D	30	3131
	35mm	B35D	30	3131

⊗ Non-adhesive sheath without liner.
⊙ Sheath with self-adhesive liner.
≐ Sheath with separate single-sided adhesive strip.

INCONTINENCE SHEATHS cont

Manufacturer	Appliance	Order No.	Quantity	List Price p
Coloplast Ltd	☉ Conveen Security + self-sealing Urisheath (non-latex) with Anti-kink Design			
	extra small	5221	30	4449
	small	5225	30	4449
	medium	5230	30	4449
	large	5235	30	4449
	extra large	5240	30	4449
	↕ Conveen Security + Sheath (non-latex) with Anti-kink Design (including Uriliner adhesive strip)			
	extra small	5021	30	4494
	small	5025	30	4494
	medium	5030	30	4494
	large	5035	30	4494
	extra large	5040	30	4494
	☉ Conveen self-sealing Urisheath			
	extra small	5212	30	4425
	small	5200	30	4425
	medium	5205	30	4425
	large	5210	30	4425
	extra large	5215	30	4425
	☉ Conveen self-sealing Urisheath short			
	20mm	23001	30	4425
	25mm	23002	30	4425
	30mm	23003	30	4425
	35mm	23004	30	4425
	40mm	23005	30	4425
	↕ Conveen Urisheath/Uriliner			
	very small	5120	30	4473
	small	5125	30	4473
	medium	5130	30	4473
	large	5135	30	4473
	ex-large	5140	30	4473

DePuy Healthcare - see Seton Continence Care

Downs Surgical Ltd - see SIMS Portex Ltd

Eschmann Bros and Walsh Ltd - see SIMS Portex Ltd

Fry Surgical International Ltd	↕ Uridom (including adhesive strip)	476-413-130	30	2707

☉ Sheath with self-adhesive liner.
↕ Sheath with separate double-sided adhesive strip.

INCONTINENCE SHEATHS cont

Manufacturer	Appliance		Order No.	Quantity	List Price p
Hollister Ltd ⊙	InCare Incontinence Sheath (Self-adhesive)				
	22-25mm		9636	30	4289
	26-30mm		9637	30	4289
	31-35mm		9639	30	4289
	36-39mm		9638	30	4289
Hospital Management and Supplies Ltd ≐	Macrodom (including adhesive strip)				
	with ✚ 51mm tube		GS7654	30	2230
	with ✚ 127mm tube		GS7655	25	2333
† ↕	Macrodom Plus (including adhesive strip)				
	small		GS7656	30	2300
	medium		GS7657	30	2300
	large		GS7658	30	2300
Jade-Euro-Med Ltd ⊙	Jade Ultra Flex Clear Sheath (Self-adhesive)				
	small		M510	30	4243
	medium		M520	30	4243
	intermediate		M530	30	4243
	large		M540	30	4243
	ex-large		M550	30	4243
Manfred Sauer ⊗	Comfort Sheath (in 11 sizes) + Residual Free removal and Anti-Blow-Back system				
	Paediatric	(dia 18mm)	53.18	30	2174
	Small -	(dia 20mm)	53.20	30	2174
	Small	(dia 22mm)	53.22	30	2174
	Small +	(dia 24mm)	53.24	30	2174
	Medium -	(dia 26mm)	53.26	30	2174
	Medium	(dia 28mm)	53.28	30	2174
	Medium +	(dia 30mm)	53.30	30	2174
	Large -	(dia 32mm)	53.32	30	2174
	Large	(dia 35mm)	53.35	30	2174
	Large +	(dia 37mm)	53.37	30	2174
	Extra Large	(dia 40mm)	53.40	30	2174
⊗	Comfort Sheath Extra Thin for male retraction + Residual Free removal and Anti-Blow-Back system.				
	Medium -	(dia 26mm)	53.26D	30	2174
	Medium +	(dia 30mm)	53.30D	30	2174
	Large	(dia 35mm)	53.35D	30	2174
	Extra Large	(dia 40mm)	53.40D	30	2174

†   to be deleted 1 January 2001
⊗   Non-adhesive sheath without liner
⊙   Sheath with self-adhesive liner.
↕   Sheath with separate double-sided adhesive strip.
≐   Sheath with separate single-sided adhesive strip.

INCONTINENCE SHEATHS - cont

Manufacturer	Appliance	Order No.	Quantity	List Price p

Manfred Sauer - cont

⊗   K + ICS Sheath (plus 5 Sheath tip connectors) have special removable tips which enable the sheath to be expanded over the penis with a special sheath expander tool, to allow for clean intermittent self catheterisation (see Tubing and Accessories section of this publication for Manfred Sauer Sheath Expander order no. 100.01).

		Order No.	Quantity	List Price p
	18mm	103.18	30	4450
	20mm	103.20	30	4450
	22mm	103.22	30	4450
	24mm	103.24	30	4450
	26mm	103.26	30	4450
	28mm	103.28	30	4450
	30mm	103.30	30	4450
	32mm	103.32	30	4450
	35mm	103.35	30	4450
	37mm	103.37	30	4450
	40mm	103.40	30	4450

IXB

⊗   Non-adhesive sheath without liner

INCONTINENCE SHEATHS - cont

Manufacturer	Appliance	Order No.	Quantity	List Price p
North West Medical ⊗ Supplies Ltd	Uridrop Incontinence Sheath			
	Size 1 (70mm)	30/80	30	1270
	Size 2 (80mm)	30/81	30	1270
	Size 3 (100mm)	30/82	30	1270
	Size 4 (107mm)	30/83	30	1270
	Size Paed 42mm	30/60	30	1270
	Size Paed 55mm	30/61	30	1270
↕	Uridrop Incontinence Sheath and Uristrip Adhesive Strip			
	Size 1 (70mm)	8480	30	2540
	Size 2 (80mm)	8481	30	2540
	Size 3 (100mm)	8482	30	2540
	Size 4 (107mm)	8483	30	2540
	Size Paed 42mm	8460	30	2540
	Size Paed 55mm	8461	30	2540
Rochester Medical ⊙ Corporation	Natural Silicone Sheath (self-adhesive)			
	25mm	31301	30	4170
	29mm	31302	30	4170
	32mm	31303	30	4170
	36mm	31304	30	4170
	41mm	31305	30	4170
⊙	Pop-On Silicone Sheath (self-adhesive)			
	25mm	32301	30	4170
	29mm	32302	30	4170
	32mm	32303	30	4170
	36mm	32304	30	4170
	41mm	32305	30	4170
⊙	Wide Band Silicone Sheath (self-adhesive)			
	25mm	36301	30	4170
	29mm	36302	30	4170
	32mm	36303	30	4170
	36mm	36304	30	4170
	41mm	36305	30	4170
S G & P Payne ⊗ Supplies Ltd	Incontiaid Penile Sheath			
	20mm	1111	1	87
	25mm	1112	1	87
	30mm	1113	1	87
	35mm	1114	1	87
	40mm	1115	1	87
↕	with adhesive strip			
	20mm	1116	10	1385
	25mm	1117	10	1385
	30mm	1118	10	1385
	35mm	1119	10	1385
	40mm	1120	10	1385

⊗   Non-adhesive sheath without liner.
↕   Sheath with separate double-sided adhesive strip.
⊙   Sheath with self-adhesive liner.

INCONTINENCE SHEATHS - cont

Manufacturer		Appliance	Order No.	Quantity	List Price p
Rüsch Uk Ltd	↕	Dryaid Penile Sheath (including adhesive strip)			
		small	834021	20	2708
		medium	834022	20	2708
		large	834023	20	2708
		ex-large	834024	20	2708
	⊗	Dryaid Penile Sheath (without strip)			
		small	861021	20	1569
		medium	861022	20	1569
		large	861023	20	1569
		ex-large	861024	20	1569
	↕	Portasheath			
		25mm	800046	25	2202
		30mm	800047	25	2202
		35mm	800048	25	2202
	≐	Secure external catheter kit (including adhesive strip)			
		25mm diameter	4000025	10	902
		30mm diameter	4000030	10	902
		35mm diameter	4000035	10	902
Salts Healthcare	↕	Heritage Cohesive/Sheath Pack			
		17mm	ZL0023	30	3550
		22mm	ZL0024	30	3550
		25mm	ZL0025	30	3550
		32mm	ZL0026	30	3550
		34mm	ZL0027	30	3550
	⊗	Male Continence Sheath			
		17mm	ZL0028	10	800
		22mm	ZL0029	10	800
		25mm	ZL0030	10	800
		32mm	ZL0031	10	800
		34mm	ZL0032	10	800

Sherwood Medical Industries Ltd - see The Kendall Company (UK) Ltd

Simcare - see SIMS Portex Ltd

Simpla Continence Care					
	⊗	Aquadry Penile Sheath			
		small - (dia. 22mm)	570508	10	1059
		medium - (dia. 26mm)	570516	10	1059
		large - (dia. 28mm)	570524	10	1059
		ex-large - (dia 32mm)	570532	10	1059

IXB

⊗   Non-adhesive sheath without liner.
↕   Sheath with separate double-sided adhesive strip.
≐   Sheath with separate single-sided adhesive strip.

INCONTINENCE SHEATHS - cont

Manufacturer	Appliance	Order No.	Quantity	List Price p
Simpla Continence Care - cont				
⊙	Aquadry Freedom Sheath (Self-adhesive)			
	small (dia 21mm)	786268	30	4338
	medium (dia 25mm)	786276	30	4338
	standard (dia 31mm)	786280	30	4338
	large (dia 35mm)	786284	30	4338
	extra large (dia 40mm)	786288	30	4338
⊙	Aquadry Freedom Plus Sheath (Self-adhesive) (Shorter length)			
	small (dia 21mm)	786292	30	4338
	medium (dia 25mm)	786306	30	4338
	standard (dia 31mm)	786310	30	4338
	large (dia 35mm)	786314	30	4338
	extra large (dia 40mm)	786318	30	4338
⊙	Clear Advantage Silicone Sheath (Self-adhesive)			
	small (dia 23mm)	786187	30	4317
	medium (dia 28mm)	786195	30	4317
	standard (dia 31mm)	786225	30	4317
	large (dia 35mm)	786233	30	4317
	extra large (dia 40mm)	786241	30	4317
≏	Simpla U-Sheath Plus (with External Liner) - Non-Latex			
	Small	380820	30	2977
	Medium	380821	30	2977
	Large	380822	30	2977
	Ex-large	380823	30	2977
↕	Simpla U-Sheath Plus (with Uriseal Liner) - Non-Latex			
	Small	380910	30	4199
	Medium	380911	30	4199
	Large	380912	30	4199
	Ex-large	380913	30	4199
↕	Simpla U-Sheath (with Uriseal Liner) - Latex			
	Small	386131	30	3859
	Medium	386132	30	3859
	Large	386133	30	3859
	Ex-large	386134	30	3859

⊙   Sheath with self-adhesive liner.
≏   Sheath with separate single-sided adhesive strip.
↕   Sheath with separate double-sided adhesive strip.

INCONTINENCE SHEATHS - cont

Manufacturer	Appliance	Order No.	Quantity	List Price p
SIMS Portex Ltd ⊗	Incontinence Sheath			
	Small	WS165-01-F	1	147
	Medium	WS165-03-K	1	147
	Large	WS165-05-P	1	147
	Ex-large	WS165-07-T	1	147
⊙	Transfix Silicone Sheath, standard self adhering			
	25mm	TF12530	30	4170
	29mm	TF12930	30	4170
	32mm	TF13230	30	4170
	36mm	TF13630	30	4170
	41mm	TF14130	30	4170
⊙	Transfix Silicone Sheath, shorter with a narrow band of adhesive			
	25mm	TF22530	30	4170
	29mm	TF22930	30	4170
	32mm	TF23230	30	4170
	36mm	TF23630	30	4170
	41mm	TF24130	30	4170
⊙	Transfix Silicone Sheath, with a wide band of adhesive			
	25mm	TF32530	30	4170
	29mm	TF32930	30	4170
	32mm	TF33230	30	4170
	36mm	TF33630	30	4170
	41mm	TF34130	30	4170
↕	Uro Flo Sheath (including adhesive strip)			
	Small	WS166-01-K	30	3999
	Medium	WS166-02-M	30	3999
	Large	WS166-03-P	30	3999
↕	Uro Flo Sheath Mk 2			
	Small	WR166-01-N	30	3999
	Medium	WR166-02-Q	30	3999
	Large	WR166-03-S	30	3999
⊗	Male Incontinence Sheath	48-232-14	100	6625
The Kendall Company (UK) Ltd				
↕	Texas Catheter (including adhesive strip)	8884-731300	12	864
↕	Uri Drain Sheath double sided adhesive strap			
	Medium (30mm)	1814-736700	10	800

Warne Franklin Medical Ltd - See Rüsch UK Ltd

⊗   Non-adhesive sheath without liner.
↕   Sheath with separate double-sided adhesive strip.
⊙   Sheath with self-adhesive liner.

INCONTINENCE SHEATH FIXING STRIPS & ADHESIVES
(Available separately from sheaths)

Manufacturer		Appliance	Order No.	Quantity	List Price p
Aldington Laboratories Ltd - see Rüsch UK Ltd					
Associated Hospital Supply - see Bio Diagnostics					
Bio Diagnostics	↕	Urifix Tape 5m	SU1	1	490
Camp Ltd	≠	Posey Sheath Holder			
		Adult	90500	12	1325
		Paediatric	6555	12	1020
CliniMed Ltd	↕	CliniFlex Medimates Adhesive Security Strips	A30D	30	1000
	≐	CliniFlex Medimates Adhesive Security Strips	A30S	30	800
ConvaTec Ltd	↕	Urihesive Strips	S120	15	655
DePuy Healthcare - see Simpla Continence Care					
Dow Corning Ltd	•⋈	Adhesive B (Silicone Adhesive Aerosol)	895-6	150mL/ 207g	1002
	•⋈	355 Medical Adhesive (brush-on silicone adhesive)	DC355	20mL	303
EMS Medical Ltd - see Simpla Continence Care					
JLJ Healthcare Ltd	↕	Urifix Tape 5m (formerly a Seton Continence Care product)	T115	1	634
Manfred Sauer	*	Original Latex Skin Adhesive in a 28g tube with a long pipette/nozzle applicator	50.01	2	809
	*	Pure Latex Skin Adhesive without any skin care components giving a stronger bond, in a 28g tube with a long pipette/nozzle applicator.	50.00	2	809
	*	Lanolin Free Latex Skin Adhesive for people allergic to lanolin, in a 28g tube with a long pipette/nozzle applicator.	50.03	2	809
	*	50% reduction in skin care components, in a 28g tube with a long pipette/nozzle applicator.	50.05	2	809

≐   Single-sided adhesive strip
↕   Double-sided adhesive strip
≠   Foam and Velcro
⋈   For use with urinal systems (see page 197)
•   Temporarily unavailable
*   Safe for direct application on the skin

INCONTINENCE SHEATH FIXING STRIPS & ADHESIVES
(Available separately from sheaths)

Manufacturer		Appliance	Order No.	Quantity	List Price p
Manfred Sauer - cont	*	2% Resin giving a stronger bond than the original adhesive 50.01, in a 28g tube with a long pipette/nozzle applicator. Should only be tried after 50.01 is found to be too weak.	50.20	2	809
	*	12% Resin giving a stronger bond than the 2% resin adhesive 50.20, in a 28g tube with a long pipette/nozzle applicator. Should only be tried after 50.20 is found to be too weak.	50.22	2	809
	*	Synthetic Skin Adhesive in a 28g tube with a long pipette/nozzle applicator	50.36-2	2	1419
	*	Synthetic Skin Adhesive in a 45mL bottle with brush in the lid	50.36	1	1419
North West Medical Supplies Ltd	⇕	Uristrip Adhesive Strip	30/84	30	1270
S G & P Payne	≠	Incontiaid Sheath Holder	1123	1	101
	⇕	Adhesive Strips	1002	10	450
Rehab Products - see Camp Ltd					
Rüsch UK Ltd	⇕	Dryaid Strip	832025	20	1139
Salts Healthcare	≠	Heritage Sheath Collar Pack	ZL0022	30	401
Simpla Continence Care					
	⇕	Aquadry Penile Liners	781649	20	867
Squibb Surgicare Ltd - see ConvaTec Ltd					

IXB

*   Safe for direct application on the skin
⇕   Double-sided adhesive strip
≠   Foam and Velcro

LEG BAGS

The leg bags listed are suitable for collection of urine from indwelling catheters or incontinence sheaths. They are intended for daytime use although the larger bags may have adequate capacity for overnight use by some patients. The bags may be worn in different positions on the leg and the intended position (eg thigh, knee or calf) will determine the length of the inlet tube. The bags are attached to the leg by means of straps (included with each pack) which are generally either latex or foam with velcro fasteners.

Note: *Plastic leg bags identified in the list with an asterisk* may on average be used for 5-7 days. With proper care and cleansing rubber leg bags are re-usable for 4-6 months.*

Manufacturer	Appliance	Order No.	Quantity	List Price p
Aldington Laboratories Ltd - see Rüsch UK Ltd				
Bard Ltd S *	Uriplan Range:			
	Shaped Leg Bags with tap outlet,			
	overnight connector and elastic velcro straps			
*	350mL, direct inlet	D3S	10	2562
*	350mL, 30cm inlet tube	D3L	10	2539
*	500mL, direct inlet	D5S	10	2581
*	500mL, 10cm inlet tube	D5M	10	2591
*	500mL, 30cm inlet tube	D5L	10	2591
*	750mL, direct inlet	D7S	10	2600
*	750mL, 10cm inlet tube	D7M	10	2600
*	750mL, 30cm inlet tube	D7L	10	2600
*	750mL, 38cm adjustable inlet tube	D7LX	10	2600
S *	Urisac Range:			
	Leg Bags with push/pull outlet and foam velcro straps			
*	350mL, long tube	7660	10	1359
*	350mL, short tube	7661	10	1319
*	500mL, long tube	7662	10	1477
*	500mL, short tube	7663	10	1436
*	750mL, long tube	7664	10	1579
*	750mL, short tube	7665	10	1515
Body's Surgical Company - see Jade-Euro-Med Ltd				
Bradgate Unitech Ltd - see Pharma-Plast Ltd				
Coloplast Ltd *	Conveen Security+ leg bag 350mL			
	25cm tube	5164	10	2134
	50cm tube	5165	10	2134
*	Conveen Security+ leg bag 500mL			
	25cm tube	5160	10	2134
	50cm tube	5161	10	2134
S	25cm tube	5162	10	2269
S	50cm tube	5163	10	2269
*	Conveen Security+ leg bag 750mL			
	25cm tube	5166	10	2134
	50cm tube	5167	10	2134

S   These leg bags are supplied sterile. This does not affect the guidance given in the note on page 181.
*   Plastics

LEG BAGS - cont

Manufacturer	Appliance	Order No.	Quantity	List Price p
Coloplast Ltd - cont *	Conveen Contour 600mL leg bag			
	(adjustable tube)	5170	10	2591
S	5cm inlet tube	5172	10	2591
S	30cm inlet tube	5173	10	2591
*	Conveen Contour 800mL leg bag			
S	45cm tube	5175	10	2591
ConvaTec Ltd *	500mL Accuseal leg bag	S450	10	1919

DePuy Healthcare - see Simpla Continence Care

Downs Surgical Ltd - see SIMS Portex Ltd

EMS Medical Ltd - see Simpla Continence Care

Flexicare Medical Ltd	Flexicare leg bag with lever tap outlet,			
	night drainage connector and velcro anti slip straps			
S*	350mL, short tube	00-1352	10	2220
S*	500mL, short tube	00-1502	10	2220
S*	750mL, short tube	00-1752	10	2220
S*	350mL, long tube	00-2352	10	2220
S*	500mL, long tube	00-2502	10	2220
S*	750mL, long tube	00-2752	10	2220
S*	500mL, (60cm adjustable tube)	00-3502	10	2260
*	500mL, (60cm adjustable tube)	00-3501	10	2150

GU Manufacturing Ltd - see S G & P Payne

Hollister Ltd	Incare Leg Bag 500ml/	9620	10	2500
	direct inlet (Regular)			
	Incare Leg Bag 500ml/	9621	10	2500
	10cm inlet (Regular)			
	Incare Leg Bag 500ml/	9624	10	2500
	50cm inlet (Regular)			
	Incare Leg Bag 800ml/	9630	10	2509
	direct inlet (Regular)			
	Incare Leg Bag 800ml/	9631	10	2509
	10cm inlet (Regular)			
	Incare Leg Bag 800ml/	9632	10	2509
	50cm variable inlet (Regular)			
*	Urinary Leg Bag 540mL with 37cm			
	extension tube	9820	10	2537
S *	Urinary Leg Bag 540mL with direct			
	inlet connector	9814	10	2476

Incare Medical - see Hollister Ltd

IXB

S   These leg bags are supplied sterile. This does not affect the guidance given in the note on page 181
*   Plastics

LEG BAGS - cont

Manufacturer	Appliance	Order No.	Quantity	List Price p
Jade-Euro-Med Ltd	Kipper bag, black	KB	1	2592
	Kipper bag, trans	KBT	1	2592
S*	Leg Drainage bag/Direct Inlet			
	350mL S	LBWT/350	10	2223
S*	Leg Drainage bag/30cm Inlet tube			
	350mL L	LBWT/350	10	2223
S*	Leg Drainage bag/Direct Inlet			
	500mL S	LBWT/500	10	2223
S*	Leg Drainage bag/10cm Inlet tube			
	500mL M	LBWT/500	10	2223
S*	Leg Drainage bag/30cm Inlet tube			
	500mL L	LBWT/500	10	2223
S*	Leg Drainage bag/Direct Inlet			
	750mL S	LBWT/750	10	2320
S*	Leg Drainage bag/10cm Inlet tube			
	750mL M	LBWT/750	10	2320
S*	Leg Drainage bag/30cm Inlet tube			
	750mL L	LBWT/750	10	2320
S*	Leg Drainage bag/38cm Inlet tube			
	750mL XL	LBWT/750	10	2320
Leyland Medical Ltd (Peoplecare) - see Rüsch UK Ltd				
Maersk Medical Ltd S	Careline Leg Bag with tap outlet,			
	overnight connection tube			
	and elasticated velcro straps			
	(1 pair per box of 10)			
*	350mL short tube	45-01 SVC	10	2312
*	350mL long tube	45-02 LVC	10	2312
*	500mL short tube	45-05 SVC	10	2373
*	500mL long tube	45-06 LVC	10	2373
*	750mL short tube	45-09 SVC	10	2423
*	750mL long tube	45-10 LVC	10	2423
	Careline Leg Bag with lever tap			
S *	500mL short tube	46-05-SVC	10	2373
S *	500mL long tube	46-06-LVC	10	2373
S *	750mL short tube	46-09-SVC	10	2423
S *	750mL long tube	46-10-LVC	10	2423
Manfred Sauer	Discreet Thigh Bag,			
	overnight connector tube and			
	fabric/velcro leg straps			
	(1 pair per box of 10)			
S *	450mL diagonal direct inlet tube suitable for			
	suprapubic catheter connection	70.04S	10	2162
S *	400mL straight direct inlet tube	70.06S	10	2162

S   These leg bags are supplied sterile. This does not affect the guidance given in the note on page 181.
*   Plastics

LEG BAGS - cont

Manufacturer	Appliance	Order No.	Quantity	List Price p
Manfred Sauer - cont	Bendi Bag leg bag with tap outlet, overnight connector tube and fabric/velcro leg straps (1 pair per box of 10)			
*	700mL short inlet tube	70.33-12	10	2014
*	700mL long inlet tube	70.33-20	10	2014
W *	1300mL short inlet tube	70.47-12	10	2014
W *	1300mL long inlet tube	70.47-20	10	2014
S *	700mL short inlet tube	70.33-12S	10	2326
S *	700mL long inlet tube	70.33-20S	10	2326
W S *	1300mL short inlet tube	70.47-12S	10	2326
W S *	1300mL long inlet tube	70.47-20S	10	2326
	600mL Sauer Urinary Leg Bag with universal adapter, 2 straps and 1 latex connector			
	Direct inlet glued adapter, swing tap	710.1104	10	2208
	15cm inlet adjustable, swing tap	710.1315adj	10	2208
	45cm inlet adjustable, swing tap	710.1345adj	10	2208
	Direct inlet glued adapter, push valve/sliding tap	710.2104	10	2208
	15cm inlet adjustable, push valve/sliding tap	710.2315adj	10	2208
	45cm inlet adjustable, push valve/sliding tap	710.2345adj	10	2208
	600mL Sauer Urinary Leg Bag, with universal adapter, 1x 4cm wide top strap & 1 x 2cm wide bottom strap and 3 latex connectors.			
S*	Direct inlet glued adapter, swing tap	710.1204S	10	2382
S*	15cm inlet adjustable, swing tap	710.1415Sadj	10	2382
S*	45cm inlet adjustable, swing tap	710.1445Sadj	10	2382
S*	Direct inlet glued adapter, push valve/sliding tap	710.2204S	10	2382
S*	15cm inlet adjustable, push valve/sliding tap	710.2415Sadj	10	2382
S*	45cm inlet adjustable, push valve/sliding tap	710.2445Sadj	10	2382
S G & P Payne *	Incontiaid leg bag			
	500mL	0830	1	259
	750mL	0831	1	259

IXB

W   Due to the size and weight of the 1300mL bags when full, this capacity of bag should be prescribed only for wheelchair-bound patients.
S   These leg bags are supplied sterile. This does not affect the guidance given in the note on page 181.
✦   Approximate Conversion
*   Plastics

LEG BAGS - cont

Manufacturer	Appliance	Order No.	Quantity	List Price p
S G & P Payne - cont	GU Black Butyl (or Latex) Rubber Kipper (SP, St. Peter's) Bags			
	Standard single chambered bag			
	✚ 568mL	0922/GU532	1	4098
	Ross type. As above, but with reinforced patches	0926/GU532/R	1	4678
	Standard ✚ 568mL bag with box outlet tap	0924/GU532/LT	1	5051
	Standard ✚ 568mL bag with short neck for females	0925/GU532/F	1	4098
	Standard ✚ 1136mL bag for night use	0923/GU532/40	1	5517
	Rubber bag for catheter drainage, short neck leg strap	SP/1	1	2809
	As above with ✚ 51mm web belt and bag support strap	SP/1a	1	3287
	Female rubber drainage bag with conical mount	SP/5	1	2666
	As above with web belt and looped support strap	SP/5a	1	3143
Pharma-Plast Ltd - see Maersk Medical Ltd				
Redland Medical Ltd - see Bard Ltd				
Rüsch UK Ltd S *	350mL long tube leg bag	240013	10	1493
S *	350mL short tube leg bag	240012	10	1397
S *	500mL long tube leg bag	240015	10	1493
S *	500mL short tube leg bag	240014	10	1397
S *	Portasystem leg bag 750mL	800100	10	999
	Kipper bag			
	Trans/white without strap and buckle	886000	1	2229
	Trans/white	886001	1	2719
	All black rubber	886002	1	2719
	All black plastic	886003	1	2719
Salts Healthcare *	Heritage leg bag pack	ZL0020	5	1056
S *	500mL short tube	ZL0407	10	1479
S *	500mL long tube	ZL0408	10	1505
S *	750mL short tube	ZL0409	10	1648
S *	750mL long tube	ZL0410	10	1687

S   These leg bags are supplied sterile. This does not affect the guidance given in the note on page 181.
✚   Approximate Conversion
*   Plastics

LEG BAGS - cont

Manufacturer	Appliance	Order No.	Quantity	List Price p
Simcare - see SIMS Portex Ltd				
Simpla Continence Care				
S *	Aquadry leg bag			
*	350mL short tube	783463	10	2365
*	350mL long tube Adjustable	783501	10	2365
*	500mL short tube	783471	10	2365
*	500mL long tube Adjustable	783528	10	2365
*	750mL short tube	783498	10	2365
*	750mL long tube Adjustable	783536	10	2365
S	Simpla Trident T1			
*	350mL short tube	370802	10	2574
*	500mL long tube	370817	10	2594
*	500mL short tube	370807	10	2594
*	750mL long tube	370819	10	2606
*	750mL short tube	370809	10	2606
*	750mL adjustable long tube	370904	10	2606
S	Simpla Trident T2			
*	350mL bag, short tube	376137	10	2605
*	500mL bag, short tube	376138	10	2634
*	500mL bag, long tube	376139	10	2634
*	750mL bag, short tube	376140	10	2646
*	750mL bag, long tube	376142	10	2646
*	750mL bag, adjustable long tube	376141	10	2646
Simpla Plastics Ltd - see Seton Continence Care				
SIMS Portex Ltd *	Catheter drainage bag -			
	Large	WP205-01-S	1	388
	Small	WP205-05-B	1	388
	Rubber bag with leg strap	WS111-05-U	1	3731
S	Leg bag with valve outlet and natural latex straps			
*	350mL short tube	350 EM-TY	10	2449
*	350mL long tube	350 V 30	10	2499
*	500mL short tube	500 EM-TY	10	2502
*	500mL long tube	500 V 30	10	2567
*	750mL short tube	750 EM-TY	10	2539
*	750mL long tube	750 V 30	10	2554

S   These leg bags are supplied sterile. This does not affect the guidance given in the note on page 181.
*   Plastics

IXB

LEG BAGS - cont

Manufacturer	Appliance	Order No.	Quantity	List Price p
SIMS Portex Ltd - cont				
	S Leg bag with twist cap and elastic straps			
	* 750mL short tube	E 750 V	10	2543
	* 750mL long tube (30cm)	E 750 V 30	10	2558
	S Tri-Form leg Bag			
	* 500mL short tube	TF 500	10	2475
	* 500mL medium tube	TF 500 M	10	2504
	* 500mL long tube	TF 500 L	10	2526
Squibb Surgicare Ltd - see ConvaTec Ltd				
Universal Hospital Supplies	S Unicorn leg bag			
	* 350mL short tube	UN222V	10	1760
	* 500mL short tube	UN333V	10	1780
	* 500mL long tube	UN333VL	10	1780
	* 750mL short tube	UN444V	10	1800
	* 750mL long tube	UN444VL	10	1800
H G Wallace Ltd - see SIMS Portex Ltd				
Ward Surgical Appliance Co	Kipper bag, black trans or white rubber	WM64	1	2332
	* Leg drainage bag			
	350mL	WM65	10	1126
	500mL	WM66	10	1161
	750mL	WM67	10	1230
	St. Peters Pattern SP bag	WM76	5	3117
	Ward's Comfort Range * Leg drainage bag			
	350mL	WM68	10	1131
	500mL	WM69	10	1163
	750mL	WM70	10	1223
Warne-Franklin Medical Ltd - see Rüsch UK Ltd				

S   These leg bags are supplied sterile. This does not affect the guidance given in the note on page 181.
*   Plastics

NIGHT DRAINAGE BAGS

These bags are suitable for night-time use for the collection of urine from indwelling catheters or incontinence sheaths. They are generally used in conjunction with a bag hanger which, being a nursing aid, is not prescribable. Supply arrangements for bag hangers tend to vary throughout the country but they are normally supplied through the community nursing service.

Note: *The drainage bags listed below except non-drainable bags, have a life-in-use of, on average 5-7 days.*

Manufacturer	Appliance	Order No.	Quantity	List Price p
Aldington Laboratories Ltd - see Rüsch UK Ltd				
Bard Ltd #	Uriplan collection bag,2 litre with 90cm inlet tube and non-return valve	D8420	10	231
	Uriplan drainage bag, 2 litre with 98cm inlet tube, non-return valve and tap outlet	D81-3131	10	1162
Body's Surgical Company - see Jade-Euro-Med Ltd				
Bradgate Unitech - see Pharma-Plast Ltd				
Coloplast Ltd	Conveen drainage bag1.5 litre	5062	10	1309
ConvaTec Ltd	Accuseal drainage bag	S500	5	772
	Night drainage bag	S320	5	772
Dansac Ltd	Dansac night drainage bag 2 litre	420-00	10	1116
DePuy Healthcare - see Simpla Continence Care				
Downs Surgical Ltd - see SIMS Portex Ltd				
Flexicare Medical Ltd	Flexicare F4, sterile 2 litre drainage bag with 100cm inlet tube, non return valve and tap outlet	00-1200	10	950
	Flexicare F4L, sterile 2 litre drainage bag with 100cm inlet tube, non return valve and lever tap outlet	00-1201	10	970
#	Flexicare F2, sterile 2 litre drainage bag with 100cm inlet tube and non return valve	00-2202C	10	210
Holister Ltd	Incare night drainage bag 2000ml (Non-Drainable) #	9651	10	221
	Incare night drainage bag 2000ml (Drainable)	9650	10	1120
	Hollister urostomy night drainage bag	5550	10	1055
Jade-Euro-Med Ltd S	2 litre drainage bag with tap outlet	2LNB	1	151

\#   Non-drainable bags.
S   These Night Drainage Bags are supplied sterile

IXB

NIGHT DRAINAGE BAGS - cont

Manufacturer	Appliance	Order No.	Quantity	List Price p
Maersk Medical Ltd				
#	Careline E1, 2 litre urine drainage bag with 90cm inlet tube	45-30-LBC	10	203
#	Careline E2, 2 litre urine drainage bag with 90cm inlet tube and non-return valve	45-40-LBC	10	218
	Careline E4, 2 litre urine drainage bag with 90cm inlet tube and non-return valve and tap outlet	45-20-IDC	10	1066
S	Careline E4 Night Bag, 2 litre with lever tap	46-20-IDC	10	1066
Pharma-Plast Ltd - see Maersk Medical Ltd				
Rand Rocket Ltd	Urine drainage bag			
#	Long tube	9777	25	387
Redland Medical Ltd - see Bard Ltd				
Rüsch UK Ltd	2 litre urine drainage bags	C	10	1075
		CV	10	1193
		CVT	10	1236
	2 litre urine drainage bags	DVT	10	1140
Salts Healthcare	2 litre urine drainage bags	ZL0400	10	1206

S   These Night Drainage Bags are supplied sterile
Non-drainable bags

NIGHT DRAINAGE BAGS - cont

Manufacturer	Appliance	Order No.	Quantity	List Price p
Simcare - see SIMS Portex Ltd				
Simpla Continence Care	Aqua 4 urine drainage bag			
	2 litre	783560	10	1023
#	Aqua 2 urine drainage bag			
	2 litre	783552	10	217
	Simpla 2 litre S5 (formerly S4 Plus)			
	Urine drainage bag	346145	10	1115
	Simpla 2 litre S4 Urine drainage bag -			
	long tube	340805	10	1235
	short tube	340801	10	1195
#	Simpla 2 litre S1 Urine drainage bag			
	with standard size connector	311102	10	236
	with slim size connector	311103	10	236
#	Simpla 2 litre S2 Urine drainage bag with non-return valve			
	with standard size connector	320902	10	248
	with slim size connector	321103	10	248
SIMS Portex Ltd	Mirage night drainage bag			
	2 litre	32-540-10	10	1067
	Uro-flo night drainage bag			
	male	WS167-45-K	10	1474
	female	WS167-47-Q	10	1474
	Inbeds 2 litre drainage bag with			
	twist tap	IB2000C	10	1361
Squibb Surgicare Ltd - see ConvaTec Ltd				
H G Wallace Ltd - see SIMS Portex Ltd				
Ward Surgical Appliance Co	2 litre drainage bag with outlet and non outlet	WM71	10	1224

IXB

\#   Non-drainable bags

SUSPENSORY SYSTEMS

These appliances should not be confused with leg bag garments which are not prescribable. Each system comprises a drainage bag with its means of support.

Note: The bags may be used for 5-7 days, sometimes longer, but the support systems will have a much longer life.

Manufacturer	Appliance	Order No.	Quantity	List Price p
Bard Ltd	Urisac Portabag belt	7681	1	722
	* Urisac Portabag	7680	10	1233
EMS Medical Ltd - see Simpla Continence Care				
Rüsch UK Ltd	Portabelt for Portabag	800210	1	894
	* Portabag	800200	10	1601
Simcare - see SIMS Portex Ltd				
Simpla Continence Care				
	Shepheard Sporran belt	T130	1	839
	* Drainage bag for use with above belt	T121	10	1681
SIMS Portex Ltd				
	Leg bag holster			
	Small ✚ 61cm-76cm	WH6176	1	895
	Medium ✚ 76cm-91.5cm	WH7691	1	895
	Large ✚ 91.5cm - 112cm	WH91112	1	895
	* 400mL Holster bag	400 H	10	1916
H G Wallace Ltd - see SIMS Portex Ltd				
Warne-Franklin Medical Ltd - see Rüsch UK Ltd				

*   Plastics
✚   Approximate Conversion

TUBING AND ACCESSORIES

Manufacturer	Appliance	Order No.	Quantity	List Price p
Bard Ltd	Adaptor for Uro sheath ✤ 203mm (penile sheath to leg bag)	0538	1	110
	Leg bag straps (washable)	15LS	10	1281
	Leg bag straps, Latex	8440	20	262
	Leg bag straps, foam/velcro	8441	20	498
	Urisleeve leg bag holder			
	Small (24-39cm)	150111	4	715
	Medium (36-55cm)	150121	4	715
	Large (40-70cm)	150131	4	715
Beambridge Medical	Beambridge Funnel Male Urinal Director/ Positioner	6-35	1	1200
Body's Surgical Company - see Jade-Euro-Med Ltd				
Coloplast Ltd	Velcrobands (washable)	5050	20	3652
ConvaTec Ltd	Accuseal leg bag extension tube	S455	10	708
DePuy Healthcare - see Simpla Continence Care				
Downs Surgical Ltd - see SIMS Portex Ltd				
EMS Medical Ltd - see Simpla Continence Care				
Eschmann Bros and Walsh Ltd - see SIMS Portex Ltd				
Flexicare Medical Ltd	Leg bag straps (pairs); washable, anti slip with velcro fastening	00-0032	10	1150
GU Manufacturing Ltd - see S G & P Payne				
Hollister Ltd	Leg bag straps ✤ 35.5cm (calf)	9342	2	288
	Leg bag straps ✤ 58.5cm (thigh)	9343	2	288
Incare Medical - see Hollister Ltd				

IXB

✤　Approximate Conversion

TUBING AND ACCESSORIES - cont

Manufacturer	Appliance	Order No.	Quantity	List Price p
Jade-Euro-Med Ltd	Euro J-strap	JEJS	5	1175
	Eurosleeve			
	Small (24-33cm)	JES1	4	700
	Standard (34-39cm)	JES2	4	700
	Medium (40-46cm)	JES3	4	700
	Large (47-64cm)	JES4	4	700
	Leg bag connecting tube with mount	LBCTM	1	243
	Leg bag connecting tube	LBCT	1	141
	Velcro leg straps	VLS	2	182
Leyland Medical Ltd (Peoplecare) - see Rüsch UK Ltd				
Maersk Medical Ltd	Careline leg bag straps	45-85-EX	10	1293
Manfred Sauer	K + ICS Sheath Expander	100.01	1	6317
	(can only be used to expand Manfred Sauer K + ICS Sheaths over the penis to allow for clean intermittant self catheterisation - see Incontinence Sheaths section this publication for Manfred Sauer K + ICS Sheaths, order no. 103.nn).			
	K + ICS Sheath Tips	100.05	10	1577
	(can only be used with Manfred Sauer K + ICS Sheaths - see Incontinence Sheaths section of this publication for Manfred Sauer K + ICS Sheaths, order no. 103.nn.)			
MMG (Europe) Ltd - see Simpla Plastics Ltd				
S G & P Payne	✢ 152mm Rubber extension tube	1201	1	347
	Velcro leg strap	1001	1	95
	Rubber leg strap	1003	1	121
Pharma-Plast Ltd - see Maersk Medical Ltd				
Portex Ltd - See SIMS Portex Ltd				
Redland Medical - see Bard Ltd				
Rüsch UK Ltd	Connecting tubes for Kipper bag	886104	1	270
	✢ 35.5cm connecting tube for drip urinal	754136	1	269
	Connecting tube for all urinals with female connector	754135	1	411
Salts Healthcare	Heritage leg bag extension tube	ZL0021	2	211

✢   Approximate Conversion

TUBING AND ACCESSORIES - cont

Manufacturer	Appliance	Order No.	Quantity	List Price p
Sherwood Medical Industries Ltd - see The Kendall Company (UK) Ltd				
Simcare - see SIMS Portex Ltd				
Simpla Continence Care	Aquasleeve			
	Small (leg circum. 24-33cm)	783678	4	728
	Standard (leg circum. 34-39cm)	783680	4	728
	Medium (leg circum. 40-46cm)	783686	4	728
	Large (leg circum. 47-64cm)	783694	4	728
	Leg bag extension tube	380303	10	482
	Elasticated leg bag straps (washable)	380812	10	1350
	Simpla G-Strap			
	short	383002	5	1236
	adult	383001	5	1236
	abdominal	383003	5	1363
SIMS Portex Ltd	Stepped tapered adaptor	700/110/100	10	895
	Tapered adaptor (catheter to leg bag)	700/150/634	10	634
	Stopcock for use on chiron plastic urinal bags in place of screw cap	WS155-20-E	1	460
	Rubber extension tube (with mounts)	WS152-01-M	1	476
	Rubber tubing (1.5m long)	WS152-20-R	1	1111
	Plastic connector with tube	WS152-25-C	1	316
	Female connector for Mitcham bag	WH566-01-G	1	212
	Night bag connector	WH533-01-C	1	129

IXB

TUBING AND ACCESSORIES - cont

Manufacturer	Appliance	Order No.	Quantity	List Price p
SIMS Portex Ltd	Spare "O" rings for pp urinal	WR045-01-R	5	121
	Uro-Flo Elastic Velcro Leg Straps	WS167-35-H	10	436
	Leg bag extension tube			
	30cm	ET30	10	2480
	60cm	ET60	10	2728
	Silgrip Elasticated leg strap	EC1	10	1262
	Silgrip side-fix leg strap (thigh fitting)	SF1	10	1262
	Silgrip side-fix leg strap (calf fitting)	SF2	10	1200
Squibb Surgicare Ltd - see ConvaTec Ltd				
The Kendall Company (UK) Ltd	Argyle Foam and Velcro leg strap 75cm (washable)	8887-600149	1	169
	Argyle Foam and Velcro Abdomen strap 150cm (washable)	8887-600156	1	317
	Argyle Suregrip General purpose tube 7mm ID, length 2.7m	8888-301226	50	3600
	Argyle Penrose Tubing			
	6mm ID, length 44cm	8888-514604	50	3075
	8mm ID, length 44cm	8888-514802	50	3075
	10mm ID, length 44cm	8888-515007	50	3075
	13mm ID, length 44cm	8888-515205	50	3075
	16mm ID, length 44cm	8888-515403	50	3075
	19mm ID, length 44cm	8888-515601	50	3075
	25mm ID, length 44cm	8888-515809	50	3075

H G Wallace Ltd - See SIMS Portex Ltd

URINAL SYSTEMS

The devices listed below are specialist appliances which comprise several components and need to be correctly fitted by someone competent to do so. Generally patients should have 2 appliances, one to wear and one to wash.

Note: In general the individual components can be prescribed separately for replacement purposes. With proper care and cleansing, each appliance should last for 6 months.

Manufacturer	Appliance	Order No.	Quantity	List Price p
Bard Ltd	Maguire urinal and adaptor waist sizes			
	66-81cm	050802	1	6258
	81-96cm	050803	1	6258
	96-112cm	050804	1	6258
	Mobile paraplegic day/ night urinal	0019	1	5107
	Maguire adaptor & tubing	600532		845
Beambridge Medical	Bridge Saddle urinal	6-26	1	1299
	Bridge urinal	6-18	1	1299
	Bridge urinal with tap	6-18T	1	1299
John Bell & Croyden	Fridjohn male urinal	U50	1	4061
	Male urinal - long bag day & night use	U51	1	3735
	Male urinal - short bag day & night use	U52	1	3735
Body's Surgical Company - see Jade-Euro-Med Ltd				
C S Bullen Ltd	Male urinal with large size long bag	LU412	1	7463

IXB

URINAL SYSTEMS - cont

Manufacturer	Appliance	Order No.	Quantity	List Price p
DePuy Healthcare - see Seton Continence Care				
Downs Surgical Ltd - see SIMS Portex Ltd				
Ellis, Son & Paramore Ltd	Hallam Modular Urinals	NS200	1	3163
	Spare bag	NS200(a)	1	168
	Spare belt	NS200(b)	1	375
GU Manufacturing Ltd - see S G & P Payne				
Hollister Ltd	Incare Retracted Penis Pouch	9811	10	2500
Jade-Euro-Med Ltd	Male urinals - all fitted with taps			
	Day and night use urinal with diaphragm, Scrotal support and bag. STATE SIZE OF DIAPHRAGM	Fig 4A	1	5370
	Urinal with waistband, Scrotal support complete with inner sheath and bag	Fig 5	1	6535
	Urinal with waistband, connection tube, rubber understraps, complete with tapered inner sheath and bag	Fig 6A	1	6350
	Adult male urinal with double bag, air vent, pressure ring suspensory band and understraps. STATE SHEATH SIZE	Fig 19	1	6726
	Adult male urinal with pressure ring, diaphragm, rubber understraps. STATE SIZE OF DIAPHRAGM	Fig 101	1	5811
	Day and night urinal with pressure ring, inner sheath, waistband and understraps. STATE SIZE OF SHEATH	Fig 104	1	6379
	As above with extension tube	Fig 104ET	1	6732
	Day and night urinal with sheath, waistbelt, understraps and plastic bag	Fig 105	1	6187

URINAL SYSTEMS - cont

Manufacturer	Appliance	Order No.	Quantity	List Price p
Jade-Euro-Med Ltd - cont				
	Urinal with inner sheath, rubber understraps and plastic bag. STATE SIZE OF SHEATH	Fig 106	1	5734
	Day and night urinal, scrotal support and plastic bag	Fig 107	1	5510
	Day and night urinal to contain penis and scrotum, fitted with inner sheath and diaphragm complete with bag	Fig 111A	1	5397
	Male jockey appliance with bag. STATE WAIST SIZE	M200	1	5747
	Replacement belt for above. STATE WAIST SIZE	JB/200	1	1128
	Outer receiver	O/R	1	1315
	Inner sheath	I/S	5	1315
	Plastic bags	OLBWT(L)	5	1448
	Rubber bag	RB/M200	1	2414
	Ring	SP/M200	1	96
	Stoke Mandeville replacement sheath (state size of sheath)	SMS	1	602
	Stoke Mandeville male urinal with double bag (state size of sheath)	SMDB	1	7325
	Male PP urinal with rubber bag (state size of sheath)	PP1	1	6523
	Male PP urinal with 5 plastic bags (state size of sheath)	PP2	1	6140

IXB

URINAL SYSTEMS - cont

Manufacturer	Appliance	Order No.	Quantity	List Price p
Jade-Euro-Med Ltd - cont	Spare parts for PP Urinals:			
	Flange with sheaths, state size	PP3	1	3048
	Cone - small straight	PP4	1	1209
	Cone - small curved	PP5	1	1209
	Cone - medium straight	PP6	1	1209
	Cone - medium curved	PP7	1	1209
	Cone - large straight	PP8	1	1209
	Cone - large curved	PP9	1	1209
	Cone - ex-large straight	PP10	1	1209
	Plastic bag small	OLBWT(S)	5	1448
	Plastic bag large	OLBWT(L)	5	1448
	Rubber bag with air vent for use with all Jade-Euro-Med urinals	PP13	1	2366
	Rubber belt	RB	1	433
	Progress long life plastic urinal bags pk 10	M700	1	2577
	Progress long life plastic scrotal urinal bags pk 10	M800	1	2577
	Fridjohn urinal	M600	1	7706
	Y.B. Wet. A complete urinal system STATE SHEATH SIZE 25mm/29mm/32mm/36mm/41mm	M500	1	6254
	Essex appliance. A complete urinal system. STATE SHEATH SIZE 21mm/25mm/ 31mm/35mm/40mm	M400	1	5220
	1-piece belt, incorporating double based flange and bag	KM28	1	5225
	1-piece belt, with flange and 5 plastic bags	KM29	1	5225
Leyland Medical Ltd (Peoplecare) - see Rüsch UK Ltd				
LRC Products Ltd	Dry Sheaths		144	1442
S G & P Payne	Male Incontinence Appliance with rubber belt			
	MK1 - with combined rubber flange & understraps	0001	1	6412
	MK2 -with rubber flange & fabric facepiece	0002	1	6894
	MK3 - with combined rubber flange understraps and coned top	0003	1	5690
	Lightweight male Incontinence Appliance MK4 - with fabric face- piece & separate long flanged plastic bag with foam pad	0004	1	4065

URINAL SYSTEMS - cont

Manufacturer	Appliance	Order No.	Quantity	List Price p
S G & P Payne - cont	Lightweight male Incontinence Appliance			
	MK5 - with fabric facepiece separate flange & long flanged plastic bag with material face-piece and belt	0005	1	5710
	MK6 - with combined flange & understraps & long flanged plastic bag & rubber belt	0006	1	5007
	MK7 - with flange material flange support reinforced coned top and plastic or rubber bag	0007	1	7184
	MK8 - with flange material flange support long plastic bag	0008	1	6001
	MK9 - with rubber flange & wide belt with scrotal support	0009	1	7184
	MK10 - with flange support with wide belt & scrotal support separate flange & long flanged plastic bag	0010	1	6001
	MK11 - with flange soft replaceable diaphragm material facepiece with belt and adjustable rubber understraps soft coned top plastic or rubber bag	0011	1	7184
	MK12 - with flange soft replaceable diaphragm material facepiece with belt and adjustable rubber understraps long plastic bag	0012	1	6001
	Replacements for above appliances			
	Rubber flange with - feathered diaphragm (MK2,MK5,MK9,MK10)			
	Medium 32mm	0511	1	1857
	Large 38mm	0512	1	1857
	Ex-large 45mm	0513	1	1857
	and understrap (MK1,MK6)			
	Small 25mm	0501	1	2874
	Medium 32mm	0502	1	2874
	Large 38mm	0503	1	2874
	Ex-large 45mm	0504	1	2874
	Feathered diaphragm & combined reinforced top (MK3)	0560	1	3260
	Rubber flange 38mm (MK11, MK12)	0516	1	1857
	Rubber flange 45mm (MK11, MK12)	0517	1	1857
	Soft replaceable rubber diaphragms (MK11, MK12)	0519	3	463

IXB

URINAL SYSTEMS - cont

Manufacturer	Appliance	Order No.	Quantity	List Price p
S G & P Payne - cont	Material facepiece with belt & loop (MK2,MK4,MK5)	0430	1	2152
	Reinforced cone top (MK1,MK2,MK9)			
	Small - to fit 25mm flange	0601	1	1249
	Medium - to fit any size flange	0602	1	1249
	Large - to fit any size flange	0603	1	1249
	Soft coned top (MK11)	0619	1	1249
	Plastic bag (MK1,MK2,MK3,MK7,MK9,MK11)	0801	1	314
	Rubber bag (MK1,MK2,MK3,MK7,MK9,MK11)	0901	1	1889
	Rubber belt (MK1,MK3,MK6)	0101	1	405
	Elastic belt (MK1,MK3,MK6)			
	Waist size 70cm	0201	1	857
	Waist size 75cm	0202	1	857
	Waist size 80cm	0203	1	857
	Waist size 85cm	0204	1	857
	Waist size 90cm	0205	1	857
	Waist size 95cm	0206	1	857
	Web belt (MK1,MK3,MK6)	0301	1	599
	Flange support with wide belt & scrotal support (MK9,MK10)			
	Small			
	Waist size 70/80cm	0420	1	2442
	Medium			
	Waist size 80/90cm	0421	1	2442
	Large			
	Waist size 90/100cm	0422	1	2442
	Material flange support (MK7, MK8)			
	70cm	0401	1	2442
	75cm	0402	1	2442
	80cm	0403	1	2442
	85cm	0404	1	2442
	90cm	0405	1	2442
	95cm	0406	1	2442
	100cm	0407	1	2442
	105cm	0408	1	2442
	110cm	0409	1	2442
	Night connector (MK1,MK2,MK3,MK7,MK9,MK11)	0701	1	405

URINAL SYSTEMS - cont

Manufacturer	Appliance	Order No.	Quantity	List Price p
S G & P Payne - cont	Long flanged plastic bag (MK5,MK6,MK8,MK10,MK12)			
	38mm - to fit 32/38mm flange	0811	1	424
	45mm - to fit 45mm flange	0812	1	424
	with foam pad (MK4)			
	38mm - to fit 32/38mm flange	0821	1	481
	48mm - to fit 45mm flange	0822	1	481
	Material facepiece with belt and adjustable rubber understraps (MK11, MK12)			
	Small	0414	1	2442
	Medium	0415	1	2442
	Large	0416	1	2442
	Material facepiece with support belt, loop and scrotal (MK2,MK4,MK5)	0441	1	2442
	Payne's Urine Director	0630	1	2294
	PP Urinal Complete with rubber bag/plastic bag	0019	1	6412
	Pubic Pressure Flange			
	25mm with -			
	13mm sheath	0520	1	2874
	17mm sheath	0521	1	2874
	19mm sheath	0522	1	2874
	22mm sheath	0523	1	2874
	32mm with			
	22mm sheath	0524	1	2874
	25mm sheath	0525	1	2874
	38mm with			
	29mm sheath	0526	1	2874
	32mm sheath	0527	1	2874
	45mm with			
	35mm sheath	0528	1	2874
	38mm sheath	0529	1	2874
	42mm sheath	0530	1	2874
	Coned Top			
	Straight			
	Small for 25mm flange	0620	1	1249
	Medium for any size flange	0621	1	1249
	Large for any size flange	0622	1	1249
	Curved			
	Small for 25mm flange	0623	1	1249
	Medium for any size flange	0624	1	1249
	Large for any size flange	0625	1	1249

IXB

URINAL SYSTEMS - cont

Manufacturer	Appliance	Order No.	Quantity	List Price p
S G & P Payne - cont	Rubber bag with vent tube (MK1,MK2,MK3,MK7,MK9,MK11)	0910	1	2267
	Reinforced cone top with vent tube			
	Small	0610	1	1643
	Medium	0611	1	1643
	Large	0612	1	1643
	Stoke Mandeville condom urinal complete	0020	1	5291
	Spares for above:			
	Kipper bags	0920	1	2977
	Rubber tube & connector	0712	1	231
	Dry incontinence sheaths			
	plain end	1101	100	1540
	teated end	1106	100	1540
	Rubber tubing			
	latex 8mm	1203	per metre	476
	red 8mm	1204	per metre	476
	latex 10mm	1205	per metre	476
	red 10mm	1206	per metre	476
	Nylon connectors			
	GU	0711	1	135
	SM	0710	1	135
	Latex tubing (per metre)			
	8mm bore	1203	1	476
	10mm bore	1205	1	476
	GU Pattern Stoke Mandeville Condom Set	0021	1	5517
	As above with ✤ 1136mL bag	0022	1	6844
	Replacement parts for above urinals			
	Kipper bags - see Leg Bags			
	Nylon studs - GU	0711	1	135
	- SM	0710	1	135
	Nylon stud with latex tube	0712	1	231
	Adjustable web belt			
	Waist size up to 95cm	0304	1	632
	Waist size up to 115cm	0305	1	632
	Waist size up to 150cm	0306	1	632

✤   Approximate Conversion

URINAL SYSTEMS - cont

Manufacturer	Appliance	Order No.	Quantity	List Price p
S G & P Payne - cont	Male urinal for day and night use, air tube to bag, inner sheath and diaphragm to receiver, web belt and cotton suspensory bag	IU/9	1	5190
	Male urinal with long narrow bag, web belt and cotton suspensory bag	IU/365	1	5402
	Male urinal for day use, the receiver to contain the penis and scrotum, web waist band and tape under-straps	IU/11	1	4957
	Male urinal for night use, similar to IU/11 but the receiver designed for use in bed	IU/12	1	4957
	Male urinal to contain penis and scrotum (for the small built man) web belt and tape understraps	IU/11B/893C	1	4957
	Male urinal for day and night use, long rubber bag with two leg straps loops and straps, flanged receiver, air tube, diaphragm and short conical inner sheath, web band and cotton suspensory bag	IU/15/3977	1	5128
	Male urinal for day and night use, short rubber bag, detachable bag and night tube, web belt and cotton suspensory bag	IU/43	1	4132
	Replacement suspension bag - small, medium & large	IU/1458	1	522
Rüsch UK Ltd	Thames urinal with standard bag and connecting tube	751100	1	7901
	Thames urinal with long bag and connecting tube	751102	1	7901
	Severn urinal with standard bag and connecting tube	752120	1	7901
	Severn urinal with long bag and connecting tube	752122	1	7901
	Severn urinal with 5 plastic bags and connecting tube	752124	1	7901

IXB

URINAL SYSTEMS - cont

Manufacturer	Appliance	Order No.	Quantity	List Price p
Rüsch UK Ltd - cont	Severn spare sheaths	758300	5	3098
	Mersey urinal with standard bag and connecting tube	753220	1	7901
	Mersey urinal with long bag and connecting tube	753222	1	7901
	Mersey urinal with 5 plastic bags and connecting tube	753224	1	7901
	Wye urinal with separate connecting tube & on/off valve	751300	1	2554
	Wye urinal with long night extension tube	751301	1	2976
	Wye urinal with short bag	751120	1	4252
	Wye urinal with long bag	751175	1	4252
	Arizona male urinal	751400	1	7901
	'55' male urinal	756200	1	7782
	Spare sheaths for '55' urinal	756212	6	3529
	Stoke Mandeville Pattern Male urinal			
	20mm sheath	754001	1	7901
	24mm sheath	754002	1	7901
	25mm sheath	754003	1	7901
	28mm sheath	754004	1	7901
	32mm sheath	754005	1	7901
	35mm sheath	754006	1	7901
	38mm sheath	754007	1	7901
	42mm sheath	754008	1	7901
	45mm sheath	754009	1	7901
	48mm sheath	754010	1	7901
	51mm sheath	754011	1	7901
	54mm sheath	754012	1	7901
	57mm sheath	754013	1	7901
	60mm sheath	754014	1	7901
	63mm sheath	754015	1	7901
	Spare sheaths on request		1	703

URINAL SYSTEMS - cont

Manufacturer	Appliance	Order No.	Quantity	List Price p
Rüsch UK Ltd - cont	Sahara one-piece top PP urinal			
	- with small rubber collection bag			
	Paed	755109	1	7532
	- with 5 small plastic collection bags			
	Paed	755110	1	7532
	- with standard collection bag and connection tube			
	Standard	755120	1	7532
	- with long collection bag and connection tube			
	Standard	755130	1	7532
	- with five medium collection bags and connection tube			
	Standard	755140	1	7532
	- with standard rubber bag and connection tube			
	Large	755150	1	7532
	- with long rubber bag and connection tube			
	Large	755160	1	7532
	- with five medium plastic bags and connection tube			
	Large	755170	1	7532
	Peoplecare PP Male urinal:			
	PP flange 25mm child Sheath size			
	13mm	844113	1	2446
	16mm	844116	1	2446
	19mm	844119	1	2446
	22mm	844122	1	2446

IXB

URINAL SYSTEMS - cont

Manufacturer	Appliance	Order No.	Quantity	List Price p
Rüsch UK Ltd - cont	PP Flange 29mm child			
	Sheath size			
	22mm	845122	1	2446
	25mm	845125	1	2446
	PP Flange 32mm child			
	Sheath size			
	19mm	845219	1	2446
	22mm	845222	1	2446
	25mm	845225	1	2446
	PP Flange 38mm adult			
	Sheath size			
	19mm	846319	1	2446
	22mm	846322	1	2446
	25mm	846325	1	2446
	29mm	846329	1	2446
	32mm	846332	1	2446
	PP Flange 44mm adult			
	Sheath size			
	35mm	847435	1	2446
	38mm	847438	1	2446
	41mm	847441	1	2446
	PP Standard bag			
	Medium	881002	1	1262
	Large	881003	1	1565
	PP Curved Top			
	Small	874101	1	952
	Medium	874102	1	952
	Large	874103	1	952
	PP Straight Top			
	Small	875211	1	952
	Medium	875212	1	952
	Large	875213	1	952
	Ex-large	875214	1	952
	Transverse rubber bag with tap for above urinal	881001	1	2585
	Double based PP Flange for above urinal	846350	1	2446
	Rubber pubic flange, adult, for above urinal	854229	1	2820
	Kipper inco set	886100	1	4232

URINAL SYSTEMS - cont

Manufacturer	Appliance	Order No.	Quantity	List Price p
Salts Healthcare	Male PP urinal			
	- rubber bag	ZL0001	1	5245
	- plastic bag (4)	ZL0001	1	5245
	Spare parts for above urinal			
	✚ 25mm flange			
	† - ✚ 12mm sheath	ZL0051	1	2493
	† - ✚ 15mm sheath	ZL0052	1	2493
	- ✚ 18mm sheath	ZL0053	1	2493
	† - ✚ 22mm sheath	ZL0054	1	2493
	✚ 32mm flange			
	† - ✚ 18mm sheath	ZL0057	1	2493
	† - ✚ 22mm sheath	ZL0058	1	2493
	- ✚ 25mm sheath	ZL0059	1	2493
	✚ 38mm flange			
	- ✚ 18mm sheath	ZL0060	1	2493
	- ✚ 22mm sheath	ZL0061	1	2493
	- ✚ 25mm sheath	ZL0062	1	2493
	- ✚ 29mm sheath	ZL0063	1	2493
	- ✚ 32mm sheath	ZL0064	1	2493
	✚ 44mm flange			
	- ✚ 35mm sheath	ZL0065	1	2493
	- ✚ 38mm sheath	ZL0066	1	2493
	† - ✚ 41mm sheath	ZL0067	1	2493
	Cone - small straight	ZL0100	1	1110
	Cone - small curved	ZL0101	1	1110
	Cone - medium straight	ZL0102	1	1110
	Cone - medium curved	ZL0103	1	1110
†	Cone - large straight	ZL0104	1	1110
	Cone - large curved	ZL0105	1	1110
	Cone - ex-large straight	ZL0106	1	1110
	Pubic Pressure Flange Belt	ZL0034	1	2190
	- plastic bags			
	child	ZL0151	4	1220
	adult	ZL0152	4	1220
	- rubber bag			
	adult	ZL0155	1	1220
	child	ZL0154	1	1220
	transverse	ZL0153	1	1220
	- belt	ZL0010	1	371

✚   Approximate Conversion
†   to be deleted 1 February 2001

URINAL SYSTEMS - cont

Manufacturer	Appliance	Order No.	Quantity	List Price p
Simcare - see SIMS Portex Ltd				
Simpla Continence Care	Aquadry cones for use with pubic pressure flanges			
	Straight			
	Small	787140	1	1183
	Medium	787159	1	1183
	Large	787167	1	1183
	Curved			
	Small	787175	1	1183
	Medium	787183	1	1183
	Large	787191	1	1183
	Aquadry pubic pressure flange with rubber understraps			
	Child			
	✤ 12mm	787000	1	2736
	✤ 15mm	787019	1	2736
	✤ 18mm	787027	1	2736
	✤ 22mm	787035	1	2736
	✤ 25mm	787043	1	2736
	Adult			
	✤ 25mm	787078	1	2819
	✤ 29mm	787086	1	2819
	✤ 32mm	787094	1	2819
	✤ 35mm	787108	1	2819
	✤ 38mm	787116	1	2819
	✤ 41mm	787124	1	2819
	✤ 44mm	787132	1	2819
	Aquadry pubic pressure urinal 1 all-in-one appliance with pressure ring, tapered inner sleeve trimmed to fit and rubber understraps	470856	1	5723
	Aquadry pubic pressure urinal 2 all-in-one appliance with pressure ring, diaphragm and rubber straps			
	✤ 25mm	785709	1	5723
	✤ 32mm	785717	1	5723
	✤ 38mm	785725	1	5723

✤   Approximate Conversion

URINAL SYSTEMS - cont

Manufacturer	Appliance	Order No.	Quantity	List Price p
Simpla Continence Care - cont	Aquadry pubic pressure urinal 3 all-in-one appliance with pressure ring, diaphragm and scrotal support			
	✚ 25mm	785733	1	5723
	✚ 32mm	785741	1	5723
	✚ 38mm	785768	1	5723
	Aquadry rubber belt			
	✚ 61cm, 71cm, 91.5cm, 112cm	787205	1	330
	Aquadry urinal all-in-one appliance with inner sheath and rubber under-straps			
	✚ 29mm	784001	1	5723
	✚ 32mm	784028	1	5723
	✚ 35mm	784036	1	5723
	✚ 38mm	784044	1	5723
	✚ 41mm	784052	1	5723
	Rubber leg bag connecting tube with female attach-ment for urinal	785776	1	288
SIMS Portex Ltd	Male PP urinal, child, with with integral flange Rubber bag: Straight cone			
	Medium	WR007-01-D	1	6293
	Plastic bag: Curved cone			
	Small	WR011-01-H	1	6152
	Medium	WR013-01-R	1	6152
	Replacement PP flange with integral sheath for child pp urinals:			
	Sheath 13mm Flange 25mm	WS025-13-K	1	3463
	Sheath 16mm Flange 25mm	WS025-16-R	1	3463
	Sheath 19mm Flange 25mm	WS025-19-X	1	3463
	Sheath 22mm Flange 25mm	WS025-22-L	1	3463
	Sheath 25mm Flange 29mm	WS029-25-K	1	3463
	Sheath 25mm Flange 32mm	WS032-25-K	1	3463

IXB

✚ Approximate Conversion

URINAL SYSTEMS - cont

Manufacturer	Appliance	Order No.	Quantity	List Price p
SIMS Portex Ltd - cont	Replacement curved rubber cone top for above urinals			
	Small	WS130-01-S	1	1464
	Medium	WS130-03-W	1	1464
	Large	WS130-05-B	1	1464
	Replacement straight rubber cone top for above urinals			
	Small	WS135-01-P	1	1464
	Medium	WS135-03-T	1	1464
	Large	WS135-05-X	1	1464
	Ex-large	WS135-07-C	1	1464
	Replacement double-based PP flange			
	child 32mm opening	WS160-32-V	1	3095
	adult 38mm opening	WS160-38-J	1	3095
	adult 44mm opening	WS160-44-D	1	3095
	Chailey male urinal, child with plastic bag	WR105-01-B	1	6475
	Chailey male urinal, adolescent/adult with			
	rubber bag	WP100-01-P	1	5805
	plastic bag	WP105-01-L	1	7354
	Spares for Chailey urinals 1 piece curved top with integral sheath and under-straps			
	child 22mm sheath	WS200-22-R	1	3874
	adult 22mm sheath	WS202-22-A	1	3874
	adult 25mm sheath	WS202-25-G	1	3874
	adult 29mm sheath	WS202-29-Q	1	3874
	adult 32mm sheath	WS202-32-D	1	3874
	adult 35mm sheath	WS202-35-K	1	3874
	adult 38mm sheath	WS202-38-R	1	3874
	adult 44mm sheath	WS202-44-L	1	3874
	- rubber belt			
	61cm	WS101-61-A	1	571
	91cm	WS101-91-K	1	571
	- rubber bags (suitable	WS110-01-G	1	1843
	also for PP and Chiron	WS110-05-Q	1	2524
	urinals)			
	- plastic bags (suitable also for PP urinals & Chiron urinals)			
	wide neck	WS120-10-N	1	380
	adult	WS120-05-V	1	380
	child	WS120-01-M	1	380

URINAL SYSTEMS - cont

Manufacturer	Appliance	Order No.	Quantity	List Price p
SIMS Portex Ltd - cont	Male PP urinal, adult, with integral flange rubber bag - various sizes	WP001-01-M	1	7290
		WP003-01-V	1	7290
		WP005-01-E	1	7290
	plastic bag - various sizes	WP011-01-S	1	6793
		WP013-01-B	1	6793
		WP015-01-K	1	6793
	Replacement PP flange for above	WS038	1	3463
	Male PP urinal, adult, with double-based flange - rubber bag - various sizes	WP025-01-Q	1	7291
		WP028-01-D	1	7291
		WP031-01-D	1	7291
	- plastic bag - various sizes	WP035-01-V	1	6793
		WP038-01-J	1	6793
		WP041-01-J	1	6793
	Replacement sheath for above urinals	WS160-01-J	10	133
	Rubber bag with vent tube for PP urinals adult	WS140-05-G	1	3022
	Rubber double bag, adult, for PP urinals	WS140-08-N	1	3236
	Stoke Mandeville sheath type urinal	WP110-01-U	1	6642
	Stoke Mandeville double rubber bag urinal	WP113-01-H	1	8632
	Replacement sheaths	WS160-02-L	10	398
	Replacement bag for WP113	WS140-07-L	1	3236
	Replacement sheath for WP113	WS162	1	906
	Chiron male rubber urinal with webbing belt	WP124-01-S	1	5978
	Male one-piece urinal	WP125-01-W	1	5690

IXB

URINAL SYSTEMS - cont

Manufacturer	Appliance	Order No.	Quantity	List Price p
SIMS Portex Ltd - cont	* Surrey model L/weight urinal			
	L - MK I	WP130	1	5407
	L - MK II	WP133	1	5407
	Replacement foam pads for Surrey urinal			
	76mm dia/32mm opening	WJ275-32-W	5	671
	Chiron male plastic urinal (rubber sheaths)	WP145-01-H	1	3093
	Chiron geriatric urinal (film type sheaths)	WP148-01-V	1	4491
	Chiron urinal (rubber sheaths)	WP151-01-V	1	4491
	Replacement sheaths for WP145 & WP151	WS168	1	571
	Replacement net suspensory for WP107, WP129 & WP145	WS107-08-W	1	1343
	Male urinal for bed use	WP136-01-G	1	5046
	Pubic flange - large opening	WS001-05-H	1	2320
	Transverse rubber bag & stopcock (child)	WS145-01-U	1	3415
	Non allergic film type sheath	WS161-01-N	10	105

Steeper (Orthopaedic) Ltd - incorporating Donald Rose Ltd - see Ward Surgical Appliance Co

* Replacement bags for the Surrey Urinal can be found on page 372.

URINAL SYSTEMS - cont

Manufacturer	Appliance	Order No.	Quantity	List Price p
Ward Surgical Appliance Co	Jockey Male Urinal	WM27	1	7314
	Varsity Male Urinal	WM14	1	5646
	Day use, covered bag complete with belt suspensory and thigh strap	Fig 4	1	4671
	Male urinal Day and Night use covered bag air vent, belt suspensory	Fig 4A	1	4834
	Male urinal Day and Night use with short bag and belt	Fig 104	1	5004
	As above with covered bag	Fig 104a	1	5424
	As above with double chamber bag	Fig 104b	1	5638
	Male urinal Day and night use with long bag and belt	Fig 105	1	5004
	Paraplegic male urinal	Fig 110	1	6839
	Stoke Mandeville Pattern	WM18	1	6571
	Stoke Mandeville removeable rubber sheath, double chamber rubber bag, thigh strap and belt	WM18a	1	5902
	Male PP urinal rubber bag	WM19	1	6123
	Stoke Mandeville spare sheaths - rubber	WM20	1	609
	Male PP urinal plastic bag (4)	WM21	1	5425
	Replacement for above PP flange	WM22	1	2809
	PP cone	WM23	1	1110
	Rubber bag	WM24	1	1521
	Plastic bag	WM26	1	304

IX

URINAL SYSTEMS - cont

Manufacturer	Appliance	Order No.	Quantity	List Price p
Ward Surgical Appliance Co - cont	Day use, covered bag complete with belt	Fig 2	1	4446
	Night use, covered bag complete with belt suspensory and thigh strap	Fig 5	1	5874
	Day and night use, covered bags, air vent complete with belt, suspensory and thigh strap	Fig 5a	1	5874
	Day and night use, long tube rubber bag with air vent, complete with belt and thigh strap	Fig 6	1	5333
	Male dribbling bag and tapes	Fig 9	1	2170
	Day and night use, short covered bag	Fig 101	1	5004
	Day and night use, short bag & belt	Fig 106	1	5004
	Male urinal - sheath and disc type with long rubber belt	WM53	1	5457
	Male urinal - sheath and suspensory with short covered bag	WM56	1	5457
	Male urinal - sheath and suspensory with long covered bag	WM57	1	5457
	Night urinal with long tube	WM59	1	2637
	Stoke Mandeville sheath type urinal, with 30 rubber film sheaths, rubber bag and thigh strap and belt	WM49	1	5224

URINAL SYSTEMS - cont

Manufacturer	Appliance	Order No.	Quantity	List Price p
Ward Surgical Appliance Co - cont	Webbing Belt	WM102	1	924
	Elastic leg strap	WM103	10	528
	Net Suspensory	WM104	1	1215
	Spare rubber bag with vent	WM105	1	2639
	Spare Receiver	WM106	1	3800

IX

CROSS REFERENCE INDEX
(INCONTINENCE APPLIANCES)

APPLIANCE RANGE	MANUFACTURER
"55"	Rüsch UK Ltd
Accuseal	ConvaTec Ltd
Aldon	Rüsch UK Ltd
Aqua	Simpla Continence Care
Aquadry	Simpla Continence Care
Aquasleeve	Simpla Continence Care
Argyle Range	The Kendall Company (UK) Ltd
Penrose	
Suregrip	
Arizona	Rüsch UK Ltd
Bendi	Manfred Sauer
Careline	Maersk Medical Ltd
Chailey	SIMS Portex Ltd
Chiron	SIMS Portex Ltd
Clear Advantage	Simpla Continence Care
CliniFlex Medimates	CliniMed Ltd
Comfort	Manfred Sauer
Contour	Coloplast Ltd
Conveen	Coloplast Ltd
Discreet	Manfred Sauer
Dribblet	C S Bullen Ltd
Dryaid	Rüsch UK Ltd
Essex	Jade-Euro-Med Ltd
Flip-Flo	Bard Ltd
Freedom	Simpla Continence Care
Fridjohn	John Bell & Croydon
Fridjohn	Jade-Euro-Med
Hallam	Ellis, Son & Paramore Ltd
Heritage	Salts Healthcare
Incare	Hollister Ltd
Incontiaid	S G & P Payne
I.n.b.e.d.s	SIMS Portex Ltd
Integrity	Bard Ltd
Jockey	Ward Surgical Applicances Co Ltd
K+ICS	Manfred Sauer
Macrodom	Hospital Management & Supplies Ltd
Macquire	Bard Ltd
Mersey	Rüsch UK Ltd
Mirage	SIMS Portex Ltd
Mitcham	SIMS Portex Ltd
MK	S G & P Payne

CROSS REFERENCE INDEX - cont
(INCONTINENCE APPLIANCES)

APPLIANCE RANGE	MANUFACTURER
Paul (Penrose)	SIMS Portex Ltd
Penrose	The Kendall Company (UK) Ltd
Peoplecare	Rüsch UK Ltd
Portabag	Rüsch UK Ltd
Portabelt	Rüsch UK Ltd
Portasheath	Rüsch UK Ltd
Posey	Camp Ltd
Progress	Jade-Euro-Med Ltd
Reliacath	Bard Ltd
Reliasheath	Bard Ltd
S	Simpla Continence Care
S4 Plus	Simpla Continence Care
S5	Simpla Continence Care
Sahara	Rüsch UK Ltd
Sauer	Manfred Sauer
Secure	Rüsch UK Ltd
Severn	Rüsch UK Ltd
Shepheard	Simpla Continence Care
Silgrip	SIMS Portex Ltd
Simpla G-Strap	Simpla Continence Care
St Peters	Wards Surgical Appliances
Surrey	SIMS Portex Ltd
Texas Catheter	The Kendall Company (UK) Ltd
Thames	Rüsch UK Ltd
Tri-Form	SIMS Portex Ltd
Trident T1	Simpla Continence Care
Trident T2	Simpla Continence Care
U-Sheath	Simpla Continence Care
U-Sheath Plus	Simpla Continence Care
Unicorn	Universal Hospital Supplies
Uridom	Fry Surgical International Ltd
Uri-Drain	The Kendall Company (UK) Ltd
Uridrop	North West Medical Supplies Ltd
Urifix Tape	Bio Diagnostics
Urifix	Seton Continence Care
Urihesive	ConvaTec Ltd
Uriplan	Bard Ltd
Urisac	Bard Ltd
Uristrip	North West Medical Supplies Ltd
Uro-flo	SIMS Portex Ltd
Uro-sheath	Bard
Varsity	Wards Surgical Appliances
Wye	Rüsch UK Ltd
YB	Jade-Euro-Med Ltd

IXB

MANUFACTURER'S ADDRESSES AND TELEPHONE NUMBERS
(INCONTINENCE APPLIANCES)

Aldington Laboratories Ltd: see Rüsch UK Ltd

Associated Hospital Supply: see Bio Diagnostic

Astra Tech Ltd, Stroud Water Business Park, Brunel Way, Stonehouse, Gloucester
  GL10 35W (01453 791763)

Bard Ltd, Forest House, Brighton Road, Crawley, West Sussex RH11 9BP (01293 527888)

Beambridge Medical, 46 Merrow Lane, Burpham, Guildford, Surrey GU4 7LQ
  (01483 827696/01483 571928)

John Bell and Croyden, 54 Wigmore Street, London W1H 0AU (0207 9355555)

Bio Diagnostics, Upton Industrial Estate, Rectory Road, Upton-upon-Severn, Worcestershire WR8 0LX
  (01684 592262)

Body's Surgical Company: see Jade-Euro-Med Ltd

Bradgate Unitech Ltd: see Maersk Medical Ltd

C S Bullen Ltd, 3-7 Moss Street, Liverpool L6 1EY (0151 2076995/6/7/8)

Camp Ltd, Northgate House, Staple Gardens, Winchester, Hampshire SO23 8ST (01962 855248)

CliniMed Ltd, Cavell House, Knaves Beech Way, Loudwater, High Wycombe, Bucks, HP10 9QY
  (01628 850100)

Coloplast Ltd, Peterborough Business Park, Peterborough PE2 6FX (01733 392000)

ConvaTec Ltd, Unit 20, First Avenue, Deeside Industrial Park, Deeside, Clywd CH5 2NU
  (01244 586244)

DePuy Healthcare: see Simpla Continence Care

Dow Corning Ltd, Kings Court, 185 Kings Road, Reading, Berkshire RG1 4EX (01734 596888)

Downs Surgical Ltd: see SIMS Portex Ltd

Ellis, Son & Paramore Ltd, Spring Street Works, Sheffield S3 8PD (0114 2738921/221269)

EMS Medical Ltd: see Simpla Continence Care

Eschmann Bros & Walsh Ltd: see SIMS Portex Ltd

Flexicare Medical Ltd, Cynon Valley Business Park, Mountain Ash, Mid-Glamorgan, CF45 4ER
  (01443 474647)

Fry Surgical International Ltd, Unit 17, Goldsworth Park Trading Estate, Woking, Surrey
  GU21 3BA (01483 721404)

G U Manufacturing Co Ltd: see S G & P Payne

Hollister Ltd, Rectory Court, 42 Broad Street, Wokingham, Berkshire, RG40 1AB
  (0118 989 5000) (Retail Pharmacy Order Line 0800 521392)

Hospital Management & Supplies Ltd, Salthouse Road, Brackmills, Northampton NN4 0U4
  (01604 704600)

MANUFACTURER'S ADDRESSES AND TELEPHONE NUMBERS - cont
(INCONTINENCE APPLIANCES)

Incare Medical Products: see Hollister Ltd

Jade-Euro-Med Ltd, Unit 14, East Hanningfield Industrial Estate, Old Church Road, East Hanningfield, Chelmsford, Essex, CM3 8BG (01245 400413)

JLJ Healthcare Ltd, Number One 61 Whitehall Road, Halesowen, West Midlands, B63 3JS (0121 6023943)

L.I.N.C Medical Systems Ltd, Stoughton Lodge Farm, Stoughton Lane, Stoughton, Leicester LE2 2FH (0116 2721061)

Leyland Medical Ltd: see Rüsch UK Ltd

LRC Products Ltd, North Circular Road, London E4 8QA (0208 5272377)

Maersk Medical Ltd, Thornhill Road, North Moons Moat, Redditch, Worcestershire B98 9NL (01527 64222)

Manfred Sauer UK: KG/D to KG/E, KG Business Centre, Kingsfield Way, Gladstone Industry, Dallington, Northampton, NN5 7QS (01604 588090)

Medasil (Surgical) Ltd, Medasil House, Hunslet Road, Leeds LS10 1AU (0113 2433491)

Medical-Assist Ltd (Wallace Products): see SIMS Portex Ltd

Mediplus Ltd: see Cliniflex Ltd

Mentor Medical Systems Ltd, The Woolpack, Church Street, Wantage, Oxon, OX12 8BL (01235 768758)

MMG (Europe) Ltd: see Simpla Continence Care

North West Medical Supplies Ltd, Premier House, Southgate Way, Orton Southgate, Peterborough, PE2 6YG (01733 361336)

S G & P Payne, Percy House, Brook Street, Hyde, Cheshire SK14 2NS (0161 3678561)

Pennine Healthcare, Pontefract Street, Ascot Drive Industrial Estate, Derby DE2 8JD (01332 384489)

Peoplecare: see Leyland Medical

Pharma-Plast Ltd : see Maersk Medical Ltd

Porges Ltd, 1 Onslow Street, Guildford, Surrey, GU1 4YS (01483 554120)

Portex Ltd: see SIMS Portex Ltd

Rand Rocket Ltd, ABCare House, Walsworth Road, Hitchin, Herts SG4 9SX (01462 58871)

Redland Medical PLC: see Bard Ltd

Rehab Products: see Camp Ltd

Rochester Medical Corporation: distributed by Jade Euro-Med Ltd

Donald Rose Ltd: see Steeper (Orthopaedic) Ltd

Rüsch UK Ltd, PO Box 138, Turnpike Road, Cressex Industrial Estate, High Wycombe, Bucks HP12 3NB (01494 532761)

Salts Healthcare, Saltair House, Lord Street, Birmingham B7 4DS (0121 3595123)

Sherwood Medical Industries Ltd: see The Kendall Company (UK) Ltd

MANUFACTURER'S ADDRESSES AND TELEPHONE NUMBERS - cont
(INCONTINENCE APPLIANCES)

Simcare: see SIMS Portex Ltd

Simpla Continence Care: A division of SSL International Plc, Toft Hall, Knutsford, Cheshire WA16 9PD (0161 6543000)

SIMS Portex Ltd, Hythe, Kent CT21 6JL (01303 260551)

Squibb Surgicare Ltd: see ConvaTec Ltd

Steeper (Orthopaedic) Ltd: see Ward Surgical Appliance Company Ltd

The Kendall Company (UK) Ltd: 154 Fareham Road, Gosport, Hampshire, PO13 0AS (01329 224280)

Universal Hospital Supplies, 313 Chase Road, London N14 6JA (0208 8826444)

UnoPlast: see Maersk Medical Ltd

H G Wallace Ltd: see SIMS Portex Ltd

Ward Surgical Appliance Company Ltd, 57A Brightwell Avenue, Westcliffe-on-Sea, Essex, SS0 9EB (01702 354064)

Warne-Franklin Medical Ltd: see Rüsch UK Ltd

S R Willis & Sons Ltd: see S G & P Payne

STOMA APPLIANCES
(Colostomy, Ileostomy, Urostomy)

1. Prescribers and suppliers should note that products not included in the list are not prescribable (See Part I Clause 2).

2. Where the information is available, the "**Reference Capacity**" of a stoma bag will be given. This is intended to give a guide of comparison between different bag sizes, but *should not be taken to indicate actual usable capacity*. "Reference Capacity" shall be measured according to BS 7127:Part 101:1991, Appendix M, with the level of water set at the lower edge of the opening of wafer or flange.

3. Only basic information has been provided and prescribers may on occasions wish to seek further information about certain products eg when assessing a patient for the first time. If so this is always available from the manufacturers (addresses and telephone numbers are given at the end of the entry). Information may also be sought from stoma nurses and community pharmacists.

4. Where the prescriber has not specified the type of appliance or part thereof or accessory, the pharmacy or appliance contractor must endorse the prescription form stating the type supplied and submit the invoice if requested by the Prescription Pricing Authority.

List of components and accessories	Page
Adhesive Discs/Rings/Pads/Plasters	224
Adhesives (Pastes, sprays, solutions)	227
Adhesive Removers (Sprays/liquid)	228
Bag Closures	229
Bag Covers	230
Belts	233
Colostomy Bags - see also Two Piece Ostomy Systems	242
Colostomy Sets	275
Deodorants	276
Filters/Bridges	277
Flanges	278
Ileostomy (Drainable) Bags - see also Two Piece Ostomy Systems	283
Ileostomy Sets	321
Irrigation/Wash-Out Appliances	322
Pressure Plates/Shield	323
Skin Fillers and Protectives (Barrier creams, pastes, aerosols, lotions, gels, wipes)	326
Skin Protectors (Wafers, blankets, foam pads, washers)	328
Stoma Caps/Dressings	333
Tubing	335
Two Piece Ostomy Systems	336
Urostomy Bags - see also Two Piece Ostomy Systems	360
Urostomy Sets	374

IXC

Cross Reference Index of Product Ranges and Manufacturers (Page 375)
Manufacturers' Addresses and Telephone Numbers (Page 378)

ADHESIVE DISCS/RINGS/PADS/PLASTERS

Manufacturer	Appliance	Order No.	Quantity	List Price p

For a list of adhesive tapes prescribable under Drug Tariff see page 154-155

Manufacturer	Appliance	Order No.	Quantity	List Price p
C S Bullen Ltd	Double Sided Adhesive Plaster Zinc Oxide			
	✢ 89mm x 89mm	UF 33	10	419
	✢ 102mm x 102mm	UF 34	10	516
	✢ 127mm x 127mm	UF 35	10	872
	Double Sided Adhesive Plastic Acrylic Base			
	✢ 89mm x 89mm	UF 62	10	375
	✢ 102mm x 102mm	UF 63	10	482
	✢ 127mm x 127mm	UF 64	10	811
	Flange Retention Strips			
	✢ 102mm x 25mm	UF440	100	374
	✢ 102mm x 51mm	UF441	100	507

Downs Surgical Ltd - see SIMS Portex Ltd

Eschmann Bros & Walsh Ltd - see SIMS Portex Ltd

Leyland Medical Ltd - see Rüsch UK Ltd

Manufacturer	Appliance	Order No.	Quantity	List Price p
Rüsch UK Ltd	Ostomy Double Sided Plasters			
	25mm opening	LM721031	25	673
	No opening	LM721035	25	673

✢   Approximate Conversion

ADHESIVE DISCS/RINGS/PADS/PLASTERS - cont

Manufacturer	Appliance	Order No.	Quantity	List Price p
Salts Healthcare	Transacryl Double Sided Plaster			
	25mm	833018	10	580
	32mm	833019	10	580
	38mm	833020	10	580
	Zopla D/S Plasters			
	Square			
	25mm	833078	10	435
	32mm	833079	10	435
	38mm	833080	10	435
	Circular			
	25mm	833081	10	506
	32mm	833082	10	506
	38mm	833083	10	506
	Kidney Seals	833087	10	455
	Reliaseal Double-sided hypo-allergic adhesive disc			
	13mm round	906009	10	1763
	19mm round	906011	10	1763
	22mm round	906012	10	1763
	25mm round	906013	10	1763
	29mm round	906014	10	1763
	32mm round	906015	10	1763
	38mm round	906016	10	1763
T J Shannon Ltd	Easychange spare plasters with rings		5	611
	Rubber retaining ring	TJS 948h	5	617
	Plastic locking ring	TJS 962c	1	230
	Double sided plasters	TJS 948a	25	1544
A H Shaw & Partners Ltd	Double Side plasters			
	128mm x 128mm hole cut to size	NSI 46	10	805
	102mm x 102mm hole cut to size	NSI 49	10	776

IXC

ADHESIVE DISCS/RINGS/PADS/PLASTERS - cont

Manufacturer	Appliance	Order No.	Quantity	List Price p
Simcare - see SIMS Portex Ltd				
SIMS Portex Ltd	Chiron Clearseal Plasters			
	100mm square -			
	19mm opening	WJ050-19-K	10	729
	35mm opening	WJ050-34-F	10	729
	Kidney Seals - Adhesive			
	Flange Retaining Strips			
	Small	WJ250-51-T	10	495
	Large	WJ250-75-J	10	495
	Double Sided - Adhesive Discs			
	76mm diam -			
	19mm opening	WJ002-19-R	10	467
	25mm opening	WJ002-25-L	10	467
	90mm diam -			
	32mm opening	WJ005-32-V	10	467
	38mm opening	WJ005-38-J	10	467
	Chiron Double-Sided Plasters			
	90mm square -			
	19mm opening	WJ010-19-N	10	634
	35mm opening	WJ010-35-L	10	634
	102mm square -			
	19mm opening	WJ011-19-S	10	729
	35mm opening	WJ011-35-Q	10	729
	127mm square -			
	19mm opening	WJ012-19-W	10	803
	35mm opening	WJ012-35-U	10	803
	150mm square -			
	19mm opening	WJ013-19-B	10	897
	102mm x 76mm -			
	19mm opening	WJ014-19-F	10	897
	102mm square -			
	25mm opening	WJ016-25-J	10	897
	125mm square -			
	25mm opening	WJ018-01-C	10	985
	Elastic Rings for use with			
	spout bags	WD600-12-E	3	230
	Carshalton Plasters Acrylic			
	25mm	48-530-40	10	496
	32mm	48-530-59	10	496
	38mm	48-530-67	10	496
	Carshalton Plasters Zinc Oxide			
	25mm	48-538-49	10	787
	32mm	48-538-57	10	787
	38mm	48-538-65	10	787
Ward Surgical Appliance Co	Double-Sided Plasters with			
	opening	WM17	10	450
	Single-Sided Waterproof			
	Plaster Strips			
	100mm x 25mm	WM17a	10	123
	100mm x 50mm	WM17b	10	185

ADHESIVE (PASTES, SPRAYS, SOLUTIONS)

Manufacturer	Appliance	Order No.	Quantity	List Price p
Dow Corning Ltd	● DC 355 Adhesive	DC 355	20mL	303
	● Medical Adhesive Spray B	895-6 207g	150mL/	1002
Hollister Ltd	Medical Adhesive Aerosol	7730	90g	1471
Manfred Sauer	* Original Skin Latex Adhesive in a 28g tube with a long pipette/nozzle applicator.	50.01	2	809
	* Pure Latex Skin Adhesive without any skin care components giving a stronger bond, in a 28g tube with a long pipette/nozzle applicator.	50.00	2	809
	* Lanolin Free Latex Skin Adhesive for people allergic to lanolin, in a 28g tube with a long pipette/nozzle applicator.	50.03	2	809
	* 50% reduction in skin care components, in a 28g tube with a long pipette/nozzle applicator.	50.05	2	809
	* 2% Resin giving a stronger bond than the original adhesive 50.01, in a 28g tube with a long pipette/nozzle applicator. Should only be tried after 50.01 is found to be too weak.	50.20	2	809
	* 12% Resin giving a stronger bond than the 2% resin adhesive 50.20, in a 28g tube with a long pipette/ nozzle applicator. Should only be tried after 50.20 is found to be too weak.	50.22	2	809
	* Synthetic Skin Adhesive in a 28g tube with a long pipette/nozzle applicator	50.36-2	2	1419
	* Synthetic Skin Adhesive in a 45mL bottle with brush in the lid	50.36	1	1419
Salts Healthcare	Latex Adhesive Solution	833005	✚ 28mL	203

● Temporarily Unavailable

✚ Approximate Conversion

* Safe for direct application on the skin

IXC

ADHESIVE REMOVERS (SPRAYS, LIQUIDS)

Manufacturer	Appliance	Order No.	Quantity	List Price p
Clinimed Ltd	Clear Peel Adhesive Remover	3910	50mL	285
Dow Corning Ltd	● Adhesive B Remover	896-6	150mL/ 227g	789
Hollister Ltd	Adhesive Remover	7731	76g	1254
Salts Healthcare	Lift Medical Adhesive Remover	5500	30 sachets	809
		5501	100ml bottle	570
	Plaster Remover SPR (Rezolve)	812010	60mL	303

●   Temporarily Unavailable

BAG CLOSURES
(Available separately from the bags)

Manufacturer	Appliance	Order No.	Quantity	List Price p
B. Braun Biotrol	Biotrol Closure Clamps (Post-op Bags)	3740	1	103
Clinimed Ltd	Closure Clamps (Drainable Bags)	3750	1	107
	Soft-end Ties White	9760	30	260
	Beige	9770	30	260
Coloplast Ltd	Coloplast Clamp	9503	20	1864
ConvaTec Ltd	Clips †(White) (System 2)	S206	10	298
	(Beige) (1-pce pouch)	S207	10	298
	Soft Wire Ties	S205	50	525
	Curved Clip for Drainable Pouches	S202	10	528
Dansac Ltd	Opaque Soft Wire Ties	095-01	50	524
	Opaque Longer Soft Wire Ties	095-02	50	600
Downs Surgical Ltd - see SIMS Portex Ltd				
John Drew Ltd	Clips	OSTO14	10	60
Eschmann Bros & Walsh Ltd - see SIMS Portex Ltd				
EuroCare - see Salts Healthcare				
Hollister Ltd	Premium Bag Clamp	7770	1	112
			20	1898
Pelican Healthcare Ltd	Drainable Pouch Clips	130406	20	618
Salts Healthcare	Closure Clips	833044	5	193
	Drainable Pouch Clips	CL1	10	677
T J Shannon Ltd	Closing Tape		reel	149
A H Shaw & Partners Ltd	Rubber Bag Fastening Ring	NSI 54	1	112
Simcare - see SIMS Portex Ltd				
SIMS Portex Ltd	Carshalton Clamp	48-540-12	5	1012
	Closure Clips for Odourproof Bags	WN110-01-E	10	673
	Bag Clamp	32-285-17	10	871
Squibb Surgicare Ltd - see ConvaTec Ltd				

△
|
IXC

†   to be deleted 1 January 2001

BAG COVERS

Note:
These stoma bag covers can be washed and reused many times. Cloth fabric ♦ types are more durable than those made of non-woven fabric ◊. Refer to the manufacturer's instructions.

Manufacturer	Appliance	Order No.	Quantity	List Price p
Body's Surgical Company - see Jade-Euro-Med Ltd				
C S Bullen Ltd	♦ Night Bag Cover	UF 57	1	841
	♦ Day Bag Cover	UF 58	1	841
Clinimed Ltd	♦ Stoma Bag			
	Covers	32-100	5	847
Coloplast Ltd	♦ Closed MC2000/MC2002			
	White	9011	5	2305
	Flesh	9021	5	2305
	♦ Open MC2000/MC2002			
	White	9012	5	2305
	Flesh	9022	5	2305
	♦ Mini Decorated Open MC2000			
	White	9013	5	2305
	Flesh	9023	5	2305
	♦ URO 2002 4260 White	9014	5	2305
	URO 2002 4240	9015	5	2305
	URO 2002 4241	9016	5	2305
	♦ ILEO B (Standard)	9003	5	2305
ConvaTec Ltd Surgicare System 2 Pouch Covers - see Cover Care				
Cover Care	♦ Cover Care Pouch Covers			
	Mini 32/38mm pouches	L198	3	693
	45/57mm pouches	L199	3	693
	Large Urostomy pouches	L200	3	734
	Standard Drainable pouches & urostomy pouches	L201	3	734
	Small 38/45 mm closed pouches small drainable pouches, combihesive closed pouches	L203	3	734
	Medium 57 & 70mm closed pouches	L204	3	734
Downs Surgical Ltd - see SIMS Portex Ltd				
John Drew Ltd	♦ Cotton bag covers	OST011	1	134

♦ Cloth Fabric
◊ Non-woven Fabric   } See note above.

BAG COVERS - cont

Manufacturer	Appliance	Order No.	Quantity	List Price p
Eschmann Bros & Walsh Ltd - see SIMS Portex Ltd				
Hollister Ltd	◊ Closed Bag	7036	5	460
	Drainable Bag	7038	5	460
Impharm Nationwide Ltd	♦ Ostocovers (white or coloured)		3	698
Jade-Euro-Med Ltd	♦ Bag Cover	KM 51	1	447
Nationwide Ostomy Supplies Ltd - see Impharm Nationwide Ltd				
Pelican Health-care Ltd	♦ Closed Pouch Covers			
	Normal	130207	5	1118
	Casual	130206	5	1112
	♦ Drainable Pouch Covers	130209	5	1156
Respond Plus Ltd	♦ Coversure Custom - made Covers Appliance to be stated	Res C1	1	827
Rüsch UK Ltd	♦ Ostopore Pouch Covers			
	Small	749040	5	1768
	Large	749050	5	1768
Salts Healthcare	♦ Salts Cotton Bag Cover (appliance to be stated)	833029	1	377
	♦ Eakin Cotton Bag Covers Size of opening			
	Small			
	32mm	839030	1	438
	45mm	839031	1	438
	64mm	839032	1	438
	Large			
	32mm	839033	1	438
	45mm	839034	1	438
	64mm	839035	1	438
A H Shaw & Partners Ltd	♦ Day Bag Cover			
	Cotton	NSI 48	1	510
	Lycra	NSI 44	1	538
	♦ Night Bag Cover			
	Cotton	NSI 47	1	538
	Lycra	NSI 45	1	577

IXC

♦ Cloth Fabric   }
◊ Non-woven Fabric   }   See note on page 230.

BAG COVERS - cont

Manufacturer	Appliance	Order No.	Quantity	List Price p
Simcare - see SIMS Portex Ltd				
SIMS Portex Ltd	♦ Cotton Bag Cover			
	Day Size	WN124-01-C	1	1095
	Night Size	WN125-04-N	1	1095
	♦ Cotton Cover to fit Redifit			
	Bags			
	25mm & 32mm			
	opening	WN103-01-M	1	781
	38mm, 44mm & 51mm			
	opening	WN103-04-T	1	781
	64mm & 75mm			
	opening	WN103-07-A	1	781
	♦ Cotton Stomabag Covers			
	White	32-238-84	5	2458
	Coloured	32-239-81	5	2458
	◊ "Symphony" Polythene			
	Bag Cover	32-286-06	5	455
Squibb Surgicare Ltd - see ConvaTec Ltd				
Steeper (Orthopaedic) Ltd incorporating Donald Rose Ltd - see Ward Surgical Appliance Co				
Ward Surgical Appliance Co				
	♦ White Linen Cover	15	1	652
Warne-Franklin Medical Ltd - see Rüsch UK Ltd				
Welland Medical Ltd	◊ Bag Shields spunbonded			
	Polypropylene			
	Small (25-44mm)	FSA 200	10	326
	Large (10,51,60mm)	FSA 301	10	326

♦   Cloth fabric   }
◊   Non-woven fabric   See note on page 230

BELTS

Manufacturer	Appliance	Order No.	Quantity	List Price p
Body's Surgical Company - see Jade-Euro-Med Ltd				
B. Braun Biotrol	Biotrol Waist Belt	3780	1	429
Bullen & Smears Ltd - see C S Bullen Ltd				
C S Bullen Ltd	Elastic Belt, ✚ 102mm deep with wire ring retainer			
	Small	UF 70	1	1446
	Medium	UF 71	1	1446
	Large	UF 72	1	1446
	✚ 38mm Elastic Belt with wire ring retainer			
	Small	UF 44	1	1017
	Medium	UF 45	1	1017
	Large	UF 46	1	1017
	✚ 25mm Elastic Belt with plastic retainer ring shield	UF 47	1	1076
	Waterproof Canvas retaining shield			
	Small	UF 48	1	1560
	Medium	UF 49	1	1560
	Large	UF 50	1	1560
	St Mark's Belt	UF 551	1	4174
	Fitting windows in Stoma belt for use with Ileostomy bags or colostomy cups	UF 561	1	492
	Camilla Panty Girdle	BS210	1	1927
	Cloe Roll-on Girdle	BS225	1	1605
	Constance Panty Girdle	BS200	1	2546
Cambac Instruments Ltd - see Dansac Ltd				
J. Chawner Surgical Belts Ltd	Made to Measure Ostomy Girdle with hole over stoma right and or left including steels; suspenders & zip as standard made in Lycra	CG1	1	3195
	Made to Measure Ostomy/Pantie/Girdle with hole over stoma right and or left including steels; suspenders & zip as standard made in Lycra	LG1	1	2890
	Made to Measure Colostomy Belt with hole over stoma right and or left including steels; understraps, suspenders & zip as standard made in Lycra	FC1	1	3130
	(A measuring chart is available for the above products on application)			

IXC

✚ Approximate Conversion

BELTS - cont

Manufacturer	Appliance		Order No.	Quantity	List Price p
Coloplast Ltd	Ileo Belt		0402	1	791
	K Flex Belt		0420	1	603
	Assura Seal Belt		0421	1	603
ConvaTec Ltd	System 2 Belt		S210	1	298
CoverCare	Male Support Belt Waist Size:				
	✦ Small 65-75cm		L100	1	2656
	✦ Medium 77.5-87.5cm		L101	1	2656
	✦ Large 90-100cm		L102	1	2656
	✦ Ex- Large 102.5-112.5cm		L103	1	2656
	Provision for hole aperture		HOLE	1	509

(Patients who require a hole in belt should ensure belt fits correctly and with it on, ask stoma care nurse to mark central position of stoma with a cross (X); and return belt to supplier with sample of pouch used so that hole in belt can be customised to fit individual requirements).

Dansac Ltd	Dansac Belt & Plate Pack 1 adjustable elasticated belt with 5 plates suitable for one and two piece appliances				
	50-63mm		09075-0000	1	3748
	Dansac Belt Pack 5 adjustable elasticated belts				
	50-63mm		09000-0000	5	3748

DePuy Healthcare - see Simpla Continence Care

Downs Surgical Ltd - see SIMS Portex Ltd

John Drew Ltd	Waistband	Metal ends	OST009A	1	262
		Plastic ends	OST009B	1	817
	Day Belts		OST018	1	1914
	Night Belts		OST019	1	1302
	Belt ✦ 102mm Deep Stoma				
		Hole	OST020A	1	624
		Stoma/Bones	OST020B	1	685

Eschmann Bros & Walsh - see SIMS Portex Ltd

Hollister Ltd	Adjustable Ostomy Belt				
	Small		7098	1	703
				10	5851
	Medium		7100	1	703
				10	5851
	Large		7099	1	703
				10	5851

✦ Approximate Conversion

BELTS - cont

Manufacturer	Appliance	Order No.	Quantity	List Price p
Jade-Euro-Med Ltd	Belt/double cotton face peice for St. Marks flange.			
	STATE HOLE SIZE	KM 22	1	1506
	Belt/double cotton face piece with elastic fixing for St. Marks flange.			
	STATE HOLE SIZE	KM 23	1	1965
	Belt/double cotton face peice with tapes fixing for St. Marks flange.			
	STATE HOLE SIZE	KM 24	1	1986
	St Mark's Pattern Col. Belt			
	Male	KM 30	1	5756
	Female	KM 31	1	5756
	St Mark's Coutil Ostomy Belt	KM 32	1	3939
	Ostomy Web and Elastic Belt with Button & Buckle			
	Fastening ✚ 25mm	KM 25	1	835
	Fastening ✚ 51mm	KM 26	1	989
	Fastening ✚ 76mm	KM 27	1	1140
	Ostomy Girdle and Panti Brief, Hole over Stoma			
	with Suspenders & under-strap	KM 21	1	4876
Leyland Medical Ltd - see Rüsch UK Ltd				
Marlen USA	Adjustable Elastic Waist Belt	5004	1	265
Omex Medical Ltd	Schacht Belt ✚ 91.5cm	780251	1	536
Orthotic Services Ltd	Made to Measure Ostomy Girdle in white - hole or panel over stoma as required; zips and suspenders as standard			
		OSL-012	1	3195
	(A measuring chart is available on application)			
J C Peacock & Son Ltd	St Marks Pattern Belt	Peak 1	1	3815
Respond Plus Ltd	Lightweight Support Belt 13cm wide, Small, Medium, Large, Ex Large Hook & Eye or Velcro Fastening			
	With hole over stoma	Res 3	1	2456
	Lightweight Support Belt (long) 23cm wide Small, Medium, Large, Ex Large Hook & Eye or Velcro Fastening			
	With hole over stoma	Res 4	1	2850
	Ladies Ostomy belt Including hole over stoma			
	With detachable suspenders	Res 5	1	3400
	Medium control Ostomy Girdle/Pantie Brief including hole over stoma			
	With suspenders as required	Res 2	1	3831
	Ostomy Girdle/Pantie Brief including hole over stoma, with			
	suspenders as required	Res 1	1	3898

✚   Approximate Conversion

IXC

BELTS - cont

Manufacturer	Appliance	Order No.	Quantity	List Price p
Respond Plus Ltd - cont	Ostoshield (without belt)	Res50	1	620
	Ostoshield Belt Small/Medium 45cm/85cm	Res40	1	320
	Ostoshield Belt Large/Extra Large 66cm/124cm	Res45	1	320
Rüsch UK Ltd	Birkbeck Elastic Waistband & Shield			
	19mm	LM725219	5	4614
	38mm	LM725238	5	4614
	54mm	LM725254	5	4614
	Birkbeck Retaining ring - for use with above			
	19mm	LM725319	5	875
	38mm	LM725338	5	875
	54mm	LM725354	5	875
	Birkbeck Elastic Waist Band	LM725100	5	3507
	Ostopore Belt Normal Width Waist			
	✚ 43cm x 86cm	749000	1	564
	✚ 71cm x 142cm	749010	1	564
	Narrow Width Waist			
	✚ 43cm x 86cm	749020	1	564
	✚ 71cm x 142cm	749030	1	564
	White Rubber Belting			
	28mm wide	LM810063	per metre	383
	72mm wide	LM811001	per metre	792
	White Sausage Belt	LM810004	per metre	789
	Waist & Support Strap	LM886103	1	651
E Sallis Ltd	Colostomy Belt for			
	Night use	14b	1	1118
		14c	1	583
	Day use	15a	1	3080
	Ostomy Girdle/Pantie Brief including hole over stoma, with suspenders as required			
	Made in elastane	Fit 15c	1	3902
	St Mark's Hospital Pattern			
	Colostomy Belt	16	1	2824
	Colostomy Shield	17	1	1023
	Zipped Pocket (fitted to 15a, 16 and Fit 15c)	21	1	523

✚   Approximate Conversion

BELTS - cont

Manufacturer	Appliance	Order No.	Quantity	List Price p
Salts Healthcare	Salger Adjustable Elastic Belt	600600	1	359
	With Velcro Fastening	600601	1	352
	Rubber front belt with straps & buckles	877001	1	685
	25mm Single Elastic Belt with 2 loops:			
	Standard ✚ 89cm long	877002	1	349
	Ex-large ✚ 107cm long	877024	1	349
	25mm Double Elastic Belt with 4 loops:	877003	1	593
	25mm Rubber Belt with 2 fastening studs	877004	1	402
	25mm Single Elastic Belt with suspender ends	877007	1	409
	102mm Elastic Belt with waterproof panel	877008	1	1433
	With 4 loops & retaining ring	877009	1	1884
	Saltair Ileostomy Girdle	877010	1	4585
	25mm Button Belt	877011	1	349
	Button & Loop Belt	877012	1	349
	Baby Lycra Belt	877013	1	1408
	With Velcro Fastening			
	Standard ✚ 89cm long	877022	1	355
	Ex-large ✚ 107cm long	877023	1	355
	150mm Elastic Belt with Waterproof Panel	877017	1	1745
	Colostomy Belt	877018	1	7178
	Saltair Ileostomy Elastic Night Belt	877019	1	1393
	Eakin Elasticated Belt			
	Small	839029	1	345
	Large	839036	1	345

IXC

✚   Approximate Conversion

BELTS - cont

Manufacturer	Appliance	Order No.	Quantity	List Price p
SASH	Made to Measure 50mm polyester webbing Stoma Hernia Support Belt attached to plastic flange with hole over stoma	S1	1	3184

(Patients are required to complete an Order Form obtainable from Stoma Care Nurses or SASH (Address: Woodhouse, Woodside Road, Hockley, Essex, SS5 4RU Tel 01702 206 502) detailing waist size and enclosing a sample of pouch used so that the hole within the belt flange can be customised to fit individual requirements)

Manufacturer	Appliance	Order No.	Quantity	List Price p
T J Shannon Ltd	Elastic Belt & Shield (with Velcro Fastening)	TJS 948c	1	758
	Elastic Belt(with button & buckle fastening)	TJS 962d	1	461
A H Shaw & Partners Ltd	Colostomy Belt 102mm wide elastic web made to measure	NSI 10	1	1458
	102mm Ostomy Belt			
	With groin strap	NSI 10A	1	1667
	With lace fastenings	NSI 11	1	1772
	With wire spring	NSI 12	1	1632
	Double zip panel	NSI 36	1	846
	Colostomy Belt 152mm wide made to measure			
	With under-strap	NSI 13	1	1953
	With lace fastenings	NSI 14	1	2642
	Colostomy Belt 205mm wide made to measure			
	With under-strap	NSI 15	1	2804
	With lace fastenings	NSI 16	1	3347
	255mm Belt made to measure	NSI 17	1	3184
	With zip panel	NSI 18	1	4018
	306mm Belt made to measure	NSI 19	1	3499
	With zip panel	NSI 20	1	4261
	357mm Belt made to measure	NSI 21	1	3568
	With zip panel	NSI 22	1	4460

BELTS - cont

Manufacturer	Appliance	Order No.	Quantity	List Price p
A H Shaw & Partners Ltd - cont	Colostomy/Ileostomy Adjustable Belt			
	25mm wide	NSI 23	1	846
	102mm wide 3 sections	NSI 24	1	2139
	154mm wide 3 sections	NSI 25	1	2697
	Colostomy Belt, Elastic with Nylon fronts made to measure			
	254mm wide	NSI 33	1	3736
	306mm wide	NSI 34	1	3925
	357mm wide	NSI 35	1	4175
	Colostomy Night Belt in net or rayon, no hole, for use with dressing pad	NSI 32	1	1557
Simcare - see SIMS Portex Ltd				
SIMS Portex Ltd	Web & Elastic Belt			
	25mm wide	WL002-25-B	1	1067
	51mm wide	WL002-51-C	1	1245
	75mm wide	WL002-75-S	1	1394
	Short Web End and Buckle	WL005-25-P	1	720
	Web & Elastic Belt			
	25mm wide	WL008-25-C	1	1166
	Narrow Belt Flange diam			
	32mm	WL111-32-F	1	2220
	38mm	WL111-38-T	1	2220
	51mm	WL111-51-K	1	2220
	Redifit Adjustable Belt			
	Small	WL123-01-H	1	897
	Medium	WL123-04-P	1	897
	Large	WL123-07-V	1	897
	Web & Elastic Belt Child			
	25mm wide	WL129-25-Y	1	897
	38mm wide	WL129-38-J	1	1250
	Elastic non-slip belt	WL132-25-Y	1	1250
	Non-slip belt	WL133-01-N	1	1830
	Rubber 'Sausage' Belt	WL135-12-C	1	2331
	Rubber 'Tubular' Belt	WL138-01-K	1	2331
	Narrow Rubber Belt	WL144-01-X	1	678

IXC

BELTS - cont

Manufacturer	Appliance	Order No.	Quantity	List Price p
SIMS Portex Ltd - cont	Night Belt Two Way Stretch			
	Small	WL236-01-H	1	2502
	Medium	WL236-04-P	1	2502
	Large	WL236-07-V	1	2502
	Ex-large	WL236-09-A	1	2502
	Carshalton Belt			
	Small	48-522-14	1	946
	Medium	48-522-22	1	946
	Large	48-524-19	1	946
	Stoma Belt			
	Small - ✚ 43cm - 66cm	32-247-83	1	593
	Medium -			
	✚ 66cm x 109cm	32-248-80	1	593
Squibb Surgicare Ltd - see ConvaTec Ltd				
Steeper (Orthopaedic) Ltd - incorporating Donald Rose Ltd - see Ward Surgical Appliance Co				
Ward Surgical Appliance Co				
	Day Colostomy Belt made to measure			
	All sizes	23	1	4116
	Night Colostomy Belt, made to measure, in White cellular material			
	All sizes	24	1	3030
	Nylon Elastic Colostomy belt hook & eye fastening, complete with 2 pairs suspenders or under-straps			
	All sizes	25	1	4252
	Gabriel type Colostomy belt with 2 pairs suspenders or under-straps			
	All sizes	26	1	4805
	Wide second stage rubberised ileostomy belt with 2 straps, and buttonholed ends for use with ileostomy boxes, or with celluloid hook ends for use with ileostomy bags	19	1	2415
	As above - with under-straps or suspenders	20	1	2715

✚   Approximate Conversion

BELTS - cont

Manufacturer	Appliance	Order No.	Quantity	List Price p
Ward Surgical Appliance Co - cont				
	Fitting "windows" in belt for use with ileostomy bags or colostomy cups, or 4 stitched holes for studs of colostomy cups or shields	35	1	438
	Web and Elastic Belt with button and buckle fastening			
	✚ 25mm wide	WM 25	1	783
	✚ 51mm wide	WM 51	1	1010
	✚ 76mm wide	WM 75	1	1147
	Hookend Elastic Belt	WM 86	1	1093
Warne-Franklin Medical Ltd - see Rüsch UK Ltd				

IXC

✚   Approximate Conversion

COLOSTOMY BAGS

Manufacturer	Appliance	Order No.	Quantity	List Price p
Body's Surgical Company - see Jade-Euro-Med				
B. Braun Biotrol	**Biotrol**			
	Colo S bag With skin protector adhesive			
	White			
	25mm	32-525	30	6657
	30mm	32-530	30	6657
	35mm	32-535	30	6657
	40mm	32-540	30	6657
	45mm	32-545	30	6657
	50mm	32-550	30	6657
	60mm	32-560	30	6657
	Elite bag With filter, skin protector adhesive, fabric backing			
	Beige			
	Starter hole	36-810	30	7021
	25mm	36-825	30	7021
	30mm	36-830	30	7021
	35mm	36-835	30	7021
	40mm	36-840	30	7021
	45mm	36-845	30	7021
	50mm	36-850	30	7021
	60mm	36-860	30	7021
	70mm	36-870	30	7021
	Transparent			
	Starter hole	30-810	30	6613
	25mm	30-825	30	6522
	30mm	30-830	30	6522
	35mm	30-835	30	6522
	40mm	30-840	30	6522
	45mm	30-845	30	6522
	50mm	30-850	30	6522
	60mm	30-860	30	6522
	70mm	30-870	30	6522
	White			
	Starter hole	32-815	30	7021
	25mm	32-825	30	7021
	30mm	32-830	30	7021
	35mm	32-835	30	7021
	40mm	32-840	30	7021
	45mm	32-845	30	7021
	50mm	32-850	30	7021
	60mm	32-860	30	7021
	70mm	32-870	30	7021
	Elite Petite bag with filter, skin protector adhesive, fabric backing			
	Beige			
	starter hole	37-310	30	5969
	25mm	37-325	30	5969
	30mm	37-330	30	5969
	35mm	37-335	30	5969
	40mm	37-340	30	5969
	45mm	37-345	30	5969

COLOSTOMY BAGS - cont

Manufacturer	Appliance	Order No.	Quantity	List Price p
B. Braun Biotrol - cont				
Biotrol - cont	Mini S size (reference capacity : 75-69mL (see Note 2, page 223))			
	with filter, skin protector adhesive, fabric backing			
	Beige			
	25mm	33-025	30	5492
	30mm	33-030	30	5492
	35mm	33-035	30	5492
	40mm	33-040	30	5492
	Integrale bag with filter & skin protector adhesive			
	White			
	starter hole	32-415	30	7021
	25mm	32-425	30	7021
	30mm	32-430	30	7021
	35mm	32-435	30	7021
	40mm	32-440	30	7021
	45mm	32-445	30	7021
	50mm	32-450	30	7021
	60mm	32-460	30	7021
	70mm	32-470	30	7021
	Preference bag			
	With filter, skin protector adhesive, fabric backing			
	Beige			
	starter hole	36-615	30	6678
	25mm	36-625	30	6678
	30mm	36-630	30	6678
	35mm	36-635	30	6678
	40mm	36-640	30	6678
	45mm	36-645	30	6678
	50mm	36-650	30	6678
	60mm	36-660	30	6678
	White			
	starter hole	32-610	30	6678
	25mm	32-625	30	6678
	30mm	32-630	30	6678
	35mm	32-635	30	6678
	40mm	32-640	30	6678
	45mm	32-645	30	6678
	50mm	32-650	30	6678
	60mm	32-660	30	6678
	Almarys bag with filter, Interface adhesive and all over soft			
	non-woven cover			
	Transparent			
	starter hole	76-015	30	6051
	Beige starter hole	76-115	30	6051
	25mm	76-025	30	6051
	30mm	76-030	30	6051
	35mm	76-035	30	6051
	40mm	76-040	30	6051
	45mm	76-045	30	6051
	50mm	76-050	30	6051
	60mm	76-060	30	6051

IXC

COLOSTOMY BAGS - cont

Manufacturer	Appliance	Order No.	Quantity	List Price p
B. Braun Biotrol - cont				
	Biotrol - cont			
	Almarys Petite bag with filter, Interface adhesive and all over soft non-woven cover			
	Beige starter hole	79-020	30	5354
	25mm	79-025	30	5354
	30mm	79-030	30	5354
	35mm	79-035	30	5354
	40mm	79-040	30	5354
	Almarys Optima Closed bag with filter and all over soft non-woven cover Transparent			
	starter hole 10mm	018610	30	5830
	Beige starterhole 10mm	008610	30	5830
	25mm	008625	30	5830
	30mm	008630	30	5830
	35mm	008635	30	5830
	40mm	008640	30	5830
	45mm	008645	30	5830
	50mm	008650	30	5830
	60mm	008660	30	5830
	Almarys Optima Mini Closed bag with filter and all over soft non woven cover			
	Beige 20mm	008920	30	5159
	25mm	008925	30	5159
	30mm	008930	30	5159
	35mm	008935	30	5159
	40mm	008940	30	5159
	Almarys Quiet Closed bag with filter and all over soft non-woven cover Transparent			
	starter hole 10mm	018110	30	5830
	Beige starter hole 10mm	008110	30	5830
	25mm	008125	30	5830
	30mm	008130	30	5830
	35mm	008135	30	5830
	40mm	008140	30	5830
	45mm	008145	30	5830
	50mm	008150	30	5830
	60mm	008160	30	5830
	Almarys Preference Closed bag with filter, skin protector and microporous adhesive and all over soft non-woven cover Transparent			
	starter hole 10mm	018310	30	5830
	Beige starter hole 10mm	008310	30	5830
	25mm	008325	30	5830
	30mm	008330	30	5830
	35mm	008335	30	5830
	40mm	008340	30	5830
	45mm	008345	30	5830
	50mm	008350	30	5830
	60mm	008360	30	5830

COLOSTOMY BAGS - cont

Manufacturer	Appliance	Order No.	Quantity	List Price p
Cambmac Instruments Ltd - see Dansac Ltd				
Coloplast Ltd	**Assura** Inspire Closed Bag with Integral Filter, Oval Adhesive and Soft Backing.			
	Midi Transparent			
	starter hole 20-65mm	12130	30	6717
	ready-cut 25mm	12134	30	6717
	30mm	12135	30	6717
	35mm	12136	30	6717
	Maxi Transparent			
	starter hole 20 - 75mm	12160	30	6717
	Inspire Closed Bag with Integral Filter, Oval Adhesive and Opaque Soft Cover Front and Back.			
	Midi Soft Cover			
	starter hole 20 - 65mm	12140	30	6717
	ready-cut 25mm	12144	30	6717
	30mm	12145	30	6717
	35mm	12146	30	6717
	40mm	12147	30	6717
	45mm	12148	30	6717
	50mm	12149	30	6717
	Maxi Soft Cover			
	starter hole 20-75mm	12170	30	6717
	Inspire Closed Bag with Integral Filter, Oval Adhesive and Soft Cover Front and Back.			
	Midi Design			
	starter hole 20 - 65mm	12150	30	6717
	ready-cut 25mm	12154	30	6717
	30mm	12155	30	6717
	35mm	12156	30	6717
	40mm	12157	30	6717
	45mm	12158	30	6717
	50mm	12159	30	6717
	Maxi Design			
	starter hole 20 - 75mm	12180	30	6717
	Closed Bag with Integral Filter and Soft Backing			
	Mini Opaque			
	starter hole 20mm	2421	30	5478
	ready-cut 25mm	2424	30	5478
	30mm	2425	30	5478
	35mm	2426	30	5478
	40mm	2427	30	5478
	Midi Clear			
	starter hole 20mm	2471	30	6717
	ready-cut 25mm	2474	30	6717
	30mm	2475	30	6717
	35mm	2476	30	6717
	40mm	2477	30	6717
	45mm	2478	30	6717
	50mm	2479	30	6717

IXC

245

COLOSTOMY BAGS - cont

Manufacturer	Appliance	Order No.	Quantity	List Price p
Coloplast Ltd - cont				
	Assura Closed Bag with Integral Filter and Soft Backing - cont			
	Midi Opaque			
	starter hole 20mm	2461	30	6717
	ready-cut 25mm	2464	30	6717
	30mm	2465	30	6717
	35mm	2466	30	6717
	40mm	2467	30	6717
	45mm	2468	30	6717
	50mm	2469	30	6717
	Maxi Clear			
	starter hole 20mm	2481	30	6717
	ready-cut 25mm	2484	30	6717
	30mm	2485	30	6717
	35mm	2486	30	6717
	40mm	2487	30	6717
	45mm	2488	30	6717
	50mm	2489	30	6717
	Maxi Opaque			
	starter hole 20mm	2511	30	6717
	ready-cut 25mm	2514	30	6717
	30mm	2515	30	6717
	35mm	2516	30	6717
	40mm	2517	30	6717
	Maxi Clear			
	starter hole 10-70mm	2482	30	6717
	Maxi Opaque			
	starter hole 10-70mm	2512	30	6717
	Paediatric Opaque			
	starter hole 10-35mm	2120	30	5853
	Closed Bag with Integral Filter and Opaque Soft Cover front and back			
	Mini			
	starter hole 20-55mm	12420	30	5379
	Midi			
	starter hole 20-55mm	12460	30	6717
	pre-cut 25mm	12464	30	6717
	30mm	12465	30	6717
	35mm	12466	30	6717
	40mm	12467	30	6717
	45mm	12468	30	6717
	50mm	12469	30	6717
	Maxi			
	starter hole 10-70mm	12580	30	6717
	starter hole 20-55mm	12480	30	6717

COLOSTOMY BAGS - cont

Manufacturer	Appliance	Order No.	Quantity	List Price p
Coloplast Ltd - cont				
	Assura			
	Seal Integral Convexity Closed Bags with Filter and Soft Backing			
	Important: This product with Integral Convexity should only be used after prior assessment of suitability by an appropriate medical professional			
	Midi Clear			
	21mm	12863	10	2237
	25mm	12864	10	2237
	28mm	12865	10	2237
	31mm	12866	10	2237
	35mm	12867	10	2237
	Midi Opaque			
	starter hole 15-33mm	12562	10	2237
	15-43mm	12563	10	2237
	Maxi Clear			
	21mm	12883	10	2237
	25mm	12884	10	2237
	28mm	12885	10	2237
	31mm	12886	10	2237
	35mm	12887	10	2237
	38mm	12888	10	2237
	Maxi Opaque			
	starter hole 15-33mm	12572	10	2237
	15-43mm	12573	10	2237
	Assura Conseal 1 Piece Plug			
	Important: This product should only be used after prior assessment of suitability by an appropriate medical professional.			
	Length Size			
	35mm stoma size 20-35mm	1435	10	2199
	stoma size 35-45mm	1485	10	2199
	45mm stoma size 20-35mm	1445	10	2199
	stoma size 35-45mm	1495	10	2199
	K-Flex Opaque 30mm	2923	30	6981
	40mm	2924	30	6981
	Extra			
	No. 2 - 30mm	0102	100	11650
	No. 2 - 40mm	0114	100	11650
	No. 3 - 30mm	0103	100	13980

IXC

COLOSTOMY BAGS - cont

Manufacturer	Appliance			Order No.	Quantity	List Price p
Coloplast Ltd - cont						
	MC2000					
	Clear	25mm		5625	30	7224
		30mm		5630	30	7224
		35mm		5635	30	7224
		40mm		5640	30	7224
		45mm		5645	30	7224
		50mm		5650	30	7224
		55mm		5655	30	7224
		60mm		5660	30	7224
	Opaque	25mm		5725	30	7224
		30mm		5730	30	7224
		35mm		5735	30	7224
		40mm		5740	30	7224
		45mm		5745	30	7224
		50mm		5750	30	7224
		55mm		5755	30	7224
		60mm		5760	30	7224
	PC 3000					
	Clear	25mm		8725	30	6822
		30mm		8730	30	6822
		35mm		8735	30	6822
		40mm		8740	30	6822
		45mm		8745	30	6822
		50mm		8750	30	6822
	Opaque	25mm		8825	30	6822
		30mm		8830	30	6822
		35mm		8835	30	6822
		40mm		8840	30	6822
		45mm		8845	30	6822
		50mm		8850	30	6822
		55mm		8855	30	6822
ConvaTec Ltd	**Colodress Plus** (Stomahesive Wafer) Closed Pouches					
	Opaque					
	starter hole -					
		19mm		S861	30	6551
	precut	25mm		S862	30	6551
		32mm		S863	30	6551
		38mm		S864	30	6551
		45mm		S865	30	6551
		50mm		S866	30	6551
		64mm		S867	30	6551

COLOSTOMY BAGS - cont

Manufacturer	Appliance		Order No.	Quantity	List Price p
ConvaTec Ltd - cont	**Colodress Plus** (Stomahesive Wafer) Closed Pouches cont.				
	Clear				
	starter hole -				
		19mm	S871	30	6551
	precut	25mm	S872	30	6551
		32mm	S873	30	6551
		38mm	S874	30	6551
		45mm	S875	30	6551
		50mm	S876	30	6551
		64mm	S877	30	6551
	Mini	19mm	S901	30	5910
		25mm	S902	30	5910
		32mm	S903	30	5910
		38mm	S904	30	5910
		45mm	S905	30	5910
	Colodress (Wafer plus microporous ring) Closed pouches				
	Opaque				
	starter hole -				
		19mm	S801	30	6518
	precut	32mm	S803	30	6518
		38mm	S805	30	6518
		45mm	S806	30	6518
		50mm	S807	30	6518
	Colodress Plus Lite Closed Pouches				
	Standard - opaque				
	starter hole -				
		19mm	S941	30	6021
	precut	25mm	S942	30	6021
		32mm	S943	30	6021
		38mm	S944	30	6021
		45mm	S945	30	6021
		50mm	S946	30	6021
	Esteem Closed Pouches with Malodour Counteractant Insert and Integral filter				
	Small - opaque				
	starter hole				
		20mm - 60mm	S5001	30	5456
	precut	25mm	S5002	30	5456
		30mm	S5003	30	5456
		40mm	S5004	30	5456
		50mm	S5005	30	5456
	Medium - clear				
	starter hole				
		20mm - 80mm	S5006	30	6138
	precut	25mm	S5007	30	6138
		30mm	S5008	30	6138
		40mm	S5009	30	6138
		50mm	S5010	30	6138

IXC

COLOSTOMY BAGS - cont

Manufacturer	Appliance	Order No.	Quantity	List Price p
ConvaTec Ltd - cont				
	Esteem Closed Pouches with Malodour Counteractant Insert and Integral filter - cont			
	Medium - opaque			
	starter hole			
	20mm-80mm	S5013	30	6138
	precut 25mm	S5014	30	6138
	30mm	S5015	30	6138
	40mm	S5016	30	6138
	50mm	S5017	30	6138
	Large - clear			
	starter hole			
	20mm-80mm	S5020	30	6138
	Large-opaque			
	starter hole			
	20mm-80mm	S5027	30	6138
	precut 25mm	S5028	30	6138
	30mm	S5029	30	6138
	40mm	S5030	30	6138
	50mm	S5031	30	6138
	60mm	S5032	30	6138
	70mm	S5033	30	6138
	Naturess Closed pouches			
	Standard - opaque			
	starter hole			
	19mm-50mm	S918	50	10229
	pre-cut 25mm	S919	50	10229
	32mm	S920	50	10229
	38mm	S921	50	10229
	45mm	S922	50	10229
	50mm	S923	50	10229
	Standard - clear			
	starter hole			
	19mm	S925	50	10229
	Small - opaque			
	starter hole			
	19mm-50mm	S926	50	9092
	pre-cut 25mm	S927	50	9092
	32mm	S928	50	9092
	38mm	S929	50	9092
	45mm	S930	50	9092

COLOSTOMY BAGS - cont

Manufacturer	Appliance	Order No.	Quantity	List Price p
ConvaTec Ltd - cont				
†	**Naturess D** Closed pouches with Malodour Counteractant Insert Standard-opaque starter hole			
	19mm-50mm	S9180	50	10053
	pre-cut 25mm	S9190	50	10053
	32mm	S9200	50	10053
	38mm	S9210	50	10053
	45mm	S9220	50	10053
	50mm	S9230	50	10053
	Standard-clear starter hole			
	19mm	S9250	50	9880
	Naturess A Closed pouches Standard Opaque with Superabsorbent Pad starter hole			
	19mm	S990	50	9979
	pre-cut 25mm	S991	50	9979
	32mm	S992	50	9979
	38mm	S993	50	9979
	45mm	S994	50	9979
	50mm	S995	50	9979
Dansac Ltd	**Combi Colo F**			
††	Opaque 25mm	01525-1000	100	17403
	30mm	01530-1000	100	17403
	38mm	01538-1000	100	17403
	44mm	01544-1000	100	17403
	50mm	01550-1000	100	17403
	63mm	01563-1000	100	17403
††	Clear 25mm	01525-2000	100	17403
	30mm	01530-2000	100	17403
	38mm	01538-2000	100	17403
	44mm	01544-2000	100	17403
	50mm	01550-2000	100	17403
	63mm	01563-2000	100	17403
††	Small - Opaque			
	25mm	01625-1000	100	17403
	30mm	01630-1000	100	17403
	38mm	01638-1000	100	17403
††	Small - Clear			
	25mm	01625-2000	100	17403
	30mm	01630-2000	100	17403
	38mm	01638-2000	100	17403
††	Standard			
	Colo 1 - 22mm	11122-4000	100	15622
	Colo 2 - 30mm	11230-4000	100	15622
	Colo 3 - 32mm	11332-4000	100	15622
	Colo 4 - 38mm	11438-4000	100	15622

IXC

† to be deleted 1 December 2000
†† to be deleted 1 February 2001

COLOSTOMY BAGS - cont

Manufacturer	Appliance	Order No.	Quantity	List Price p
Dansac Ltd				
	CombiMicro C & S			
	† Opaque			
	25mm	22025-1300	30	7137
	32mm	22032-1300	30	7137
	38mm	22038-1300	30	7137
	44mm	22044-1300	30	7137
	50mm	22050-1300	30	7137
	63mm	22063-1300	30	7137
	† Cut to Fit			
	starter hole			
	10mm - 38mm	22110-1300	30	7137
	38mm - 63mm	22138-1300	30	7137
	† Clear			
	25mm	22025-2300	30	7137
	32mm	22032-2300	30	7137
	38mm	22038-2300	30	7137
	44mm	22044-2300	30	7137
	50mm	22050-2300	30	7137
	63mm	22063-2300	30	7137
	† Cut to Fit			
	starter hole			
	10mm - 38mm	22110-2300	30	7137
	38mm - 63mm	22138-2300	30	7137

Dansac Light Convex
Integral convexity closed bag with filter and soft cover front and back
Important: This product with integral convexity should only be used after prior assessment of suitability by an appropriate medical professional.

		Order No.	Quantity	List Price p
Opaque				
starter hole	15-24mm	257-24	10	2177
	15-37mm	257-37	10	2177
	15-46mm	257-46	10	2177
Opaque				
pre-cut	20mm	257-20	10	2177
	25mm	257-25	10	2177
	30mm	257-30	10	2177
	35mm	257-35	10	2177
	40mm	257-40	10	2177
	45mm	257-45	10	2177
Clear				
starter hole	15-24mm	258-24	10	2177
	15-37mm	258-37	10	2177
	15-46mm	258-46	10	2177

† to be deleted 1 February 2001

COLOSTOMY BAGS - cont

Manufacturer	Appliance		Order No.	Quantity	List Price p
Dansac Ltd - cont					
	Dansac Light Convex - cont				
	Clear				
	pre-cut	20mm	258-20	10	2177
		25mm	258-25	10	2177
		30mm	258-30	10	2177
		35mm	258-35	10	2177
		40mm	258-40	10	2177
		45mm	258-45	10	2177
	Unique				
	Opaque				
		starter hole	227-20	30	6229
		25mm	225-25	30	6229
		30mm	225-30	30	6229
		35mm	225-35	30	6229
		40mm	225-40	30	6229
		45mm	225-45	30	6229
		50mm	225-50	30	6229
		60mm	225-60	30	6229
	Clear				
		starter hole	228-20	30	6229
		25mm	226-25	30	6229
		30mm	226-30	30	6229
		35mm	226-35	30	6229
		40mm	226-40	30	6229
		45mm	226-45	30	6229
		50mm	226-50	30	6229
		60mm	226-60	30	6229
	Mini opaque (reference capacity: 220mL (see Note 2, page 223))				
	cut to fit				
		20mm-50mm	231-20	30	5744
	pre-cut				
		25mm	231-25	30	5744
		30mm	231-30	30	5744
		35mm	231-35	30	5744
		40mm	231-40	30	5744
	Oval Flange				
	Opaque - starter hole		223-15	30	6229
	Clear - starter hole		224-15	30	6229
	Dansac Nova				
	Opaque				
	starter hole				
		20-60mm	801-20	30	6600
	pre-cut				
		25mm	801-25	30	6600
		30mm	801-30	30	6600
		35mm	801-35	30	6600
		40mm	801-40	30	6600
		45mm	801-45	30	6600
		50mm	801-50	30	6600
	Clear				
	starter hole				
		20-60mm	802-20	30	6600

IXC

COLOSTOMY BAGS - cont

Manufacturer	Appliance	Order No.	Quantity	List Price p
Dansac Ltd - cont				
	Dansac Nova Mini			
	Opaque			
	starter hole			
	20-50mm	803-20	30	5400
	pre-cut			
	25mm	803-25	30	5400
	30mm	803-30	30	5400
	35mm	803-35	30	5400
	40mm	803-40	30	5400
	Unique Light			
	Closed pouch			
	Opaque-soft lining on both sides, tapered barrier and fully activated filter			
	cut-to-fit			
	20mm-60mm	255-20	30	6240
	pre-cut			
	25mm	255-25	30	6240
	30mm	255-30	30	6240
	35mm	255-35	30	6240
	40mm	255-40	30	6240
	45mm	255-45	30	6240
	50mm	255-50	30	6240
	60mm	255-60	30	6240

DePuy Healthcare - see Simpla Continence Care

Downs Surgical Ltd - see SIMS Portex Ltd

Eschmann Bros & Walsh Ltd - see SIMS Portex Ltd

EuroCare - see Salts Healthcare

COLOSTOMY BAGS - cont

Manufacturer	Appliance	Order No.	Quantity	List Price p
Hollister Ltd	**Compact**			
	Closed Pouch			
	Clear-with filter and white comfort backing on body-worn side			
	cut-to-fit			
	13 - 64mm	3460	30	6647
	Beige-with filter and beige comfort backing on both sides			
	cut-to-fit			
	13 - 64mm	3470	30	6647
	pre-cut			
	25mm	3472	30	6647
	32mm	3478	30	6647
	38mm	3473	30	6647
	44mm	3479	30	6647
	51mm	3474	30	6647
	64mm	3475	30	6647
	Transparent - with filter and white comfort backing on body-worn side			
	cut-to-fit			
	13-64mm	3520	30	6647
	pre-cut			
	25mm	3522	30	6647
	32mm	3528	30	6647
	38mm	3523	30	6647
	44mm	3529	30	6647
	51mm	3524	30	6647
	64mm	3525	30	6647
	Karaya 5 seal only with filter			
	Opaque			
	✚ 25mm	2112	30	5957
	✚ 32mm	2118	30	5957
	✚ 38mm	2113	30	5957
	✚ 44mm	2119	30	5957
	✚ 51mm	2114	30	5957
	✚ 64mm	2115	30	5957
	✚ 76mm	2116	30	5957
	Karaya 5 seal without filter			
	Transparent			
	✚ 25mm	7162	30	5957
	✚ 32mm	7168	30	5957
	✚ 38mm	7163	30	5957
	✚ 44mm	7169	30	5957
	✚ 51mm	7164	30	5957
	✚ 64mm	7165	30	5957
	✚ 76mm	7166	30	5957
	Karaya 5 seal with microporous adhesive and filter			
	Opaque			
	✚ 25mm	3312	30	7064
	✚ 32mm	3318	30	7064
	✚ 38mm	3313	30	7064
	✚ 44mm	3319	30	7064
	✚ 51mm	3314	30	7064
	✚ 64mm	3315	30	7064
	✚ 76mm	3316	30	7064

IXC

✚   Approximate Conversion

COLOSTOMY BAGS - cont

Manufacturer	Appliance	Order No.	Quantity	List Price p
Hollister Ltd - cont				
	Karaya 5 seal with microporous adhesive and filter - cont			
	Transparent			
	✚ 25mm	3322	30	7064
	✚ 32mm	3328	30	7064
	✚ 38mm	3323	30	7064
	✚ 44mm	3329	30	7064
	✚ 51mm	3324	30	7064
	✚ 64mm	3325	30	7064
	✚ 76mm	3326	30	7064
	Microporous Adhesive only with filter			
	Transparent			
	✚ 25mm	3142	50	7579
	✚ 32mm	3148	50	7579
	✚ 38mm	3143	50	7579
	✚ 44mm	3149	50	7579
	✚ 51mm	3144	50	7579
	✚ 64mm	3145	50	7579
	✚ 76mm	3146	50	7579
	Premium Bag with Karaya 5 seal microporous adhesive and filter			
	Opaque			
†	✚ 25mm	3532	15	3563
	✚ 32mm	3538	15	3563
	✚ 38mm	3533	15	3563
	✚ 44mm	3539	15	3563
	✚ 51mm	3534	15	3563
	✚ 64mm	3535	15	3563
	✚ 76mm	3536	15	3563
	Transparent			
	✚ 25mm	3552	15	3563
	✚ 32mm	3558	15	3563
	✚ 38mm	3553	15	3563
	✚ 44mm	3559	15	3563
	✚ 51mm	3554	15	3563
	✚ 64mm	3555	15	3563
	✚ 76mm	3556	15	3563

✚   Approximate Conversion
†   to be deleted 1 December 2000

COLOSTOMY BAGS - cont

Manufacturer	Appliance	Order No.	Quantity	List Price p	
Hollister Ltd - cont	**Impression "C"** with convex wafer Beige with filter and beige Comfort backing on both sides				
	19mm	3490	10	2313	
	22mm	3491	10	2313	
	25mm	3492	10	2313	
	29mm	3493	10	2313	
	32mm	3494	10	2313	
	35mm	3495	10	2313	
	38mm	3496	10	2313	
	41mm	3497	10	2313	
	44mm	3498	10	2313	
	51mm	3499	10	2313	
	Impression "C" with convex wafer, Transparent front with filter and beige Comfort backing on body worn side				
	19mm	3590	10	2271	
	22mm	3591	10	2271	
	25mm	3592	10	2271	
	29mm	3593	10	2271	
	32mm	3594	10	2271	
	35mm	3595	10	2271	
	38mm	3596	10	2271	
	41mm	3597	10	2271	
	44mm	3598	10	2271	
	51mm	3599	10	2271	
	Moderma				
	Closed Pouch with skin-resting barrier, filter and beige comfort backing on body worn side, Quiet Film				
	Transparent				
	Starter Hole				
	15-50mm	23000	30	6169	Δ
	Closed Pouch with skin-resting barrier, filter and beige comfort backing on both sides, Quiet Film				
	Opaque				
	Starter Hole				
	15-50mm	22000	30	6169	Δ
	20mm	22020	30	6169	Δ
	25mm	22025	30	6169	Δ
	30mm	22030	30	6169	Δ
	35mm	22035	30	6169	Δ
	40mm	22040	30	6169	Δ
	45mm	22045	30	6169	Δ
	50mm	22050	30	6169	Δ

IXC

COLOSTOMY BAGS - cont

Manufacturer	Appliance	Order No.	Quantity	List Price p
Hollister Ltd - cont				
	Moderma - Flex			
	Closed Pouch with skin-resting barrier, filter and beige comfort backing on bodyworn side.			
	Transparent			
	Starter Hole			
	15-55mm	22500	30	6062
	Closed pouch with skin-resting barrier, filter and beige comfort backing on both sides.			
	Beige			
	Starter Hole			
	15-55mm	22100	30	6062
	20mm	22120	30	6062
	25mm	22125	30	6062
	30mm	22130	30	6062
	35mm	22135	30	6062
	40mm	22140	30	6062
	45mm	22145	30	6062
	Moderma L.C.			
	Closed Pouch with skin-resting barrier, filter and beige comfort backing on both sides			
	Starter Hole			
	15mm-50mm	2000	30	6169
	20mm	2020	30	6169
	25mm	2025	30	6169
	30mm	2030	30	6169
	35mm	2035	30	6169
	40mm	2040	30	6169
	45mm	2045	30	6169
	50mm	2050	30	6169
Jade-Euro-Med Ltd	**Black Butyl** Screw-cap outlet			
	Day bag	KM 38	1	2891
	Night bag	KM 40	1	3372
	White Rubber Screw-cap outlet			
	Day bag	KM 44	1	1607
	Night bag	KM 46	1	1841
Leyland Medical Ltd - see Rüsch UK Ltd				
Marlen USA	**Ultra** Closed Bag			
	Opaque			
	Flat Starter hole	801312	15	2880
	Transparent			
	Flat Starter Hole	861312	15	2880

COLOSTOMY BAGS - cont

Manufacturer	Appliance	Order No.	Quantity	List Price p
Marlen USA - cont	**Ultra Closed Bag**			
	Flat Pre-Cut			
	Opaque			
	12mm	801412	15	2880
	16mm	801416	15	2880
	19mm	801419	15	2880
	22mm	801422	15	2880
	25mm	801425	15	2880
	29mm	801429	15	2880
	32mm	801432	15	2880
	34mm	801434	15	2880
	38mm	801438	15	2880
	41mm	801441	15	2880
	44mm	801444	15	2880
	48mm	801448	15	2880
	50mm	801450	15	2880
	54mm	801454	15	2880
	57mm	801457	15	2880
	60mm	801460	15	2880
	63mm	801463	15	2880
	67mm	801467	15	2880
	70mm	801470	15	2880
	73mm	801473	15	2880
	76mm	801476	15	2880
	Flat Pre-Cut			
	Transparent			
	12mm	861412	15	2880
	16mm	861416	15	2880
	19mm	861419	15	2880
	22mm	861422	15	2880
	25mm	861425	15	2880
	29mm	861429	15	2880
	32mm	861432	15	2880
	34mm	861434	15	2880
	38mm	861438	15	2880
	41mm	861441	15	2880
	44mm	861444	15	2880
	48mm	861448	15	2880
	50mm	861450	15	2880
	54mm	861454	15	2880
	57mm	861457	15	2880
	60mm	861460	15	2880
	63mm	861463	15	2880
	67mm	861467	15	2880
	70mm	861470	15	2880
	73mm	861473	15	2880
	76mm	861476	15	2880

STOMA APPLIANCES

COLOSTOMY BAGS - cont

Manufacturer	Appliance	Order No.	Quantity	List Price p
Marlen USA - cont	**Ultra Closed Bag**			
	Shallow Convex Pre-Cut			
	Opaque			
	12mm	801512	15	2880
	16mm	801516	15	2880
	19mm	801519	15	2880
	22mm	801522	15	2880
	25mm	801525	15	2880
	29mm	801529	15	2880
	32mm	801532	15	2880
	34mm	801534	15	2880
	38mm	801538	15	2880
	41mm	801541	15	2880
	44mm	801544	15	2880
	48mm	801548	15	2880
	50mm	801550	15	2880
	54mm	801554	15	2880
	57mm	801557	15	2880
	60mm	801560	15	2880
	63mm	801563	15	2880
	67mm	801567	15	2880
	70mm	801570	15	2880
	73mm	801573	15	2880
	76mm	801576	15	2880
	Transparent			
	12mm	861512	15	2880
	16mm	861516	15	2880
	19mm	861519	15	2880
	22mm	861522	15	2880
	25mm	861525	15	2880
	29mm	861529	15	2880
	32mm	861532	15	2880
	34mm	861534	15	2880
	38mm	861538	15	2880
	41mm	861541	15	2880
	44mm	861544	15	2880
	48mm	861548	15	2880
	50mm	861550	15	2880
	54mm	861554	15	2880
	57mm	861557	15	2880
	60mm	861560	15	2880
	63mm	861563	15	2880
	67mm	861567	15	2880
	70mm	861570	15	2880
	73mm	861573	15	2880
	76mm	861576	15	2880
Oakmed Ltd	**Option** - Mini Pouch with Soft Covering to one side			
	Cut-to-fit 10mm-50mm			
	Clear	0910K	30	5159
	Opaque	1010K	30	5159

COLOSTOMY BAGS - cont

Manufacturer	Appliance	Order No.	Quantity	List Price p
Oakmed Ltd - cont	**Option** - Colostomy with Soft Covering to one side			
	Clear			
	starter hole			
	20mm	0120K	30	5698
	25mm	0125K	30	5698
	30mm	0130K	30	5698
	35mm	0135K	30	5698
	40mm	0140K	30	5698
	45mm	0145K	30	5698
	50mm	0150K	30	5698
	55mm	0155K	30	5698
	60mm	0160K	30	5698
	Opaque			
	starter hole			
	20mm	0220K	30	5698
	25mm	0225K	30	5698
	30mm	0230K	30	5698
	35mm	0235K	30	5698
	40mm	0240K	30	5698
	45mm	0245K	30	5698
	50mm	0250K	30	5698
	55mm	0255K	30	5698
	60mm	0260K	30	5698
	Option - Colostomy Plus with Soft Covering to one side			
	Clear starter hole			
	20mm	0520K	30	5835
	25mm	0525K	30	5835
	30mm	0530K	30	5835
	35mm	0535K	30	5835
	40mm	0540K	30	5835
	45mm	0545K	30	5835
	50mm	0550K	30	5835
	55mm	0555K	30	5835
	60mm	0560K	30	5835
	Opaque starter hole			
	20mm	0620K	30	5835
	25mm	0625K	30	5835
	30mm	0630K	30	5835
	35mm	0635K	30	5835
	40mm	0640K	30	5835
	45mm	0645K	30	5835
	50mm	0650K	30	5835
	55mm	0655K	30	5835
	60mm	0660K	30	5835

IXC

COLOSTOMY BAGS - cont

Manufacturer	Appliance	Order No.	Quantity	List Price p
Oakmed Ltd - cont				
	Option - Mini Pouch with Filter and Soft Covering to both sides			
	Opaque			
	cut to fit 10mm - 50mm	1110k	30	5349
	Option - Colostomy with Filter and Soft Covering to both sides			
	Opaque			
	starter hole			
	20mm	0320k	30	6048
	25mm	0325k	30	6048
	30mm	0330k	30	6048
	35mm	0335k	30	6048
	40mm	0340k	30	6048
	45mm	0345k	30	6048
	50mm	0350k	30	6048
	55mm	0355k	30	6048
	60mm	0360k	30	6048
	Option - Colostomy Plus with Filter and Soft Covering to both sides			
	Opaque			
	starter hole			
	20mm	0420k	30	6195
	25mm	0425k	30	6195
	30mm	0430k	30	6195
	35mm	0435k	30	6195
	40mm	0440k	30	6195
	45mm	0445k	30	6195
	50mm	0450k	30	6195
	55mm	0455k	30	6195
	60mm	0460k	30	6195
	Option - Colostomy Maxi with Filter and Soft Covering to one side			
	Clear			
	cut to fit 20mm-100mm	0720k	30	6564
	Option - Colostomy Maxi with Filter and Soft Covering to both sides			
	Opaque			
	cut to fit 20mm-100mm	0820k	30	6698
Omex Medical Ltd	Schacht Colostomy Pouches	785474	100	3426

Palex - see Salts Healthcare

COLOSTOMY BAGS - cont

Manufacturer	Appliance	Order No.	Quantity	List Price p
Pelican Healthcare Ltd - cont				
	Phoenix Closed pouches			
	Opaque - normal size			
	32mm	101425	100	16962
	40mm	101426	100	16962
	45mm	101427	100	16962
	Opaque - casual size			
	32mm	101420	100	15778
	40mm	101421	100	15778
	45mm	101422	100	15778
	Sassco Closed pouches			
	Opaque - normal size			
	32mm	100806	100	16155
	40mm	100807	100	16155
	45mm	100808	100	16155
	Pelican Pouches with skin protector, adhesive, filter, comfort backing			
	Closed pouches			
	Opaque - normal size			
	starter hole	100500	30	7466
	26mm	100524	30	7466
	32mm	100525	30	7466
	40mm	100526	30	7466
	45mm	100527	30	7466
	50mm	100528	30	7466
	Opaque - casual size			
	32mm	100520	30	7084
	40mm	100521	30	7084
	45mm	100522	30	7084
	Pelican Select			
	with skin protector, fabric both sides, filter			
	Closed pouches			
	Clear			
	cut-to-fit			
	20-65mm	100700	30	6486
	pre-cut			
	27mm	101727	30	6486
	34mm	101734	30	6486
	41mm	101741	30	6486
	48mm	101748	30	6486
	55mm	101755	30	6486
	Opaque			
	cut-to-fit			
	20-65mm	100720	30	6486
	pre-cut			
	27mm	100727	30	6486
	34mm	100734	30	6486
	41mm	100741	30	6486
	48mm	100748	30	6486
	55mm	100755	30	6486

IXC

COLOSTOMY BAGS - cont

Manufacturer	Appliance	Order No.	Quantity	List Price p
Pelican Healthcare Ltd - cont				
	Mini Closed Pouches			
	Clear cut-to-fit			
	20-65mm	100600	30	5441
	Opaque cut-to-fit			
	20-65mm	100620	30	5441
	Opaque pre-cut			
	27mm	100627	30	5441
	34mm	100634	30	5441
	41mm	100641	30	5441
	48mm	100648	30	5441
	55mm	100655	30	5441
Rüsch UK Ltd	**Ostopore** Colo with adhesive & vent			
	Opaque			
	25mm	742025	30	4203
	32mm	742032	30	4203
	38mm	742038	30	4203
	45mm	742045	30	4203
	Colo with Karaya adhesive & vent			
	Opaque			
	25mm	744025	30	5723
	32mm	744032	30	5723
	38mm	744038	30	5723
	45mm	744045	30	5723
	51mm	744051	30	5723
	Transparent			
	32mm	740032	30	7307
	38mm	740038	30	7307
	45mm	740045	30	7307
	51mm	740051	30	7307
	White Rubber Spout outlet			
	Day bag			
	19mm	LM 885101	1	1193
	25mm	LM 885102	1	1193
	28mm	LM 885103	1	1193
	Night bag			
	19mm	LM 885111	1	1287
	25mm	LM 885112	1	1287
	28mm	LM 885113	1	1287
Salts Healthcare	**Cohflex - with filter**			
	Closed			
	starter hole (10-60mm)			
	Flesh/Flesh	515410	30	6086
	Flesh/Clear	515420	30	6086
	pre-cut Flesh/Flesh			
	25mm	515425	30	6086
	30mm	515430	30	6086
	35mm	515435	30	6086
	40mm	515440	30	6086
	45mm	515445	30	6086
	50mm	515450	30	6086
	55mm	515455	30	6086
	60mm	515460	30	6086

COLOSTOMY BAGS - cont

Manufacturer	Appliance	Order No.	Quantity	List Price p
Salts Healthcare - cont				
	Coloset			
	Closed bag			
	Medium starter	713655	30	1613
	Small starter	713656	30	1061
	Large starter	713658	30	1337
	Medium starter	713659	30	1220
	Confidence			
	Closed pouches			
	Opaque			
	starter hole			
	13mm	C13	30	6156
	pre-cut			
	25mm	C25	30	6156
	32mm	C32	30	6156
	38mm	C38	30	6156
	45mm	C45	30	6156
	52mm	C52	30	6156
	Mini Closed pouches			
	starter hole			
	13mm	CM13	30	4850
	pre-cut			
	25mm	CM25	30	4850
	32mm	CM32	30	4850
	38mm	CM38	30	4850
	45mm	CM45	30	4850
	52mm	CM52	30	4850
	Closed pouches - transparent/overlap film			
	Standard			
	starter hole			
	13mm	CT13	30	5894
	Closed pouches-transparent/no overlap			
	Standard			
	starter hole			
	13mm	CTT13	30	5894
	Closed pouches-transparent/overlap film			
	pre-cut			
	25mm	CT25	30	6072
	32mm	CT32	30	6072
	38mm	CT38	30	6072
	45mm	CT45	30	6072
	52mm	CT52	30	6072
	Closed pouches-transparent/overlap film			
	Large			
	starter hole			
	13mm	CLT13	30	5967
	Closed pouches - transparent/no overlap			
	Large			
	starter hole			
	13mm	CLTT13	30	5967

IXC

COLOSTOMY BAGS - cont

Manufacturer	Appliance	Order No.	Quantity	List Price p
Salts Healthcare - cont				
	Confidence Gold			
	with hypoallergenic hydrocolloid and soft beige			
	comfort backing on both sides, filter			
	Closed Pouches			
	Opaque			
	starter hole			
	13mm	CNW13	30	6050
	pre-cut			
	25mm	CNW25	30	6050
	32mm	CNW32	30	6050
	35mm	CNW35	30	6050
	38mm	CNW38	30	6050
	45mm	CNW45	30	6050
	52mm	CNW52	30	6050
	Mini Closed Pouches			
	starter hole			
	13mm	CMNW13	30	4767
	pre-cut			
	25mm	CMNW25	30	4767
	32mm	CMNW32	30	4767
	35mm	CMNW35	30	4767
	38mm	CMNW38	30	4767
	45mm	CMNW45	30	4767
	52mm	CMNW52	30	4767
	Closed Pouches - Transparent			
	Film/Beige Overlap Comfort Backing			
	Standard			
	starter hole			
	13mm	CTNW13	30	5792
	pre-cut			
	25mm	CTNW25	30	5967
	32mm	CTNW32	30	5967
	35mm	CTNW35	30	5967
	38mm	CTNW38	30	5967
	45mm	CTNW45	30	5967
	52mm	CTNW52	30	5967
	Large			
	starter hole			
	13mm	CLTNW13	30	5967
	Eakin			
	Closed bag			
	Clear			
	32mm	839130	20	4500
	45mm	839131	20	4500
	64mm	839132	20	4500

COLOSTOMY BAGS - cont

Manufacturer	Appliance	Order No.	Quantity	List Price p
Salts Healthcare - cont				
	Simplicity 1 - with filter			
	Closed			
	starter hole (10mm-60mm)			
	White/White	511310	30	7143
	White/Clear	511311	30	7143
	Flesh/Flesh	511410	30	6934
	Flesh/Clear	511411	30	6934
	pre-cut			
	White/White			
	30mm	511330	30	7143
	40mm	511340	30	7143
	50mm	511350	30	7143
	60mm	511360	30	7143
	Flesh/Flesh			
	30mm	511430	30	6934
	40mm	511440	30	6934
	50mm	511450	30	6934
	60mm	511460	30	6934
	† Paediatric			
	13mm starter	621212	20	4697
	Simplicity 1 Anatomical			
	Closed			
	Clear - starter hole	541311	30	6772
	Opaque - starter hole	541310	30	6772
	30mm	541330	30	6772
	40mm	541340	30	6772
	50mm	541350	30	6772
	60mm	541360	30	6772
	Supasac			
	Closed bag			
	Medium starter	713644	30	2515
T J Shannon Ltd	Night bags	TJS 948e	1	2621
	Day bags	TJS 948f	1	2291
	Disposable bags	TJS 948g	100	1135
	Day bags tap outlet	TJS 948j	1	2621
	Night bags tap outlet	TJS 948k	1	2858
	Easychange spare bags		100	4578
	Bags with elastic necks		50	2289
	Disposable bags and plasters sealed both ends		12	626

† to be deleted 1 February 2001

IXC

COLOSTOMY BAGS - cont

Manufacturer	Appliance	Order No.	Quantity	List Price p
A H Shaw & Partners Ltd	Hainsworth bags with body mould adhesive hole size 25mm, 32mm, 38mm, and 51mm	NSI 63	20	4367
	Hainsworth bags with Healwell adhesive hole size 25mm, 32mm, 38mm, and 51mm	NSI 39	20	2292
	Stick on bags with plasters	NSI 62	10	868
	Shaw double seal 280mm x 154mm	NSI 64	100	1045
	Colostomy bags 350mm x 204mm	NSI 65	100	1143
Simcare - see SIMS Portex Ltd				
SIMS Portex Ltd	**Adhesive Stoma Bag**			
	25mm	32-232-80	90	13085
	32mm	32-233-88	90	13085
	38mm	32-234-85	90	13085
	44mm	32-240-07	90	13085
	51mm	32-235-82	90	13085
	64mm	32-237-87	90	13085
	With filter			
	25mm	32-242-87	90	14705
	32mm	32-243-84	90	14705
	38mm	32-244-81	90	14705
	44mm	32-241-04	90	14705
	51mm	32-245-89	90	14705
	64mm	32-246-86	90	14705
	Chiron			
	Disposable bags for 19mm stoma			
	305mm x 102mm	WD119-01-L	10	1027
	305mm x 127mm	WD119-02-N	10	1027
	Chiron Clearseal			
	Disposable bags sealed both ends for			
	22mm Stoma - small	WD222-02-U	10	1541
	38mm Stoma - small	WD238-02-B	10	1541
	38mm Stoma - medium	WD238-03-D	10	1541
	Chironseal			
	Disposable bags for 22mm Stoma			
	305mm x 102mm	WD022-01-E	10	1157
	305mm x 127mm	WD022-02-G	10	1157
	230mm x 127mm	WD022-03-J	10	1157
	305mm x 150mm	WD022-04-L	10	1157
	305mm x 205mm	WD022-05-N	10	1328
	305mm x 255mm	WD022-06-Q	10	1328

COLOSTOMY BAGS - cont

Manufacturer	Appliance	Order No.	Quantity	List Price p
SIMS Portex Ltd - cont	**Chironseal** - cont			
	Disposable bags for 38mm Stoma			
	305mm x 102mm	WD038-01-L	10	1157
	305mm x 127mm	WD038-02-N	10	1157
	230mm x 127mm	WD038-03-Q	10	1157
	305mm x 150mm	WD038-04-S	10	1157
	305mm x 205mm	WD038-05-U	10	1328
	305mm x 255mm	WD038-06-W	10	1328
	Reinforced Disposable bags			
	Sealed at both ends	WD525-01-A	10	1541
		WD538-02-V	10	1541
	Spout outlet bag PVC	WD600-10-A	10	3169
	EC1 Range			
	Beige			
	starter hole 15-64mm	32-330-06	30	7027
	fixed size - 25mm	32-330-14	30	7027
	fixed size - 32mm	32-330-22	30	7027
	fixed size - 38mm	32-330-30	30	7027
	fixed size - 44mm	32-330-49	30	7027
	fixed size - 51mm	32-330-57	30	7027
	fixed size - 64mm	32-330-65	30	7027
	Clear			
	starter hole 15-64mm	32-334-05	30	7027
	fixed size - 25mm	32-334-13	30	7027
	fixed size - 32mm	32-334-21	30	7027
	fixed size - 38mm	32-334-48	30	7027
	fixed size - 44mm	32-334-56	30	7027
	fixed size - 51mm	32-334-80	30	7027
	fixed size - 64mm	32-334-99	30	7027
	Mirage Closed Pouches			
	Beige			
	starter hole 19-44mm	32-510-10	30	5938
	starter hole 19-64mm	32-510-15	30	5938
	25mm	32-510-25	30	5938
	32mm	32-510-32	30	5938
	38mm	32-510-38	30	5938
	44mm	32-510-44	30	5938
	51mm	32-510-51	30	5938
	64mm	32-510-64	30	5938
	Large Outline cut 19-90mm			
		32-510-90	10	2145
	Clear			
	starter hole 19-44mm	32-515-10	30	5938
	starter hole 19-64mm	32-515-15	30	5938
	25mm	32-515-25	30	5938
	32mm	32-515-32	30	5938
	38mm	32-515-38	30	5938
	44mm	32-515-44	30	5938
	51mm	32-515-51	30	5938
	64mm	32-515-64	30	5938
	Large Outline cut 19-90mm			
		32-515-90	10	2145

IXC

COLOSTOMY BAGS - cont

Manufacturer	Appliance	Order No.	Quantity	List Price p
SIMS Portex Ltd - cont				
	Mirage Flushable Soft-backed Closed Pouches			
	Beige			
	starter hole 19-44mm	32-610-19	30	6427
	25mm	32-610-25	30	6427
	32mm	32-610-32	30	6427
	38mm	32-610-38	30	6427
	44mm	32-610-44	30	6427
	51mm	32-610-51	30	6427
	Clear			
	starter hole 19-44mm	32-615-19	30	6427
	25mm	32-615-25	30	6427
	32mm	32-615-32	30	6427
	38mm	32-615-38	30	6427
	44mm	32-615-44	30	6427
	51mm	32-615-51	30	6427
	Omni 1-piece closed bag			
	Beige			
	starter hole 15-44mm	32-311-86	30	7129
	fixed size 25mm	32-311-00	30	7129
	fixed size 32mm	32-311-19	30	7129
	fixed size 38mm	32-311-27	30	7129
	fixed size 44mm	32-311-35	30	7129
	fixed size 51mm	32-311-43	30	7129
	Clear			
	starter hole 15-44mm	32-319-09	30	7129
	Redifit			
	Continuation bags with Karaya			
	32mm	WA009-32-N	20	7450
	38mm	WA009-38-B	20	7450
	44mm	WA009-44-V	20	7450
	51mm	WA009-51-S	20	7450
	64mm	WA009-64-C	20	7450
	75mm	WA009-75-H	20	7450
	Non-adhesive bags with Karaya			
	44mm	WA010-44-M	20	7450
	Without Karaya			
	38mm	WA012-38-B	20	5654
	Hospital bags (closed)			
	with Karaya			
	44mm	WA033-44-L	20	7450
	51mm	WA033-51-H	20	7450
	64mm	WA033-64-S	20	7450
	Rediseal			
	Opaque fronted			
	38mm	WB005-38-R	10	1455
	44mm	WB005-44-L	10	1455

COLOSTOMY BAGS - cont

Manufacturer	Appliance	Order No.	Quantity	List Price p
SIMS Portex Ltd - cont	**Symphony** 'WC Disposable' Closed bag Beige			
	starter hole 15-44mm	32-336-18	30	7353
	fixed size 25mm	32-336-26	30	7353
	fixed size 32mm	32-336-34	30	7353
	fixed size 38mm	32-336-42	30	7353
	fixed size 44mm	32-336-50	30	7353
	fixed size 51mm	32-336-69	30	7353
	Clear			
	fixed size 25mm	32-335-10	30	7353
	fixed size 32mm	32-335-29	30	7353
	fixed size 38mm	32-335-37	30	7353
	fixed size 44mm	32-335-45	30	7353
	fixed size 51mm	32-335-53	30	7353
	Symphony Classic Soft-backed "WC Disposable" Closed Bag Beige			
	starter hole 15 - 51mm	32-340-15	30	7353
	fixed size 25mm	32-340-25	30	7353
	"　　" 32mm	32-340-32	30	7353
	"　　" 38mm	32-340-38	30	7353
	"　　" 44mm	32-340-44	30	7353
	"　　" 51mm	32-340-51	30	7353
Squibb Surgicare Ltd - see ConvaTec Ltd				
Ward Surgical Appliance Co	Colostomy Disposable bags, sealed both ends			
	✚ 30.5cm x 102mm with 102mm x 76mm plasters	WM 15	10	887
	✚ 30.5cm x 127mm with 102mm x 102mm plasters	WM 16	10	887
	Rubber colostomy bag for above with mount outlet	WM 12	1	1531
Warne-Franklin Medical Ltd - see Rüsch Ltd				
Welland Medical Ltd	Silhouette Standard Length Closed Pouches Beige			
	10mm	SCS 510	30	5952
	25mm	SCS 525	30	5952
	29mm	SCS 529	30	5952
	32mm	SCS 532	30	5952
	35mm	SCS 535	30	5952
	38mm	SCS 538	30	5952
	44mm	SCS 544	30	5952
	51mm	SCS 551	30	5952
	60mm	SCS 560	30	5952

IX

✚ Approximate Conversion

COLOSTOMY BAGS - cont

Manufacturer	Appliance	Order No.	Quantity	List Price p
Welland Medical Ltd - cont	Silhouette Standard Length Closed Pouches			
	Clear			
	10mm	SCS 710	30	5952
	25mm	SCS 725	30	5952
	29mm	SCS 729	30	5952
	32mm	SCS 732	30	5952
	35mm	SCS 735	30	5952
	38mm	SCS 738	30	5952
	44mm	SCS 744	30	5952
	51mm	SCS 751	30	5952
	60mm	SCS 760	30	5952
	Silhouette Vogue Shorter Length Closed Pouches			
	Beige			
	10mm	SCV 510	30	5281
	25mm	SCV 525	30	5281
	29mm	SCV 529	30	5281
	32mm	SCV 532	30	5281
	35mm	SCV 535	30	5281
	38mm	SCV 538	30	5281
	44mm	SCV 544	30	5281
	51mm	SCV 551	30	5281
	Clear			
	10mm	SCV 710	30	5281
	25mm	SCV 725	30	5281
	29mm	SCV 729	30	5281
	32mm	SCV 732	30	5281
	35mm	SCV 735	30	5281
	38mm	SCV 738	30	5281
	44mm	SCV 744	30	5281
	51mm	SCV 751	30	5281
	Vogue Mini Bags			
	Beige			
	starter hole 10mm	VOG 910	30	5631
	25mm	VOG 925	30	5631
	29mm	VOG 929	30	5631
	32mm	VOG 932	30	5631
	35mm	VOG 935	30	5631
	38mm	VOG 938	30	5631
	44mm	VOG 944	30	5631
	51mm	VOG 951	30	5631
	Clear			
	starter hole 10mm	VOG 710	30	5631
	25mm	VOG 725	30	5631
	29mm	VOG 729	30	5631
	32mm	VOG 732	30	5631
	35mm	VOG 735	30	5631
	38mm	VOG 738	30	5631
	44mm	VOG 744	30	5631
	51mm	VOG 751	30	5631

COLOSTOMY BAGS - cont

Manufacturer	Appliance	Order No.	Quantity	List Price p
Welland Medical Ltd - cont	Welland Colostomy Bags with filter			
	Beige			
	starter hole 10mm	FSC 110	30	6245
	25mm	FSC 125	30	6245
	32mm	FSC 132	30	6245
	38mm	FSC 138	30	6245
	44mm	FSC 144	30	6245
	51mm	FSC 151	30	6245
	60mm	FSC 160	30	6245
	† Clear			
	starter hole 10mm	FSC 410	30	6245
	25mm	FSC 425	30	6245
	32mm	FSC 432	30	6245
	38mm	FSC 438	30	6245
	44mm	FSC 444	30	6245
	51mm	FSC 451	30	6245
	60mm	FSC 460	30	6245
	Welland Colostomy Bags with soft backing			
	Beige			
	starter hole 10mm	FSC 910	30	6351
	25mm	FSC 925	30	6351
	29mm	FSC 929	30	6351
	32mm	FSC 932	30	6351
	35mm	FSC 935	30	6351
	38mm	FSC 938	30	6351
	44mm	FSC 944	30	6351
	51mm	FSC 951	30	6351
	60mm	FSC 960	30	6351
	Clear			
	starter hole 10mm	FSC 710	30	6351
	25mm	FSC 725	30	6351
	29mm	FSC 729	30	6351
	32mm	FSC 732	30	6351
	35mm	FSC 735	30	6351
	38mm	FSC 738	30	6351
	44mm	FSC 744	30	6351
	51mm	FSC 751	30	6351
	60mm	FSC 760	30	6351

IXC

†   to be deleted 1 January 2001

COLOSTOMY BAGS - cont

Manufacturer	Appliance	Order No.	Quantity	List Price p
Welland Medical Ltd - cont	Welland Ovation Closed Pouch with oval skin protector.			
	Clear			
	starter hole 10mm	FCO 710	30	6566
	Beige			
	starter hole 10mm	FCO 910	30	6566
	Welland Ovation Colostomy Pouch with large oval skin protector			
	Clear			
	starter hole 10mm	FLO 710	30	6453
	Beige			
	starter hole 10mm	FLO 910	30	6453
	Welland Impact Colostomy Bags with Toilet disposable liner and soft backing			
	Mini			
	Beige			
	19mm	IMP 219	30	5373
	25mm	IMP 225	30	5373
	29mm	IMP 229	30	5373
	32mm	IMP 232	30	5373
	35mm	IMP 235	30	5373
	38mm	IMP 238	30	5373
	44mm	IMP 244	30	5373
	51mm	IMP 251	30	5373
	Standard			
	Beige			
	19mm	IMP 919	30	6539
	25mm	IMP 925	30	6539
	29mm	IMP 929	30	6539
	32mm	IMP 932	30	6539
	35mm	IMP 935	30	6539
	38mm	IMP 938	30	6539
	44mm	IMP 944	30	6539
	51mm	IMP 951	30	6539
	Maxi			
	Beige			
	19mm	IMP 319	30	6539
	25mm	IMP 325	30	6539
	29mm	IMP 329	30	6539
	32mm	IMP 332	30	6539
	35mm	IMP 335	30	6539
	38mm	IMP 338	30	6539
	44mm	IMP 344	30	6539
	51mm	IMP 351	30	6539

COLOSTOMY SETS

Manufacturer	Appliance	Order No.	Quantity	List Price p
DePuy Healthcare - see Seton Continence Care				
Downs Surgical Ltd - see SIMS Portex Ltd				
Omex Medical Ltd	Schacht Odourproof Colostomy Appliance	785466	1	2955
T J Shannon Ltd	Colostomy Appliance	TJS 962	1	1740
	Easychange Colostomy Appliance 27mm, 40mm, 57mm		1	459
	Colostomy Outfit	TJS 948A	1	7736
	" "	TJS 948NA	1	7491
	" "	TJS 948T	1	4102
	Adhesive Appliance	TJS 948B	1	4995
A H Shaw & Partners Ltd	Complete Colostomy outfit comprising of a 102mm wide elastic web belt with groin-strap 660mm, 715mm etc. to 107cm, 1 Colostomy facepiece (flange), 100 Colostomy bags 280mm x 154mm	NSI 6	1	4047
	Complete Colostomy outfit comprising of a 102mm wide elastic web belt with groin-strap 660mm, 715mm etc. to 107cm, 76cm inner diameter facepiece, 100 Colostomy bags 350mm x 204mm	NSI 7	1	4128
	Complete Colostomy outfit comprising of an adjustable 102mm wide elastic web belt with groin-strap 660mm, 715mm etc. to 107cm, 1 Colostomy facepiece, 100 Colostomy bags 280mm x 154mm	NSI 8	1	4419
Simcare - see SIMS Portex Ltd				
SIMS Portex Ltd	Chiron Appliances Adhesive model with spout bag			
	MK I	WE001-38-W	1	7102
	MK III	WE007-38-X	1	7102

DEODORANTS

Manufacturer	Appliance	Order No.	Quantity	List Price p
Adams Healthcare	Atmocol Pocket Spray	785911	25mL	205
AlphaMed Ltd	NaturCare	1100	50mL	369
Anglo Venture 2000 Ltd	Friends Ostomy Deodorant Spray			
	Cinnamon	012345	75mL	355
	Victorian Rose	012346	75mL	355
	Lemon	012347	75mL	355
C S Bullen Ltd - see Coloplast Ltd				
Clinimed Ltd	Limone Ostomy Deodorant Spray	3905	50mL	433
Coloplast Ltd	Coloplast OAD	1523	✤ 36mL	431
	Ostobon Deodorising Powder Tube	4750	22g	424
Dansac Ltd	Nodor S	080-00	50mL	378
		080-01	250mL	774
Downs Surgical Ltd - see SIMS Portex Ltd				
Loxley Products	Day-drop	LL04	7.5mL	109
		LL05	15mL	181
		LL06	30mL	309
	Lemon Day-drop	LL07	7.5mL	109
		LL08	15mL	181
	Lemon Day-drop Spray	LL010	50mL	345
Pelican Healthcare Ltd	Dor Pouch Deodorant	130103	7mL	195
	Citrus Fresh Pouch Deodorant Spray	2200	50mL	362
Rüsch UK Ltd	Translet			
	Plus One Male	703001	7mL	298
	Plus Two Female	703002	7mL	298
Salts Healthcare	Noroma	833021	✤ 28mL	241
		833056	✤ 227mL	788
T J Shannon Ltd	Colostomy Plus		7mL	277
A H Shaw & Partners Ltd	Forest Breeze	NSI 61	✤ 14mL	346
Simcare - see SIMS Portex Ltd				
SIMS Portex Ltd	Chironair Odour Control Liquid	WN003-01-F	110mL	595
Warne-Franklin Medical Ltd - see Rüsch UK Ltd				

✤   Approximate Conversion

FILTERS/BRIDGES

Manufacturer	Appliance	Order No.	Quantity	List Price p
B. Braun Biotrol	Biotrol Flatus Filters	35-500	50	1221
Coloplast Ltd	Filtrodor Filters	0509	50	1975
	Maclet Filter Washers	0502	20	2796
ConvaTec Ltd †	System 2 Closed Pouch Filters	S208	30	838
Cuxson Gerrard	Flatus Patches 3.8cm x 3.8cm	FLA 830 (T33)	50	312
Downs Surgical Ltd - see SIMS Portex Ltd				
Eschmann Bros & Walsh Ltd - see SIMS Portex Ltd				
Hollister Ltd	Replacement Filter elements for series 366 drainable bags	7766	20 100	308 1512
Salts Healthcare	Metal Bridges ready- fixed to lightweight & LWU disposable bags	833052	20	926
	- for use with other disposable bags	833053	30	1389
Simcare - see SIMS Portex Ltd				
SIMS Portex Ltd	Doublesure Flatus Filter (pack)	WJ130-11-N	10	359
	Stoma Bridge	32-298-07	20	321
	Spare filters for Beta & Omni range	32-297-34	20	757
	Spare filters for Mirage drainable pouches	32-560-20	20	415
Squibb Surgicare Ltd - see ConvaTec Ltd				

IXC

---

†   to be deleted 1 January 2001

FLANGES

Manufacturer	Appliance	Order No.	Quantity	List Price p
Body's Surgical Company - see Jade-Euro-Med Ltd				
C S Bullen Ltd	Lenbul			
	✤ 25mm diameter 51mm base	UF 24	1	917
	✤ 38mm diameter 76mm base	UF 25	1	1395
	✤ 51mm diameter 102mm base	UF 26	1	1628
DePuy Healthcare - see Simpla Continence Care				
Downs Surgical Ltd - see SIMS Portex Ltd				
John Drew Ltd	Kapok Flanges ✤ 25mm-38mm	OST021	1	1401
Eschmann Bros & Walsh Ltd - see SIMS Portex Ltd				
Jade-Euro-Med Ltd	Colostomy flange St Mark's pattern, state size	KM54	1	1364
	Colostomy flange St Mark's pattern with diaphragm, state size	KM55	1	1364
Omex Medical Ltd	Schacht Colo Flanges and Locking Rings	784583	1	540
	Schacht Ileo Flanges and Locking Rings	784575	1	540

✤   Approximate Conversion

FLANGES - cont

Manufacturer	Appliance	Order No.	Quantity	List Price p
Rüsch UK Ltd	St Mark's Flanges made in two Rubbers with Hard Centre			
	22mm int diam, 16mm deep, 76mm base	LM 841101	2	3472
	32mm int diam, 16mm deep, 76mm base	LM 841103	2	3472
	32mm int diam, 10mm deep, 76mm base	LM 841104	2	3472
	38mm int diam, 16mm deep, 76mm base	LM 841105	2	3472
	38mm int diam, 10mm deep, 76mm base	LM 841106	2	3472
	44mm int diam, 16mm deep, 102mm base	LM 841107	2	3472
	25mm int diam, 13mm deep, 76mm base	LM 841110	2	3472
	51mm int diam, 16mm deep, 102mm base	LM 841109	2	3472
	St Mark's Flanges made in Soft Honey Coloured Rubber			
	25mm int diam, 13mm deep, 51mm base	LM 842101	2	2025
	32mm int diam, 16mm deep, 76mm base	LM 842103	2	2025
	32mm int diam, 10mm deep, 76mm base	LM 842104	2	2025
	38mm int diam, 16mm deep, 76mm base	LM 842105	2	2025
	38mm int diam, 10mm deep, 76mm base	LM 842106	2	2025
	44mm int diam, 16mm deep, 102mm base	LM 842107	2	2025
	51mm int diam, 16mm deep, 102mm base	LM 842109	2	2025
	25mm int diam, 13mm deep, 76mm base	LM 842111	2	2025
	Any of the above Flanges are available with a Diaphragm, or Cowl, or Dressing Retainer at the extra cost of:			324
	St Mark's Flanges, Black Firm Rubber			
	22mm int diam, 13mm deep, 51mm base	LM 843101	2	2317
	32mm int diam, 16mm deep, 76mm base	LM 843103	2	2317
	32mm int diam, 10mm deep, 76mm base	LM 843104	2	2317
	38mm int diam, 16mm deep, 76mm base	LM 843105	2	2317
	38mm int diam, 10mm deep, 76mm base	LM 843106	2	2317
	44mm int diam, 16mm deep, 102mm base	LM 843107	2	2317
	51mm int diam, 16mm deep, 102mm base	LM 843109	2	2317

IXC

FLANGES - cont

Manufacturer	Appliance	Order No.	Quantity	List Price p
Rüsch UK Ltd - cont	Birkbeck Flanges, White Rubber			
	20mm int diam, 16mm			
	deep, 75mm base	LM 722019	2	2317
	38mm int diam, 16mm			
	deep, 90mm base	LM 722038	2	2317
	58mm int diam, 16mm			
	deep, 110mm base	LM 722054	2	2317
Salts Healthcare	Latex Foam Diaphragm with			
	Rigid Face Piece			
	Flanges 38mm	811002	1	4187
	Latex Sheath for use with			
	811002 Flanges	811003	1	696
	SF1 Soft Rubber Flanges			
	25mm	822001	1	738
†	SF2 Semi-Rigid Flange			
	25mm	822002	1	1186
†	SF3 Hard Rubber Flange			
	25mm	822003	1	843
	SF4 Soft Rubber Flange			
	38mm	822004	1	749
	SF5 Semi-Rigid Flange			
	38mm	822005	1	1284
	SF6 Semi-Rigid Hard			
	Rubber Flange 38mm	822006	1	856
†	SF7 Soft Rubber Flange			
	51mm	822007	1	942
	SF8R Flexible (recessed)			
	Flange 32mm	822008	1	1186
	Baby Flange with Diaphragm			
	19mm	822009	1	981
	Salger Polythene Flange			
	40mm	600340	1	207
	Salger Polythene Flange			
	57mm	600357	1	207

† to be deleted 1 February 2001

FLANGES - cont

Manufacturer	Appliance	Order No.	Quantity	List Price p
T J Shannon Ltd	Flange Ring	TJS 962e	1	231
A H Shaw & Partners Ltd	Rubber Adhesive Flange	NSI 1	1	611
	Rubber Non-Stick Flange	NSI 2	1	740
	Adhesive Flange & Diaphragm	NSI 3	1	963
	Non-Stick Inner Diaphragm	NSI 4	1	287
	Colostomy facepiece rubber-foam face, hole diameter 45mm,			
	65mm, 77mm	NSI 9	1	1119
Simcare - see SIMS Portex Ltd				
Simpla Continence Care				
	St Mark's Flange with Inner Cuff			
	25mm diam, 16mm deep			
	76mm base	781704	1	1342
	32mm diam, 16mm deep			
	76mm base	781705	1	1342
	35mm diam, 16mm deep			
	100mm base	781706	1	1342
	38mm diam, 16mm deep			
	100mm base	781707	1	1342
	45mm diam, 16mm deep			
	100mm base	781708	1	1342
	50mm diam, 16mm deep			
	100mm base	781709	1	1342
SIMS Portex Ltd	Chiron Flanges,			
	38mm int diam,			
	10mm deep	WK102-38-K	1	1667
	22mm 13mm deep	WK103-25-E	1	1667
	32mm 16mm deep	WK104-32-F	1	1667
	38mm 16mm deep	WK104-38-T	1	1667
	Rubber Flange			
	38mm int diam,			
	16mm deep	WK108-38-L	1	1667
	St Mark's Pattern Flanges			
	25mm diam, 13mm deep			
	51mm base	WK111-25-B	1	1421
	76mm base	WK113-25-K	1	1421
	32mm diam, 10mm deep			
	76mm base	WK115-32-Q	1	1421
	32mm diam, 16mm deep			
	76mm base	WK117-32-Y	1	1421
	38mm diam, 10mm deep			
	76mm base	WK119-38-V	1	1421
	38mm diam, 16mm deep			
	76mm base	WK121-38-R	1	1421
	44mm diam, 16mm deep			
	102mm base	WK123-44-U	1	1421
	51mm diam, 16mm deep			
	102mm base	WK125-51-A	1	1421

IXC

FLANGES - cont

Manufacturer	Appliance	Order No.	Quantity	List Price p
SIMS Portex Ltd - cont	St Mark's Pattern Flanges			
	38mm with dressing retainer	WK126-01-N	1	1794
	38mm with 16mm canopy	WK126-02-Q	1	1794
	Flanges all Blue Rubber			
	25mm int diam, 13mm deep, 51mm base	WK132-25-R	1	1509
	38mm int diam, 10mm deep, 76mm base	WK135-38-P	1	1509
	38mm int diam, 16mm deep, 76mm base	WK138-38-C	1	1509
	Flanges Blue and Brown			
	25mm int diam, 13mm deep, 76mm base	WK141-25-S	1	2190
	38mm int diam, 10mm deep, 76mm base	WK144-38-Q	1	2190
	38mm int diam, 16mm deep, 76mm base	WK147-38-D	1	2190
	Chiron Plastic Flanges flexible without diaphragm			
	32mm int diam, 13mm deep	WK155-32-M	1	834
	38mm int diam, 13mm deep	WK155-38-A	1	834
	Rubber Flanges, double base hole			
	38mm int diam	WK160-38-J	1	2210
	Belt Flanges			
	19mm	32-269-80	1	28
	25mm	32-270-81	1	28
	32mm	32-271-89	1	28
	38mm	32-272-86	1	28
	44mm	32-275-88	1	28
	51mm	32-273-83	1	28
	64mm	32-274-80	1	28
	Redifit belt flange	WL124-01-M	1	67
Ward Surgical Appliance Co	Plastic/Rubber airfilled Flange	WM 88	1	1784
	St Mark's standard flange	WM 100	1	1174
	St Mark's flange with diaphragm	WM 101	1	1435

ILEOSTOMY (DRAINABLE) BAGS

Manufacturer	Appliance	Order No.	Quantity	List Price p
Body's Surgical Company - See Jade-Euro-Med Ltd				
B. Braun Biotrol	**Biotrol**			
	Elite bag with skin protector adhesive and fabric backing			
	Beige			
	Starter hole	38-810	30	7185
	20mm	38-820	30	7185
	25mm	38-825	30	7185
	30mm	38-830	30	7185
	35mm	38-835	30	7185
	40mm	38-840	30	7185
	45mm	38-845	30	7185
	50mm	38-850	30	7185
	60mm	38-860	30	7185
	70mm	38-870	30	7185
	Transparent			
	Starter hole	31-810	30	6778
	20mm	31-820	30	6655
	25mm	31-825	30	6655
	30mm	31-830	30	6655
	35mm	31-835	30	6655
	40mm	31-840	30	6655
	45mm	31-845	30	6655
	50mm	31-850	30	6655
	60mm	31-860	30	6655
	70mm	31-870	30	6655
	White			
	Starter hole	34-815	30	7185
	20mm	34-820	30	7185
	25mm	34-825	30	7185
	30mm	34-830	30	7185
	35mm	34-835	30	7185
	40mm	34-840	30	7185
	45mm	34-845	30	7185
	50mm	34-850	30	7185
	60mm	34-860	30	7185
	70mm	34-870	30	7185
	Elite Petite bag with skin protector adhesive and fabric backing			
	Beige			
	Starter hole	37-710	30	6165
	25mm	37-725	30	6165
	30mm	37-730	30	6165
	35mm	37-735	30	6165
	40mm	37-740	30	6165
	45mm	37-745	30	6165

IXC

ILEOSTOMY (DRAINABLE) BAGS - cont

Manufacturer	Appliance		Order No.	Quantity	List Price p
B. Braun Biotrol - cont	**Biotrol** - cont				
	Ileo S Bag with skin protector				
	White	Starter hole	32-715	30	7185
		20mm	32-720	30	7185
		25mm	32-725	30	7185
		30mm	32-730	30	7185
		35mm	32-735	30	7185
		40mm	32-740	30	7185
		45mm	32-745	30	7185
		50mm	32-750	30	7185
		60mm	32-760	30	7185
		70mm	32-770	30	7185
	Post-op Bag				
	Clear	Small	32-210	30	7486
		Large	32-215	30	10516
	Preference Bag with skin protector, microporous adhesive and fabric backing				
	Beige	Starter hole	34-615	30	7185
		20mm	34-620	30	7185
		25mm	34-625	30	7185
		30mm	34-630	30	7185
		35mm	34-635	30	7185
		40mm	34-640	30	7185
		45mm	34-645	30	7185
		50mm	34-650	30	7185
		60mm	34-660	30	7185
	Almarys bag with Interface adhesive and all over, soft non-woven cover.				
	Transparent				
		Starter hole	77-015	30	6494
	Beige	Starter hole	77-115	30	6494
		25mm	77-025	30	6494
		30mm	77-030	30	6494
		35mm	77-035	30	6494
		40mm	77-040	30	6494
		45mm	77-045	30	6494
		50mm	77-050	30	6494
		60mm	77-060	30	6494
	Almarys Optima Drainable bag with all over soft non-woven cover				
	Transparent				
		Starter hole 10mm	018710	30	6258
	Beige	Starter hole 10mm	008710	30	6258
		25mm	008725	30	6258
		30mm	008730	30	6258
		35mm	008735	30	6258
		40mm	008740	30	6258
		45mm	008745	30	6258
		50mm	008750	30	6258
		60mm	008760	30	6258

ILEOSTOMY (DRAINABLE) BAGS - cont

Manufacturer	Appliance	Order No.	Quantity	List Price p
B. Braun Biotrol - cont	**Biotrol** - cont			
	Almarys Optima Mini Drainable bag with all over soft non woven cover			
	Beige			
	20mm	008820	30	5820
	25mm	008825	30	5820
	30mm	008830	30	5820
	35mm	008835	30	5820
	40mm	008840	30	5820
	Almarys Optima Drainable bag with filter and soft cover			
	Transparent			
	Starter hole 10mm	019510	30	6258
	Beige			
	Starter hole 10mm	009510	30	6258
	25mm	009525	30	6258
	30mm	009535	30	6258
	35mm	009535	30	6258
	40mm	009540	30	6258
	45mm	009545	30	6258
	50mm	009550	30	6258
	60mm	009560	30	6258
	Almarys Preference Drainable bag with skin protector and microporous adhesive and all over soft non-woven cover			
	Transparent			
	Starter hole 10mm	018410	30	6258
	Beige			
	Starter hole 10mm	008410	30	6258
C S Bullen Ltd	**Lenbul**			
	With screw outlet			
	Day Bag	F 5	1	1297
	Night Bag	F 6	1	1429
Coloplast Ltd	**Assura**			
	Inspire Drainable Bag with Integral Filter and Soft Backing			
	Mini Transparent			
	Starter hole 10-55mm	13300	30	6795
	Midi Transparent			
	Starter hole 10-55mm	13330	30	6795
	Maxi Transparent			
	Starter hole 10-70mm	13360	30	6795
	Inspire Drainable Bag with Integral Filter and Opaque Soft Cover Front and Back.			
	Mini Soft Cover			
	Starter hole 10-55mm	13310	30	6795
	Midi Soft Cover			
	Starter hole 10-55mm	13340	30	6795
	Ready Cut 25mm	13344	30	6795
	30mm	13345	30	6795
	35mm	13346	30	6795
	Maxi Soft Cover			
	Starter hole 10-70mm	13370	30	6795

IXC

ILEOSTOMY (DRAINABLE) BAGS - cont

Manufacturer	Appliance	Order No.	Quantity	List Price p
Coloplast Ltd - cont	**Assura**			
	Inspire Drainable Bag with Integral Filter and Soft Cover Front and Back.			
	Mini Design			
	Starter hole 10-55mm	13320	30	6795
	Midi Design			
	Starter hole 10-55mm	13350	30	6795
	Maxi Design			
	Starter hole 10-70mm	13380	30	6795
	Drainable Bag with soft backing			
	Mini Opaque			
	Starter hole 10mm	2400	30	6795
	Midi Clear			
	Starter hole 10mm	2450	30	6795
	25mm	2454	30	6795
	30mm	2455	30	6795
	35mm	2456	30	6795
	40mm	2457	30	6795
	Midi Opaque			
	Starter hole 10mm	2440	30	6795
	25mm	2444	30	6795
	30mm	2445	30	6795
	35mm	2446	30	6795
	40mm	2447	30	6795
	Maxi Clear			
	Starter hole 10mm	2490	30	6795
	25mm	2494	30	6795
	30mm	2495	30	6795
	35mm	2496	30	6795
	40mm	2497	30	6795
	Maxi Opaque			
	Starter hole 10mm	2520	30	6795
	25mm	2524	30	6795
	30mm	2525	30	6795
	35mm	2526	30	6795
	40mm	2527	30	6795
	Paediatric Clear			
	Starter hole 10-35mm	2115	30	5874
	Paediatric Opaque			
	Starter hole 10-35mm	2110	30	5874
	Large Post-Op for high output			
	Clear Starter hole 10-70mm	12805	10	2591

ILEOSTOMY (DRAINABLE) BAGS - cont

Manufacturer	Appliance	Order No.	Quantity	List Price p
Coloplast Ltd - cont	**Assura** - cont			
	Drainable Bag with opaque Soft Cover front and back			
	Mini			
	Starter hole			
	10-55mm	12400	30	6795
	Midi			
	Starter hole			
	10-55mm	12440	30	6795
	Pre-cut 25mm	12444	30	6795
	30mm	12445	30	6795
	35mm	12446	30	6795
	40mm	12447	30	6795
	45mm	12448	30	6795
	50mm	12449	30	6795
	Maxi			
	Starter hole			
	10-70mm	12490	30	6795
	Seal Integral Convexity Drainable Bags with Soft Backing			
	Important:This product with Integral Convexity should only be used after prior assessment of suitability by an appropriate medical professional.			
	Maxi Clear			
	21mm	12953	10	2346
	25mm	12954	10	2346
	28mm	12955	10	2346
	31mm	12956	10	2346
	35mm	12957	10	2346
	38mm	12958	10	2346
	41mm	12959	10	2346
	Maxi Opaque			
	Starter hole			
	15-33mm	12582	10	2346
	15-43mm	12583	10	2346
	Maxi Opaque			
	18mm	12962	10	2346
	21mm	12963	10	2346
	25mm	12964	10	2346
	28mm	12965	10	2346
	31mm	12966	10	2346
	35mm	12967	10	2346
	38mm	12968	10	2346
	41mm	12969	10	2346
	Ileo B			
	Clear 22mm	0401	100	17350
	Decorated White			
	20mm	0405	100	17350
	Mini Decorated White			
	20mm	0404	100	17250
	K-Flex			
	Transparent			
	10mm	2900	30	7755
	40mm	2904	30	7755

IXC

ILEOSTOMY (DRAINABLE) BAGS - cont

Manufacturer	Appliance		Order No.	Quantity	List Price p
Coloplast Ltd - cont	**MC 2000**				
	Clear	20mm	5920	30	7653
		25mm	5925	30	7653
		30mm	5930	30	7653
		35mm	5935	30	7653
		40mm	5940	30	7653
		45mm	5945	30	7653
		50mm	5950	30	7653
		55mm	5955	30	7653
		60mm	5960	30	7653
	Opaque				
		25mm	6325	30	7653
		30mm	6330	30	7653
		35mm	6335	30	7653
		40mm	6340	30	7653
		45mm	6345	30	7653
	Large Open Adjustable				
		10mm-80mm	6100	30	7653
	Mini Opaque				
		20mm	5820	30	7224
		25mm	5825	30	7224
		30mm	5830	30	7224
		35mm	5835	30	7224
		40mm	5840	30	7224
	PC 3000				
	Clear	20mm	8520	30	6990
		25mm	8525	30	6990
		30mm	8530	30	6990
		35mm	8535	30	6990
		40mm	8540	30	6990
		45mm	8545	30	6990
		50mm	8550	30	6990
	Opaque	20mm	8620	30	6990
		25mm	8625	30	6990
		30mm	8630	30	6990
		35mm	8635	30	6990
		40mm	8640	30	6990
	Mini starter hole				
		15mm	8980	30	6333
		20mm	8981	30	6333
		30mm	8983	30	6333
	Sterile Post-Op Bag		2200	20	5224
			2202	20	3402

ILEOSTOMY (DRAINABLE) BAGS - cont

Manufacturer	Appliance	Order No.	Quantity	List Price p
ConvaTec Ltd	**Esteem** Drainable Pouches with Integral Filter			
	Small - clear			
	starter hole			
	20mm	S5040	10	1923
	Small - opaque			
	starter hole			
	20mm	S5041	10	1923
	pre-cut			
	25mm	S5042	10	1923
	30mm	S5043	10	1923
	40mm	S5044	10	1923
	50mm	S5045	10	1923
	Medium - clear			
	starter hole			
	20mm	S5047	10	2137
	Medium - opaque			
	starter hole			
	20mm	S5048	10	2137
	pre-cut			
	25mm	S5049	10	2137
	30mm	S5050	10	2137
	40mm	S5051	10	2137
	50mm	S5052	10	2137
	60mm	S5053	10	2137
	Large - clear			
	starter hole			
	20mm	S5055	10	2137
	pre-cut			
	25mm	S5056	10	2137
	30mm	S5057	10	2137
	40mm	S5058	10	2137
	50mm	S5059	10	2137
	60mm	S5060	10	2137
	70mm	S5061	10	2137
	Large - opaque			
	starter hole			
	20mm	S5062	10	2137
	pre-cut			
	25mm	S5063	10	2137
	30mm	S5064	10	2137
	40mm	S5065	10	2137
	50mm	S5066	10	2137
	60mm	S5067	10	2137
	70mm	S5068	10	2137

IXC

ILEOSTOMY (DRAINABLE) BAGS - cont

Manufacturer	Appliance	Order No.	Quantity	List Price p
ConvaTec Ltd - cont	**Ileodress** Pouches			
	Small Size			
	Opaque			
	19mm starter hole	S851	10	2254
	25mm starter hole	S852	10	2254
	32mm starter hole	S853	10	2254
	38mm starter hole	S855	10	2254
	45mm starter hole	S856	10	2254
	50mm starter hole	S857	10	2254
	64mm starter hole	S860	10	2254
	Standard Size			
	Clear			
	19mm starter hole	S841	10	2280
	38mm precut	S845	10	2280
	45mm precut	S846	10	2280
	50mm precut	S847	10	2280
	64mm precut	S850	10	2280
	Standard Size			
	Opaque			
	19mm starter hole	S831	10	2280
	25mm precut	S832	10	2280
	32mm precut	S833	10	2280
	38mm precut	S835	10	2280
	45mm precut	S836	10	2280
	50mm precut	S837	10	2280
	64mm precut	S840	10	2280
	Ileodress Plus			
	- with modified Stomahesive wafer, perforated plastic backing and beige clip pouches			
	Standard Size			
	Clear			
	19mm starter hole	S420	10	2280
	38mm precut	S423	10	2280
	45mm precut	S424	10	2280
	50mm precut	S425	10	2280
	64mm precut	S426	10	2280
	Opaque			
	19mm starter hole	S411	10	2280
	25mm precut	S412	10	2280
	32mm precut	S413	10	2280
	38mm precut	S414	10	2280
	45mm precut	S415	10	2280
	50mm precut	S416	10	2280
	64mm precut	S417	10	2280
	Small Size			
	Opaque			
	19mm starter hole	S430	10	2014
	25mm	S431	10	2014
	32mm	S432	10	2014
	38mm	S433	10	2014
	45mm	S434	10	2014
	50mm	S436	10	2014
	Little-Ones			
	Mini Size			
	8mm starter hole	S880	15	3137

ILEOSTOMY (DRAINABLE) BAGS - cont

Manufacturer	Appliance	Order No.	Quantity	List Price p
ConvaTec Ltd - cont	**Naturess**			
	Drainable pouch with Integral Filter			
	Standard Size			
	Opaque			
	19mm starter hole	S947	20	4348
	pre-cut			
	25mm	S948	20	4348
	32mm	S949	20	4348
	38mm	S950	20	4348
	45mm	S951	20	4348
	50mm	S952	20	4348
	Clear			
	19mm starter hole	S960	20	4348
	Drainable pouch with Integral Filter			
	Small Size			
	Opaque			
	starter hole			
	19mm	S954	20	3913
	pre-cut			
	25mm	S955	20	3913
	32mm	S956	20	3913
	38mm	S957	20	3913
	45mm	S958	20	3913
	50mm	S959	20	3913
	Drainable pouch			
	Standard Size			
	Clear			
	starter hole			
	19mm	S953	20	4348
	Stomadress Pouches			
	Clear			
	8mm starter hole	S439	10	2218
Dansac Ltd	**CombiMicro**			
†	Infant			
	Clear			
	cut to fit 10-25mm	31010-2320	30	6343
	Opaque			
	cut to fit 10-25mm	31010-1320	30	6343
	CombiMicro D + S			
†	Clear			
	starter hole 25mm diam	34525-2	30	7274
	precut 32mm diam	34532-2	30	7274
	38mm diam	34538-2	30	7274
	44mm diam	34544-2	30	7274
	50mm diam	34550-2	30	7274
	63mm diam	34563-2	30	7274
†	starter hole - clear			
	Stoma hole, range			
	10-38mm	32010-2310	30	7274
	38-63mm	32038-2310	30	7274

† to be deleted 1 February 2001

ILEOSTOMY (DRAINABLE) BAGS - cont

Manufacturer	Appliance		Order No.	Quantity	List Price p
Dansac Ltd - cont	**CombiMicro D + S** - cont				
	† Opaque				
	starter hole				
		25mm diam	32125-1310	30	7339
	precut	32mm diam	32132-1310	30	7339
		38mm diam	32138-1310	30	7339
		44mm diam	32144-1310	30	7339
		50mm diam	32150-1310	30	7339
		63mm diam	32163-1310	30	7339
	† starter hole - Opaque				
	Stoma hole, range				
		10-38mm	32010-1310	30	7274
		38-63mm	32038-1310	30	7274
	Invent Drainable with filter, soft spunlace material on both sides anatomically shaped				
	Opaque				
	Cut-to-fit	15-60mm	339-15	30	6643
	Precut	20mm	339-20	30	6643
		25mm	339-25	30	6643
		30mm	339-30	30	6643
		35mm	339-35	30	6643
		40mm	339-40	30	6643
		45mm	339-45	30	6643
		50mm	339-50	30	6643
	InVent Mini Drainable with filter, soft spunlace material on both sides, anatomically shaped				
	Opaque				
	Cut-to-fit	15-50mm	335-15	30	6529
	Precut	20mm	335-20	30	6529
		25mm	335-25	30	6529
		30mm	335-30	30	6529
		35mm	335-35	30	6529
	InVent Symmetrical Drainable with filter, soft spunlace cover front and back (opaque) and back only (clear), symmetrically shaped				
	Clear				
	Cut-to-fit	15-60mm	338-15	30	6522
	Precut	20mm diam	338-20	30	6522
		25mm diam	338-25	30	6522
		30mm diam	338-30	30	6522
		35mm diam	338-35	30	6522
		40mm diam	338-40	30	6522
		45mm diam	338-45	30	6522
		50mm diam	338-50	30	6522
	Opaque				
	Cut-to-fit	15-60mm	337-15	30	6522
	Precut	20mm diam	337-20	30	6522
		25mm diam	337-25	30	6522
		30mm diam	337-30	30	6522
		35mm diam	337-35	30	6522
		40mm diam	337-40	30	6522
		45mm diam	337-45	30	6522
		50mm diam	337-50	30	6522

† to be deleted 1 February 2001

ILEOSTOMY (DRAINABLE) BAGS - cont

Manufacturer	Appliance	Order No.	Quantity	List Price p

Dansac Ltd - cont

Dansac InVent Convex
Integral convexity drainable bag with filter, soft spunlace cover front and back, anatomically shaped
Important: This product with integral convexity should only be used after prior assessment of suitability by an appropriate medical professional.

		Order No.	Quantity	List Price p
Opaque				
starter hole 15-24mm		341-24	10	2340
15-37mm		341-37	10	2340
15-46mm		341-46	10	2340
Opaque				
pre-cut	20mm	341-20	10	2340
	25mm	341-25	10	2340
	30mm	341-30	10	2340
	35mm	341-35	10	2340
	40mm	341-40	10	2340
	45mm	341-45	10	2340

Dansac InVent Symm Convex
Integral convexity drainable bag with filter, soft spunlace cover front and back (opaque) and back only (clear) symmetrically shaped
Important: This product with integral convexity should only be used after prior assessment of suitability by an appropriate medical professional.

		Order No.	Quantity	List Price p
Opaque				
starter hole 15-24mm		343-24	10	2340
15-37mm		343-37	10	2340
15-46mm		343-46	10	2340
Opaque				
pre-cut	20mm	343-20	10	2340
	25mm	343-25	10	2340
	30mm	343-30	10	2340
	35mm	343-35	10	2340
	40mm	343-40	10	2340
	45mm	343-45	10	2340
Clear				
starter hole 15-24mm		344-24	10	2340
15-37mm		344-37	10	2340
15-46mm		344-46	10	2340
Clear				
pre-cut	20mm	344-20	10	2340
	25mm	344-25	10	2340
	30mm	344-30	10	2340
	35mm	344-35	10	2340
	40mm	344-40	10	2340
	45mm	344-45	10	2340

IXC

ILEOSTOMY (DRAINABLE) BAGS - cont

Manufacturer	Appliance	Order No.	Quantity	List Price p
Dansac Ltd - cont	**Unique**			
	Maxi Clear			
	Cut-to-fit			
	10mm-90mm	324-10	10	2262
	Opaque			
	Starter hole	321-15	30	6428
	20mm	319-20	30	6428
	25mm	319-25	30	6428
	30mm	319-30	30	6428
	35mm	319-35	30	6428
	40mm	319-40	30	6428
	45mm	319-45	30	6428
	50mm	319-50	30	6428
	60mm	319-60	30	6428
	Clear			
	Starter hole	322-15	30	6428
	20mm	320-20	30	6428
	25mm	320-25	30	6428
	30mm	320-30	30	6428
	35mm	320-35	30	6428
	40mm	320-40	30	6428
	45mm	320-45	30	6428
	50mm	320-50	30	6428
	60mm	320-60	30	6428
	Mini opaque (reference capacity: 250mL (see Note 2, page 223))			
	Cut-to fit			
	15mm-50mm	315-15	30	6223
	Precut			
	20mm	315-20	30	6223
	25mm	315-25	30	6223
	30mm	315-30	30	6223
	35mm	315-35	30	6223
	Mini clear (reference capacity: 250mL (see Note 2, page 223))			
	Cut-to-fit			
	15mm-50mm	316-15	30	6223
	Infant opaque (reference capacity: 190mL (see Note 2, page 223))			
	Cut-to-fit			
	10mm-40mm	313-10	30	6214
	Infant clear (reference capacity: 190mL (see Note 2, page 223))			
	cut-to-fit			
	10mm-40mm	314-10	30	6214
	Oval flange			
	Opaque Starter hole	317-15	30	6428
	Clear Starter hole	318-15	30	6428

ILEOSTOMY (DRAINABLE) BAGS - cont

Manufacturer	Appliance	Order No.	Quantity	List Price p
DePuy Healthcare - see Seton Continence Care				
Downs Surgical Ltd - see SIMS Portex Ltd				
John Drew Ltd	Ileostomy Bags			
	D1/1	OST002	50	6185
	D1/6	OST004	50	4415
Eschmann Bros & Walsh Ltd - see SIMS Portex Ltd				
EuroCare - see Salts Healthcare				
Hollister Ltd	**Compact**			
	Drainable Pouch			
	Clear-with beige comfort backing on body-worn side			
	cut-to-fit			
	13-64mm	3250	10	2326
	Beige-with beige comfort backing on both sides			
	cut-to-fit			
	13-64mm	3251	10	2326
	pre-cut			
	19mm	3257	10	2326
	25mm	3252	10	2326
	32mm	3258	10	2326
	38mm	3253	10	2326
	44mm	3259	10	2326
	51mm	3254	10	2326
	64mm	3255	10	2326
	Mini-Drainable Pouch			
	Beige-with beige comfort backing on both sides			
	cut-to-fit			
	13-51mm	3241	10	2128
	pre-cut			
	19mm	3247	10	2128
	25mm	3242	10	2128
	32mm	3248	10	2128
	38mm	3243	10	2128
	44mm	3249	10	2128
†	51mm	3244	10	2128
	Karaya 5 seal			
	with microporous adhesive			
	✤ 229mm Length			
	Opaque			
	✤ 25mm	3132	30	7803
	✤ 32mm	3138	30	7803
	✤ 38mm	3133	30	7803
	✤ 44mm	3139	30	7803
	✤ 51mm	3134	30	7803

IXC

✤   Approximate Conversion
†   to be deleted 1 December 2000

ILEOSTOMY (DRAINABLE) BAGS - cont

Manufacturer	Appliance	Order No.	Quantity	List Price p
Hollister Ltd - cont	**Karaya 5 seal**			
	✚ 30.5cm Length			
	Opaque			
	✚ 25mm	3112	30	7588
	✚ 32mm	3118	30	7588
	✚ 38mm	3113	30	7588
	✚ 44mm	3119	30	7588
	✚ 51mm	3114	30	7588
	✚ 64mm	3115	30	7588
	✚ 76mm	3116	30	7588
	✚ 30.5cm Length			
	Transparent			
	✚ 25mm	3222	30	7803
	✚ 32mm	3228	30	7803
	✚ 38mm	3223	30	7803
	✚ 44mm	3229	30	7803
	✚ 51mm	3224	30	7803
	✚ 64mm	3225	30	7803
	✚ 76mm	3226	30	7803
	✚ 41cm Length			
	Transparent			
	✚ 25mm	3272	30	7803
	✚ 32mm	3278	30	7803
	✚ 38mm	3273	30	7803
	✚ 44mm	3279	30	7803
	✚ 51mm	3274	30	7803
	✚ 64mm	3275	30	7803
	✚ 76mm	3276	30	7803
	Karaya 5 seal			
	with microporous adhesive			
	and quiet film			
	Transparent			
	✚ 25mm	3602	15	3829
	✚ 32mm	3608	15	3829
	✚ 38mm	3603	15	3829
	✚ 44mm	3609	15	3829
	✚ 51mm	3604	15	3829
	✚ 64mm	3605	15	3829
	✚ 76mm	3606	15	3829
	Karaya 5 seal			
	with regular adhesive			
	✚ 30.5cm Length			
	Transparent			
	✚ 25mm	7222	30	7803
	✚ 32mm	7228	30	7803
	✚ 38mm	7223	30	7803
	✚ 44mm	7229	30	7803
	✚ 51mm	7224	30	7803
	✚ 64mm	7225	30	7803
	✚ 76mm	7226	30	7803

✚   Approximate Conversion

ILEOSTOMY (DRAINABLE) BAGS - cont

Manufacturer	Appliance	Order No.	Quantity	List Price p
Hollister Ltd - cont				
	Premium			
	with synthetic seal			
	25mm	3642	15	3829
	32mm	3648	15	3829
	38mm	3643	15	3829
	44mm	3649	15	3829
	51mm	3644	15	3829
	64mm	3645	15	3829
	with integral filter holder and twenty replacement filters			
	25mm	3662	15	4175
	32mm	3668	15	4175
	38mm	3663	15	4175
	44mm	3669	15	4175
	51mm	3664	15	4175
	64mm	3665	15	4175
	Impression with Convex wafer			
	Transparent			
	19mm	3610	10	2514
	22mm	3611	10	2514
	25mm	3612	10	2514
	29mm	3613	10	2514
	32mm	3614	10	2514
	35mm	3615	10	2514
	38mm	3616	10	2514
	41mm	3617	10	2514
	44mm	3618	10	2514
	51mm	3619	10	2514
	Opaque			
	19mm	3680	10	2514
	22mm	3681	10	2514
	25mm	3682	10	2514
	29mm	3683	10	2514
	32mm	3684	10	2514
	35mm	3685	10	2514
	38mm	3686	10	2514
	41mm	3687	10	2514
	44mm	3688	10	2514
	51mm	3689	10	2514

IXC

ILEOSTOMY (DRAINABLE) BAGS - cont

Manufacturer	Appliance	Order No.	Quantity	List Price p
Hollister Ltd - cont	**Impression "C"** with convex wafer Beige with beige Comfort backing on both sides			
	19mm	3260	10	2414
	22mm	3261	10	2414
	25mm	3262	10	2414
	29mm	3263	10	2414
	32mm	3264	10	2414
	35mm	3265	10	2414
	38mm	3266	10	2414
	41mm	3267	10	2414
	44mm	3268	10	2414
	51mm	3269	10	2414
	Transparent with beige Comfort backing on body worn side			
	19mm	3280	10	2370
	22mm	3281	10	2370
	25mm	3282	10	2370
	29mm	3283	10	2370
	32mm	3284	10	2370
	35mm	3285	10	2370
	38mm	3286	10	2370
	41mm	3287	10	2370
	44mm	3288	10	2370
	51mm	3289	10	2370
	Moderma - Flex Drainable Pouch with skin resting barrier, filter, transparent front. Anatomical shape. Beige comfort backing on body worn side. Starter Hole			
	15-55mm	26500	30	6678
	Drainable Pouch with skin-resting barrier, filter. Anatomical shape. Beige comfort backing on both sides.			
	Starter Hole 15-55mm	26200	30	6678
	20mm	26220	30	6678
	25mm	26225	30	6678
	30mm	26230	30	6678
	35mm	26235	30	6678
	40mm	26240	30	6678
	Mini Drainable Pouch with skin resting barrier, filter. Beige comfort backing on both sides.			
	Starter Hole 15-55mm	26100	30	6678
	20mm	26120	30	6678
	25mm	26125	30	6678
	30mm	26130	30	6678
	35mm	26135	30	6678
	40mm	26140	30	6678

ILEOSTOMY (DRAINABLE) BAGS - cont

Manufacturer	Appliance	Order No.	Quantity	List Price p
Jade-Euro-Med Ltd	**Black Butyl**			
	Spout outlet			
	Day Bag	KM 42	1	3053
	Night Bag	KM 43	1	3053
	White Rubber			
	Spout outlet			
	Day Bag	KM 48	1	1444
	Night Bag	KM 49	1	1444
Leyland Medical Ltd - see Rüsch Ltd				
Marlen USA	**Ultra**			
	Small Bag			
	Transparent			
	Starter hole	561312	15	3225
	Opaque			
	Starter hole	501312	15	3225
	12mm	501412	15	3225
	16mm	501416	15	3225
	19mm	501419	15	3225
	22mm	501422	15	3225
	25mm	501425	15	3225
	29mm	501429	15	3225
	32mm	501432	15	3225
	34mm	501434	15	3225
	38mm	501438	15	3225
	41mm	501441	15	3225
	44mm	501444	15	3225
	48mm	501448	15	3225
	50mm	501450	15	3225
	54mm	501454	15	3225
	57mm	501457	15	3225
	60mm	501460	15	3225
	63mm	501463	15	3225
	67mm	501467	15	3225
	70mm	501470	15	3225
	73mm	501473	15	3225
	76mm	501476	15	3225

IXC

ILEOSTOMY (DRAINABLE) BAGS - cont

Manufacturer	Appliance	Order No.	Quantity	List Price p
Marlen USA - cont	**Ultra**			
	Large Bag			
	Transparent			
	Starter hole	562312	15	3225
	Opaque			
	Starter hole	502312	15	3225
	12mm	502412	15	3225
	16mm	502416	15	3225
	19mm	502419	15	3225
	22mm	502422	15	3225
	25mm	502425	15	3225
	29mm	502429	15	3225
	32mm	502432	15	3225
	34mm	502434	15	3225
	38mm	502438	15	3225
	41mm	502441	15	3225
	44mm	502444	15	3225
	48mm	502448	15	3225
	50mm	502450	15	3225
	54mm	502454	15	3225
	57mm	502457	15	3225
	60mm	502460	15	3225
	63mm	502463	15	3225
	67mm	502467	15	3225
	70mm	502470	15	3225
	73mm	502473	15	3225
	76mm	502476	15	3225
	Small Bag with Convex Flange			
	Opaque 12mm	501512	15	3300
	16mm	501516	15	3300
	19mm	501519	15	3300
	22mm	501522	15	3300
	25mm	501525	15	3300
	29mm	501529	15	3300
	32mm	501532	15	3300
	34mm	501534	15	3300
	38mm	501538	15	3300
	41mm	501541	15	3300
	44mm	501544	15	3300
	48mm	501548	15	3300
	50mm	501550	15	3300
	54mm	501554	15	3300
	57mm	501557	15	3300
	60mm	501560	15	3300
	63mm	501563	15	3300
	67mm	501567	15	3300
	70mm	501570	15	3300
	73mm	501573	15	3300
	76mm	501576	15	3300

ILEOSTOMY (DRAINABLE) BAGS - cont

Manufacturer	Appliance	Order No.	Quantity	List Price p
Marlen USA -cont	**Ultra** - cont			
	Large Bag with Convex Flange			
	Opaque 12mm	502512	15	3300
	16mm	502516	15	3300
	19mm	502519	15	3300
	22mm	502522	15	3300
	25mm	502525	15	3300
	29mm	502529	15	3300
	32mm	502532	15	3300
	34mm	502534	15	3300
	38mm	502538	15	3300
	41mm	502541	15	3300
	44mm	502544	15	3300
	48mm	502548	15	3300
	50mm	502550	15	3300
	54mm	502554	15	3300
	57mm	502557	15	3300
	60mm	502560	15	3300
	63mm	502563	15	3300
	67mm	502567	15	3300
	70mm	502570	15	3300
	73mm	502573	15	3300
	76mm	502576	15	3300
Oakmed Ltd	**Option** - Mini Ileostomy with Soft Covering to one side			
	cut-to-fit 10mm-50mm			
	Clear	2410K	30	5464
	Opaque	2510K	30	5464
	Option - Ileostomy with Soft Covering to one side			
	Clear			
	starter hole 20mm	2020K	30	5835
	25mm	2025K	30	5835
	30mm	2030K	30	5835
	35mm	2035K	30	5835
	40mm	2040K	30	5835
	45mm	2045K	30	5835
	50mm	2050K	30	5835
	55mm	2055K	30	5835
	60mm	2060K	30	5835
	Opaque			
	starter hole 20mm	2120K	30	5835
	25mm	2125K	30	5835
	30mm	2130K	30	5835
	35mm	2135K	30	5835
	40mm	2140K	30	5835
	45mm	2145K	30	5835
	50mm	2150K	30	5835
	55mm	2155K	30	5835
	60mm	2160K	30	5835

IXC

ILEOSTOMY (DRAINABLE) BAGS - cont

Manufacturer	Appliance	Order No.	Quantity	List Price p
Oakmed Ltd - cont				
	Option - Ileostomy Midi with Filter and Soft Covering to one side			
	Clear			
	starter hole 20mm	3220k	30	5897
	25mm	3225k	30	5897
	30mm	3230k	30	5897
	35mm	3235k	30	5897
	40mm	3240k	30	5897
	45mm	3245k	30	5897
	50mm	3250k	30	5897
	55mm	3255k	30	5897
	60mm	3260k	30	5897
	Opaque			
	starter hole 20mm	3320k	30	5897
	25mm	3325k	30	5897
	30mm	3330k	30	5897
	35mm	3335k	30	5897
	40mm	3340k	30	5897
	45mm	3345k	30	5897
	50mm	3350k	30	5897
	55mm	3355k	30	5897
	60mm	3360k	30	5897
	Option - Ileostomy with Filter and Soft Covering to one side			
	Clear			
	starter hole 20mm	3020k	30	6235
	25mm	3025k	30	6235
	30mm	3030k	30	6235
	35mm	3035k	30	6235
	40mm	3040k	30	6235
	45mm	3045k	30	6235
	50mm	3050k	30	6235
	55mm	3055k	30	6235
	60mm	3060k	30	6235
	Opaque			
	starter hole 20mm	3120k	30	6235
	25mm	3125k	30	6235
	30mm	3130k	30	6235
	35mm	3135k	30	6235
	40mm	3140k	30	6235
	45mm	3145k	30	6235
	50mm	3150k	30	6235
	55mm	3155k	30	6235
	60mm	3160k	30	6235

ILEOSTOMY (DRAINABLE) BAGS - cont

Manufacturer	Appliance	Order No.	Quantity	List Price p
Oakmed Ltd - cont				
	Option - Ileostomy Midi with Filter and Soft Covering to both sides			
	Opaque			
	starter hole 20mm	4320k	30	6182
	25mm	4325k	30	6182
	30mm	4330k	30	6182
	35mm	4335k	30	6182
	40mm	4340k	30	6182
	45mm	4345k	30	6182
	50mm	4350k	30	6182
	55mm	4355k	30	6182
	60mm	4360k	30	6182
	Option - Ileostomy with Filter and Soft Covering to both sides			
	Opaque			
	starter hole 20mm	4120k	30	6512
	25mm	4125k	30	6512
	30mm	4130k	30	6512
	35mm	4135k	30	6512
	40mm	4140k	30	6512
	45mm	4145k	30	6512
	50mm	4150k	30	6512
	55mm	4155k	30	6512
	60mm	4160k	30	6512
Omex Medical Ltd	Schacht	470511	50	2100

IXC

ILEOSTOMY (DRAINABLE) BAGS - cont

Manufacturer	Appliance		Order No.	Quantity	List Price p
Pelican Healthcare Ltd	**Sassco**				
	Size	26mm	110801	100	18547
		32mm	110802	100	18547
	Pelican Pouch - with Skin Protector, Adhesive, Comfort Backing, Opaque				
	Size	26mm	110524	30	7544
		32mm	110525	30	7544
		40mm	110526	30	7544
		45mm	110527	30	7544
		50mm	110528	30	7544
	Paediatric/Neonatal Pouch				
	Size	7mm - 40mm	120705	30	6759
	† Post-Op Pouch				
	Size	20mm - 80mm	140501	10	4153
	Pelican Select - with skin protector, fabric both sides				
	Drainable Pouch				
	Clear				
	cut-to-fit	20-65mm	110620	30	6596
	pre-cut	13mm	110613	30	6596
		27mm	110627	30	6596
		34mm	110634	30	6596
		41mm	110641	30	6596
		48mm	110648	30	6596
		55mm	110655	30	6596
	Opaque				
	cut-to-fit	20-65mm	110720	30	6596
	pre-cut	13mm	110713	30	6596
		27mm	110727	30	6596
		34mm	110734	30	6596
		41mm	110741	30	6596
		48mm	110748	30	6596
		55mm	110755	30	6596
	Paediatric Pouch - with skin protector, plain fabric both sides				
	Clear				
	cut-to-fit 10mm-50mm		101600	30	5900
	Opaque				
	cut-to-fit 10mm-50mm		101602	30	5900
	Paediatric Pouch - with skin protector, fabric both sides with printed motif				
	Clear				
	cut-to-fit 10mm-50mm		101601	30	5900
	Opaque				
	cut-to-fit 10mm-50mm		101603	30	5900
	Select Drainable DuoVent - with two filters, easy access outlet, skin protector, fabric both sides				
	Clear - Standard				
	cut-to-fit 15-65mm		110215	30	6500
	pre-cut	20mm	110220	30	6500
		27mm	110227	30	6500
		34mm	110234	30	6500
		41mm	110241	30	6500
		48mm	110248	30	6500
		55mm	110255	30	6500

† to be deleted 1 February 2001

ILEOSTOMY (DRAINABLE) BAGS - cont

Manufacturer	Appliance	Order No.	Quantity	List Price p
Pelican Healthcare Ltd - cont				
	Select Drainable DuoVent - with two filters, easy access outlet, skin protector, fabric both sides - Cont			
	Opaque - Standard			
	cut-to-fit 15-65mm	110315	30	6500
	pre-cut 20mm	110320	30	6500
	27mm	110327	30	6500
	34mm	110334	30	6500
	41mm	110341	30	6500
	48mm	110348	30	6500
	55mm	110355	30	6500
	Clear - Mini			
	cut-to-fit 15-65mm	111200	30	6300
	Opaque - Mini			
	cut-to-fit 15-65mm	111215	30	6300
	pre-cut 20mm	111220	30	6300
	27mm	111227	30	6300
	34mm	111234	30	6300
	41mm	111241	30	6300
	48mm	111248	30	6300
	55mm	111255	30	6300
Rüsch UK Ltd	**Birkbeck**			
	with Screwcap outlet			
	Black Rubber			
	Day Bag			
	19mm	LM 723225	1	2763
	38mm	LM 723230	1	2763
	54mm	LM 723235	1	2763
	Night Bag			
	19mm	LM 723275	1	3160
	38mm	LM 723280	1	3160
	54mm	LM 723295	1	3160
	Disposable Plastic Bag	LM 724000	100	1610
	Pink Rubber			
	Day Bag			
	19mm	LM 724225	1	2763
	38mm	LM 724230	1	2763
	54mm	LM 724235	1	2763
	Night Bag			
	19mm	LM 724275	1	3160
	38mm	LM 724280	1	3160
	54mm	LM 724295	1	3160
	White Rubber			
	with Screwcap outlet			
	Day Bag			
	38mm	LM 882111	1	1237
	44mm	LM 882112	1	1237
	51mm	LM 882113	1	1237
	with air vent			
	38mm	LM 882114	1	1480
	on body side			
	38mm	LM 882115	1	1336

IXC

ILEOSTOMY (DRAINABLE) BAGS - cont

Manufacturer	Appliance	Order No.	Quantity	List Price p
Rüsch UK Ltd - cont	**White Rubber**			
	Child's			
	Day Bag			
	19mm	LM 882101	1	1193
	25mm	LM 882102	1	1193
	28mm	LM 882103	1	1193
	Night Bag			
	19mm	LM 882121	1	1459
	25mm	LM 882122	1	1459
	28mm	LM 882123	1	1459
	Ostopore			
	Ileo Karaya adhesive and vent			
	Opaque 25mm	746025	30	6402
	32mm	746032	30	6402
	38mm	746038	30	6402
Salts Healthcare	**Cohflex**			
	Drainable			
	starter hole 10-60mm			
	Flesh/Flesh	514410	30	6533
	Flesh/Clear	514420	30	6533
	pre-cut			
	Flesh/Flesh			
	25mm	514425	30	6533
	30mm	514430	30	6533
	35mm	514435	30	6533
	40mm	514440	30	6533
	45mm	514445	30	6533
	50mm	514450	30	6533
	55mm	514455	30	6533
	60mm	514460	30	6533
	Paediatric			
	10mm starter	632310	30	5789
	Paediatric (Flesh)			
	10mm starter	632410	30	5789
	Coloset			
	Medium starter	713689	30	2263
	Confidence			
	Drainable pouches			
	Opaque			
	starter hole			
	13mmD13		30	5976
	pre-cut			
	25mmD25		30	5976
	32mmD32		30	5976
	38mmD38		30	5976
	45mmD45		30	5976
	52mmD52		30	5976
	Small Drainable pouches			
	starter hole			
	13mm	DS13	30	4768
	pre-cut			
	25mm	DS25	30	4768
	32mm	DS32	30	4768
	38mm	DS38	30	4768
	45mm	DS45	30	4768
	52mm	DS52	30	4768

ILEOSTOMY (DRAINABLE) BAGS - cont

Manufacturer	Appliance	Order No.	Quantity	List Price p
Salts Healthcare - cont	**Confidence**			
	Drainable pouches - transparent/overlap film			
	Standard			
	starter hole			
	13mm	DT13	30	5723
	Drainable pouches - transparent/no overlap			
	Standard			
	starter hole			
	13mm	DTT13	30	5723
	Drainable pouches - transparent /overlap film			
	Large			
	starter hole			
	13mm	DLT13	30	5976
	Drainable pouches - transparent/no overlap			
	Large			
	starter hole			
	13mm	DLTT13	30	5976
	Drainable pouch - transparent/overlap film			
	pre-cut			
	25mm	DT25	30	6072
	32mm	DT32	30	6072
	38mm	DT38	30	6072
	45mm	DT45	30	6072
	52mm	DT52	30	6072
	Confidence Gold			
	with hypoallergenic hydrocolloid and soft beige comfort backing on both sides			
	Drainable Pouches			
	Opaque			
	starter hole			
	13mm	DNW13	30	5874
	pre-cut			
	25mm	DNW25	30	5874
	32mm	DNW32	30	5874
	35mm	DNW35	30	5874
	38mm	DNW38	30	5874
	45mm	DNW45	30	5874
	52mm	DNW52	30	5874
	Small Drainable Pouches			
	starter hole			
	13mm	DSNW13	30	4686
	pre-cut			
	25mm	DSNW25	30	4686
	32mm	DSNW32	30	4686
	35mm	DSNW35	30	4686
	38mm	DSNW38	30	4686
	45mm	DSNW45	30	4686
	52mm	DSNW52	30	4686

IXC

ILEOSTOMY (DRAINABLE) BAGS - cont

Manufacturer	Appliance	Order No.	Quantity	List Price p
Salts Healthcare - cont	**Confidence Gold**			
	Drainable Pouches - Transparent Film/Beige			
	Overlap Comfort Backing			
	Standard			
	starter hole			
	13mm	DTNW13	30	5624
	pre-cut			
	25mm	DTNW25	30	5967
	32mm	DTNW32	30	5967
	35mm	DTNW35	30	5967
	38mm	DTNW38	30	5967
	45mm	DTNW45	30	5967
	52mm	DTNW52	30	5967
	Large			
	starter hole			
	13mm	DLTNW13	30	5874
	Eakin			
	Clear			
	Large			
	32mm	839120	20	5199
	45mm	839121	20	5199
	64mm	839122	20	5199
	Small			
	32mm	839110	20	5199
	45mm	839111	20	5199
	64mm	839112	20	5199
	White			
	Large			
	32mm	839006	20	5199
	45mm	839007	20	5199
	64mm	839008	20	5199
	Small			
	32mm	839012	20	5199
	45mm	839013	20	5199
	64mm	839014	20	5199
	Eakin Fistula			
	Infant	839210	10	3811
	Small	839211	10	5409
	Medium	839212	10	6996
	Large	839213	10	12863
	Large (Open)	839214	10	12863
	Wide 90mm opening	839230	20	10692
	with remote drainage			
	Infant	839220	10	3811
	Small	839221	10	5409
	Medium	839222	10	6996
	Large	839223	10	12863
	Large (Open)	839224	10	12863
	Large (Vertical)	839225	10	12863

ILEOSTOMY (DRAINABLE) BAGS - cont

Manufacturer	Appliance	Order No.	Quantity	List Price p
Salts Healthcare - cont	**Koenig Rutzen**			
	All Rubber Black Screw Outlet			
	Large			
	25mm	161125	1	3215
	29mm	161129	1	3215
	32mm	161132	1	3215
	35mm	161135	1	3215
	38mm	161138	1	3215
	44mm	161144	1	3215
	51mm	161151	1	3215
	Small			
	25mm	161225	1	3215
	32mm	161232	1	3215
	38mm	161238	1	3215
	† 44mm	161244	1	3215
	† 51mm	161251	1	3215
	Special	161099	1	3339
	Spout Outlet			
	Large			
	25mm	171125	1	2404
	29mm	171129	1	2404
	32mm	171132	1	2404
	38mm	171138	1	2404
	44mm	171144	1	2404
	51mm	171151	1	2404
	Small			
	25mm	171225	1	2404
	32mm	171232	1	2404
	38mm	171238	1	2404
	† 44mm	171244	1	2404
	† 51mm	171251	1	2404
	Special	171099	1	2493

IXC

† to be deleted 1 February 2001

ILEOSTOMY (DRAINABLE) BAGS - cont

Manufacturer	Appliance	Order No.	Quantity	List Price p
Salts Healthcare - cont				
	Koenig Rutzen - cont			
	MB with Bridge			
	Screw Outlet			
	Large			
	25mm	165125	1	4313
	32mm	165132	1	4313
	38mm	165138	1	4313
	44mm	165144	1	4313
†	51mm	165151	1	4313
	Small			
	25mm	165225	1	4273
	32mm	165232	1	4273
	38mm	165238	1	4273
	Special	165099	1	4479
	MB with Bridge			
	Spout Outlet			
	Large			
	25mm	175125	1	3115
	32mm	175132	1	3115
	38mm	175138	1	3115
†	44mm	175144	1	3115
	51mm	175151	1	3115
†	Small			
	25mm	175225	1	3115
	32mm	175232	1	3115
	38mm	175238	1	3115
	Special	175099	1	3236
	WP Reinforced Rubber, Black			
	Screw Outlet			
	Large			
	25mm	163125	1	4313
	32mm	163132	1	4313
	38mm	163138	1	4313
	Small			
	25mm	163225	1	4313
	32mm	163232	1	4313
	38mm	163238	1	4313
	Special	163099	1	4338

† to be deleted 1 February 2001

ILEOSTOMY (DRAINABLE) BAGS - cont

Manufacturer	Appliance	Order No.	Quantity	List Price p
Salts Healthcare - cont				
	Koenig Rutzen - cont			
	WP Reinforced Rubber, Black			
	Spout Outlet			
	Large			
	25mm	173125	1	3231
	32mm	173132	1	3231
	38mm	173138	1	3231
	Small			
	25mm	173225	1	3231
	32mm	173232	1	3231
	38mm	173238	1	3231
	Special	173099	1	3388
	WP MB with Bridge			
	Screw Outlet			
	Large			
	25mm	168125	1	5026
	32mm	168132	1	5026
	38mm	168138	1	5026
	44mm	168144	1	5026
	51mm	168151	1	5026
	WP MB with Bridge			
	Screw Outlet - cont			
	Small			
	25mm	168225	1	5026
	32mm	168232	1	5026
	38mm	168238	1	5026
	Special	168099	1	5219
	Spout Outlet			
	Large			
	† 25mm	178125	1	3979
	32mm	178132	1	3979
	38mm	178138	1	3979
	† 44mm	178144	1	3979
	† 51mm	178151	1	3979
	† Small			
	25mm	178225	1	3979
	32mm	178232	1	3979
	38mm	178238	1	3979
	Special	178099	1	4174

IXC

† to be deleted 1 February 2001

ILEOSTOMY (DRAINABLE) BAGS - cont

Manufacturer	Appliance		Order No.	Quantity	List Price p
Salts Healthcare - cont					
	Light White				
	Opaque				
	Large				
		25mm	273125	30	5125
		32mm	273132	30	5125
		38mm	273138	30	5125
	Medium				
		25mm	273325	30	5125
		32mm	273332	30	5125
		38mm	273338	30	5125
	Small				
		25mm	273225	30	5125
		32mm	273232	30	5125
†		38mm	273238	30	5125
	Adhesive Bag				
	Opaque				
	Large				
		25mm	274125	30	5800
		32mm	274132	30	5800
		38mm	274138	30	5800
		44mm	274144	30	5800
	Medium				
		25mm	274325	30	5800
		32mm	274332	30	5800
		38mm	274338	30	5800
	Small				
		25mm	274225	30	5800
		32mm	274232	30	5800
		38mm	274238	30	5800
	Salger				
	Clear				
	Medium				
		40mm	600240	10	1194
		57mm	600257	10	1194

† to be deleted 1 February 2001

ILEOSTOMY (DRAINABLE) BAGS - cont

Manufacturer	Appliance	Order No.	Quantity	List Price p
Salts Healthcare - cont				
	Simplicity 1			
	Drainable			
	starter hole (10mm-60mm)			
	White/White	510310	30	7450
	White/Clear	510311	30	7450
	Flesh/Flesh	510410	30	7234
	Flesh/Clear	510411	30	7234
	pre-cut			
	White/White			
	30mm	510330	30	7450
	40mm	510340	30	7450
	50mm	510350	30	7450
	60mm	510360	30	7450
	Flesh/Flesh			
	30mm	510430	30	7234
	40mm	510440	30	7234
	50mm	510450	30	7234
	60mm	510460	30	7234
	† Paediatric			
	13mm starter hole	622212	30	4697
	Simplicity 1 Anatomical			
	Clear - starter hole	540311	30	7262
	Opaque - starter hole	540310	30	7262
	30mm	540330	30	7262
	40mm	540340	30	7262
	50mm	540350	30	7262
	60mm	540360	30	7262

IXC

† to be deleted 1 February 2001

ILEOSTOMY (DRAINABLE) BAGS - cont

Manufacturer	Appliance	Order No.	Quantity	List Price p
A H Shaw & Partner Ltd	Black Rubber Day Bag (with screw cap)			
	22mm	NSI 66	1	2455
	29mm		1	2455
	38mm		1	2455
	Black Rubber Night Bag (with screw cap)			
	22mm	NSI 67	1	2601
	29mm		1	2601
	38mm		1	2601
Simcare - see SIMS Portex Ltd				
SIMS Portex Ltd	**Adhesive Stoma Bag**			
	19mm	32-250-89	60	9565
	25mm	32-251-86	60	9565
	32mm	32-252-83	60	9565
	38mm	32-253-80	60	9565
	51mm	32-254-88	60	9565
	Cavendish Clear PVC Bag			
	25mm	WD650-25-R	10	3243
	32mm	WD650-32-N	10	3243
	38mm	WD650-38-B	10	3243
	Plastic Bag			
	25mm	WC010-25-X	10	3223
	32mm	WC010-32-U	10	3223
	38mm	WC010-38-H	10	3223
	with adhesive flange			
	25mm	WC013-25-L	10	3882
	32mm	WC013-32-H	10	3882
	38mm	WC013-38-V	10	3882
	Chiron Black Butyl Screw Cap Outlet Day Bag			
	38mm	WF005-38-W	1	3353
	44mm	WF005-44-R	1	3353
	51mm	WF005-51-N	1	3353
	Night Bag			
	38mm	WF025-38-H	1	4024
	44mm	WF025-44-C	1	4024
	Latex Rubber Screw cap outlet Day Bag			
	38mm	WF003-38-N	1	1704
	Night Bag			
	38mm	WF023-38-Y	1	2254

ILEOSTOMY (DRAINABLE) BAGS - cont

Manufacturer	Appliance		Order No.	Quantity	List Price p
SIMS Portex Ltd - cont					
	Chiron - cont				
	White Rubber Screw cap outlet				
	Day Bag				
		38mm	WF001-38-E	1	1931
		44mm	WF001-44-Y	1	1931
		51mm	WF001-51-V	1	1931
	Night Bag				
		38mm	WF021-38-Q	1	2254
		51mm	WF021-51-G	1	2254
	Children's Bag				
		38mm	WF012-38-P	1	1687
	Screw cap outlet on body side				
	Day Bag				
		38mm	WF002-38-J	1	1931
	Night Bag				
		38mm	WF031-01-V	1	1845
	Children's Bag				
		38mm	WF011-38-K	1	1523
	Spout Outlet				
	Day Bag				
		38mm	WF051-38-G	1	1659
	Night Bag				
		38mm	WF061-38-M	1	1802
	EC1 Range				
		10-64mm	32-331-62	30	7362
		19mm	32-331-03	30	7362
		25mm	32-331-11	30	7362
		32mm	32-331-38	30	7362
		38mm	32-331-46	30	7362
		44mm	32-331-54	30	7362
	Mini	(Clear)	32-333-08	30	7362
		(Opaque)	32-333-16	30	7362
	Post Op				
		Large outline 10-90mm	32-338-12	30	10745
		Small outline 10-64mm	32-338-04	30	7593

IXC

ILEOSTOMY (DRAINABLE) BAGS - cont

Manufacturer	Appliance	Order No.	Quantity	List Price p
SIMS Portex Ltd - cont				
	Mirage Drainable Pouches			
	Beige			
	starter hole 19-44mm	32-520-10	30	6373
	starter hole 19-64mm	32-520-15	30	6373
	25mm	32-520-25	30	6373
	32mm	32-520-32	30	6373
	38mm	32-520-38	30	6373
	44mm	32-520-44	30	6373
	51mm	32-520-51	30	6373
	Large Outline cut 19-90mm			
		32-520-90	10	2220
	Clear			
	starter hole 19-44mm	32-525-10	30	6373
	starter hole 19-64mm	32-525-15	30	6373
	25mm	32-525-25	30	6373
	32mm	32-525-32	30	6373
	38mm	32-525-38	30	6373
	44mm	32-525-44	30	6373
	51mm	32-525-51	30	6373
	Mirage Mini - Drainable Pouches			
	Beige			
	starter hole to 44mm	32-550-10	30	5876
	25mm	32-550-25	30	5876
	32mm	32-550-32	30	5876
	38mm	32-550-38	30	5876
	44mm	32-550-44	30	5876
	51mm	32-550-51	30	5876
	Clear			
	starter hole to 44mm	32-555-10	30	5876
	Omni-1-Piece			
	with flatus filter and			
	20 replacement filters			
	Beige			
	Starter hole 10-44mm	32-299-55	20	4904
	25mm	32-299-12	20	4904
	32mm	32-299-20	20	4904
	38mm	32-299-39	20	4904
	44mm	32-299-47	20	4904
	Clear			
	Starter hole 10-44mm	32-318-79	20	4904

ILEOSTOMY (DRAINABLE) BAGS - cont

Manufacturer	Appliance	Order No.	Quantity	List Price p
SIMS Portex Ltd - cont	**Redifit**			
	with Karaya			
	Clear			
	Medium			
	25mm	WA027-25-T	20	7201
	44mm	WA027-44-X	20	7201
	64mm	WA027-64-E	20	7201
	Opaque			
	Medium			
	25mm	WA018-25-S	20	7201
	32mm	WA018-32-P	20	7201
	38mm	WA018-38-C	20	7201
	44mm	WA018-44-W	20	7201
	51mm	WA018-51-T	20	7201
	64mm	WA018-64-D	20	7201
	Small			
	25mm	WA020-25-N	20	7201
	32mm	WA020-32-K	20	7201
	38mm	WA020-38-X	20	7201

Squibb Surgicare Ltd - see ConvaTec Ltd

Steeper (Orthopaedic) Ltd - incorporating Donald Rose Ltd - see Ward Surgical Appliance Co

Ward Surgical Appliance Co	**Black Rubber**			
	with screw outlet			
	19mm, 35mm or 54mm			
	Day Size	WM 08	1	1849
	Night Size	WM 09	1	1932
	White Rubber			
	with screw outlet			
	Day Size	WM 01	1	1264
	Night Size	WM 02	1	1421
	with spout outlet			
	Day Size	WM 03	1	1264
	Night Size	WM 04	1	1421
	with tap outlet			
	Day Size	WM 05	1	1851
	Night Size	WM 06	1	2052
	with flange attached	WM 99	1	2795

IXC

ILEOSTOMY (DRAINABLE) BAGS - cont

Manufacturer	Appliance		Order No.	Quantity	List Price p
Ward Surgical Appliance Co - cont	Transverse bag tap and mount outlet all sizes black and white rubber		WM 07	1	2954
	Donald Rose registered design rubber bags with celluloid collars, solid, flat or fluid rims.		9	1	1977
	New improved rubber bag only, complete with collar.		12	1	2146
	Extra tap outlet and skirt (also extra for Donald Rose RD bag)		13	1	252
	Shaped rubber night bag with long vertical spring vulcanite screw outlet		18	1	1967
Warne-Franklin Medical Ltd - see Rüsch UK Ltd					
Welland Medical Ltd	Silhouette Plus Drainable Pouches with filter				
	Beige	19mm	SDF 519	30	6410
		25mm	SDF 525	30	6410
		29mm	SDF 529	30	6410
		32mm	SDF 532	30	6410
		35mm	SDF 535	30	6410
		38mm	SDF 538	30	6410
		44mm	SDF 544	30	6410
		51mm	SDF 551	30	6410
	Clear	19mm	SDF 719	30	6410
		25mm	SDF 725	30	6410
		29mm	SDF 729	30	6410
		32mm	SDF 732	30	6410
		35mm	SDF 735	30	6410
		38mm	SDF 738	30	6410
		44mm	SDF 744	30	6410
		51mm	SDF 751	30	6410
	Silhouette Standard Length Drainable Pouches				
	Beige	19mm	SDS 519	30	6410
		25mm	SDS 525	30	6410
		29mm	SDS 529	30	6410
		32mm	SDS 532	30	6410
		35mm	SDS 535	30	6410
		38mm	SDS 538	30	6410
		44mm	SDS 544	30	6410
		51mm	SDS 551	30	6410

ILEOSTOMY (DRAINABLE) BAGS - cont

Manufacturer	Appliance		Order No.	Quantity	List Price p
Welland Medical Ltd - cont	Silhouette Standard Length Drainable Pouches - cont				
	Clear	19mm	SDS 719	30	6410
		25mm	SDS 725	30	6410
		29mm	SDS 729	30	6410
		32mm	SDS 732	30	6410
		35mm	SDS 735	30	6410
		38mm	SDS 738	30	6410
		44mm	SDS 744	30	6410
		51mm	SDS 751	30	6410
	Silhouette Vogue Shorter Length Drainable Pouches				
	Beige	19mm	SDV 519	30	5537
		25mm	SDV 525	30	5537
		29mm	SDV 529	30	5537
		32mm	SDV 532	30	5537
		35mm	SDV 535	30	5537
		38mm	SDV 538	30	5537
		44mm	SDV 544	30	5537
		51mm	SDV 551	30	5537
	Clear	19mm	SDV 719	30	5537
		25mm	SDV 725	30	5537
		29mm	SDV 729	30	5537
		32mm	SDV 732	30	5537
		35mm	SDV 735	30	5537
		38mm	SDV 738	30	5537
		44mm	SDV 744	30	5537
		51mm	SDV 751	30	5537
	Vogue Shorter Drainable Bag				
	Beige				
		Starter hole 19mm	VOD 919	30	5634
		25mm	VOD 925	30	5634
		29mm	VOD 929	30	5634
		32mm	VOD 932	30	5634
		35mm	VOD 935	30	5634
		38mm	VOD 938	30	5634
		44mm	VOD 944	30	5634
		51mm	VOD 951	30	5634
	Clear				
		Starter hole 19mm	VOD 719	30	5634
		25mm	VOD 725	30	5634
		29mm	VOD 729	30	5634
		32mm	VOD 732	30	5634
		35mm	VOD 735	30	5634
		38mm	VOD 738	30	5634
		44mm	VOD 744	30	5634
		51mm	VOD 751	30	5634

IXC

ILEOSTOMY (DRAINABLE) BAGS - cont

Manufacturer	Appliance	Order No.	Quantity	List Price p
Welland Medical Ltd - cont	Standard Length Drainable Bags with softbacking			
	Beige			
	Starter hole 19mm	FSI 919	30	6584
	25mm	FSI 925	30	6584
	29mm	FSI 929	30	6584
	32mm	FSI 932	30	6584
	35mm	FSI 935	30	6584
	38mm	FSI 938	30	6584
	44mm	FSI 944	30	6584
	51mm	FSI 951	30	6584
	Clear			
	Starter hole 19mm	FSI 719	30	6584
	25mm	FSI 725	30	6584
	29mm	FSI 729	30	6584
	32mm	FSI 732	30	6584
	35mm	FSI 735	30	6584
	38mm	FSI 738	30	6584
	44mm	FSI 744	30	6584
	51mm	FSI 751	30	6584
	Welland Ovation Drainable Pouch with oval skin protector			
	Beige Starter hole 10mm	FSI 910	30	6932
	Clear Starter hole 10mm	FSI 710	30	6932
	Welland Ovation Drainable Pouch with large vertical oval skin protector			
	Clear			
	Starter hole 10mm	FVI 710	10	2271
	Beige			
	Starter hole 10mm	FVI 910	10	2271
	Large Post-Op Drainable Bag with Softbacking			
	Clear Starter hole 10mm	FSP700	30	6786
	Beige Starter hole 10mm	FSP900	30	6786
	Welland Ovation Mini Drainable Pouch with oval skin protector			
	Clear Starter hole 10mm	FSM710	30	6034 Δ
	Beige Starter hole 10mm	FSM910	30	6034 Δ
	Welland Ovation Mini Drainable with Vertical Skin Protector			
	Clear Starter hole 10mm	FVM 710	10	1976 Δ
	Beige Starter hole 10mm	FVM 910	10	1976 Δ

ILEOSTOMY SETS

Manufacturer	Appliance	Order No.	Quantity	List Price p
DePuy Healthcare - see Simpla Continence Care				
John Drew Ltd	Ileostomy Appliance			
	D1/1	OST001	1	3252
	D1/6	OST003	1	2786
Leyland Medical Ltd - see Rüsch UK Ltd				
Oakmed Ltd	The SR-F Set	SR-F	1	5560
	The OPR-F Appliance	OPR-F	1	8069
	The LOP-F7 Appliance	LOP-F7	1	3868
Omex Medical Ltd	Schacht Odourproof Ileostomy Appliance	470538	1	3103
Rüsch UK Ltd	**Birkbeck**			
	Appliance "A"			
	19mm	LM 720119	1	9645
	38mm	LM 720138	1	9645
	54mm	LM 720154	1	9645
	Appliance "B"			
	19mm	LM 720519	1	6224
	38mm	LM 720538	1	6224
	54mm	LM 720554	1	6224
Steeper (Orthopaedic) Ltd - incorporating Donald Rose Ltd - see Ward Surgical Appliance Co				
Ward Surgical Appliance Co	Donald Rose Ileostomy Appliance			
	First Stage	1	1	4838
	Second Stage	8	1	4786
	New Improved	11	1	5079

IXC

IRRIGATION/WASH - OUT APPLIANCES - (Replacement Parts)
(SLEEVES/DRAINS/BAGS/CONES/LUBRICATION)
NB. Complete Appliances are not prescribable

Manufacturer	Appliance	Order No.	Quantity	List Price p
Astra Tech Ltd	Medena Ileostomy Catheter	M8730	5	468
B. Braun Biotrol	Biotrol Irrigation			
	Sleeves	3061	50	3935
	Cone	3062	1	273
Cambmac Instruments Ltd - see Dansac Ltd				
Coloplast Ltd	Disposable Sleeve	1540	30	3426
	Disposable Sleeve	1560	30	3426
	Colotip	1110	1	650
	Irrigator Bag	1511	1	1230
	Supporting Plate	1120	1	619
	Irrigation Belt	0420	1	603
Dansac Ltd	Irri-Drain with Ring Holder			
	for Silicone Ring	950-20	20	2315
	Silicone Ring	09547-0000	1	465
	Irri-Drain Adhesive	950-35	20	2258
	Water Container	95200-0000	1	1811
	Clamp	95210-0000	1	783
	Cone	95205-0000	1	1163
	Brush	95220-0000	1	197
	Tube	95215-0000	1	138
	Unique 2 Irri-Drain			
	for use with Dansac Unique 2			
	36mm Flange	506-36	10	1146
	43mm Flange	506-43	10	1146
	55mm Flange	506-55	10	1146
Hollister Ltd	Stoma Cone/Irrigator Kit	7718	1	2050
	Irrigator Drain	7724	20	2827
	Replacement Cones	7723	10	7270
			1	889
	Stoma Lubricant	7740	1	503
Medicina Ltd	Medicina Caecostomy and ACE Washout sets			
	For Caecostomy Button	AS01	1	880
	For Caecostomy Tube or			
	ACE Catheter	AS02	1	880
Ward Surgical Appliance Co	Belt	WM 79	1	838

PRESSURE PLATES/SHIELDS

Manufacturer	Appliance	Order No.	Quantity	List Price p
Coloplast Ltd	Supporting Plate	1120	1	619
	Assura Convex Inserts (for use with Assura 2 Piece Base Plates)			
	40mm (stoma size 10-23mm)	4043	5	133
	40mm (stoma size 23-26mm)	4044	5	133
	40mm (stoma size 26-30mm)	4045	5	133
	50mm (stoma size 30-33mm)	4052	5	133
	50mm (stoma size 33-36mm)	4053	5	133
	50mm (stoma size 36-40mm)	4054	5	133
	60mm (stoma size 40-43mm)	4062	5	133
	60mm (stoma size 43-46mm)	4063	5	133
ConvaTec Ltd †	**System 2** Convex Inserts (for use with Combihesive, Stomahesive & Flexible flanges)			
	38mm (✦ 25mm internal dia)	S624	5	137
	45mm (✦ 32mm internal dia)	S626	5	137
	45mm (✦ 35mm internal dia)	S627	5	137
	57mm (✦ 41mm internal dia)	S629	5	137
	Combihesive Natura Convex Inserts (for use with Combihesive Natura flanges)			
	38mm (25mm internal dia)	S7624	5	134
	45mm (32mm internal dia)	S7626	5	134
	45mm (35mm internal dia)	S7627	5	134
	57mm (41mm internal dia)	S7629	5	134
DePuy Healthcare - see Simpla Continence Care				
Downs Surgical Ltd - see SIMS Portex Ltd				
John Drew Ltd	Pressure Plates			
	Oval	OST010A	1	268
	Round	OST010B	1	268
	4 Slot	OST010C	1	402
Eschmann Bros & Walsh Ltd - see SIMS Portex Ltd				
Respond Plus Ltd	Ostoshield (without belt)	Res50	1	620
	Ostoshield Belt Small/Medium 45cm/85cm	Res40	1	320
	Ostoshield Belt Large/Extra Large 66cm/124cm	Res45	1	320

IXC

✦ Approximate Conversion
† to be deleted 1 December 2000

PRESSURE PLATES/SHIELDS - cont

Manufacturer	Appliance	Order No.	Quantity	List Price p
Salts Healthcare	Plastic Retaining Shield			
	Single	833008	1	326
	Double	833009	1	504
	SS Wire Retaining Ring			
	Large	833010	1	326
	Medium	833011	1	311
	Small	833012	1	303
	Plastic Retaining Shield			
	Large	833030	1	399
	Light White Anti-Sag Ring			
	For Belt use	833038	1	147
	For Velcro Belt Fastening	833086	1	168
	Light White Stabilising Ring	833039	1	130
	Convex Plate for Light			
	White Bag 32mm	833046	5	1408
	† 38mm	833047	5	1408
	44mm	833048	5	1408
	Pressure Plate for Simplicity, Kombo & Solo			
	30mm	833057	1	203
	40mm	833058	1	203
	50mm	833059	1	203
	60mm	833060	1	203
	Pressure Plate			
	Kombo 30mm	833088	1	192
	40mm	833089	1	192
	50mm	833090	1	192
	60mm	833091	1	192
	Eakin Support Frame			
	32mm	839037	1	126
	45mm	839038	1	126
	64mm	839039	1	126
	90mm	839040	1	126
	Second Nature			
	Convex Inserts (for use with Second Nature Adhesive Flanges)			
	38mm (19mm internal dia)	CI3819	5	127
	38mm (22mm internal dia)	CI3822	5	127
	38mm (25mm internal dia)	CI3825	5	127
	45mm (29mm internal dia)	CI4529	5	127
	45mm (32mm internal dia)	CI4532	5	127
	45mm (35mm internal dia)	CI4535	5	127
	57mm (38mm internal dia)	CI5738	5	127
	57mm (41mm internal dia)	CI5741	5	127

† to be deleted 1 February 2001

PRESSURE PLATES/SHIELDS - cont

Manufacturer	Appliance	Order No.	Quantity	List Price p
T J Shannon Ltd	Facepiece	TJS 948b	1	780
Simcare - see SIMS Portex Ltd				
Simpla Continence Care				
	Cotton Face Piece with attached non-slip belt (for use with St Mark's flange)			
	45mm diam	781710	1	1898
SIMS Portex Ltd	Surrey Model Plastic Pressure Plate			
	25mm	WK001-25-P	1	751
	32mm	WK001-32-L	1	751
	Standard Plastic Pressure Plates to use with Lightweight Bag attached Flange			
	25mm int diameter	WK004-25-C	1	751
	32mm int diameter	WK004-32-Y	1	751
	38mm int diameter	WK004-38-M	1	751
	Stainless Wire Pressure Frames, Hook and Lug To fit			
	25mm Flange	WK012-25-Y	1	915
	32mm "	WK012-32-V	1	915
	38mm "	WK012-38-J	1	915
	44mm "	WK012-44-D	1	915
	51mm "	WK012-51-A	1	915
	Cotton Facepiece	WS300-01-P	1	2277
	Body Plates			
	25mm	48-526-48	1	526
	32mm	48-526-56	1	526
	38mm	48-526-64	1	526
Ward Surgical Appliance Co				
	Celluloid Colostomy Cup			
	With sponge or solid rim, Small, Medium or Large	WM10	1	3683
	With Sponge Rubber or Solid Rim, Belt Fitting	WM11	1	4201
	St Mark's Shields (celluloid)			
	4 studs	WM13	1	800

IXC

SKIN FILLERS AND PROTECTIVES
(Barrier Creams, Pastes, Aerosols, Lotions, Powders, Gels and Wipes)

Manufacturer	Appliance	Order No.	Quantity	List Price p
3M Health Care Ltd	3M Cavilon No Sting Barrier Film			
	Pump Spray (Sterilised)	3346P	28mL	599
	Foam Applicators (Sterile)	3343P	1mL	89
		3345P	3mL	143
C S Bullen Ltd	Balspray Aerosol	UF 95	1	700
	Karaya Gum Powder	UF 65	70g	464
Cambmac Instruments Ltd - see Dansac Ltd				
Clinimed Ltd	Clinishield Wipes	3800	50	1250
Coloplast Ltd	Coloplast Strip Paste	2655	10 strips	679
	Comfeel Barrier Cream	4720	60g	416
	Comfeel Protective Film			
	Sachets	4735	30	951
	Applicator	4731	1	451
ConvaTec Ltd	Orabase Paste	S103	30g	181
		S104	100g	403
	Orahesive Powder	S106	25g	209
	Stomahesive Paste	S105	60g	683
Dansac Ltd	Soft Paste	77550-0	50g	318
DePuy Healthcare - see Simpla Continence Care				
Downs Surgical Ltd - see SIMS Portex Ltd				
Eschman Bros & Walsh Ltd - see SIMS Portex Ltd				
Hollister Ltd	Karaya Paste	7910	128g	742
	Karaya Powder	7905	71g	855
	Premium Paste	7930	57g	332
	Skin Gel	7916	28g	644
Loxley Products	Day-Drop Barrier Cream	LL09	50g	219
Manfred Sauer	Preventox Skin Protecting Film Individually Packed Wipes	50.50	50	809
	Preventox Skin Protecting Film with Roll-on applicator	50.58	50mL	663
Medlogic Global Ltd	SuperSkin	SS0001	2g	700
S G & P Payne	Payne's Barrier Cream	1320	50g	365
Pelican Healthcare Ltd	Pelican Paste	130101	100g	681

SKIN FILLERS AND PROTECTIVES- cont
(Barrier Creams, Pastes, Aerosols, Lotions, Powders, Gels and Wipes)

Manufacturer	Appliance	Order No.	Quantity	List Price p
Rüsch UK Ltd	Translet Barrier Wipes	732730	30	584
Salts Healthcare	Stoma Paste	SP60	60g	323
	Karaya Powder 4oz Puffer Pack	833004	1	456
	Ostomy Cleaning Soap (Saltair Soap)	833007	110mL	274
	Peri-Prep Wipes	840001	50	1482
Simpla Continence Care	Skin Shield Wipes	781630	50	866
Simcare - see SIMS Portex Ltd				
SIMS Portex Ltd	Chiron Barrier Cream	WM102-01-A	52g	497
	Karaya Powder	WM083-01-R	100g	721
	Derma-gard Skin Wipes	32-291-06	50	1457

Squibb Surgicare Ltd - see ConvaTec Ltd

Warne-Franklin Medical Ltd - see Rüsch UK Ltd

IXC

SKIN PROTECTORS (Wafers, Blankets, Foam Pads, Washers)

Manufacturer	Appliance	Order No.	Quantity	List Price p
B. Braun Biotrol	Biotrol Skin Protectors			
	10cm x 10cm	32-075	10	1720
	10cm dia	32-076	10	1720
C S Bullen Ltd	Karaya Gum Washers in tins			
	✦ 51mm diameter			
	Regular			
	✦ 51mm x 22mm opening	UF 601	10	1262
	✦ 51mm x 29mm opening	UF 602	10	1262
	Extra Hard			
	✦ 51mm x 22mm opening	UF 6601	10	1262
	✦ 51mm x 29mm opening	UF 6602	10	1262
	✦ 64mm diameter			
	Regular			
	✦ 64mm x 32mm opening	UF 603	10	1463
	Extra Hard			
	✦ 64mm x 38mm opening	UF 6603	10	1463
	✦ 76mm diameter			
	Regular			
	✦ 76mm x 22mm opening	UF 604	10	1678
	✦ 76mm x 29mm opening	UF 605	10	1678
	✦ 76mm x 38mm opening	UF 606	10	1678
	✦ 76mm x 51mm opening	UF 607	10	1678
	Extra Hard			
	✦ 76mm x 22mm opening	UF 6604	10	1678
	✦ 76mm x 29mm opening	UF 6605	10	1678
	✦ 76mm x 38mm opening	UF 6606	10	1678
	✦76mm x 51mm opening	UF 6607	10	1678

Cambmac Instruments Ltd - see Dansac Ltd

✦   Approximate Conversion

SKIN PROTECTORS (Wafers, Blankets, Foam Pads, Washers) - cont

Manufacturer	Appliance	Order No.		Quantity	List Price p
Coloplast Ltd	Coloplast Protective Sheets Non Sterile				
	10cm x 10cm	3210		10	2110
	15cm x 15cm	3215		5	2499
	20cm x 20cm	3220		5	4546
	Coloplast Protective Rings				
	10mm	2310		30	3660
	15mm	2315		30	3660
	20mm	2320		30	3660
	25mm	2325		30	3660
	30mm	2330		30	3660
	40mm	2340		30	3660
	50mm	2350		30	3660
ConvaTec Ltd	Stomahesive Wafers				
	100mm x 100mm	S100		5	1030
	200mm x 200mm	S101		3	2525
	Varihesive Wafers				
	100mm x 100mm	S108		5	901
Dansac Ltd	Dansac GX-tra Seals				
	Washers				
	20mm (50mm outer diameter)	725-20	†	25	3163
				30	3731
	30mm (60mm outer diameter)	725-30	†	25	3163
				30	3731
	40mm (70mm outer diameter)	725-40	†	25	3163
				30	3731
	50mm (80mm outer diameter)	725-50	†	25	3163
				30	3731
DePuy Healthcare - see Simpla Continence Care					
Downs Surgical Ltd - see SIMS Portex Ltd					
John Drew Ltd	K Seal Karaya Gum				
	Washers Small	OST013B		20	853
	Large	OST013A		20	1009
Eschman Bros & Walsh Ltd - see SIMS Portex Ltd					
Hollister Ltd	Hollister Skin Barrier				
	✚ 102mm x 102mm	7700		5	1061
	✚ 203mm x 203mm	7701		4	3336
Omex Medical Ltd					
	Schacht Foam Rings				
	Colostomy	784885		10	752
	Ileostomy	784893		10	752
Pelican Healthcare Ltd	Pelican Skin Proctector				
	100mm x 100mm	130320		10	1974

✚   Approximate Conversion
†   to be deleted 1 February 2001

IXC

SKIN PROTECTORS (Wafers, Blankets, Foam Pads, Washers) - cont

Manufacturer	Appliance	Order No.	Quantity	List Price p
Salts Healthcare	Salger Karaya Washers with Foam			
	† 40mm	600440	5	1356
	57mm	600457	5	1356
	Salts Saltair Twin Pack			
	Small	833001	1	958
	Large	833002	1	1340
	Salts Small Karaya Washers	833003	10	782
†	Foam Cushions			
	25mm	833014	5	259
	32mm	833015	5	259
	38mm	833016	5	259
	51mm	833017	5	259
	Salts Dri Pads 40mm	833024	5	248
	Foam Seals as in small twin pack	833031	10	195
	Salts Large Karaya Washers	833084	10	1275
	Foam Seals as in large twin pack	833085	10	195
	Cohesive Washers			
	Small 48mm	839002	20	3293
	Large 98mm	839001	10	2199
	Protective Wafer			
	10cm x 10cm	PW1010	10	2010
	15cm x 15cm	PW1515	5	2194
	Realistic Washers			
	13mm	833070	10	1597
	19mm	833071	10	1597
	22mm	833072	10	1597
	25mm	833073	10	1597
	29mm	833074	10	1597
	32mm	833075	10	1597
	38mm	833076	10	1597
	United Skin Barrier Wafer			
	10cm x 10cm	840040	5	1055
	20cm x 20cm	840041	3	2449

†   to be deleted 1 February 2001

SKIN PROTECTORS (Wafers, Blankets, Foam Pads, Washers) - cont

Manufacturer	Appliance	Order No.	Quantity	List Price p
T J Shannon Ltd	Foam Sponge Rings	TJS 962b	1	76
	Kaygee Washers			
	✤ 64mm base			
	(✤ 29mm or 22mm hole)		10	683
	✤ 70mm base			
	(✤ 35mm or 22mm hole)		10	683
A H Shaw & Partners Ltd	Shaw Healwell Squares hole sizes 25mm, 32mm and 38mm	NSI 53	12	1068
	Body Mould Squares hole sizes 25mm, 32mm and 38mm	NSI 56	5	1126
	Washers hole sizes 25mm, 32mm	NSI 59	10	1032
	Rings hole sizes 25mm, 32mm and 38mm	NSI 55	5	1032
	Shaw Healwell Rings hole sizes 25mm, 32mm and 38mm	NSI 52	12	923
Simcare - see SIMS Portex Ltd				
SIMS Portex Ltd	White Foam Pads			
	76mm diam			
	25mm opening	WJ275-25-A	5	490
	29mm opening	WJ275-29-J	5	671
	32mm opening	WJ275-32-W	5	671
	38mm opening	WJ275-38-K	5	671
	90mm diam			
	32mm opening	WJ290-32-L	5	671
	38mm opening	WJ290-38-Y	5	671

IXC

✤   Approximate Conversion

SKIN PROTECTORS (Wafers, Blankets, Foam Pads, Washers) - cont

Manufacturer	Appliance	Order No.	Quantity	List Price p
SIMS Portex Ltd - cont	Black Foam Pads 76mm diam			
	25mm opening	WJ475-25-N	5	627
	Karaya Washers to fit (Redifit) Bag			
	25mm	WM080-25-T	10	1447
	32mm	WM080-32-Q	10	1447
	38mm	WM080-38-D	10	1447
	44mm	WM080-44-X	10	1447
	51mm	WM080-51-U	10	1447
	Downs Adhesive Karaya Gum Washers			
	22mm centre opening 51mm base	WM051-23-C	10	1173
	29mm centre opening 51mm base	WM051-28-N	10	1173
	22mm centre opening 70mm base	WM070-23-J	10	1447
	29mm centre opening 70mm base	WM070-28-U	10	1447
	Karaya Gum Sheets			
	300mm x 100mm	WM089-01-S	1	722
	Karaya Rings			
	19mm	32-263-87	20	2634
	25mm	32-264-84	20	2634
	32mm	32-265-81	20	2634
	38mm	32-266-89	20	2634
	51mm	32-267-86	20	2634
	Seel-a-Peel Squares			
	100mm sq	32-292-03	20	4061
	150mm sq	32-292-11	5	2501
	Rings			
	19mm	32-293-00	20	2409
	25mm	32-293-19	20	2409
	32mm	32-293-27	20	2409
	38mm	32-293-35	20	2409
	44mm	32-293-43	20	2409
Squibb Surgicare - see ConvaTec Ltd				
Welland Medical Ltd	Welland Hyperseal Washers			
	Small	HWA 300	25	3000
	Large	HWA 350	10	2000

STOMA CAPS/DRESSINGS

Manufacturer	Appliance	Order No.	Quantity	List Price p
B. Braun Biotrol	Biotrol Petite	F00015	30	3258
Cambmac Instrument Ltd - see Dansac Ltd				
Coloplast Ltd	Colocap	1014	100	11650
	Assura Minicap Opaque			
	20mm Starter hole	2501	30	3474
ConvaTec Ltd	Colodress Plus Stoma Cap			
	19mm Starter hole	S821	30	3368
Dansac Ltd	Dansac Minicap			
	(Opaque)			
	30mm	01930-1000	50	5727
	44mm	01944-1000	50	5727
	Dansac Unique Mini Cap			
	(Opaque)			
	cut-to-fit			
	20mm-50mm	229-20	30	3390
	pre-cut			
	30mm	229-30	30	3390
	40mm	229-40	30	3390
	50mm	229-50	30	3390
Downs Surgical Ltd - see SIMS Portex Ltd				
EuroCare - see Salts Healthcare				
Eschmann Bros & Walsh Ltd - see SIMS Portex Ltd				
Hollister Ltd	Hollister Stoma Cap			
	51mm	7184	50	5854
	76mm	7186	50	5854
Oakmed Ltd	Option Stoma Cap	1320K	50	4976
	Option Stoma Cap with Soft Covering and Filter			
	(Opaque)			
	cut to fit 20mm-50mm	1420k	50	5498
Salts Healthcare	Confidence Stomacap with filter			
	starter hole			
	13mm	SC13	30	3115
	Second Nature Stoma Cap with filter			
	32mm	2SC32	30	2900
	38mm	2SC38	30	2900
	45mm	2SC45	30	2900
	57mm	2SC57	30	2900
	Simplicity 1.			
	Stoma caps	510250	30	3506

IXC

STOMA CAPS/DRESSINGS - cont

Manufacturer	Appliance	Order No.	Quantity	List Price p
Simcare - see SIMS Portex Ltd				
SIMS Portex Ltd	Leisure Pouch	32-287-11	20	2371
Squibb Surgicare - see ConvaTec Ltd				
Steeper (Orthopaedic) Ltd - incorporating Donald Rose Ltd - see Ward Surgical Appliance Co				
Ward Surgical Appliance Co	Two zip fasteners fitted to colostomy belt	36	1	795
	Waterproof front, fitted to colostomy belt	37	1	656
	Donald Rose rubber ileo/ colostomy bath belt with internal chamber for dressings, with stud fastenings for adjustment	51	1	1970
	Woven understraps with buttonhold ends	21	1 pair	304

TUBING

Manufacturer	Appliance	Order No.	Quantity	List Price p
Eschmann Bros & Walsh Ltd - see SIMS Portex Ltd				
Hollister Ltd	Urostomy Drain Tube	7328	10	2555
	Urostomy Drain Tube for fitting to LO-Profile Urostomy Bags	7330	8	2377
	Premium Urostomy drain tube adaptor	7331	10	2039
Salts Healthcare	Salts Night Tube Adaptor	833043	2	98
	Urostomy Night Drainage Adaptor	NDA6	6	1099
Simcare - see SIMS Portex Ltd				
SIMS Portex Ltd	Carshalton Connector	11-110-19	10	423
Steeper (Orthopaedic) Ltd - incorporating Donald Rose Ltd - see Ward Surgical Appliance Co				
Ward Surgical Appliance Co	Metal Spring Tubing Clip	48	1	221

IXC

TWO PIECE OSTOMY SYSTEMS

Manufacturer	Appliance		Order No.	Quantity	List Price p
B. Braun Biotrol	Biotrol LockRing 2				
	Flange	35mm	22-135	5	1291
		50mm	22-150	5	1291
		75mm	22-175	5	1291
	Biotrol LockRing 2 Hydrocolloid Flange				
		35mm	24-235	5	1266
		50mm	24-250	5	1266
		62mm	24-262	5	1266
		75mm	24-275	5	1266
	Closed Bag				
	Beige	35mm	22-835	30	3216
		50mm	22-850	30	3216
		62mm	22-862	30	3216
		75mm	22-875	30	3216
	White	35mm	22-335	30	3216
		50mm	22-350	30	3216
	Transparent				
		75mm	22-375	30	3216
	Drainable Bag				
	Beige	35mm	22-535	30	3216
		50mm	22-550	30	3216
		62mm	22-562	30	3216
		75mm	22-575	30	3216
	White	35mm	22-435	30	3216
		50mm	22-450	30	3216
	Transparent				
		75mm	22-475	30	3216
	Paediatric				
	Flange	35mm	23-035	5	1275
	Paediatric Closed Bag				
	Beige	35mm	23-435	30	2819
	Drainable Bag				
	Beige	35mm	23-735	30	3111
	Urostomy Bag - Transparent				
	Baby	35mm	23-835	10	2418
	Child	35mm	23-935	10	2418
	Urostomy Bag				
	Transparent	35mm	22-635	10	2418
		50mm	22-650	10	2418
		75mm	22-775	10	2418

TWO PIECE OSTOMY SYSTEMS

Manufacturer	Appliance	Order No.	Quantity	List Price p
Cambmac Instruments Ltd - see Dansac Ltd				
Coloplast Ltd	**Assura**			
	Base Plates with 10mm starter hole:			
	40mm for 10-35mm stoma	2894	5	1463
	50mm for 30-45mm stoma	2895	5	1463
	60mm for 40-55mm stoma	2896	5	1463
	Convex inserts for use with the above - see "Pressure Plates"			
	Base Plates			
	40mm for paediatric bags	2180	5	1455
	Assura Seal Integral Convexity Baseplates			
	Important: This product with Integral Convexity should only be used after prior assessment of suitability by an appropriate medical professional.			
	40mm flange 15mm pre cut	12701	5	1419
	40mm flange 18mm pre cut	12702	5	1419
	40mm flange 21mm pre cut	12703	5	1419
	50mm flange starter hole 15-33mm	12716	5	1419
	50mm flange 25mm pre cut	12704	5	1419
	50mm flange 28mm pre cut	12705	5	1419
	50mm flange 31mm pre cut	12706	5	1419
	60mm flange starter hole 15-43mm	12719	5	1419
	60mm flange 35mm pre cut	12707	5	1419
	60mm flange 38mm pre cut	12708	5	1419
	60mm flange 41mm pre cut	12709	5	1419
	Assura Closed Bags:			
	Paediatric Opaque			
	40mm	2160	30	2766
	Mini Opaque			
	40mm	2724	30	3045
	50mm	2725	30	3045
	Midi Clear			
	40mm	2774	30	3705
	50mm	2775	30	3705
	60mm	2776	30	3705
	Midi Opaque			
	40mm	2764	30	3705
	50mm	2765	30	3705
	60mm	2766	30	3705
	Maxi Clear			
	40mm	2784	30	3705
	50mm	2785	30	3705
	60mm	2786	30	3705
	Maxi Opaque			
	40mm	2814	30	3705
	50mm	2815	30	3705
	60mm	2816	30	3705
	Minicap Opaque			
	40mm	2804	30	2964
	50mm	2805	30	2964

IXC

TWO PIECE OSTOMY SYSTEMS - cont

Manufacturer	Appliance	Order No.	Quantity	List Price p
Coloplast Ltd - cont				
	Assura Drainable Bag:			
	Paediatric Opaque			
	40mm	2150	30	3204
	Midi Clear			
	40mm	2754	30	3705
	50mm	2755	30	3705
	60mm	2756	30	3705
	Midi Opaque			
	40mm	2744	30	3705
	50mm	2745	30	3705
	60mm	2746	30	3705
	Maxi Clear			
	40mm	2794	30	3705
	50mm	2795	30	3705
	60mm	2796	30	3705
	Maxi Opaque			
	40mm	2824	30	3705
	50mm	2825	30	3705
	60mm	2826	30	3705
	Closed Bag with Integral Filter and Opaque Soft Cover front and back			
	Midi			
	40mm	12461	30	3705
	50mm	12462	30	3705
	60mm	12463	30	3705
	Maxi			
	40mm	12481	30	3705
	50mm	12482	30	3705
	60mm	12483	30	3705
	Drainable Bag with Opaque Soft Cover front and back			
	Midi			
	40mm	12441	30	3705
	50mm	12442	30	3705
	60mm	12443	30	3705
	Urostomy Bag (include 4 drain tube adaptors per pack)			
	Midi Clear with soft backing on body-worn side			
	40mm	2854	30	7401
	50mm	2855	30	7401
	Maxi Clear with soft backing on body-worn side			
	40mm	2874	30	7401
	50mm	2875	30	7401
	60mm	2876	30	7401
	Paediatric Clear with soft backing on body-worn side			
	40mm	2175	30	7401
	Maxi Opaque with soft backing on body-worn side			
	40mm	2864	30	7401
	50mm	2865	30	7401
	60mm	2866	30	7401
	Paediatric Opaque with soft backing on body-worn side			
	40mm	2170	30	7401

TWO PIECE OSTOMY SYSTEMS - cont

Manufacturer	Appliance	Order No.	Quantity	List Price p
Coloplast Ltd - cont	Assura:**Inspire**			
	Closed Bag with integral filter and soft backing			
	Midi Transparent			
	40mm	12344	30	3780
	50mm	12345	30	3780
	60mm	12346	30	3780
	Maxi Transparent			
	40mm	12374	30	3780
	50mm	12375	30	3780
	60mm	12376	30	3780
	Closed Bag with integral filter and opaque soft cover front and back			
	Midi Soft Cover			
	40mm	12354	30	3780
	50mm	12355	30	3780
	60mm	12356	30	3780
	Maxi Soft Cover			
	40mm	12384	30	3780
	50mm	12385	30	3780
	60mm	12386	30	3780
	Closed Bag with integral filter and soft cover front and back			
	Midi Design			
	40mm	12364	30	3780
	50mm	12365	30	3780
	60mm	12366	30	3780
	Maxi Design			
	40mm	12394	30	3780
	50mm	12395	30	3780
	60mm	12396	30	3780
	Drainable Bag with integral filter and soft backing			
	Midi Transparent			
	40mm	13444	30	3780
	50mm	13445	30	3780
	60mm	13446	30	3780
	Maxi Transparent			
	40mm	13474	30	3780
	50mm	13475	30	3780
	60mm	13476	30	3780
	Drainable Bag with integral filter and opaque soft cover front and back			
	Midi Soft Cover			
	40mm	13454	30	3780
	50mm	13455	30	3780
	60mm	13456	30	3780
	Maxi Soft Cover			
	40mm	13484	30	3780
	50mm	13485	30	3780
	60mm	13486	30	3780
	Drainable Bag with integral filter and soft cover front and back			
	Midi Design			
	40mm	13464	30	3780
	50mm	13465	30	3780
	60mm	13466	30	3780
	Maxi Design			
	40mm	13494	30	3780
	50mm	13495	30	3780
	60mm	13496	30	3780

IX

TWO PIECE OSTOMY SYSTEMS - cont

Manufacturer	Appliance	Order No.	Quantity	List Price p
Coloplast Ltd - cont	**MC 2002**			
	Base Plates			
	40mm flanges 15mm stoma	6742	5	1507
	40mm flanges 25mm stoma	6743	5	1507
	60mm flanges 35mm stoma	6764	5	1507
	60mm flanges 45mm stoma	6765	5	1507
	Closed Pouches			
	Clear 40mm	6641	30	4080
	60mm	6661	30	4080
	Opaque 40mm	6642	30	4080
	60mm	6662	30	4080
	Open Pouches			
	Clear 40mm	6541	30	4503
	60mm	6561	30	4503
	Opaque 40mm	6542	30	4503
	60mm	6562	30	4503
	Belt Plates 40mm	4270	1	61
	60mm	4271	1	61
	URO2002			
	Base Plates			
	40mm flange	4245	5	1545
	60mm flange	4265	5	1545
	Bags			
	40mm Large	4240	20	5984
	Small	4241	20	5984
	60mm Large	4260	20	5984
	Conseal			
	Base Plates			
	40mm	1200	5	1444
	50mm	1250	5	1444
	Colostomy Plug			
	40 x 35mm	1235	10	1315
	40 x 45mm	1245	10	1315
	50 x 35mm	1285	10	1315
	50 x 45mm	1295	10	1315
	Closed Bag			
	40mm	1210	30	3903
	50mm	1260	30	3903
	Discharge Bag			
	40mm	1220	50	285
	50mm	1270	50	285

TWO PIECE OSTOMY SYSTEMS - cont

Manufacturer	Appliance	Order No.	Quantity	List Price p
ConvaTec Ltd	**Combihesive Natura**			
	Durahesive with Convex-IT Flange			
	Important: This product with deep convexity should only be used after prior assessment of suitability by an appropriate medical professional			
	13mm/45mm	S7325	5	1425
	16mm/45mm	S7326	5	1425
	19mm/45mm	S7327	5	1425
	22mm/45mm	S7328	5	1425
	25mm/45mm	S7329	5	1425
	28mm/45mm	S7330	5	1425
	32mm/45mm	S7331	5	1425
	35mm/45mm	S7332	5	1425
	38mm/57mm	S7335	5	1425
	41mm/57mm	S7336	5	1425
	45mm/57mm	S7337	5	1425
	50mm/57mm	S7338	5	1425
	Flexible Flange with Micropore surround			
	32mm	S7244	5	1400
	38mm	S7245	5	1400
	45mm	S7246	5	1400
	57mm	S7247	5	1400
	70mm	S7248	5	1400
	Stomahesive Flange			
	32mm	S7294	10	2449
	38mm	S7295	10	2449
	45mm	S7296	10	2449
	57mm	S7297	10	2449
	70mm	S7298	10	2449
	100mm	S7299	10	2449
	Stomahesive Flexible Flange			
	32mm	S7340	10	2646
	38mm	S7341	10	2646
	45mm	S7342	10	2646
	57mm	S7343	10	2646
	70mm	S7344	10	2646
	Flange Cap with filter			
	Opaque			
	38mm	S7250	25	2313
	45mm	S7251	25	2313
	57mm	S7252	25	2313

Convex inserts for use with above - see Pressure Plates

TWO PIECE OSTOMY SYSTEMS - cont

Manufacturer	Appliance	Order No.	Quantity	List Price p
ConvaTec Ltd - cont	**Combihesive Natura**			
	Closed Pouch with filter			
	Standard Size - Opaque			
	32mm	S7254	30	3386
	38mm	S7255	30	3386
	45mm	S7256	30	3386
	57mm	S7257	30	3386
	70mm	S7258	30	3386
	Mini Size - Opaque			
	32mm	S7290	20	1856
	38mm	S7291	20	1856
	45mm	S7292	20	1856
	57mm	S7293	20	1856
	Closed pouch no filter			
	Standard size - Opaque			
	32mm	S7215	30	3239
	38mm	S7216	30	3239
	45mm	S7217	30	3239
	57mm	S7218	30	3239
	70mm	S7219	30	3239
	Drainable Pouch			
	Standard Size - Opaque			
	32mm	S7269	10	1121
	38mm	S7270	10	1121
	45mm	S7271	10	1121
	57mm	S7272	10	1121
	70mm	S7273	10	1121
	Small Size - Opaque			
	32mm	S7279	10	1121
	38mm	S7280	10	1121
	45mm	S7281	10	1121
	57mm	S7282	10	1121
	70mm	S7283	10	1121
	Standard Size - Clear			
	32mm	S7228	10	1121
	38mm	S7229	10	1121
	45mm	S7230	10	1121
	57mm	S7231	10	1121
	70mm	S7232	10	1121
	100mm	S7233	10	1987
	Drainable Pouch with Filter			
	Standard Size - Opaque for:-			
	32mm flange	S7400	10	1099
	38mm flange	S7401	10	1099
	45mm flange	S7402	10	1099
	57mm flange	S7403	10	1099
	70mm flange	S7404	10	1099
●	Small Size - Opaque for:-			
	32mm flange	S7406	10	1099
	38mm flange	S7407	10	1099
	45mm flange	S7408	10	1099
	57mm flange	S7409	10	1099
	70mm flange	S7410	10	1099

● Temporarily Unavailable

TWO PIECE OSTOMY SYSTEMS - cont

Manufacturer	Appliance	Order No.	Quantity	List Price p
ConvaTec Ltd - cont	**Combihesive Natura**			
	Urostomy Pouch with Improved Accuseal Tap			
	Standard Size -			
	Clear for:-			
	32mm flange	S7380	10	2456
	38mm flange	S7381	10	2456
	45mm flange	S7382	10	2456
	57mm flange	S7383	10	2456
	70mm flange	S7384	10	2456
	Urostomy Pouch with Improved Accuseal Tap			
	Standard Size - Opaque for:-			
	32mm flange	S7370	10	2456
	38mm flange	S7371	10	2456
	45mm flange	S7372	10	2456
	57mm flange	S7373	10	2456
	Small Size - Opaque for:-			
	32mm flange	S7390	10	2456
	38mm flange	S7391	10	2456
	45mm flange	S7392	10	2456
	57mm flange	S7393	10	2456
	Urostomy Pouch with Standard Tap			
	Standard Size - Clear for:-			
	32mm flange	S7350	10	2397
	38mm flange	S7351	10	2397
	45mm flange	S7352	10	2397
	57mm flange	S7353	10	2397
	70mm flange	S7354	10	2596
	100mm flange	S7355	10	3600
	Small Size - Clear for:			
	32mm flange	S7360	10	2397
	38mm flange	S7361	10	2397
	45mm flange	S7362	10	2397
	57mm flange	S7363	10	2397
	Combihesive Natura High Output			
	Drainable Pouch with Filter			
	Opaque for:-			
	45mm	S7467	5	1793
	57mm	S7468	5	1793
	70mm	S7469	5	1793
	Consecura Low Profile			
	Locking flange with Micropore surround			
	35mm	S601LP	5	1298
	45mm	S602LP	5	1298
	57mm	S603LP	5	1298
	70mm	S604LP	5	1298
	Stomahesive Flexible Locking Flange			
	35mm	S590LP	5	1298
	45mm	S591LP	5	1298
	57mm	S592LP	5	1298
	70mm	S593LP	5	1298

IXC

TWO PIECE OSTOMY SYSTEMS - cont

Manufacturer	Appliance	Order No.	Quantity	List Price p
ConvaTec Ltd - cont	**Consecura Low Profile**			
	Closed Pouch with Filter			
	Standard Size			
	Opaque for:-			
	35mm flange	S616LP	30	3263
	45mm Flange	S617LP	30	3263
	57mm flange	S618LP	30	3263
	70mm flange	S619LP	30	3263
	Clear for:-			
	35mm flange	S630LP	30	3263
	45mm flange	S631LP	30	3263
	57mm flange	S632LP	30	3263
	70mm flange	S633LP	30	3263
	Drainable Pouch			
	Standard Size			
	Opaque for:-			
	35mm flange	S606LP	10	1081
	45mm flange	S607LP	10	1081
	57mm flange	S608LP	10	1081
	70mm flange	S609LP	10	1081
	Clear for:-			
	35mm flange	S611LP	10	1081
	45mm flange	S612LP	10	1081
	57mm flange	S613LP	10	1081
	70mm flange	S614LP	10	1081
	100mm flange	S615LP	10	1852

TWO PIECE OSTOMY SYSTEMS - cont

Manufacturer	Appliance	Order No.	Quantity	List Price p
ConvaTec Ltd - cont	**Consecura Low Profile**			
	Urostomy Pouch with Accuseal Tap			
	Standard Size			
	Clear for:-			
	35mm flange	S640LP	10	2356
	45mm flange	S641LP	10	2356
	57mm flange	S642LP	10	2356
	Opaque for:-			
	35mm flange	S655LP	10	2356
	45mm flange	S656LP	10	2356
	57mm flange	S657LP	10	2356
	70mm flange	S658LP	10	2356
	Urostomy Pouch with Fold-up Tap			
	Standard Size			
	Clear for:-			
	35mm flange	S635LP	10	2356
	45mm flange	S636LP	10	2356
	57mm flange	S637LP	10	2356
Dansac Ltd	**Unique 2 Flexi Flange**			
	36mm Flange (100mm x 100mm)			
	Starter hole (15-28mm)	536-15	5	1412
	Precut 20mm	536-20	5	1412
	Precut 25mm	536-25	5	1412
	43mm Flange (100mm x 100mm)			
	Starter hole (15-35mm)	543-15	5	1412
	Precut 30mm	543-30	5	1412
	55mm Flange (100mm x 100mm)			
	Starter hole (15-47mm)	555-15	5	1412
	Precut 35mm	555-35	5	1412
	Precut 40mm	555-40	5	1412
	80mm Flange (125mm x 125mm)			
	Starter hole (15-70mm)	580-15	5	1440
	Precut 45mm	580-45	5	1440
	Precut 50mm	580-50	5	1440

IXC

TWO PIECE OSTOMY SYSTEMS - cont

Manufacturer	Appliance	Order No.	Quantity	List Price p
Dansac Ltd - cont	**Unique 2 S Flange**			
	30mm Flange (100mm x 100mm)			
	Starter hole (10-22mm)	430-10	5	1367
	Precut 15mm	430-15	5	1367
	36mm Flange (100mm x 100mm)			
	Starter hole (15-28mm)	436-15	5	1367
	Precut 20mm	436-20	5	1367
	Precut 25mm	436-25	5	1367
	43mm Flange (100mm x 100mm)			
	Starter hole (15-35mm)	443-15	5	1367
	Precut 30mm	443-30	5	1367
	55mm Flange (100mm x 100mm)			
	Starter hole (15-47mm)	455-15	5	1367
	Precut 35mm	455-35	5	1367
	Precut 40mm	455-40	5	1367
	80mm Flange (125mm x 125mm)			
	Starter hole (15-70mm)	480-15	5	1365
	Precut 45mm	480-45	5	1365
	Precut 50mm	480-50	5	1365

Unique 2 Convex Flange

Important: This product with deep convexity should only be used after prior assessment of suitability by an appropriate medical professional.

	36mm Flange (100mm x 100mm)			
	Starter hole (15-25mm)	736-15	5	1415
	Precut 20mm	736-20	5	1415
	Precut 25mm	736-25	5	1415
	43mm Flange (100mm x 100mm)			
	Starter hole (15-32mm)	743-15	5	1415
	Precut 25mm	743-25	5	1415
	Precut 30mm	743-30	5	1415
	55mm Flange (115mm x 115mm)			
	Starter hole (15-44mm)	755-15	5	1415
	Precut 35mm	755-35	5	1415
	Precut 40mm	755-40	5	1415

Manufacturer	Appliance	Order No.	Quantity	List Price p
Dansac Ltd - cont	**Urostomy Drainable Pouch** (includes 1 Dansac Drain Tube Adaptor and 3 caps)			
	Opaque with spunlace backing for:			
	30mm Flange	401-30	10	2458
	36mm Flange	401-36	10	2458
	43mm Flange	401-43	10	2458
	55mm Flange	401-55	10	2458
	Clear with spunlace backing for:			
	30mm Flange	402-30	10	2458
	36mm Flange	402-36	10	2458
	43mm Flange	402-43	10	2458
	55mm Flange	402-55	10	2458
	Unique 2 Closed Pouch			
	Opaque with spunlace cover next to skin for:			
	36mm Flange	501-36	30	3451
	43mm Flange	501-43	30	3451
	55mm Flange	501-55	30	3451
	80mm Flange	501-80	30	3451
	Clear with spunlace cover next to skin for:			
	36mm Flange	502-36	30	3451
	43mm Flange	502-43	30	3451
	55mm Flange	502-55	30	3451
	80mm Flange	502-80	30	3451
	Unique 2 Plus Closed Pouch			
	Opaque with spunlace cover front and back for:			
	36mm Flange	505-36	30	3375
	43mm Flange	505-43	30	3375
	55mm Flange	505-55	30	3375
	80mm Flange	505-80	30	3375
	Unique 2 Mini Closed Pouch			
	Opaque with spunlace cover front and back for:			
	36mm Flange	503-36	30	2866
	43mm Flange	503-43	30	2866
	55mm Flange	503-55	30	2866
	Unique 2 MiniCap			
	Opaque for:			
	36mm Flange	507-36	30	3007
	43mm Flange	507-43	30	3007
	55mm Flange	507-55	30	3007

IXC

TWO PIECE OSTOMY SYSTEMS - cont

Manufacturer	Appliance	Order No.	Quantity	List Price p
Dansac Ltd - cont				
	Unique 2 Drainable Regular			
	Opaque with spunlace cover next to skin for:			
	36mm Flange	511-36	10	1141
	43mm Flange	511-43	10	1141
	55mm Flange	511-55	10	1141
	80mm Flange	511-80	10	1141
	Clear with spunlace cover next to skin for:			
	36mm Flange	512-36	10	1141
	43mm Flange	512-43	10	1141
	55mm Flange	512-55	10	1141
	80mm Flange	512-80	10	1141
	Unique 2 Drainable Large			
	Opaque with spunlace cover next to skin for:			
	36mm Flange	521-36	10	1141
	43mm Flange	521-43	10	1141
	55mm Flange	521-55	10	1141
	80mm Flange	521-80	10	1141
	Clear with spunlace cover next to skin for:			
	36mm Flange	522-36	10	1141
	43mm Flange	522-43	10	1141
	55mm Flange	522-55	10	1141
	80mm Flange	522-80	10	1141
	InVent 2 - Drainable with filter, soft spunlace backing on both sides, anatomically shaped			
	Opaque			
	36mm Flange	513-36	10	1121
	43mm Flange	513-43	10	1121
	55mm Flange	513-55	10	1121
	InVent 2 Mini Drainable with filter, soft spun lace material on both sides, anatomically shaped			
	Opaque			
	36mm Flange	519-36	10	1102
	43mm Flange	519-43	10	1102
	55mm Flange	519-55	10	1102
	InVent 2 Sym - Drainable Symmetrical pouch with filter, soft spunlace backing, symmetrically shaped			
	Opaque			
	36mm Flange	515-36	10	1121
	43mm Flange	515-43	10	1121
	55mm Flange	515-55	10	1121
	Clear			
	36mm Flange	516-36	10	1121
	43mm Flange	516-43	10	1121
	55mm Flange	516-55	10	1121
	80mm Flange	518-80	10	1121
Eschmann Bros & Walsh Ltd - see SIMS Portex Ltd				
EuroCare - see Salts Healthcare				

TWO PIECE OSTOMY SYSTEMS - cont

Manufacturer	Appliance	Order No.	Quantity	List Price p
Hollister Ltd	**Conform 2**			
	Fixed Flange			
	35mm flange 13-30mm stoma	23100	5	1323
	35mm flange 20mm stoma	23120	5	1323
	35mm flange 25mm stoma	23125	5	1323
	35mm flange 30mm stoma	23130	5	1323
	45mm flange 30mm stoma	24130	5	1323
	45mm flange 35mm stoma	24135	5	1323
	45mm flange 40mm stoma	24140	5	1323
	45mm flange 13-40mm stoma	24100	5	1323
	55mm flange 13-50mm stoma	25100	5	1323
	55mm flange 45mm stoma	25145	5	1323
	55mm flange 50mm stoma	25150	5	1323
	70mm flange 13-65mm stoma	27100	5	1323
	Floating Flange			
	45mm flange 13-30mm stoma	24200	5	1323
	55mm flange 13-40mm stoma	25200	5	1323
	70mm flange 40mm stoma	27240	5	1323
	70mm flange 13-55mm stoma	27200	5	1323
	Closed Pouch			
	with beige comfort backing			
	45mm	24400	30	3205
	55mm	25400	30	3205
	70mm	27400	30	3205
	transparent front, beige comfort backing on body worn side			
	45mm	24500	30	3205
	55mm	25500	30	3205
	70mm	27500	30	3205
	Drainable Pouch			
	transparent			
	45mm	24600	10	1079
	55mm	25600	10	1079
	70mm	27600	10	1079
	Drainable Pouch with Filter - anatomical shape			
	Beige			
	35mm	23720	30	3360
	45mm	24720	30	3360
	55mm	25720	30	3360
	Transparent			
	35mm	23820	30	3360
	45mm	24820	30	3360
	55mm	25820	30	3360
	Mini Drainable Pouch with Filter			
	Beige			
	35mm	23710	30	3360
	45mm	24710	30	3360
	55mm	25710	30	3360

IXC

TWO PIECE OSTOMY SYSTEMS - cont

Manufacturer	Appliance	Order No.	Quantity	List Price p
Hollister Ltd - cont	**Guardian Range**			
	'F' Floating Flanges			
	25mm	4402	5	1381
	38mm	4403	5	1381
	51mm	4404	5	1381
	64mm	4405	5	1381
	102mm	4406	5	1448
	Impression			
	Convex Flanges			
	13mm	4430	5	1466
	16mm	4431	5	1466
	19mm	4432	5	1466
	22mm	4433	5	1466
	25mm	4434	5	1466
	29mm	4435	5	1466
	32mm	4436	5	1466
	35mm	4437	5	1466
	38mm	4438	5	1466
	41mm	4439	5	1466
	44mm	44310	5	1466
	51mm	44311	5	1466
	Closed Pouch			
	Clear - with filter and comfort backing on body-worn side			
	25mm	4502	15	1711
	38mm	4503	15	1711
	51mm	4504	15	1711
	64mm	4505	15	1711
	Opaque - with filter and comfort backing on both sides			
	25mm	4512	15	1711
	38mm	4513	15	1711
	51mm	4514	15	1711
	64mm	4515	15	1711
	Drainable Pouch			
	Clear - with beige non-woven backing on body-worn side			
	25mm	4602	10	1140
	38mm	4603	10	1140
	51mm	4604	10	1140
	64mm	4605	10	1140
	102mm	4606	10	2386

TWO PIECE OSTOMY SYSTEMS - cont

Manufacturer	Appliance	Order No.	Quantity	List Price p
Hollister Ltd - cont	Drainable Pouch			
	Opaque - with beige non-woven backing on both sides			
	25mm	4612	10	1140
	38mm	4613	10	1140
	51mm	4614	10	1140
†	64mm	4615	10	1140
	Mini Pouch			
	Opaque - with beige non-woven backing on both sides			
	25mm	4642	10	1112
	38mm	4643	10	1112
	51mm	4644	10	1112
	64mm	4645	10	1112
	Urostomy Pouch			
	Clear - with beige non-woven backing on body-worn side			
	25mm	4702	10	2529
	38mm	4703	10	2529
	51mm	4704	10	2529
	Tandem Range			
	Floating Flange - Barrier and adhesive			
	cut-to-fit 25mm	3727	5	1349
	32mm	3722	5	1349
	44mm	3723	5	1349
	57mm	3724	5	1349
	89mm	3726	5	1398
	Floating Flange - Barrier and adhesive			
	pre-cut 19mm	3747	5	1349
	25mm	3742	5	1349
	32mm	3748	5	1349
	38mm	3743	5	1349
	44mm	3749	5	1349
	51mm	3744	5	1349
	57mm	3746	5	1349
	Floating Flange - Barrier only			
	cut-to-fit 25mm	3767	5	1349
	32mm	3762	5	1349
	44mm	3763	5	1349
	57mm	3764	5	1349
	89mm	3766	5	1398

IXC

†   to be deleted 1 December 2000

TWO PIECE OSTOMY SYSTEMS - cont

Manufacturer	Appliance	Order No.	Quantity	List Price p
Hollister Ltd - cont	**Tandem Range** - cont			
	Impression CPL			
	Convex Flange			
	pre-cut			
	13mm	3730	5	1444
	16mm	3731	5	1444
	19mm	3732	5	1444
	22mm	3733	5	1444
	25mm	3734	5	1444
	29mm	3735	5	1444
	32mm	3736	5	1444
	35mm	3737	5	1444
	38mm	3738	5	1444
	41mm	3739	5	1444
	44mm	37310	5	1444
	51mm	37311	5	1444
	Convex Flange - Barrier only			
	pre-cut			
	13mm	3780	5	1444
	16mm	3781	5	1444
	19mm	3782	5	1444
	22mm	3783	5	1444
	25mm	3784	5	1444
	29mm	3785	5	1444
	32mm	3786	5	1444
	35mm	3787	5	1444
	38mm	3788	5	1444
	41mm	3789	5	1444
	44mm	37810	5	1444
	51mm	37811	5	1444
	cut-to-fit			
	Up to 25mm	3794	5	1444
	Up to 38mm	3798	5	1444
	Up to 51mm	37911	5	1444
	Closed Pouch			
	Transparent with filter and comfort backing on body-worn side			
	38mm	3337	30	3324
	44mm	3332	30	3324
	57mm	3333	30	3324
	70mm	3334	30	3324
	Closed Pouch			
	Beige - with filter and comfort backing on both sides			
	38mm	3347	30	3324
	44mm	3342	30	3324
	57mm	3343	30	3324
	70mm	3344	30	3324

TWO PIECE OSTOMY SYSTEMS - cont

Manufacturer	Appliance	Order No.	Quantity	List Price p
Hollister Ltd - cont	**Tandem Range** - cont			
	Impression CPL - cont			
	Mini Closed Pouch with filter			
	Opaque			
	38mm	3357	30	2871
	44mm	3352	30	2871
	57mm	3353	30	2871
	70mm	3354	30	2871
	Drainable Pouch			
	Transparent - with comfort backing on body-worn side only			
	38mm	3807	10	1119
	44mm	3802	10	1119
	57mm	3803	10	1119
	70mm	3804	10	1119
	102mm	3806	10	2151
	Beige - with comfort backing on both sides			
	38mm	3817	10	1119
	44mm	3812	10	1119
	57mm	3813	10	1119
	70mm	3814	10	1119
	102mm	3816	10	2151
	Mini Drainable Pouch			
	Beige - with comfort backing on both sides			
	38mm	3847	10	1076
	44mm	3842	10	1076
	57mm	3843	10	1076
	70mm	3844	10	1076
	Urostomy Pouch			
	Transparent - with comfort backing on the body-worn side			
	38mm	3907	10	2463
	44mm	3902	10	2463
	57mm	3903	10	2463
	70mm	3904	10	2463

IXC

TWO PIECE OSTOMY SYSTEMS - cont

Manufacturer	Appliance	Order No.	Quantity	List Price p
Oakmed Ltd	**Option Range**			
	Option Flange			
	50mm	F500	5	1310
	70mm	F700	5	1310
	Colostomy with Filter and Soft Covering to one side			
	Clear for:-			
	50mm flange	CB50K	30	3256
	Colostomy with Filter and Soft Covering to both sides			
	Opaque for:-			
	50mm flange	CA50K	30	3295
	Colostomy Plus with Filter and Soft Covering to one side			
	Clear for:-			
	70mm flange	CD70K	30	3309
	Colostomy Plus with Filter and Soft Covering to both sides			
	Opaque for:-			
	70mm flange	CC70K	30	3348
	Ileostomy Midi with Filter and Soft Covering to one side			
	Clear for:-			
	50mm flange	IG50K	30	3309
	70mm flange	IG70K	30	3309
	Ileostomy with filter and Soft Covering to one side			
	Clear for:-			
	50mm flange	IB50K	30	3309
	70mm flange	IB70K	30	3309
	Ileostomy Midi with Filter and Soft Covering to both sides			
	Opaque for:-			
	50mm flange	ID50K	30	3329
	70mm flange	ID70K	30	3329
	Ileostomy with Filter and Soft Covering to both sides			
	Opaque for:-			
	50mm flange	IA50K	30	3329
	70mm flange	IA70K	30	3329
Rüsch UK Ltd	Translet Range			
	Premier Colostomy Set			
	(1 adhesive ring and			
	6 bags)			
	27mm opening	731127	15	6622
	40mm opening	731140	15	6622
	57mm opening	731157	15	6622
	Premier Spare Bags			
	28cm length	732100	10	508
	18cm length	732150	10	508

TWO PIECE OSTOMY SYSTEMS - cont

Manufacturer	Appliance	Order No.	Quantity	List Price p
Rüsch UK Ltd - cont	Royal Colostomy Set (1 adhesive ring and 6 odour proof bags)			
	27mm opening	731027	15	9203
	40mm opening	731040	15	9203
	57mm opening	731057	15	9203
	Royal Spare Bags			
	28cm length	732000	10	804
	18cm length	732050	10	804
	Translet Adhesive Rings			
	27mm	732327	5	678
	40mm	732340	5	678
	57mm	732357	5	678
	Translet Microporous Spare Adhesive Rings			
	27mm	732427	5	678
	40mm	732440	5	678
	57mm	732457	5	678
Salts Healthcare	**Black Rubber Bag** (for use with flange)			
	Screw outlet			
	Large	362129	1	3179
	Small	362229	1	3179
	Special	362099	1	3303
	Spout outlet			
	Large	372129	1	2221
	Small	372229	1	2221
	Special	372099	1	2348
	Tap outlet			
	† Large	382129	1	3918
	Medium	382229	1	3918
	Small	382329	1	3918
	Special	382099	1	4011
	White Rubber Bag (for use with flange)			
	Screw outlet			
	Large	461129	1	1058
	Small	461229	1	1058
	Spout bag			
	Large	472129	1	883
	Small	472229	1	883
	Tap outlet			
	† Large	482129	1	1145
	Medium	482329	1	1145
	Small	482229	1	1145

IXC

†   to be deleted 1 February 2001

TWO PIECE OSTOMY SYSTEMS - cont

Manufacturer	Appliance	Order No.	Quantity	List Price p
Salts Healthcare - cont				
	Second Nature			
	Wafer 110 x 100mm			
	32mm Flange	2FL32	5	1167
	38mm Flange	2FL38	5	1167
	45mm Flange	2FL45	5	1167
	Wafer 134 x 124m			
	57mm Flange	2FL57	5	1167
	Wafer 151 x 140mm			
	70mm Flange	2FL70	10	2680
	Convex inserts for use with above - see "Pressure Plates"			
	Closed Pouches			
	Opaque for:			
	32mm Flange	2C32	30	3404
	38mm Flange	2C38	30	3404
	45mm Flange	2C45	30	3404
	57mm Flange	2C57	30	3404
	Transparent/overlap film for:			
	45mm Flange	2CT45	30	3404
	57mm Flange	2CT57	30	3404
	Transparent/overlap film			
	Large 70mm Flange	2CLT70	30	3404
	Transparent/no overlap			
	Large 70mm Flange	2CLTT70	30	3404
	Drainable Pouches			
	Opaque for:			
	32mm Flange	2D32	30	3346
	38mm Flange	2D38	30	3346
	45mm Flange	2D45	30	3346
	57mm Flange	2D57	30	3346
	Transparent/overlap film for:			
	45mm Flange	2DT45	30	3346
	57mm Flange	2DT57	30	3346
	Transparent/overlap film			
	Large 70mm Flange	2DLT70	30	3346
	Transparent/no overlap			
	Large 70mm Flange	2DLTT70	30	3346
	Mini Closed Pouches			
	Opaque for:			
	32mm Flange	2CM32	30	2836
	38mm Flange	2CM38	30	2836
	45mm Flange	2CM45	30	2836
	57mm Flange	2CM57	30	2836
	Mini Drainable Pouches			
	Opaque for:			
	32mm Flange	2DM32	30	3251
	38mm Flange	2DM38	30	3251
	45mm Flange	2DM45	30	3251
	57mm Flange	2DM57	30	3251

TWO PIECE OSTOMY SYSTEMS - cont

Manufacturer	Appliance	Order No.	Quantity	List Price p
Salts Healthcare - cont	**Second Nature** - cont			
	Urostomy Pouch-transparent/overlap			
	(includes 2 drain tube connectors per pack)			
	32mm Flange	2U32	10	2371
	38mm Flange	2U38	10	2371
	45mm Flange	2U45	10	2371
	57mm Flange	2U57	10	2371
	Secuplast Circular Plasters			
	32mm	SP32	10	985
	38mm	SP38	10	985
	45mm	SP45	10	985
	57mm	SP57	10	985
	70mm	SP70	10	985
	Secu-Ring to fit:			
	32mm Flange	SR32	10	1036
	38mm Flange	SR38	10	1036
	45mm Flange	SR45	10	1036
	57mm Flange	SR57	10	1036
	70mm Flange	SR70	10	1036
	Simplicity			
	Flanges			
	Standard 30mm	500130	5	307
	40mm	500140	5	307
	50mm	500150	5	307
	60mm	500160	5	307
	Clear Closed Pouch			
	Medium 40mm	530940	30	1688
	50mm	530950	30	1688
	60mm	530960	30	1688
	70mm	530970	30	1688
	Pink Closed Pouch			
	Medium 40mm	530340	30	1671
	50mm	530350	30	1671
	60mm	530360	30	1671
†	Clear Drainable Bag			
	Medium 40mm	531340	30	1924
	50mm	531350	30	1924
	60mm	531360	30	1924
	Post-Op Closed Bag			
	Large 40mm	530240	30	1671
	50mm	530250	30	1671
	60mm	530260	30	1671
†	**Simplicity 2**			
	Flange 30mm	520130	5	1511
	40mm	520140	5	1511
	50mm	520150	5	1511
	60mm	520160	5	1511

IXC

† to be deleted 1 February 2001

TWO PIECE OSTOMY SYSTEMS - cont

Manufacturer	Appliance	Order No.	Quantity	List Price p
Salts Healthcare - cont	**Simplicity 2** - cont			
	Closed Bag			
	30mm	520330	30	3585
	† 40mm	520340	30	3585
	† 50mm	520350	30	3585
	† 60mm	520360	30	3585
	† 70mm	520370	30	3585
	† Drainable Bag			
	30mm	521330	15	1969
	40mm	521340	15	1969
	50mm	521350	15	1969
	60mm	521360	15	1969
	70mm	521370	15	1969
	Post-Op Open Bag			
	30mm	520230	30	3968
	40mm	520240	30	3968
	50mm	520250	30	3968
	60mm	520260	30	3968
	70mm	520270	30	3968
	Transverse Flange	520530	5	2205
	† Transverse Bag	520630	10	4507
Simcare - see SIMS Portex Ltd				
SIMS Portex Ltd	Beta 2 Piece kit	32-294-08	1	5407
	Beta 2 Piece spare bags	32-294-16	90	14887
	Serenade			
	"WC Disposable"			
	Closed bag with filter			
	25mm	32-350-09	30	3499
	32mm	32-350-17	30	3499
	38mm	32-350-25	30	3499
	44mm	32-350-33	30	3499
	51mm	32-350-41	30	3499
	Closed bag with soft-backing and filter			
	25mm	32-352-03	30	3639
	32mm	32-352-11	30	3639
	38mm	32-352-38	30	3639
	44mm	32-352-46	30	3639
	51mm	32-352-54	30	3639
	Mini closed bag with soft-backing and filter			
	15-51mm	32-354-08	30	2859
	Base Plate			
	25mm	32-360-05	10	2887
	32mm	32-360-13	10	2887
	38mm	32-360-21	10	2887
	44mm	32-360-48	10	2887
	51mm	32-360-56	10	2887

†   to be deleted 1 February 2001

TWO PIECE OSTOMY SYSTEMS - cont

Manufacturer	Appliance	Order No.	Quantity	List Price p

Squibb Surgicare Ltd - see ConvaTec Ltd

Warne-Franklin Medical Ltd - see Rüsch UK Ltd

Welland Medical Ltd	**Silhouette 2** closed pouch with soft backing and filter			
	Beige			
	45mm	UNC545	30	3200
	60mm	UNC560	30	3200
	Silhouette 2 drainable pouch with soft backing			
	Beige			
	45mm	UND545	30	3250
	60mm	UND560	30	3250
	Silhouette 2 drainable pouch with soft backing and filter			
	Beige			
	45mm	UNF545	30	3250
	60mm	UNF560	30	3250
	Silhouette 2 Hydrocolloid Flange			
	45mm Flange			
	Starter Hole	UNH410	5	1200
	Precut 25mm	UNH425	5	1200
	Precut 32mm	UNH432	5	1200
	Precut 38mm	UNH438	5	1200
	60mm Flange			
	Starter Hole	UNH610	5	1200
	Precut 32mm	UNH632	5	1200
	Precut 44mm	UNH644	5	1200
	Precut 51mm	UNH651	5	1200
	Precut 57mm	UNH657	5	1200
	Silhouette 2 Dual Adhesive Flange			
	45mm Flange			
	Starter hole	UNB410	5	1200
	Precut 25mm	UNB425	5	1200
	Precut 32mm	UNB432	5	1200
	Precut 38mm	UNB438	5	1200
	60mm Flange			
	Starter hole	UNB610	5	1200
	Precut 32mm	UNB632	5	1200
	Precut 44mm	UNB644	5	1200
	Precut 51mm	UNB651	5	1200
	Precut 57mm	UNB657	5	1200

IXC

STOMA APPLIANCES

UROSTOMY BAGS

Manufacturer	Appliance	Order No.	Quantity	List Price p
Body's Surgical Company - See Jade-Euro-Med				
C S Bullen Ltd	**Lenbul**			
	Bag with tap			
	Day	U 5	1	1508
	Night	U 6	1	1722
	Bag with large opening			
	Day	U 7	1	1565
	Night	U 8	1	1788
Coloplast Ltd	Stoma Urine Bag			
	Maxi	1005	30	8298
	Assura (include 4 drain tube adaptors per pack)			
	Urostomy Bag with Soft Backing			
	Midi Clear with soft backing on body-worn side			
	cut-to-fit 10-55mm	2550	30	12594
	Midi Opaque with soft backing on body-worn side			
	cut-to-fit 10-55mm	2540	30	12594
	Maxi Clear with soft backing on body-worn side			
	cut-fo-fit 10-55mm	2570	30	12594
	Maxi Opaque with soft backing on body-worn side			
	cut-to-fit 10-55mm	2560	30	12594
	Paediatric Clear with soft backing on body-worn side			
	cut-to-fit 10-35mm	2135	30	12594
	Paediatric Opaque with soft backing on body-worn side			
	cut-to-fit 10-35mm	2130	30	12594

UROSTOMY BAGS - cont

Manufacturer	Appliance	Order No.	Quantity	List Price p
Coloplast Ltd - cont	**Assura** Seal Integral Convexity Urostomy Bag			
	Important: This product with Integral Convexity should only be used after prior assessment of suitability by an appropriate medical professional.			
	Maxi Clear			
	15mm	12991	10	4017
	18mm	12992	10	4017
	21mm	12993	10	4017
	25mm	12994	10	4017
	28mm	12995	10	4017
	31mm	12996	10	4017
	Maxi Transparent			
	starter hole 15-33mm	12595	10	4017
	15-43mm	12596	10	4017
	pre-cut 35mm	12997	10	4017
	38mm	12998	10	4017
	41mm	12999	10	4017
ConvaTec Ltd	Urodress			
	19mm	S896	10	4558
	25mm	S897	10	4558
	32mm	S898	10	4558
	38mm	S899	10	4558
	45mm	S900	10	4558
	Urodress Deep Convex Urostomy Pouch			
	Important: This product with deep convexity should only be used after prior assessment of suitability by an appropriate medical professional			
	Clear Standard			
	16mm	S910	5	
	19mm	S911	5	2006
	22mm	S912	5	2006
	25mm	S913	5	2006
	28mm	S914	5	2006
	32mm	S915	5	2006
	35mm	S916	5	2006
	38mm	S917	5	2006

Downs Surgical Ltd - see SIMS Portex Ltd

IXC

UROSTOMY BAGS - cont

Manufacturer	Appliance	Order No.	Quantity	List Price p
John Drew Ltd	Urostomy Bags D1/2	OST006	50	7634
	Rubber Bags	OST016	1	1303
		OST017	1	1367
Eschmann Bros and Walsh Ltd - see SIMS Portex Ltd				
Hollister Ltd	**Compact**			
	Urostomy Pouch			
	(All include 1 drain tube per pack)			
	Clear-with beige comfort backing on body-worn side			
	cut-to-fit			
	13-64mm	1400	10	4607
	Transparent-with beige comfort backing on body-worn side			
	cut-to-fit			
	13-64mm	1401	10	4607
	pre-cut			
	13mm	1440	10	4607
	16mm	1441	10	4607
	19mm	1447	10	4607
	25mm	1442	10	4607
	32mm	1448	10	4607
	38mm	1443	10	4607
	44mm	1449	10	4607
	51mm	1444	10	4607
	Karaya 5 Seal			
	with Regular Adhesive			
	Transparent			
	✚ 229mm length			
	Gasket Size:			
	✚ 18mm	7417	20	7031
	✚ 25mm	7412	20	7031
	✚ 32mm	7418	20	7031
	✚ 38mm	7413	20	7031
	✚ 44mm	7419	20	7031
	✚ 51mm	7414	20	7031
	✚ 30.5cm length			
	Gasket Size:			
	✚ 25mm	7482	20	7031
	✚ 32mm	7488	20	7031
	✚ 38mm	7483	20	7031
	✚ 44mm	7489	20	7031
	✚ 51mm	7484	20	7031

✚   Approximate Conversion

UROSTOMY BAGS - cont

Manufacturer	Appliance	Order No.	Quantity	List Price p
Hollister Ltd - cont	With Belt Lugs, Transparent			
	✚ 30.5cm length			
	Gasket Size:			
	✚ 25mm	7472	20	5389
	✚ 32mm	7478	20	5389
	✚ 38mm	7473	20	5389
	✚ 44mm	7479	20	5389
	✚ 51mm	7474	20	5389
	Lo-Profile			
	With Microporous II Adhesive only			
	Gasket Size:			
	✚ 18mm	1427	10	4492
	✚ 25mm	1422	10	4492
	✚ 32mm	1428	10	4492
	✚ 38mm	1423	10	4492
	✚ 44mm	1429	10	4492
	✚ 51mm	1424	10	4492
	With Microporous II Adhesive and Karaya 5 Seal			
	Gasket Size:			
	✚ 18mm	1437	10	5206
	✚ 25mm	1432	10	5206
	✚ 32mm	1438	10	5206
	✚ 38mm	1433	10	5206
	✚ 44mm	1439	10	5206
	✚ 51mm	1434	10	5206

IXC

✚   Approximate Conversion

UROSTOMY BAGS - cont

Manufacturer	Appliance	Order No.	Quantity	List Price p
Hollister Ltd - cont	**First Choice** With Microporous II Adhesive and Synthetic Skin Barrier			
	13mm-64mm starter hole	1460	10	4818
	19mm	1467	10	4818
	25mm	1462	10	4818
	32mm	1468	10	4818
	38mm	1463	10	4818
	44mm	1469	10	4818
	51mm	1464	10	4818
	Impression With Convex wafer (transparent)			
	13mm	1480	10	4818
	16mm	1481	10	4818
	19mm	1482	10	4818
	22mm	1483	10	4818
	25mm	1484	10	4818
	29mm	1485	10	4818
	32mm	1486	10	4818
	35mm	1487	10	4818
	38mm	1488	10	4818
	44mm	1489	10	4818
	Impression "C" with convex wafer Transparent with beige comfort backing on body-worn side			
	13mm	1450	10	4209
	16mm	1451	10	4209
	19mm	1452	10	4209
	22mm	1453	10	4209
	25mm	1454	10	4209
	29mm	1455	10	4209
	32mm	1456	10	4209
	35mm	1457	10	4209
	38mm	1458	10	4209
	44mm	1459	10	4209
	51mm	14510	10	4209
Jade-Euro-Med Ltd	White rubber urostomy bags			
	Night bag tap outlet	KM 47	1	1841
	Day bag tap outlet	KM 45	1	1607
	Black Butyl bag odourless			
	Night bag tap outlet	KM 41	1	3372
	Day bag tap outlet	KM 39	1	3214

Leyland Medical Ltd - see Rüsch UK Ltd

UROSTOMY BAGS - cont

Manufacturer	Appliance	Order No.	Quantity	List Price p
Marlen USA	**Ultra**			
	Transparent			
	Starter hole			
	Small 12mm	761312	10	3924
	Large 12mm	762312	10	3924
	Small Bag Transparent			
	Flat Pre-cut			
	12mm	761412	10	3924
	16mm	761416	10	3924
	19mm	761419	10	3924
	22mm	761422	10	3924
	25mm	761425	10	3924
	29mm	761429	10	3924
	32mm	761432	10	3924
	34mm	761434	10	3924
	38mm	761438	10	3924
	41mm	761441	10	3924
	44mm	761444	10	3924
	48mm	761448	10	3924
	50mm	761450	10	3924
	54mm	761454	10	3924
	57mm	761457	10	3924
	60mm	761460	10	3924
	63mm	761463	10	3924
	67mm	761467	10	3924
	70mm	761470	10	3924
	73mm	761473	10	3924
	76mm	761476	10	3924
	Large Bag Transparent			
	Flat Pre-cut			
	12mm	762412	10	3924
	16mm	762416	10	3924
	19mm	762419	10	3924
	22mm	762422	10	3924
	25mm	762425	10	3924
	29mm	762429	10	3924
	32mm	762432	10	3924
	34mm	762434	10	3924
	38mm	762438	10	3924
	41mm	762441	10	3924
	44mm	762444	10	3924
	48mm	762448	10	3924
	50mm	762450	10	3924
	54mm	762454	10	3924
	57mm	762457	10	3924
	60mm	762460	10	3924
	63mm	762463	10	3924
	67mm	762467	10	3924
	70mm	762470	10	3924
	73mm	762473	10	3924
	76mm	762476	10	3924

IXC

UROSTOMY BAGS - cont

Manufacturer	Appliance	Order No.	Quantity	List Price p
Marlen USA - cont	**Ultra**			
	Small Bag Transparent			
	Shallow Convex			
	12mm	761512	10	3924
	16mm	761516	10	3924
	19mm	761519	10	3924
	22mm	761522	10	3924
	25mm	761525	10	3924
	29mm	761529	10	3924
	32mm	761532	10	3924
	34mm	761534	10	3924
	38mm	761538	10	3924
	41mm	761541	10	3924
	44mm	761544	10	3924
	48mm	761548	10	3924
	50mm	761550	10	3924
	54mm	761554	10	3924
	57mm	761557	10	3924
	60mm	761560	10	3924
	63mm	761563	10	3924
	67mm	761567	10	3924
	70mm	761570	10	3924
	73mm	761573	10	3924
	76mm	761576	10	3924
	Large Bag Transparent			
	Shallow Convex			
	12mm	762512	10	3924
	16mm	762516	10	3924
	19mm	762519	10	3924
	22mm	762522	10	3924
	25mm	762525	10	3924
	29mm	762529	10	3924
	32mm	762532	10	3924
	34mm	762534	10	3924
	38mm	762538	10	3924
	41mm	762541	10	3924
	44mm	762544	10	3924
	48mm	762548	10	3924
	50mm	762550	10	3924
	54mm	762554	10	3924
	57mm	762557	10	3924
	60mm	762560	10	3924
	63mm	762563	10	3924
	67mm	762567	10	3924
	70mm	762570	10	3924
	73mm	762573	10	3924
	76mm	762576	10	3924

UROSTOMY BAGS - cont

Manufacturer	Appliance	Order No.	Quantity	List Price p
Rüsch UK Ltd	Birkbeck Black Rubber			
	Day Bag			
	19mm	LM 723125	1	3160
	Night Bag			
	19mm	LM 723175	1	3447
	Pink Rubber			
	Day Bag			
	19mm	LM 724125	1	3160
	Night Bag			
	19mm	LM 724175	1	3447
	White Rubber Day Bag			
	19mm	LM 883111	1	1716
	25mm	LM 883112	1	1716
	28mm	LM 883113	1	1716
	White Rubber Night Bag			
	19mm	LM 883121	1	1763
	25mm	LM 883122	1	1763
	28mm	LM 883123	1	1763
	White Rubber Glasgow Bag			
	Small tap	LM 884230	1	2096
	Large tap	LM 884232	1	2096
	White Rubber Transverse			
	Bag Right			
	Small	LM 884104	1	2096
	Medium	LM 884105	1	2096
	Large	LM 884106	1	2096
	White Rubber Transverse			
	Bag Left			
	Small	LM 884114	1	2096
	Medium	LM 884115	1	2096
	Large	LM 884116	1	2096
Salts Healthcare	**Confidence** Urostomy Pouch transparent/overlap film (includes 2 drain tube connectors per pack)			
	starter hole			
	13mm	U13	10	3867
	pre-cut			
	25mm	U25	10	3867
	32mm	U32	10	3867
	38mm	U38	10	3867
	45mm	U45	10	3867

IXC

UROSTOMY BAGS - cont

Manufacturer	Appliance	Order No.	Quantity	List Price p
Salts Healthcare - cont				
	Koenig Rutzen			
	All Rubber Black			
	with Tap outlet and			
	N-R valve			
	Large			
	† 19mm	181119	1	4150
	25mm	181125	1	4150
	32mm	181132	1	4150
	† 38mm	181138	1	4150
	Medium			
	19mm	181319	1	4150
	25mm	181325	1	4150
	32mm	181332	1	4150
	38mm	181338	1	4150
	Special	181099	1	4310
	MB with Bridge, Tap			
	outlet and N-R valve			
	Large			
	† 19mm	185119	1	4853
	25mm	185125	1	4853
	† 32mm	185132	1	4853
	38mm	185138	1	4853
	Medium			
	19mm	185319	1	4853
	† 25mm	185325	1	4853
	32mm	185332	1	4853
	38mm	185338	1	4853
	Special	185099	1	5041
	All Rubber White Tap outlet			
	Large			
	† 25mm	281125	1	1718
	32mm	281132	1	1718
	† 38mm	281138	1	1718
	† 44mm	281144	1	1718
	† 51mm	281151	1	1718
	Medium			
	† 25mm	281325	1	1718
	32mm	281332	1	1718
	38mm	281338	1	1718
	Small			
	25mm	281225	1	1718
	32mm	281232	1	1718
	38mm	281238	1	1718

†   to be deleted 1 February 2001

UROSTOMY BAGS - cont

Manufacturer	Appliance	Order No.	Quantity	List Price p
Salts Healthcare - cont	Reinforced Rubber Black with Tap outlet and N-R valve			
	Large			
	19mm	183119	1	5087
	25mm	183125	1	5087
	32mm	183132	1	5087
	38mm	183138	1	5087
	Medium			
	19mm	183319	1	5087
	25mm	183325	1	5087
	32mm	183332	1	5087
	38mm	183338	1	5087
	Special	183099	1	5282
	MB with Bridge, Tap outlet and N-R valve			
	Large			
	† 19mm	188119	1	5827
	25mm	188125	1	5827
	32mm	188132	1	5827
	38mm	188138	1	5827
	Medium			
	19mm	188319	1	5827
	† 25mm	188325	1	5827
	† 32mm	188332	1	5827
	† 38mm	188338	1	5827
	Special	188099	1	6052

IXC

†   to be deleted 1 February 2001

UROSTOMY BAGS - cont

Manufacturer	Appliance	Order No.	Quantity	List Price p
Salts Healthcare - cont	**Light White**			
	Clear			
	Large			
	25mm	296125	20	8582
	32mm	296132	20	8582
	38mm	296138	20	8582
	† Small			
	25mm	296225	20	8582
	32mm	296232	20	8582
	38mm	296238	20	8582
	Opaque			
	Large			
	25mm	294125	20	8582
	32mm	294132	20	8582
	38mm	294138	20	8582
	Adhesive Bag			
	Clear			
	Large			
	25mm	299125	20	8974
	32mm	299132	20	8974
	38mm	299138	20	8974
	† Small			
	25mm	299225	20	8974
	32mm	299232	20	8974
	38mm	299238	20	8974
	Opaque			
	Large			
	25mm	298125	20	8974
	32mm	298132	20	8974
	38mm	298138	20	8974
	with Realistic Washer			
	Clear			
	Large			
	25mm	293125	20	11274
	32mm	293132	20	11274
	38mm	293138	20	11274
	Small			
	† 25mm	293225	20	11274
	32mm	293232	20	11274
	† 38mm	293238	20	11274
	Opaque			
	Large			
	25mm	292125	20	11252
	32mm	292132	20	11252
	38mm	292138	20	11252
	† **Simplicity 1**			
	Paediatric Uri-bag			
	13mm Starter	623212	15	4342

† to be deleted 1 February 2001

UROSTOMY BAGS - cont

Manufacturer	Appliance	Order No.	Quantity	List Price p
Simcare - see SIMS Portex Ltd				
SIMS Portex Ltd	**Carshalton**			
	with acrylic adhesive			
	Oval			
	25mm	48-534-58	10	2045
	32mm	48-534-66	10	2045
	38mm	48-534-74	10	2045
	Triangular			
	25mm	48-532-37	10	2045
	32mm	48-532-45	10	2045
	38mm	48-532-53	10	2045
	Chiron			
	Black Rubber			
	Day Bag			
	22mm	WF205-22-T	1	3660
	Latex Rubber			
	Day Bag			
	38mm	WF203-38-B	1	2536
	Night Bag			
	38mm	WF213-38-G	1	2876
	White Rubber			
	Day Bag			
	38mm	WF201-38-S	1	2536
	Night Bag			
	38mm	WF211-38-X	1	2876
	44mm	WF211-44-S	1	2876
	51mm	WF211-51-P	1	2876
	Childs			
	Day Bag	WF221-01-D	1	2128
	Great Ormond Street			
	Minicare Bag			
	Clear	WC100-19-E	10	1971
	Opaque	WC100-20-N	10	1971
	Mirage			
	Urostomy Pouches			
	Beige			
	starter hole to 44mm	32-530-15	10	3938
	25mm	32-530-25	10	3938
	32mm	32-530-32	10	3938
	38mm	32-530-38	10	3938
	44mm	32-530-44	10	3938
	Clear			
	starter hole to 64mm	32-535-15	10	3938

IXC

UROSTOMY BAGS - cont

Manufacturer	Appliance	Order No.	Quantity	List Price p
SIMS Portex Ltd - cont	**Mitcham**			
	Maxi			
	adhesive			
	25mm	WH119-25-G	10	4168
	32mm	WH119-32-D	10	4168
	38mm	WH119-38-R	10	4168
	non-adhesive			
	25mm	WH009-25-U	10	3403
	32mm	WH009-32-R	10	3403
	38mm	WH009-38-E	10	3403
	Mini			
	adhesive			
	19mm	WH116-19-Y	10	4168
	25mm	WH116-25-T	10	4168
	32mm	WH116-32-Q	10	4168
	non-adhesive			
	25mm	WH005-25-C	10	3403
	32mm	WH005-32-Y	10	3403
	Standard			
	adhesive			
	19mm	WH111-19-C	10	4168
	25mm	WH111-25-W	10	4168
	32mm	WH111-32-T	10	4168
	38mm	WH111-38-G	10	4168
	non-adhesive			
	19mm	WH002-19-U	10	3403
	25mm	WH002-25-P	10	3403
	32mm	WH002-32-L	10	3403
	38mm	WH002-38-Y	10	3403
	* With Foam Pads			
	non-adhesive			
	25mm	WH012-25-U	1	573
	32mm	WH012-32-R	1	573
	38mm	WH012-38-E	1	573
	Rediflow			
	adhesive			
	19mm	WG001-19-H	20	6124
	25mm	WG001-25-C	20	6124
	32mm	WG001-32-Y	20	6124
	38mm	WG001-38-M	20	6124
	44mm	WG001-44-G	20	6124
	51mm	WG001-51-D	20	6124

*   Replacement bags for Surrey Urinal on page 214.

UROSTOMY BAGS - cont

Manufacturer	Appliance	Order No.	Quantity	List Price p
Ward Surgical Appliance Co	**Ureterostomy Bag**			
	tap outlet, 19mm, 35mm			
	or 54mm opening			
	Night Size	WM 47	1	2019
	Day Size	WM 48	1	1891
Welland Medical Ltd	**Silhouette URO**			
	Urostomy pouch with soft backing			
	Clear 13mm	SUR 713	10	4070
	16mm	SUR 716	10	4070
	19mm	SUR 719	10	4070
	22mm	SUR 722	10	4070
	25mm	SUR 725	10	4070
	32mm	SUR 732	10	4070
	38mm	SUR 738	10	4070
	Beige 13mm	SUR 913	10	4070
	16mm	SUR 916	10	4070
	19mm	SUR 919	10	4070
	22mm	SUR 922	10	4070
	25mm	SUR 925	10	4070
	32mm	SUR 932	10	4070
	38mm	SUR 938	10	4070

IXC

UROSTOMY SETS

Manufacturer	Appliance	Order No.	Quantity	List Price p
John Drew Ltd	Ureterostomy Appliance			
	D1/2	OST005	1	3883
Downs Surgical Ltd - see SIMS Portex Ltd				
Eschmann Bros & Walsh Ltd - see SIMS Portex Ltd				
Oakmed Ltd	The SR-U Appliance	SR-U	1	6060
	The OPR-U Appliance	OPR-U	1	8069
	The LOP-U Appliance	LOP-U	1	3868
Simcare - see SIMS Portex Ltd				
SIMS Portex Ltd	Chiron Ileal Bladder			
	Apparatus	WE202-38-P	1	7940
	Carshalton Sets			
	Oval Bag			
	25mm	48-503-19	1	6857
	32mm	48-503-27	1	6857
	38mm	48-503-35	1	6857
	Triangle Bag			
	25mm	48-503-43	1	6857
	32mm	48-503-51	1	6857
	38mm	48-505-13	1	6857

CROSS REFERENCE INDEX
(STOMA APPLIANCES)

Appliance Range	Manufacturer
Accordion (flange)	ConvaTec Ltd
AR	Salts Healthcare
Assura	Coloplast
Atmocol	Adams Healthcare
Beta	SIMS Portex Ltd
Biopore	B. Braun Biotrol
Biotrol	B. Braun Biotrol
Camila	C S Bullen Ltd
Carshalton	SIMS Portex Ltd
Cavendish	SIMS Portex Ltd
Cavilon	3M Health Care Ltd
Chiron	SIMS Portex Ltd
Citrus Fresh	Pelican Healthcare Ltd
Clearseal	SIMS Portex Ltd
Clinishield	Clinimed Ltd
Cloe	C S Bullen Ltd
Cohesive	Salts Healthcare
Cohflex	Salts Healthcare
Colodress	ConvaTec Ltd
Coloset	Salts Healthcare
Combihesive	ConvaTec Ltd
Combi Micro	Dansac Ltd
Comfeel	Coloplast Ltd
Comfort	Coloplast Ltd
Compact	Hollister Ltd
Confidence	Salts Healthcare
Conform 2	Hollister Ltd
Conseal	Coloplast Ltd
Constance	C S Bullen Ltd
C & S	Dansac Ltd
Consecura	ConvaTec Ltd
Coversure	Respond Plus Ltd
D -	John Drew Ltd
Dansac	Dansac Ltd
Day-drop	Loxley Products
Dor	Pelican Healthcare Ltd
D & S	Dansac Ltd
Eakin	Salts Healthcare
Easy Change	T J Shannon Ltd
EC1 Range	SIMS Portex Ltd
Elite	B. Braun Biotrol
Esteem	ConvaTec Ltd
FirstChoice	Hollister Ltd
Friends Ostomy	JLR Sales And Marketing Co Ltd
Glasgow	SIMS Portex Ltd
Gt Ormond Street	SIMS Portex Ltd
Guardian	Hollister Ltd
GX-tra	Dansac Ltd
Hainsworth	Shaw AH & Partners Ltd
Healwell	Shaw AH & Partners Ltd
Holligard	Hollister Ltd

IXC

CROSS REFERENCE INDEX - cont
(STOMA APPLIANCES)

Appliance Range	Manufacturer
ILeo-B	Coloplast Ltd
Ileodress	ConvaTec Ltd
Ileo KAV	Rüsch UK Ltd
Impact	Welland Medical Ltd
Impression	Hollister Ltd
Inspire	Coloplast Ltd
Integrale	B. Braun Biotrol
InVent	Dansac Ltd
K -Flex	Coloplast Ltd
Koenig Rutzen	Salts Healthcare
Kombo	Salts Healthcare
KR	Salts Healthcare
Lenbul	C S Bullen Ltd
Light White	Salts Healthcare
Limone	Clinimed Ltd
Little-Ones	ConvaTec Ltd
LockRing 2	B. Braun Biotrol
LOP	Oakmed Ltd
LO-Profile	Hollister Ltd
MC	Coloplast Ltd
Medena	Astra Meditec Ltd
Moderma	Hollister Ltd
Moderma L.C.	Hollister Ltd
Mirage	SIMS Portex Ltd
Mitcham	SIMS Portex Ltd
Newcastle	SIMS Portex Ltd
New Freedom	T J Shannon Ltd
Omni	SIMS Portex Ltd
O.P.R.	Oakmed Ltd
Option	Oakmed Ltd
Ostocover	Impharm Nationwide Ltd
Ostopore	Rüsch UK Ltd
Ovation	Welland Medical Ltd
Peri-Prep	Salts Healthcare
Petit	Dansac Ltd
Phoenix	Pelican Healthcare Ltd
Preference	B. Braun Biotrol
Premium	Hollister Ltd
Preventox	Manfred Sauer
Realistic	Salts Healthcare
Redifit	SIMS Portex Ltd
Rediseal	SIMS Portex Ltd
Reliaseal	Salts Healthcare
Royal	Rüsch UK Ltd
Salgar	Salts Healthcare
Saltair	Salts Healthcare
Sassco	Pelican Healthcare Ltd
Schacht	Omex Medical Ltd

CROSS REFERENCE INDEX - cont
(STOMA APPLIANCES)

Appliance Range	Manufacturer
Second Nature	Salts Healthcare
Secuplast	Salts Healthcare
Secu-ring	Salts Healthcare
Select	Pelican Healthcare Ltd
Serenade	SIMS Portex Ltd
SF	Salts Healthcare
Silhouette	Welland Medical Ltd
Simplicity	Salts Healthcare
Skintone	SIMS Portex Ltd
Solo	Salts Healthcare
SR	Oakmed Ltd
Stomadress	ConvaTec Ltd
Stomahesive	ConvaTec Ltd
Supasac	Salts Healthcare
Surgicare	ConvaTec Ltd
Surrey	SIMS Portex Ltd
SuperSkin	Medlogic Global ltd
Symphony	SIMS Portex Ltd
System 2	ConvaTec Ltd
Tandem	Hollister Ltd
Transacryl	Salts Healthcare
Translet	Rüsch UK Ltd
Ultra	Marlen USA
Unique	Dansac Ltd
United	Salts Healthcare
Urisleeve	Bard Ltd
URO	Coloplast Ltd
Urodress	ConvaTec Ltd
Vogue	Welland Medical Ltd

IXC

MANUFACTURERS' ADDRESSES AND TELEPHONE NUMBERS
(STOMA APPLIANCES)

3M Health Care Ltd, 3M House, Morley Street, Loughborough, Leics, LE11 1EP (01509 611611)

Abbott Laboratories Limited: see Hollister Ltd

Adams Healthcare, Lotherton Way, Garforth, Leeds LS25 2JY (0113 2320066)

AlphaMed Ltd, Bensham House, 340 Bensham Lane, Thornton Heath, Surrey CR7 7EQ (0181 6840470)

Anglo Venture 2000 Ltd, The Mill, Hatfield Health, Bishop's Stortford, Herts, CM22 7DL
    (01279 730733)

Astra Tech Ltd, Stroud Water Business Park, Brunel Way, Stonehouse, Gloucestershire GL10 3SW
    (01453 791763)

Bard Ltd, Forest House, Brighton Road, Crawley, West Sussex, RH11 9BP (01293 527888)

Body's Surgical Company: see Jade-Euro-Med Ltd

B. Braun Biotrol, Thorncliffe Park, Sheffield, S35 2PW (0114 225 9000)

Bullen & Smears Ltd: see C S Bullen Ltd

C S Bullen Ltd, 3-7 Moss Street, Liverpool, L6 1EY (0151 2076995/6/7/8)

Cambmac Instruments Ltd: see Dansac Ltd

Cambridge Selfcare Diagnostics Ltd, Palex Ostomy Division: see Salt & Son Ltd

J. Chawner Surgical Belts Ltd, Unit 1B Mayfields, Southcrest, Redditch, B98 7DU (01527 404353)

Clinimed Ltd, Cavell House, Knaves Beech Way, Loudwater, High Wycombe, Bucks, HP10 9QY
    (01628 850100)

Coloplast Ltd, Peterborough Business Park, Peterborough, PE2 6FX (01733 392000)

ConvaTec Ltd, Unit 20, First Avenue, Deeside Industrial Park, Deeside, Clwyd CH5 2NU (01244 586244)

Cover Care, 5 Ancaster Gardens, Wollaton Park, Nottingham, NG8 1FR (0115 928 7883)

Cuxson Gerrard & Company Ltd, 26 Fountain Lane, Oldbury, Warley, West Midlands, B69 3BB
    (0121 5447117)

Dansac Ltd, Victory House, Vision Park, Histon, Cambridge CB4 4ZR (01223 235100)

DePuy Healthcare: see Simpla Continence Care

Dow Corning Ltd, Kings Court, 185 Kings Road, Reading, Berkshire RG1 4EX (01734 596888)

Downs Surgical Ltd: see SIMS Portex Ltd

John Drew (London) Ltd, 433 Uxbridge Road, Ealing, London, W5 3NT (0208 9920381)

Ellis, Son & Paramore Ltd, Spring Street Works, Sheffield, S3 8PD (0114 2738921/221269)

Eschmann Bros and Walsh Ltd: see SIMS Portex Ltd

EuroCare: see Salts Healthcare

Hollister Ltd, Rectory Court, 42 Broad Street, Wokingham, Berkshire, RG40 1AB (0118 989 5000)
    (Retail Pharmacy Order Line 0800 521392)

MANUFACTURERS' ADDRESSES AND TELEPHONE NUMBERS
(STOMA APPLIANCES) - cont

Impharm Nationwide Ltd, PWS Building, Nelson Street, Bolton, BL3 2JW (01204 371155)

Jade-Euro-Med Ltd, Unit 14, East Hanningfield Industrial Estate, Old Church Road, East Hanningfield, Chelmsford, Essex CM3 8BG (01245 400413)

Leyland Medical Ltd: see Rüsch UK Ltd

Loxley Products: Unit 8, South Lincolnshire Enterprise Agency, Station Road East, Grantham, Lincolnshire, NG31 6HX (01476 560194)

Manfred Sauer UK: KG/D to KG/E, KG Business Centre, Kingsfield Way, Gladstone Industry, Dallington, Northampton, NN5 7QS (01604 588090)

Marlen USA products: distributed by Pelican Healthcare Ltd, Cardiff Business Park, Cardiff, CF4 5WF (02920 747000)

Medicina Ltd, Oak House, Lower Road, Cookham, Berkshire, SL6 9HJ (01628 533253)

Medlogic Global Ltd, Western Wood Way, Language Science Park, Plympton, Plymouth, Devon, PL7 5BG (01752 209955)

Nationwide Ostomy Supplies Ltd: see Impharm Nationwide Ltd

North West Ostomy Suppliers (Wholesale) Ltd: see Impharm Nationwide Ltd

Oakmed Ltd, 54 Adams Avenue, Northampton, NN1 4LJ (01604 239250)

Omex Medical Ltd, 25, Sea Lane, East Preston, Littlehampton, West Sussex, BN16 1NH (01903 783744)

Orthotic Services Ltd, Heartlands House, 19 Cato Street, The Heartlands, Birmingham, B7 4TS (0121 3596323)

S G & P Payne, Percy House, Brook Street, Hyde, Cheshire, SK14 2NS (0161 3678561)

J C Peacock & Son Ltd, Friar House, Clavering Place, Newcastle upon Tyne, NE1 3NR (0191 2329917)

Pelican Healthcare Ltd, Cardiff Business Park, Cardiff, CF4 5WF (02920 747787)

Respond Plus, 1 The Carlton Business Centre, Carlton, Nottingham, NG4 3AA (0115 940 3080)

Donald Rose Ltd: see Steeper (Orthopaedic) Ltd

Rüsch UK Ltd, PO Box 138, Turnpike Road, Cressex Industrial Estate, High Wycombe, Bucks, HP12 3NB (01494 532761)

E Sallis Ltd, Vernon Works, Waterford Street, Old Basford, Nottingham, NG6 0DH (0115 9787841/2)

Salts Healthcare, Saltair House, Lord Street, Nechells, Birmingham, B7 4DS (0121 3595123)

SASH, Woodhouse, Woodside Road, Hockley, Essex, SS5 4RU (01702 206502)

IXC

MANUFACTURERS' ADDRESSES AND TELEPHONE NUMBERS
(STOMA APPLIANCES) - cont

T J Shannon Ltd, 59 Bradford Street, Bolton, BL2 1HT (01204 521789)

A H Shaw and Partners Ltd, Manor Road, Ossett, West Yorkshire, WF5 0LF (01924 273474)

Simcare Ltd: See SIMS Portex Ltd

Simpla Continence Care: A division of SSL International Plc, Toft Hall, Knutsford, Cheshire, WA16 9PD
(0161 6543000)

SIMS Portex Ltd, Hythe, Kent CT21 6JL (01303 260551)

Squibb Surgicare Ltd: see ConvaTec Ltd

Steeper (Orthopaedic) Ltd: see Ward Surgical Appliance Company Ltd

Ward Surgical Appliance Company Ltd, 57A Brightwell Avenue, Westcliffe-on-Sea, Essex SSO 9EB
(01702 354064)

Warne-Franklin Medical Ltd: see Rüsch UK Ltd

Welland Medical Ltd Products: distributed by Clinimed Ltd, Cavell House, Knaves Beech Way, Loudwater, High
Wycombe, Bucks, HP10 9QY (01628 850100)

This Page Is Intentionally Blank

This Page Is Intentionally Blank

APPROVED LIST OF CHEMICAL REAGENTS

The only chemical reagents which may be supplied as part of the pharmaceutical services are those listed in Part IXR of the Tariff. The items within Part IXR which are not prescribable on FP10(CN) and FP10(PN) are annotated Ⓧ

The price listed in respect of a chemical reagent specified in the following list is the basic price on which payment will be calculated pursuant to Part II, Clause 6A for the dispensing of that chemical reagent.

The Notes to Part IX shall also apply to Part IXR when 'chemical reagent(s)' shall be substituted for 'appliance(s)'.

Chemical reagents are listed in the order; detection tablets, reagent solutions, compounds required for cholecystographic examination, detection strips (urine), and detection strips (blood).

1. DETECTION TABLETS

		Quantity	Basic Price P

1.1 Detection tablets for Glycosuria

		Quantity	Basic Price P
Copper Solution Reagent Tablet _(Clinitest)_		36	190
Copper Sulphate anhydrous	18.75mg		
Citric Acid anhydrous	300mg		
Sodium Hydroxide	250mg		
Sodium Carbonate anhydrous	62.5mg		
Excipient			

(Supplied with an instruction sheet, analysis record and colour chart)

1.2 Detection tablets for Ketonuria

		Quantity	Basic Price P
Nitroprusside Reagent Tablets _(Acetest)_		100	336
(Syn: Rothera's Tablets)			
Aminoacetic Acid anhydrous	9.0mg		
Sodium Nitroprusside	1.0mg		
Sodium Phosphate anhydrous	94.0mg		
Sodium Borate anhydrous	73.0mg		
Lactose	20.0mg		
Starch	2.5mg		
Magnesium Stearate	0.5mg		

(Supplied with an instruction sheet and colour chart)

2. REAGENT SOLUTIONS

2.1 Ⓧ	Gerhardt's Reagent (Ferric Chloride Solution, 10%)	25mL		7
2.2 Ⓧ	Ammonia Solution Strong BP	500mL		340

3. CHOLECYSTOGRAPHIC EXAMINATION ORAL COMPOUNDS

Compounds required for oral administration for the purpose of cholecystographic examination to be supplied in a container with instructions to patient.

3.1 Ⓧ	Sodium Iopodate Capsules, 500mg _(Biloptin)_	6		407

Chemical Reagent	Quantity	Basic Price P

4.   DETECTION STRIPS, URINE

4.1 Detection strips, urine for Glycosuria

4.1.1 *Clinistix*
Strip impregnated one end with:
glucose oxidase and a peroxidase, and o-tolidine
buffered
(Supplied with an instruction sheet, analysis record
and colour chart)

| | 50 | 298 |

4.1.2 *Diabur Test 5000*
Twin zone strip impregnated one
end with: glucose oxidase/peroxidase and
tetramethylbenzidine indicator
(Supplied with an instruction sheet, analysis record
and colour chart)

| | 50 | 246 |

4.1.3 *Diastix*
Strip impregnated one end with:
glucose oxidase and a peroxidase, and potassium
iodide, buffered
(Supplied with an instruction sheet, analysis record
and colour chart)

| | 50 | 253 |

4.1.4 *Medi-Test Glucose*
Strip impregnated one end with:
glucose oxidase and a peroxidase, and o-tolidine,
(Supplied with an instruction sheet, analysis record
and colour chart)

| | 50 | 210 |

4.2 Detection Strips, Urine for Ketonuria *(Acetonuria)*

4.2.1 *Ketostix*
Strip impregnated one end with:
sodium nitroprusside, glycine and phosphate
buffer
(Supplied with an instruction sheet and colour chart)

| | 50 | 268 |

4.2.2 *Ketur Test*
Strip impregnated one end with:
sodium nitroprusside, glycine and alkaline buffer
(Supplied with an instruction sheet and colour chart)

| | 50 | 236 |

4.3 Detection Strips, urine for Proteinuria

4.3.1 *Albustix*
Strip impregnated one end with:
tetrabromophenol blue, and citrate buffer
(Supplied with an instruction sheet and colour chart)

| | 50 | 369 |

4.3.2 *Medi-Test Protein 2*
Strip impregnated one end with :
tetrabromophenol blue, and citrate buffer
(Supplied with instruction sheet and colour chart)

| | 50 | 294 |

Chemical Reagent	Quantity	Basic Price P

5. DETECTION STRIPS, BLOOD FOR GLUCOSE

Notes on the use of **Blood Glucose Testing Strips (BGTS)** are given in the Appendix to Part IXR Page 391. Lancets are listed on pages 145-146. Meters for use with BGTS are not available on prescription Form FP10.

5.1 Colorimetric Strips - visually readable

5.1.1 *BM-Test 1-44*   50   1507

(previously called *BM-Test Glycemie 1-44*)

Strip with twin pads at one end impregnated with glucose oxidase and peroxidase with chromogens.

The lower test area (nearer the "handle") gives readings in the range 1.0-7.0 mmol/L light - mid blue; the higher test area range is 7.0-44.0 mmol/L buff - green - dark green.

(Supplied with an instruction sheet, analysis record and colour chart)

5.1.2 *Glucostix*   50   1507

A plastic strip with two pads at one end impregnated with glucose oxidase and peroxidase with chromogens.

The larger of the two test areas (the low range pad) changes colour from yellow through pale green to dark green to give readings in the range of 1.0 to 6.0 mmol/L. The smaller of the two test areas (the high range pad) changes from yellow through orange to red to give readings in the range 8 to 44 mmol/L.

(Supplied with instruction sheet, analysis record and colour chart).

IXR

Chemical Reagent	Quantity	Basic Price P

5.1.3 Hypoguard *Supreme*   50   1318

Strip with single pad at one end. Colour change
from White to Blue corresponding with the 10
block colour chart. Gives a reading in the range
2.2-27.8mmol/L, 40-500mg/dL
This strip can also be used with all Supreme
Blood Glucose Meters.

(Supplied with instruction sheet, analysis
record and colour chart)

5.1.4 *Medi-Test Glycaemie C*   50   1344

Strip with twin pads at one end impregnated with
glucose oxidase with chromogens.

The upper (yellow) area (nearer the "handle") changes
from green to dark bluish green to give readings in
the range 13.3-27.8 mmol/L; the lower (white) area
(away from the "handle") changes through
shades of light blue to blue for readings in the range
1.1-13.3 mmol/L.

(Supplied with an instruction sheet, colour chart and
analysis records).

5.1.5 Hypoguard *Supreme Spectrum*   50   999

Strip with a single pad at one end. Colour change
from White to Blue corresponding with the 10
block colour chart. Gives a reading in the range
2.2-27.8 mmol/L, 40-500mg/dL

(Supplied with instruction sheet, analysis record and
colour chart)

Chemical Reagent	Quantity	Basic Price P

5.2 Biosensor strips to be read only with the appropriate meter

These meters are not available on prescription)

Biosensor strips have a target area for the blood sample at one end, impregnated with glucose oxidase. The test strip is inserted into the meter and when the blood sample is applied to the target area a current is produced proportionate to the concentration of blood glucose in the sample.

NB: ExacTech, MediSense G2 and MediSense Optium strips are not interchangeable.

5.2.1 *ExacTech*	50	1420

Gives a reading in the range 2.2 - 25.0mmol/L

(Supplied with an instruction sheet, analysis record, and meter calibrator).

5.2.2 MediSense *G2*	50	1365

Gives a reading in the range 1.1-33.3mmol/L

(Supplied with an instruction sheet, analysis record, and meter calibrator)

5.2.3 MediSense *Optium*	50	1392

MediSense Optium Electrodes for Blood glucose testing with Medisense Optium Sensor. Measurement range is 1.1 - 33.3mmol/L

(Supplied with an instruction sheet, analysis record and meter calibrator)

5.2.4 *PocketScan*	50	1417

Biosensor test strip with a target area for the blood sample at one end. The test strip is inserted into the meter and when a small blood sample is applied to the target area it is then automatically drawn into the reaction cell impregnated with glucose oxidase. The system measures an electrical current generated from the reaction, which is proportional to the level of glucose in the sample. Measurement range is 1.1-33.3 mmol/L

(Supplied with an instructions sheet).

5.2.5 *GlucoMen Sensors*	50	1393

Gives a reading in the range 1.1-33.3mmol/L

(Supplied with an instruction data sheet)

Chemical Reagent	Quantity	Basic Price P

5.3 Biosensor disc to be read only with the appropriate meter.

Biosensor test sensor disc contains 10 individually
sealed test strips. Blood is drawn by capillary action
into a strip exposed from inside the meter. The
level of glucose is measured using a mediated
electrochemical technique based on the
glucose oxidose

5.3.1 *Glucometer Esprit* **test sensor discs**	5 discs of 10 strips each	1452

Gives a reading in the range 0.6-33.3mmol/L

(Supplied with instruction sheet and analysis record).

5.4 Colorimetric strips - to be read only with appropriate meter.

5.4.1 *BM-Accutest*	50	1431

Strip with a single pad at one end, impregnated
with glucose oxidase and chromogens. The yellow
test area gives readings in the range
1.1 - 33.3 mmol/L (yellow to dark green). The
strips cannot be visually read and the use of
an "Accutrend" blood glucose meter (see Note,
page 385) is essential.

(Supplied with an instruction sheet and
analysis record).

5.4.2 *One Touch*	50	1436

Strip with a small circular test area forming
a well over a single pad impregnated with glucose
oxidase, peroxidase and chromogens. The strip
gives readings in the range 0.0 -33.3 mmol/L
(cream to blue). The strips cannot be visually
read and the use of a "*One Touch*" blood glucose
meter (see Note page 385) is essential.

(Supplied with an instruction sheet and analysis
record).

Chemical Reagent	Quantity	Basic Price P

5.4.3 *Glucotide*   50   1433

Strip with a small circular test area forming a
well over a single pad impregnated with
hexokinase, diaphorase and a
tetrazolium indicator. The strip gives
readings in the range of 0.6 - 33.3 mmol/L
(yellow to brown). The strips cannot be
visually read and the use of the *Glucometer 4*
blood glucose meter (see Note page 385)
is essential.

(Supplied with an instruction sheet and analysis record)

†   **5.4.4** *Glucotrend*   50   1476

Strip with application zone consisting of detection
film, covered by a yellow protective mesh and
featuring a reservoir to collect excess blood.
Glucose is converted by glucose-dye-oxidoreductase,
and an indicator reaction produces the colour change.
The strip gives readings in the range 0.6-33.3mmol/l.
The use of a *Glucotrend* meter is essential.

(Supplied with an instruction sheet, colour chart and coding chip).

IXR

5.4.5 *Glucotrend Plus*   50   1476

Strip with application zone consisting of detection
Film, covered by a green protective mesh and
featuring a reservoir to collect excessive blood.
Glucose is converted by glucose-dye-oxidoreductase,
and an indicator reaction produces the colour change.
The strip gives readings in the range 0.6-33.3mmol/l.
The use of a Glucotrend meter is essential.

(Supplied with an instruction sheet, colour chart and coding chip)

†   to be deleted 1 January 2001

This Page Is Intentionally Blank

APPENDIX
Notes on Blood Glucose Testing

1. Blood glucose testing strips (BGTS) are primarily intended for insulin-dependent diabetics who will normally have received consultant advice on their condition. One pack (50 strips) would normally be sufficient for two months. All strips should be kept in their original container and should not be cut or slit. Because of the differences in colour change in colorimetric types, strips are not interchangeable. **Due regard should be given to the manufacturer's instructions, and the recommendation on storage and period of use after first opening.**

2. General Practitioners should be aware that defects in colour vision may occur in diabetes and certain colorimetric BGT strips should not be prescribed for such patients for visual use. (See outline of colour changes described in entries on pages 385-389).

3. Misleading results, which could be hazardous if acted upon, might arise if users are inadequately trained. (Hazard Notice HN(87)(13)). It is therefore essential that patients should receive appropriate training before attempting to use BGTS for monitoring their blood glucose. The training may be given by suitably qualified health-care professionals. It should be noted that there are variations in technique between different makes. Some technical factors are given in paragraph 4 below.

4. Reagent strips are subject to the following limitations:

Fluoride Specimen:	The strips are not to be used with blood specimens preserved with
fluoride.	
Serum and Plasma:	The strips are not designed for use with serum or plasma.
Haematocrit:	Extremes in haematocrit levels can affect test results.

   Due regard should be given to the manufacturer's product specifications.

5. **Disposal of Lancets.** Patients should be reminded of the need to exercise caution when disposing of used lancets. These should be placed in a tin or other strong container before disposal. (The needle clipping device listed on page 146 is not generally suitable for use with lancets).

   As with single-use syringes, the arrangements outlined above are not suitable for patients where there is a risk of infection being transmitted. General Practitioners are similarly advised that blood lancets should only be prescribed for patients who are carriers of infectious diseases where suitable arrangements have been made for the disposal of the used articles as contaminated waste. Medical Officers for environmental health can advise on these arrangements.

This Page Is Intentionally Blank

1. DOMICILIARY OXYGEN

1.1 Oxygen should be prescribed for patients in the home only after careful evaluation and never on a placebo basis. Oxygen may be supplied in cylinders or where the quantity required justifies it, from a concentrator but in general the appropriate method of supply will depend on the type of therapy, intermittent or long term, to be prescribed.

2. INTERMITTENT THERAPY

2.1 The majority of patients will have oxygen prescribed for intermittent use in a variety of respiratory conditions. This type of therapy is used in patients with hypoxaemia of short duration, for example, asthma, when the condition is likely to recur over months or years. It may be prescribed for patients with advanced irreversible respiratory disorders to increase mobility and capacity for exercise and ease discomfort, for example in chronic obstructive bronchitis, emphysema, widespread fibrosis and primary or thromboemolic pulmonary hypertension. Such patients will usually be supplied with oxygen in cylinders (see also paragraph 18.1).

2.2 **Arrangements for the prescription and supply of cylinder oxygen to those patients who require intermittent therapy are set out at paragraph 3.** GPs are asked to co-operate in an effort to make this part of the oxygen service more cost effective. If more than one or two are regularly required for a particular period, prescribing in multiples of 3 cylinders would produce savings by reducing the number of journeys. It is accepted that it will not always be possible to prescribe in this way, for example, because of the infrequency of use of oxygen or because of storage problems at the patient's home.

3. OXYGEN CYLINDER SERVICE

3.1 Health Authority lists of pharmacy contractors who provide domiciliary oxygen therapy services include only those pharmacy contractors who are authorised to hold a number of light-weight single unit oxygen sets (approved sets are listed on page 395) and stands, and:

3.1.1 regularly stock oxygen equipment, as specified in the Drug Tariff, and oxygen gas on the premises;

3.1.2 are prepared, when it would not be reasonable to expect that the patient's representative could safely do so or when he is unable to do so, to deliver the oxygen set and cylinders to the patient's home, to collect empty cylinders when they are being replaced, and to collect the set and cylinders when informed that treatment has been discontinued; and

3.1.3 are prepared to erect and explain the operation of the oxygen set and cylinders at the patient's home, particularly when a patient is having oxygen therapy for the first time.

3.2 At any time a pharmacy contractor willing to provide this service may apply to the Health Authority for inclusion in the list.

3.3 A copy of the Health Authority list of oxygen contractors, with details of the services being provided, is supplied to every pharmacy contractor and doctor in the area. A copy of the list for an adjacent area will be sent on application.

3.4 If a prescription for an oxygen set or cylinders is presented to a pharmacy contractor whose name is not included in the list, he should provide the patient or his representative with the name, address and telephone number of at least two pharmacy contractors who provide oxygen therapy services at the time the need arises, and who are nearest to the patient's home.

3.5   Except where, in emergency, a set has been loaned by a distant pharmacy contractor, oxygen gas shall be supplied to a patient only by the pharmacy contractor who has loaned the set. When, exceptionally, cylinder replacements are provided by a pharmacy contractor other than the one who supplied the set, he should, at the time when cylinders are supplied, satisfy himself that the patient continues to operate the equipment satisfactorily.

3.6   Delivery and collection of sets and/or cylinders is to be undertaken by the patient's representative where he is willing, providing the pharmacy contractor can fully satisfy himself that the representative is able to transport a set and/or a cylinder, carry it and secure it in position in the house, and fit the mask after the instructions provided in the set have been explained to him. In other circumstances delivery, erection and collection of sets and/or cylinders and the explanation of the operation of oxygen equipment at the patient's home, particularly at the commencement of treatment, is to be undertaken by the pharmacy contractor.

3.7   The recovery of empty cylinders from patients, and their prompt return to the supplier for refilling, is essential if adequate supplies of oxygen for the use of patients are to be maintained.

4.   **OXYGEN EQUIPMENT WHICH MAY BE ORDERED**

4.1   The sets of equipment which may be provided by the pharmacy contractor are listed on page 395 (see also Specification 01A and 01B, page 399).

4.2   The oxygen masks which may be ordered are listed on page 396 (See also illustrations, page 397). The type of treatment they provide is indicated in paragraph 6.

4.3   One constant performance mask (either the Intersurgical 010 Mask, 28% or the Ventimask Mk IV, 28%) is supplied as part of the set, but is packaged separately on account of bulk (see list of approved masks, page 396 and figures 1 and 2 page 397). When a constant performance mask is supplied to a patient, the recommended flow rate is 2 litres per minute (the Medium setting on the control head) (see page 399, and diagrams on pages 400-403).

4.4   Where the prescriber considers that a mask different to that provided in the standard set is required for treatment, he must state which mask is to be supplied.

4.5   Every mask is supplied for the use of one patient only. All masks, therefore, are "disposable" but each is sufficiently robust to withstand usage even over a long period of treatment.

4.6   Oxygen should only be ordered in 1360 litre cylinders. When 3400 litre cylinders are prescribed, the pharmacy contractor will supply the gas in 1360 litre cylinders.

4.7   A cylinder stand may be ordered. If one is not ordered and the pharmacy contractor considers that the cylinder cannot be effectively secured to avoid the risk of accident to patient or set, a cylinder stand should be supplied on loan.

5.   **PROCEDURE TO BE FOLLOWED IN LOANING EQUIPMENT, CONFIRMING CONTINUED USE AND TERMINATION OF THE HEALTH AUTHORITY'S LIABILITY**

5.1   The pharmacy contractor shall on making the loan include a note with the set saying that "This Set is the property of the Pharmacy Contractor to whom it must be returned in good condition by the patient".

5.2   The pharmacy contractor shall endorse the prescription form with:

5.2.1   Name of set supplied;

5.2.2   Date of commencement of loan;

5.2.3   Size and number of cylinders supplied. When 3400 litre cylinders are ordered the gas is to be supplied in 1360 litre cylinders.

5.3   The pharmacy contractor shall make a monthly return to the Health Authority showing:

   5.3.1   Date of loan set;

   5.3.2   Date for return of set (when applicable) or date of notice by Health Authority (see iii below); or

   5.3.3   Confirmation that the set is still on loan (when applicable).

5.4   Where the return shows that the set has been on loan at least three months and has not been returned to the pharmacy contractor, the Health Authority shall ascertain from the doctor whether the equipment is still required; subsequent enquiries shall be made at intervals not exceeding three months during the first year of the loan.

   5.4.1   Where the Health Authority are satisfied, after making enquiries, that the equipment is no longer required by the patient, or where between enquiries the doctor informs the Authority to that effect, the Authority shall notify the contractor to arrange recovery.

5.5   Where the patient fails to return the equipment the onus of collecting it rests on the pharmacy contractor.

   Note: different local Health Authority arrangements may apply.

6.   **OXYGEN EQUIPMENT WHICH THE PHARMACY CONTRACTOR MAY SUPPLY ON LOAN TO THE PATIENT**

6.1   OXYGEN SETS

   The following sets* (See Specification 01A and 01B, page 399 and diagrams, pages 400-403) are approved for use within the Domiciliary Oxygen Therapy Service, and any one may be loaned against an order for a set:

		Price (excluding carriage)
6.1.1	Specification 01A	
	BOC Domiflow Set (888830)	8648p
	Oxylitre Set (M 210)	7660p
	Oxylitre Set (M 410)	7660p
	Puritan Bennett Set (778435)	8000p
	Sabre Medical Oxydom Set	7990p
	Therapy Equipment Dialreg Set (5120)	6300p
6.1.2	Specification 01B	
	Air Apparatus and Valve Set (D24)	8091p

   A constant performance mask (see paragraph 6.2.1, below and figures 1 and 2, page 397) shall be supplied by the manufacturer with each set.

   When supplying an oxygen set meeting Specification 01B with a constant performance mask, the pharmacy contractor should ensure that the flow selector is at the Medium setting, ie 2 litres per minute (see diagram on page 401).

   On no account should pharmacy contractor attempt to modify any oxygen set to produce a higher flow rate than that for which it has been designed. To do so could create a hazardous situation for the patient.

   * Spare O-rings may be supplied by the manufacturer with the set, but these should be removed by the pharmacy contractor before the set is supplied to the patient.

6.2 OXYGEN MASKS

The following masks are approved for use within the Domiciliary Oxygen Therapy Service:

6.2.1 Constant Performance Masks

These masks provide a nearly constant concentration of 28% oxygen in air over a wide range of oxygen supply, and irrespective of breathing pattern. The most economic oxygen flow rate is 2 litres per minute (the Medium setting on the control head).

Intersurgical 010 Mask 28% (figure 1, page 397) +
The mask comprises a soft moulded plastic facepiece, an adjustable elastic headstrap and a metal nose clip to ensure a close fit across the nose. A lightweight white venturi diluter fitted to the front of the mask ensures a near constant oxygen concentration. This can be rotated to suit varying positions of the connecting tube.

    Weight (less supply tube)   44 grams
    Supplied by Intersurgical Ltd

Ventimask Mk IV 28% (figure 2, page 397) +
The mask consists of a one piece transparent flexible moulded facepiece, incorporating a lightweight rigid clear plastic venturi device that ensures near constant concentration.

It is fitted with an adjustable elastic head-band, and has soft metal reinforcing strip to ensure a good fit over the bridge of the nose.

    Weight (less supply tube)   66 grams
    Supplied by Flexicare Medical Ltd

6.2.2 Variable Performance Masks

A flow rate of 2 litres per minute is recommended for these masks, no claim being made for the resulting oxygen concentration. They provide a variable concentration of oxygen in air. The concentration varies with the rate of flow of oxygen supplied and the breathing pattern of the patient.

Intersurgical 005 Mask (figure 3, page 397)

This mask comprises a soft moulded plastic facepiece, adjustable elastic headstrap and a metal nose clip to ensure a close fit across the nose. A swivel connector on the front of the mask, to which the oxygen tube is connected, can be rotated to suit varying position of the connecting tube.

    Weight (less supply tube)   40 grams
    Supplied by Intersurgical Ltd.

Venticaire Mask (figure 4, page 397)

This mask comprises a soft moulded clear plastic facepiece, with either an adjustable elastic headstrap, or ear loops. A swivel connector is provided on the front of the mask, this rotates to suit varying positions of the oxygen supply tube (not included).

    Weight   39 grams
    Supplied by Flexicare Medical Ltd

+   Either of these masks may be supplied with the standard set

7   ILLUSTRATIONS OF APPROVED OXYGEN MASKS
(See list on page 396)

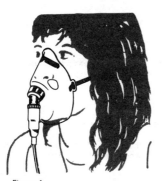

Figure 1
Inter-Surgical 010 Mask

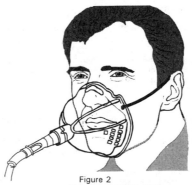

Figure 2
Ventimask Mk1V, 28%

X

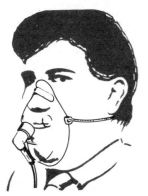

Figure 3
Inter-Surgical 005 Mask

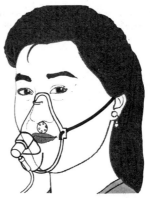

Figure 4
Venticaire Mask

8.   BASIC PRICE OF APPROVED OXYGEN EQUIPMENT

Note: Arrangements for the provision and payment of the domiciliary oxygen service are now made on a local basis.

8.1   **Basic Price for the supply of a mask,** when prescribed after the initial order on a separate prescription form (see list of approved masks, page 396 and illustrations, page 397).

Intersurgical 010 Mask, 28%	figure 1	97p
Ventimask Mk IV, 28%	figure 2	136p
Intersurgical 005 Mask	figure 3	78p
Venticaire Mask	figure 4	65p

8.2   **Basic Price for;**

Oxygen BP, cylinder	1360 litres	719p
Oxygen BP, composite cylinder with integral headset to specification 02	1360 litres	719p

Contractors are reminded of the importance of ensuring that as few empty cylinders as possible remain in circulation. They should be exchanged promptly and withdrawn (full or empty) together with other equipment should the service cease.

9.   METHOD OF CLAIMING COMPENSATION FOR FINANCIAL LOSS IN RESPECT OF OXYGEN EQUIPMENT

Where the pharmacy contractor suffers financial loss as a result of the act or default of a person causing the loss of, or damage to, oxygen equipment loaned, the pharmacy contractor should inform the Health Authority of such financial loss.

Reimbursement of the loss will depend on local Health Authority arrangements.

Necessary out-of-pocket expenses incidentally involved in the repair of or replacement of the equipment, such as postage or carriage should also be met.

In this paragraph, the expression "person" means the person supplied, the patient concerned, members of his household, or the authorities of an institution to which the equipment is delivered, as the case may be.

10. **ADDITIONAL SPECIFICATIONS**

10.1 SPECIFICATION 01A (Lightweight (Single Unit) Oxygen Set)
The set comprises:
10.1.1 The Control Head, which shall include the following features:

10.1.1.1 A valve which reduces the gas cylinder pressure from 13650 kPa. to a pressure of 70 to 415 kPa.;
10.1.1.2 A miniature contents (pressure) gauge, calibrated with 1/4, 1/2 and FULL markings;
10.1.1.3 A cap, consisting of a two flow selector, which can be turned from the ratchet position marked OFF to ratchet positions marked MED and HIGH, these being designed to correspond to flow rates of 2 litres and 4 litres respectively per minute;
10.1.1.4 An outlet, being the male portion of a bayonet type connection;
10.1.1.5 A standard bull-nose cylinder adaptor designed for finger tightening, and preferably incorporating an O-ring washer;
10.1.1.6 A safety device, such as a sintered filter, to prevent the spontaneous combustion of particulate material in the control head, or in the neck of the cylinder.

10.1.2 Connection Tubing: 150cm (approximately) plastic tubing, 5mm bore, 8mm externally (Ref. Portex 800/012/300) with at one end a bayonet fitting to the control head.

10.1.3 A Key Spanner of 100mm to 150mm length, for opening the oxygen cylinder valve.

10.1.4 One disposable plastic mask (figure 1 or figure 2 on page 397); in a closed plastic bag.

Note: The set parts 1 to 3 are packed in a strong box, with full operating instructions in the lid. The mask, being partly rigid, is packed separately and supplied with the boxed parts.

Note: Spare O-rings may be supplied by the manufacturer with the set, but these should be removed by the contractor before the set is supplied to the patient.

10.2 SPECIFICATION 01B (Lightweight (Single Unit) Oxygen Set)

The set will comply with all the requirements of Specification 01A, with the exception of clause 1c, where the following clause will apply:

"A ratchet selection device to enable the gas flow to be set at predetermined positions to give flow rates of 2 litres and 4 litres per minute respectively. The positions will be clearly indicated and labelled 2L (MED) and 4L (HIGH); and a control knob which permits the flow of gas to be turned on and off. It will be suitably labelled to indicate the ON and OFF positions and the direction of the rotation to turn ON..."

10.3 SPECIFICATION 02 (Oxygen BP, Composite Cylinder with Integral Headset)

10.3.1 The integral valve (pillar valve/pressure regulator/flow controller), shall comply with BS EN 738 part 3: 1997
With the following additions:
10.3.1.1 miniature contents (pressure) gauge with at least 1/4, 1/2 and Full markings
10.3.1.2 the flow control valve shall consist of either:
a flow selector, which can be turned from the ratchet position marked OFF to rachet positions
marked 2L(MED) and 4L(HIGH), these being designed to correspond to flow rates of 2 and 4
litres per minute respectively.
or
shall contain a control knob which permits the flow of gas to be turned on and off. It will be suitably labelled to indicate the ON and OFF positions and the direction of the rotation to turn ON.
A rachet selection device to enable the gas flow to give gas flow rates of 2 and 4 litres per minute.
The positions will be clearly indicated and labelled 2L(MED) and 4L(HIGH);
10.3.1.3 an outlet, being the male portion of a bayonet type connection;

10.3.2 All devices should be CE marked under the European Medical Device Directive

SPECIFICATION 01 - cont

Lightweight (Single Unit) Set 01A

NB: Actual Shape of Control Head varies with make

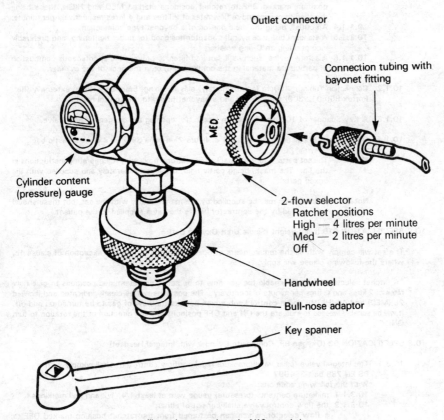

Illustration approximately 4/10 actual size

The Set is packed in a strong box

A Constant performance mask is packed separately with the boxed parts

SPECIFICATION 01 - cont

Light Weight (Single Unit) Set 01B

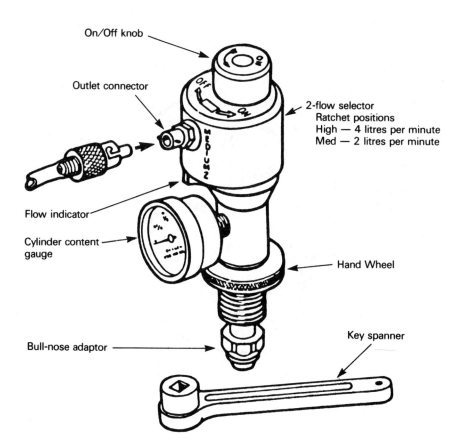

Illustration approximately 4/10 size

The Set is packed in a strong box

A Constant performance mask is packed separately and supplied with boxed parts

SPECIFICATION 02

Oxygen BP, Composite Cylinder with Integral Headset

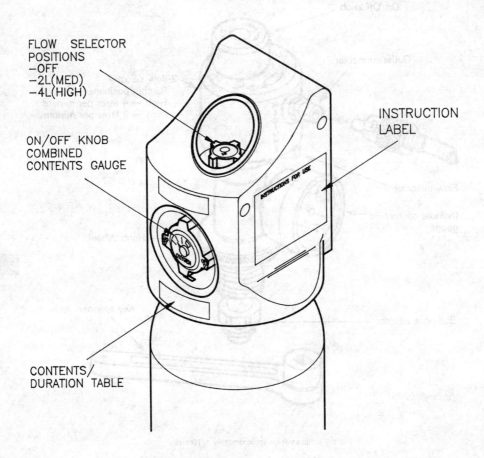

FLOW   SELECTOR
POSITIONS
–OFF
–2L(MED)
–4L(HIGH)

INSTRUCTION
LABEL

ON/OFF KNOB
COMBINED
CONTENTS GAUGE

CONTENTS/
DURATION TABLE

VIEW FROM FRONT OF CYLINDER

APPROX. SCALE 1/3 FULL SIZE

SPECIFICATION 02 - cont

Oxygen BP, Composite Cylinder with Integral Headset

CONNECTION TUBE

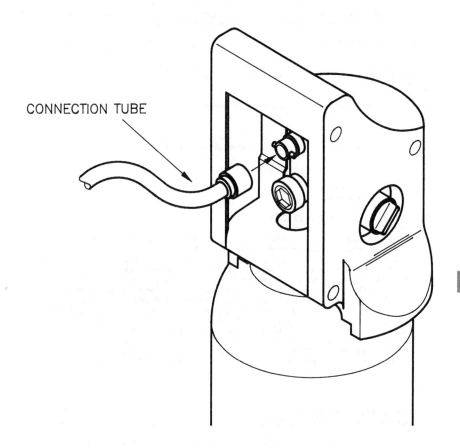

VIEW FROM REAR OF CYLINDER

APPROX. SCALE 1/3 FULL SIZE

11. LONG TERM OXYGEN THERAPY (LTOT)

11.1 Long term oxygen therapy is the provision of oxygen for 15 hours or more a day for a prolonged period and is of benefit to many patients with chronic hypoxaemia. For these patients oxygen should, where possible, be provided by a concentrator.

11.2 Since it is important to recognise that long term oxygen therapy is of benefit to a limited number of patients and that the needs of the majority of patients will continue to be met by intermittent therapy from cylinders, clinical guidelines for prescribing long term therapy have been drawn up for the benefit of general practitioners. These guidelines are set out in full below.

12. GUIDELINES FOR PRESCRIBING LONG TERM OXYGEN THERAPY (LTOT)

12.1 On present information, patients who are likely to benefit from long-term oxygen therapy will by definition have chronic hypoxaemia, but may for the purposes of these guidelines be divided into three groups:-

12.1.1 Those for whom there is an absolute indication, for which there is scientific evidence of the value of long-term oxygen therapy.

12.1.2 Those in whom there are good grounds for assuming the value of oxygen therapy, but for which there is no firm scientific evidence at present.

12.1.3 Patients in whom oxygen would have a useful palliative effect.

12.2 GPs who identify patients who might belong to any of these groups will wish to have consultant advice on the need for LTOT.

13. INDICATIONS FOR THE USE OF LTOT

13.1 Absolute indication. Patients for whom there is clear evidence of the value of LTOT will be those with chronic obstructive airways disease, hypoxaemia and oedema. Such patients will have ankle oedema or a history of an acute exacerbation when ankle oedema was observed. It will be necessary for such patients to be seen and assessed by a respiratory physician with access to respiratory function services. Suitable patients would have a forced expiratory volume (FEV_1) of less than 1.5L, a forced vital capacity (FVC) of less than 2L, an arterial oxygen tension less than 7.3kPa (55mm/mercury) and some elevation of arterial carbon dioxide tension ($PaCO_2$) greater than 6.0 kPa or 45mm/mercury. These tests are the minimum requirement and they should be made in a stable phase of the condition when all reversible factors have been adequately treated eg infection, reversible airways disease, cardiac disease etc. In order to establish stability, the spirometric measurements and the arterial blood gases should be repeated at an interval of not less than three weeks. There should be variation of no more than ± 5mm/mercury or 0.6 kPa in the arterial oxygen tension. If such variations are exceeded then a further three week interval should elapse before the tests are repeated again.

13.2 Other patients with chronic obstructive airways disease.

The second group will include all patients with chronic obstructive airways disease having the same spirometric characteristics and the same levels of arterial oxygen tension as those described in 13.1, but in whom hypercapnia is not present and oedema has not been witnessed. Many such patients were studied in American trials of long-term domiciliary oxygen therapy and benefit was clearly shown but such patients were excluded from the British studies. However, many of these patients, including refractory asthmatics and sufferers from cystic fibrosis could be expected to benefit from long-term oxygen therapy. On present evidence long-term domiciliary oxygen therapy should not be denied but the same criteria of stability should be applied to ensure that they are established cases of chronic hypoxaemia. We hope that further studies on this group of patients can be urgently carried out.

13.3 Palliative use of oxygen

This group should include patients with other respiratory conditions associated with severe arterial hypoxaemia, but without hypercapnia, for which oxygen therapy may have a useful palliative effect, without necessarily affecting survival. Examples would be severe hypoxaemia associated with the terminal stages of fibrosing alveolitis, industrial lung fibrosis, terminal stages of emphysema, and lung infiltrations such as sarcoidosis, lymphangitis carcinomatosa and certain collagen disorders.

13.4 Other conditions

There are other conditions in which palliation of chronic respiratory failure might be considered, for example in severe kyphoscoliosis, gross obesity and the end stages of irreversible peripheral neuropathies and muscle disorders. However, these conditions are associated with such serious disturbances of ventilatory drive that the abolition of hypoxaemia by providing additional inspired oxygen may be dangerous. There is also preliminary evidence that long-term oxygen therapy may help some children with pulmonary hypertension. For all these patients the initial assessment would have to be even more detailed than that already described for patients with chronic obstructive airways disease.

14. POST ASSESSMENT

14.1 If LTOT is to be prescribed and used effectively, it must be remembered that the treatment involves a minimum of 15 hours oxygen per day and whenever possible this should be provided by means of a concentrator. The patient must be fully acquainted with the installation, the working of the concentrator and the need to keep to the arduous therapeutic regimen. The initial flow rate of oxygen through standard nasal prongs will be 2L/min, but may need to be modified between 1.5 and 2.5 litres per minute when the arterial blood gases have been checked with the patient breathing oxygen. The aim is to elevate PAO_2, to 60 mmHg (8kPa) or more without excessive hypercapnia.

14.2 Full co-operation by the patient is essential and expert support will be necessary to enable the 15 hours daily treatment period to be achieved. Regular monitoring in the home by appropriately trained nurses or lung function technicians and follow-up in respiratory out-patients by theracic physicians will be necessary to ensure that the treatment is achieving optimum results.

15. PATIENTS FOR WHOM LONG TERM OXYGEN THERAPY IS NOT USEFUL

15.1 It is important to stress the circumstances under which LTOT is not indicated. Patients with respiratory conditions that merely produce breathlessness without hypoxaemia should not be treated. Long term therapy is not intended for acute conditions such as lobar pneumonia and other chest infections. Patients with lesser degrees of chronic obstructive airways disease (ie not conforming to the criteria in 13.1) or reversible obstructive airways disease including those having acute exacerbations are not candidates for this form of oxygen delivery since their hypoxaemia is likely to be only of short duration.

16. **SMOKING AND LONG TERM THERAPY**

16.1 Patients who continue to smoke are unlikely to gain much benefit from LTOT and every effort must be made to persuade them to discontinue smoking. There is also the additional hazard of fire.

17. **OXYGEN CONCENTRATOR SERVICE**

17.1 An oxygen concentrator is an electrically powered machine which separates a high proportion of nitrogen and some other components from ambient air and thus delivers oxygen enriched gases to patients. For the purposes of the concentrator service, England and Wales have been divided into 9 regional groups of Health Authorities and after a competitive tender exercise one supplier has been selected to provide the service in each group. The regional groups and the selected supplier for each one are set out in page 409. Each Health Authority will appoint an 'Authorised Officer' to whom all queries relative to the concentrator service should be addressed.

17.2 Oxygen concentrator services comprise the supply, installation with full instructions to the patient, maintenance and removal when no longer required of a concentrator and associated equipment in a patient's home on the prescription of a general practitioner. Concentrators are generally reliable and the risk of breakdown is low but in the event of a breakdown suppliers will be responsible for responding to an emergency call-out within 10 hours. However, where a doctor considers a patient to be at risk in the event of a concentrator failure, he may prescribe an emergency back-up supply of cylinder oxygen BP which the patient could use until the concentrator is repaired. Such back-up equipment should normally be prescribed along with the concentrator but the GP should review the need for back-up oxygen regularly and the supply should be withdrawn if no longer required. The emergency back-up supply will form part of the services to be provided by the concentrator supplier. The supplier will also be responsible for the payment of patients' electricity costs associated with concentrator usage.

It is anticipated that the provision of oxygen concentrators for such patients described above who have proven chronic hypoxaemia will be an additional service. It is not intended that oxygen concentrator installations will compete with intermittent oxygen therapy at present provided for patients by cylinder supplies. Patients who would benefit from LTOT from concentrators will need to be carefully selected and carefully monitored and will be relatively few in number compared with those having intermittent short burst therapy.

18. PRESCRIBING ARRANGEMENTS FOR OXYGEN CONCENTRATORS

18.1 Concentrators will normally be prescribed when a patient requires long term oxygen therapy (ie 15 hours or more a day over a prolonged period). However, it will still be cost effective to prescribe a concentrator for patients who require or are using the equivalent of 21 cylinders or more per month (ie 8 hours per day). When a general practitioner decides that a patient should receive long term oxygen therapy he should take the following action to obtain a concentrator for his patient.

18.2 Using form FP10, prescribe a concentrator and any other related equipment (eg humidifier) specifying on the form the amount of oxygen required (ie hours per day) and the flow rate. If a back-up oxygen set and cylinder are required (see paragraph 18.8 below) these should be ordered at the same time.

18.3 The GP should give the prescription form to the patient along with an explanation of what a concentrator is and advise the patient that the supplier will be in touch shortly to arrange installation. The patient should also be instructed to give the prescription form to the supplier when he visits the patient's home. If the patient moves residence a new prescription form should be issued in order that another installation can be arranged.

18.4 The GP should then advise the concentrator supplier by telephone that he has prescribed a concentrator for the patient and ask the supplier to arrange for its installation. The supplier will acknowledge receipt of the order by sending written confirmation to the GP, the patient and the Health Authority (Details of the supplier for each region, including address and telephone number are set out in the Drug Tariff (page 409). There is a Freephone arrangement).

18.5 If at any time during the patient's treatment the GP wishes to order additional equipment eg emergency back-up set and cylinder if not previously ordered, he should follow the procedure at paragraphs 18.2-18.4 above.

18.6 If for any reason the GP wishes to alter the regime he should inform the patient, complete the card which has been given to the patient by the concentrator supplier (entering the date, recommended flow rate, hours of use and his initials) and tell the patient to show it to the supplier when he next visits his home to service the machine.

18.7 It is essential that the GP notifies the Health Authority's Authorised Officer by telephone immediately the concentrator and/or emergency supply is no longer required by a particular patient.

18.8 Patients who are suitable for long term oxygen therapy are generally not clinically at risk if their oxygen supply is interrupted for a few hours but for those patients considered to be at risk, GPs may wish to prescribe emergency back-up cylinder oxygen in case of such a breakdown. (See paragraph 17.2 above).

19. UNDER-USE OF A CONCENTRATOR

19.1 Once a patient has had a concentrator installed in his home, it will be important to monitor the volume of oxygen consumption. If the patient's oxygen consumption falls below the level prescribed it may not be cost-effective for him to continue to have a concentrator. Under the terms of their contract, suppliers are required to submit to Health Authorities a statement accompanying claims for reimbursement of patients' electricity costs, setting out in respect of each patient a comparison between the patient's average daily usage of the concentrator over a period of the claim and the daily usage as prescribed by the general practitioner. In those cases where it appears that there may have been a significant under-use of the concentrator the Health Authority should bring the matter to the attention of the prescriber so that he may re-consider the prescribed regime.

19.2 In those cases where the average daily usage has fallen below the specified level at which a concentrator should be prescribed (See para 18.1) prescribers should be asked specifically to confirm that the patient has been counselled and that usage of the concentrator will increase. Where no such confirmation is obtained the Health Authority should arrange for the concentrator to be withdrawn and for the doctor to prescribe cylinder oxygen for the patient. Similar action should be taken if, after receiving a prescriber's confirmation of a continuing need for a concentrator at the first enquiry, a further statement from the supplier indicates that usage is still below the specified level. Health Authorities should discuss these arrangements with their Local Medical Committees in order to ensure that prescribers are absolutely clear about the interpretation.

20. TRANSFER OF EXISTING PATIENTS FROM CYLINDERS TO CONCENTRATORS

20.1 Some patients who have had cylinder oxygen prescribed for their treatment may reach a point where their oxygen requirements are such that supply would be more economical by concentrator. The Pricing Authority will identify such patients using the specified level at paragraph 18.1 and advise the Authority. The Health Authority will then write to each patient's general practitioner to consider whether the prescription of a concentrator would be a more appropriate form of providing oxygen therapy. If so the GP should follow the procedure at paragraph 18. In such cases a close liaison between the doctor, the concentrator supplier and the patient's existing cylinder supplier will be necessary to ensure that the patient receives sufficient cylinder oxygen to meet his needs until but only until the concentrator is installed.

20.2 Health Authorities should ensure the oxygen cylinder contractors are aware of concentrator installations and that they withdraw their equipment and any cylinders (empty or full) from the patient's home as soon as possible after the concentrator has been installed.

21. WITHDRAWAL OF A CONCENTRATOR AND/OR ASSOCIATED EQUIPMENT

21.1 Where a GP advises the Health Authority that a concentrator and/or emergency supply of cylinder oxygen is no longer required for a particular patient the Health Authority should immediately request the supplier to arrange for removal of the equipment from the patient's home. At the same time the Health Authority should inform the Pricing Authority of the details and date of removal notification.

22. SUPPLY OF EMERGENCY SUPPLY THROUGH OXYGEN CYLINDER CONTRACTORS

22.1 When emergency back-up oxygen is prescribed it will normally be supplied by the concentrator supplier. However, where exceptionally supply is made through a cylinder contractor it is important that the Health Authority identifies the patient and notifies the Pricing Authority so that the patient's records can be co-ordinated - Health Authorities should make alternative arrangements for supply to be made through the concentrator supplier as soon as possible.

23. EQUIPMENT WHICH MAY BE PRESCRIBED

Oxygen concentrator -
Accessories - face mask, nasal cannula, humidifier
Emergency back-up supply (comprising regulator, tubing, administration mask and cylinder of oxygen BP).

24. CLAIMS FOR PAYMENT

Contractors shall despatch prescription forms together with the appropriate claim forms to the Pricing Authority not later than the fifth day of the month following that in which the supply was made.

25. CONCENTRATOR SUPPLIERS

Oxygen concentrators together with face mask, nasal cannulae and humidifiers are included in the approved list of appliances and can be obtained in the area of the Health Authorities listed in column 1 in the table below from the suppliers listed in column 2 of that table opposite those Authorities.

Regional Groups of HAs   **Concentrator Supplier**

South Western

Avon	BOC Gases
Berkshire	
Buckinghamshire	Telephone
Cornwall & Isles of Scilly	Dial 0800 111333
Devon (S & W)	(Free of Charge)
Dorset	
Exeter & N Devon	
Gloucestershire	
Hampshire (N & Mid)	
IOW	
Oxfordshire	
Portsmouth & SE Hampshire	
Somerset	
Southampton & SW Hampshire	
Wiltshire	

West Midlands

Birmingham	De Vilbiss Medequip Ltd
Coventry	High Street
Derbyshire (N & Southern)	Wollaston
Dudley	DY8 4PS
Herefordshire	
Leicestershire	Telephone
Northamptonshire	Dial 0800 020202
Nottinghamshire (& N Notts)	(Free of Charge)
Sandwell	
Shropshire	
Solihull	
Staffordshire (N & S)	
Walsall	
Warwickshire	
Wolverhampton	
Worcestershire	

X

25 CONCENTRATOR SUPPLIERS - cont

Regional Groups of HAs	Concentrator Supplier

Central and South Wales

Bro Taf
Dyfed Powys
Gwent
Iechyd Morgannwg

The Oxygen Therapy Company Limited
Ocean Way
Ocean Park
Cardiff
CF1 5HF

Telephone
Dial 0800 373580
(Free of Charge)

North Western and North Wales

Bury & Rochdale
Cheshire (N & S)
Lancashire (E, NW & S)
Liverpool (St Helens & Knowsley, Sefton & Wirral)
Manchester
Morecambe Bay
North Wales
Salford & Trafford
Stockport
West Pennine
Wigan & Bolton

De Vilbiss Medequip Ltd
High Street
Wollaston
DY8 4PS
Telephone
Dial 0800 020202
(Free of Charge)

London North

Barking, Havering
Barnet
Brent & Harrow
Camden and Islington
City and E London
Enfield & Haringey
Hertfordshire (E & N and W)
Redbridge & Waltham Forest

De Vilbiss Medequip Ltd
High Street
Wollaston
DY8 4PS

Telephone
Dial 0800 020202
(Free of Charge)

Eastern

Anglia (NW)
Bedfordshire
Cambridge & Huntingdon
Essex (N & S)
Norfolk (E)
Suffolk

De Vilbiss Medequip Ltd
High Street
Wollaston
DY8 4PS

Telephone
Dial 0800 020202
(Free of Charge)

25   **CONCENTRATOR SUPPLIERS** - cont

Regional Groups of HAs   **Concentrator Supplier**

London South

Bromley	BOC Gases
Croydon	
Ealing, Hammersmith and Hounslow	Telephone
East Sussex, Brighton & Hove	Dial 0800 136603
Greenwich & Bexley	(Free of Charge)
Hillingdon	
Kensington, Chelsea and Westminster	
Kent (E & W)	
Kingston & Richmond	
Lambeth, Southwark and Lewisham	
Merton, Sutton and Wandsworth	
Surrey (E & W)	
Sussex (W)	

Yorkshire (South & West) and Humberside

Barnsley	The Oxygen Therapy Company Limited
Bradford	Ocean Way
Calderdale & Kirklees	Ocean Park
Doncaster	Cardiff
E Riding & S. Humber	CF1 5HF
Leeds	
Lincolnshire	Telephone
North Lindsey	Dial 0800 373580
Rotherham	(Free of Charge)
Sheffield	
Wakefield	

Northern

Cumbria (N)	The Oxygen Therapy Company Limited
Durham	Ocean Way
Gateshead & S Tyneside	Ocean Park
Newcastle & N Tyneside	Cardiff
Northumberland	CF1 5HF
N Yorkshire	
Sunderland	Telephone
Tees	Dial 0800 373580
	(Free of Charge)

This Page Is Intentionally Blank

The previous arrangements for out of hours services ended on 31 March 1999.

Instead, the Secretary of State for Health has issued Directions to Health Authorities authorising them from 1 April 1999 to make arrangements with pharmacy contractors to ensure access by the public to the professional services of a registered pharmacist outside normal working hours, ie

> All day Sunday, Good Friday, Christmas Day, Bank Holidays and 28th December (if 26th December falls on a Saturday)

> Before 09.00 or after 17.30 on any other day (after 13.00 on an early closing day).

These Directions are reproduced in Part XIVA. Similar Directions have been issued by the National Assembly for Wales.

In accordance with these Directions, Health Authorities will determine what Pharmacist Access Services they wish to purchase. They will also determine the terms and conditions - including the remuneration - on which arrangements for these services are to be made with pharmacy contractors.

XI

This Page Is Intentionally Blank

1. **Interpretation**

   In this Part -

   "Authority" means the Health Authority in whose locality the premises are located;

   "Contractor" means only the pharmacy contractor whose name is included in a pharmaceutical list of the Authority;

   "pharmacy" means a pharmacy at premises from which the contractor supplies pharmaceutical services;

   "premises" means the premises from which the contractor provides pharmaceutical services;

   "prescriptions" means prescriptions for supply of drugs, medicines and listed appliances under pharmaceutical services.

   "year" means the period from 1 April in any one year to 31 March of the following year.

2. **Entitlement**

   2.1 Where, in any year -

       2.1.1 the pharmacy dispenses fewer than 19,536 prescriptions; and

       2.1.2 that pharmacy is more than 1 kilometre by the nearest practicable route available to the public on foot from the next nearest pharmacy or is less than 1 kilometre but previously qualified as a special consideration case and the circumstances of the pharmacy remain unchanged; and

       2.1.3 in the case of pharmacy which has, in the year immediately preceding that year, dispensed fewer than 6,000 prescriptions, the authority certifies in writing at the beginning of that year that the pharmacy is essential to the proper provision of pharmaceutical services, the contractor shall, subject to the following sub-paragraphs, be entitled to ESPS payments calculated in accordance with paragraph 3 below.

       (Note. No new special consideration cases will be entertained).

   2.2 To qualify for payment, contractors must also have produced a practice leaflet and display up to a maximum of 8 health promotion leaflets.

   2.3 A contractor shall be entitled to claim ESP payments in any one year if, on or before 31 January in the year immediately preceding, he estimates, on the basis of the number of prescriptions dispensed in the preceding twelve months or having regard to any special circumstances, that the number of items to be dispensed in the next year will be less than 19,536

   2.4 The contractor shall apply to the Authority for ESPS payments, in the form specified (Form ESPS1 for contractors on the list not less than 10 months at 31 January and Form ESPS2 for those on list less than 10 months) on or before 31 January in the year immediately preceding the year to which the claim relates.

   2.5 On 1 April of the year to which the claim relates, or as soon as practicable thereafter, but before any payment is made, the contractor shall declare to the Authority his estimate of the number of prescriptions dispensed by the pharmacy in the year just ended, if the Authority is satisfied that -

       2.5.1 that number is less than 19,536

       2.5.2 that the number of prescriptions to be dispensed in the year to which the claim relates is unlikely to exceed 19,536 and

       2.5.3 the conditions set out in sub-paragraph 2.1.2 and 2.1.3 above are met,

       payments shall be made by the Authority in accordance with paragraph 3, subject to the conditions in sub-paragraphs 2.5 and 2.6.

XII

2.6   The Authority, will as soon in the current financial year as they have available the Prescription Pricing Authority figure of prescriptions dispensed by the contractor during the preceding financial year compare this with the contractor's declared estimated figure (sub-paragraph 2.4 above) and if the PPA figure of prescriptions dispensed in the previous financial year is 19,536 or more, the ESPS payments made so far in the current financial year shall be recovered form the contractor in the 3 months following that in which the last ESPS payment was made.

2.7   Where, at any time in any year during which ESPS payments are made to the contractor in respect of a pharmacy.

     2.7.1   the number of prescriptions dispensed by that pharmacy exceeds 19,536 the contractor shall be deemed not to have been entitled to ESPS payments for that year in respect of that pharmacy, and any such payment made to him in that year shall be recovered from the remuneration due to him in the 3 months immediately following the month in which the number of prescriptions dispensed reached 19,536.

     2.7.2   a second contractor begins to provide pharmaceutical services from a pharmacy at premises which are less than 1 kilometre by the nearest practicable route available to the public on foot from the premises of the first contractor, payment to the first contractor shall continue at the full rate during the current year and during the following year at half of the full rate but will then cease.

     2.7.3   in a case to which sub-paragraph 2.1.3 applies, the Authority decides that the pharmacy is no longer essential, it shall notify the contractor and after the date of that notification no further ESPS payments shall be paid in that year in respect of that pharmacy.

2.8   Where the provision by the contractor of pharmaceutical services from any premises has just begun, the preceding sub-paragraphs shall be modified as follows:-

     2.8.1   the contractor may apply to the Authority for ESPS payments, in the form specified (Form ESPS2) at any time during the year;

     2.8.2   he shall be entitled to ESPS payments if -

          2.8.2.1   in the case of a contractor who is providing services from premises from which, immediately before the day on which he began to provide those services, those services were provided by another contractor, the number of prescriptions dispensed in the twelve months immediately preceding that day was less than 19,536;

          2.8.2.2   in any other case, he estimates, and the Authority is satisfied that, less than 19,536 prescriptions will be dispensed in the first twelve months of the provision of pharmaceutical services, and

          2.8.2.3   in any case the condition in sub-paragraph 2.1.2 is satisfied;

     2.8.3   any entitlement shall begin -

          2.8.3.1   if the claim is made within 3 months of the entry on the list in question, from the date of entry;

          2.8.3.2   in any case, from the date on which the application is made.

3. Payments

3.1 ESPS payments shall be the difference between one-twelfth of the target payment (£37,780) and the remuneration due (i.e. professional fees as in Part IIIA and any payments made under Part VIA but excluding payments made under Part IIIA 2.I), subject to para 3.3 below. See worked example.

3.2 Payments shall be paid in arrears.

3.3 The maximum monthly payment shall be £2,630. If in any month the contractor is entitled to more than the maximum payment the amount due should be carried forward and paid in the following month, again subject to a maximum payment of £2,630.

3.4 Any over, or any under, ESPS payment shall be if necessary, corrected in the remuneration paid in the first month of the following year.

3.5 Where a contractor normally provides pharmaceutical services at a pharmacy for less than 30 hours a week, any ESPS payment shall be calculated by reference to the following formula:-

Average hours/30 x payments appropriate to a full-time pharmacy with the same prescription volume, as determined by the Secretary of State for Health as respects England and the National Assembly for Wales as respects Wales.

4. Worked Example

4.1 Month 1.

April   calculate 1/12 of target payment £37,780

make ESPS payment of the difference between calculated amount and remuneration due.

4.2 Month 2.

May   calculate 2/12 of target payment £37,780

make ESPS payment of the difference between calculated amount and sum of total payment of remuneration due plus ESPS made in month 1 and remuneration due in month 2.

XII

4.3 Month 3.

June   calculate 3/12 of target payment £37,780

make ESPS payment of difference between calculated amount and sum of total payments made in months 1 and 2 and remuneration due in month 3.

This Page Is Intentionally Blank

1. From 1 January 1997 a grant of £4,740 is payable to pharmacy contractors who provide the pre-registration training experience needed by pharmacy graduates and certain undergraduates for admission to the Royal Pharmaceutical Society of Great Britain's Register of Pharmaceutical Chemists. The grants are payable at annual rates, determined annually in respect of each pre-registration training place filled by a pharmacy graduate or an under graduate on a sandwich course recognised by the Royal Pharmaceutical Society of Great Britain as pre-registration training.

2. Pharmacy contractors who have undertaken to provide pre-registration training should submit a claim to the Health Authority (HA) at the start of the training period. HAs will arrange for the payment to be made monthly in arrears. Contractors MUST notify the HA immediately in writing if the arrangement to provide pre-registration training ceases.

XIII

This Page Is Intentionally Blank

The previous arrangements for advice to residential and nursing homes services ended on 31 March 1999.

Instead, the Secretary of State for Health has issued Directions to Health Authorities authorising them from 1 April 1999 to make new arrangements for pharmaceutical advice to care homes under the Directions.

These Directions are below. Similar Directions have been issued by the National Assembly for Wales.

In accordance with these Directions, Health Authorities will determine what arrangements to make for pharmaceutical advice to residential and nursing homes. They will also determine the terms and conditions - including the remuneration - on which arrangements for these services are to be made with pharmacy contractors.

Details of local arrangements including any training requirements will be obtainable from Health Authorities.

NATIONAL HEALTH SERVICE ACT 1977

Directions to Health Authorities concerning arrangements for providing additional pharmaceutical services

The Secretary of State in exercise of powers conferred on him by sections 17, 41A and 41B of the National Health Service Act 1977[a] hereby gives the following Directions:-

Application, commencement and interpretation

1.- (1)   These Directions are given to Health Authorities in England and shall come into force on 1st April 1999.

(2)   Words and phrases used in these Directions which appear in the National Health Service (Pharmaceutical Services) Regulations 1992[b] have the meaning they bear in those Regulations.

(3)   In these Directions, unless the context otherwise requires -

"care home" means any residential care home or nursing home registered under the Registered Homes Act 1984[c] and any residential care home that by virtue of section 1(5)(j) of that Act is not required to be registered;

"neighbouring Health Authority" means another Health Authority, which may be either in England or in Wales, with which a Health Authority in England has a common boundary;

"the PhS Regulations" means the National Health Service (Pharmaceutical Services) Regulations 1992.

Provision of a pharmaceutical advisory service to care homes   XIVA

2.- (1)   Subject to sub-paragraph (4) and paragraph 3, a Health Authority may make arrangements with any chemist, other than a supplier of appliances only, whose name is included in its pharmaceutical list or in the pharmaceutical list of a neighbouring Health Authority for the provision of such advice as is specified in the arrangements to any person other than the Health Authority in connection with any specified care home in its area.

(2)   For the purpose of this paragraph "advice" means advice given by a pharmacist approved for this purpose by the Health Authority, being advice falling within any of the following -

(a) the proper and effective ordering of drugs and appliances for the benefit of residents in the home;

(b) the proper and effective administration and use of drugs and appliances in the home;

(c) the safe and appropriate storage of drugs and appliances;

[a]   1977 c.49. Section 17 was substituted by the Health Authorities Act 1995 (c.17), paragraph 8 of Schedule 1.
[b]   S.I 1992/662; amended by S.I. 1993/2451, 1994/2402, 1995/644, 1996/698, 1998/681, and 1998/2224.
[c]   1984 c.23.

(3) A pharmacist may be approved by the Health Authority for the purposes of this paragraph if he-

(a) is either the chemist with whom the Health Authority has made an arrangement under this paragraph or an employee of that chemist, and

(b) has, in the opinion of the Health Authority, the appropriate training to provide advice.

(4) Any arrangement made by a Health Authority under this paragraph must include a term that the chemist with whom the arrangement is made either

(a) keeps a record of the services provided in such manner as may be specified by the Health Authority and makes such record available to the Health Authority on request or

(b) imposes such a condition on any employee who is approved by the Health Authority for the purpose of giving advice as mentioned in sub-paragraph (2) and assumes responsibility for securing compliance with that condition.

3.- (1) A Health Authority must determine whether there is a need in its area for the provision of the advice referred to in paragraph 2(1) and keep that determination under review.

(2) Before making any arrangement under paragraph 2(1) a Health Authority must take into account its findings under sub-paragraph (1).

4. Where the Health Authority makes any arrangements under paragraph 2(1), it must publish -

(a) the names of the chemists with whom arrangements have been made and the address of the premises in the Health Authority's area from which they are providing pharmaceutical services; and

(b) the number of care homes receiving advice under the arrangements

(whether or not it also publishes any other details).

Provision of additional pharmacist access services

5. Subject to paragraph 6 a Health Authority may make arrangements with any chemist, other than a supplier of appliances only, whose name is included in their pharmaceutical list or in the pharmaceutical list of a neighbouring Health Authority to ensure that a pharmacist is available to any person in its area for such consultation as the Health Authority may specify at such times, outside the times of noraml availability required by paragraph 4(2) of Schedule 2 to the PhS Regulations, as the Health Authority may specify.

6.- (1) A Health Authority must determine whether there is a need in its area for the availability of pharmacists outside the hours of normal availability referred to in paragraph 5 and keep that determination under review.

(2) Before making any arrangement under paragraph 5 a Health Authority must take into account its findings under sub-paragraph (1).

7. Where the Health Authority makes any arrangement under paragraph 5 it must publish -

(a) the names of the chemists with whom such arrangements have been made and the address of the premises in the Health Authority's area from which they provide pharmaceutical services:

(b) the details of the consultation specified under paragraph 5, and

(c) the times at which a registered pharmacist is to be available for consultation;

(whether or not it also publishes any other details).

Signed on behalf of the Secretary of State for Health

K J Guinness

Dated 9th March 1999

1. These arrangements cover the keeping of records of medicines supplied to patients who are on long term medication, if they are in one of two groups:-

    1.1 those who are exempt from prescription charges: men and women aged 60 and over;

    1.2 others whom the pharmacist considers may have difficulty in understanding the nature and dosage of the drug supplied and the times at which it is to be taken.

2. Each record should cover all the drugs supplied to one patient. It will be eligible for inclusion in these arrangements only if the circumstances and nature of one or more of the drugs which are being or have been supplied by the pharmacist to the patient are such that in the opinion of the pharmacist supplying them, the same or a similar drug is likely to be prescribed for that person regularly on future occasions.

3. The record keeping system should be suitable for the purpose of the arrangements and provide appropriate levels of confidentiality. It may be computer based or use a manual recording system. It must provide as a minium a record of the name and address of the person to whom the drug is supplied, the name, quantity and dosage of the drug supplied and the date on which it is supplied. Pharmacy contractors will be responsible for any necessary registration under the Data Protection Act 1984.

4. Pharmacists should have obtained a valid certificate as proof of undertaking either the original medication records training course, developed by the Royal Pharmaceutical Society of Great Britain, with the support of the Pharmaceutical Services Negotiating Committee and the National Pharmaceutical Association, or have successfully completed the revised training course, introduced on1 June 1994, (which is available for pharmacists in England from the National Administration Office, Centre for Pharmacy Postgraduate Education, Manchester, tel: 0161-778-4040; and for pharmacists in Wales from Dr D J Temple, the Welsh Centre for Postgraduate Pharmaceutical Education, Cardiff, tel: 02920-874784).

5. Pharmacy contractors who wish to take part in the scheme should apply to the Health Authority confirming that the minimum number of medication records has been reached. Application forms are available from the Health Authority. The completed application form should be returned to the Health Authority with a copy of the course completion certificate.

6. Pharmacists will be required to make all records kept as part of these arrangements available to the Health Authority for inspection on request.

7. The record keeping system shall contain records for a minimum of 100 patients. In the case of a pharmacy which qualifies for support under the Essential Small Pharmacy Scheme the minimum number of records shall be for 50 patients.

8. From 1 August 1996 pharmacy contractors who have passed for pricing 1100 prescriptions a month or less, and who do not qualify for payment under the essential small pharmacy scheme can apply for a £300 fee for setting up a new patient medication record system.

XIVB

This Page Is Intentionally Blank

Payments to chemists who claim a payment under Regulation 18B(1) of the National Health Service (Pharmaceutical Services) Regulations 1992, as amended (SI 1999/696).

The Scheme allows chemists to claim a financial reward where they have identified a fraudulent prescription form, and thereby prevented fraud. A reward is payable where there is an identified saving for the NHS and the conditions for one or both types of reward have been met.

The Scheme applies in England and Wales. Directions issued to the Prescription Pricing Authority (PPA) will allow the PPA to make reward payments on behalf of Health Authorities in England from 14 June 1999 on claims submitted after that date. Health Solutions Wales (Bro Taf Health Authority) (HSW) will make payments on behalf of Health Authorities in Wales from 14 June 1999. The PPA and HSW are referred to jointly below as "Pricing Authority".

The Basic Reward: Claims made where the chemist has not provided the drugs, medicines, or listed appliances ordered on the fraudulent prescription form.

The chemist will be eligible for a payment of 10% of the basic NHS price of the items ordered on the fraudulent prescription form, or £10, whichever is the greater, where all the conditions for payment are met.

The conditions for payment are:

i.   the drugs, medicines, or listed appliances specified on the fraudulent prescription form have not been provided, and the Health Authority was immediately informed, in accordance with Regulation 18B(1)(i);

ii.   a claim is made by returning to the Pricing Authority a duly completed claim form, provided by the Pricing Authority, within 10 days of the form having been presented;

iii.   the form presented as a prescription form was not a genuine order for the person named on the form; an order would not be a genuine order if, for example, it had been stolen or counterfeited and not signed by an authorised prescriber; or had been altered otherwise than by the authorised prescriber by whom it was issued.

The Bonus Reward: where the chemist has either not provided the drugs, medicines, or listed appliances specified on the fraudulent prescription form presented; or where the chemist has provided the drugs, medicines, or listed appliances specified, but subsequently came to have reason to believe that the order was not genuine.

The chemist will be eligible for a payment of 5% of the savings resulting from the information he provides, or £10,000, whichever is the less, where the conditions for payment are met.

The conditions for payment are:

i.   the Health Authority was immediately informed, in accordance with Regulation 18B(1)(i), or informed within 14 days of the order being presented to the chemist, in accordance with Regulation 18B(1)(ii) as appropriate;

ii.   a claim is made by returning to the Prescription Authority a duly completed claim form, provided by the Pricing Authority, within 24 days of the form having been presented;

iii.   the form presented as a prescription form was not a genuine order for the person named on the form; an order would not be a genuine order if, for example, it had been stolen or counterfeited and not signed by an authorised prescriber; or had been altered otherwise than by the authorised prescriber by whom it was issued.

XIVC

iv.   the Pricing Authority consider that the information on the claim form has contributed to the detection and prevention of a fraud, or the recovery for the NHS of sums lost through a fraud, other than the cost of the drugs or listed appliances ordered on the fraudulent prescription form which is the subject of the claim; to satisfy this condition, the Pricing Authority must consider that at least one of the following criteria is fulfilled:

-   the fraud would not have been detected or stopped without the information provided on the claim
-   the fraud would not have been detected until a later date, or would not have been stopped until a later date, without the information provided on the claim
-   the information provided on the claim was cited as evidence in criminal or civil proceedings; this is regardless of the outcome of those proceedings, provided that condition (v) below is met.

v.   the Pricing Authority consider that the fraud, about which the claim provided information, has been stopped subsequently to the claim being received.

The Pricing Authority will estimate savings resulting from the information provided, by the addition of (a) and (b) as follows:

a)   losses prevented will be calculated by reference to an estimate of whichever is the greater of:-

-   losses in the 12 months up to the stopping of the fraud, _or_
-   losses in the financial year previous to the stopping of the fraud, _or_
-   an annual rate of loss over an average of up to 5 previous financial years before the stopping of the fraud, if the data are available

b)   if previous losses to the NHS are recovered, whether or not by civil proceedings, the total sum recovered.

The level of savings must be certified by a member of the NHS Counter Fraud Operational Service.

If a number of claims, each of which fully meets the conditions for payment, lead to the prevention or detection of one fraud, or the recovery for the NHS of sums lost through one fraud, a Bonus Reward of 5% of the savings or £20,000, whichever is the smaller, in total may be shared between the claims. The Pricing Authority will decide the shares for each claim according to their contributions to the saving for the NHS, or, if this cannot reasonably be estimated, the shares will be allocated equally to each claim meeting the conditions for payment.

In certain conditions some foods and toilet preparations have characteristics of drugs and the Advisory Committee on Borderline Substances advises as to the circumstances in which such substances may be regarded as drugs. The Advisory Committee's recommendations are listed below. Prescriptons issued in accordance with the Committee's advice and endorsed "ACBS" will normally not be investigated.

LIST A

This is an alphabetical index of products which the ACBS has recommended for the management of the conditions shown under each product.

General Practitioners are reminded that the Advisory Committee on Borderline Substances recommends products on the basis that they may be regarded as drugs for the treatment of specified conditions. Doctors should satisfy themselves that the products can be safely prescribed, that patients are adequately monitored and that, where necessary, expert hospital supervision is available. Prescriptions for products recommended by the Committee should be endorsed "ACBS".

Note: The Committee has recommended a number of products as complete feeds for certain conditions. They may be prescribed both as sole sources of nutrition and as necessary nutritional supplements prescribable on medical grounds.

Definitions

1.   The Committee has defined proven lactose or sucrose intolerance as "A condition of intolerance to an intake of the relevant disaccharide confirmed by:

   (i)   demonstrated clinical benefit of the effectiveness of the disaccharide free diet; and

   (ii) the presence of reducing substances and/or excessive acid (1.00pH) in the stools, a low concentration of the correspondent disaccharidase enzyme on intestinal biopsy, or by breath tests or lactose tolerance tests."

2.   The Committee has defined proven whole protein sensitivity as "Intolerance to whole protein, proven by at least two withdrawal and challenge tests, as suggested by an accurate dietary history."

3.   The Committee has defined dysphagia as that associated with "Intrinsic disease of the oesophagus, eg. oesophagitis; neuromuscular disorders, eg. multiple sclerosis and motor neurone disease; major surgery and/or radiotherapy for cancer of the upper digestive tract; protracted severe inflammatory disease of the upper disgestive tract, eg. Stevens-Johnson Syndrome and epidermolysis bullosa."

LIST A cont

AGLUTELLA LOW-PROTEIN PRODUCTS

See: Low-Protein Products

AL110 (NESTLE)

Proven lactose intolerance in pre-school children, galactosaemia and galactokinase deficiency.

ALCOHOLIC BEVERAGES

See: Rectified Spirit

ALEMBICOL-D (MCT OIL)

Steatorrhoea associated with cystic fibrosis of the pancreas, intestinal lymphangiectasia, surgery of the intestine, chronic liver disease, liver cirrhosis, other proven malabsorption syndromes, a ketogenic diet in the management of epilepsy and in type 1 hyperlipoproteinaemia.

ALFARE

Disaccharide and/or whole protein intolerance, or where amino acids or peptides are indicated in conjunction with MCT.

AMBRE SOLAIRE TOTAL SUNSCREEN FOR SUN-SENSITIVE SKIN SPF 60

Protection from UV radiation in abnormal cutaneous photosensitivity resulting from genetic disorders or photodermatoses, including vitiligo and those resulting from radiotherapy; chronic or recurrent herpes simplex labialis.

AMINEX LOW-PROTEIN PRODUCTS

See: Low-Protein Products

AMINOGRAN FOOD SUPPLEMENT

Phenylketonuria

AMINOGRAN FOOD SUPPLEMENT TABLETS

For use in the dietary management of phenylketonuria. Not to be prescribed for any child under 8 years of age.

AMINOGRAN MINERAL MIXTURE

Phenylketonuria and as a mineral supplement in synthetic diets.

ANALOG LCP

Phenylketonuria in infants and children under two years of age

ANALOG MSUD

Maple Syrup Urine Disease

ANALOG RVHB

Hypermethioninaemia, homocystinuria

LIST A cont

ANALOG XLYS

Hyperlysinaemia

ANALOG XMET, THRE, VAL, ISOLEU

Methylmalonic acidaemia, propionic acidaemia

ANALOG XP

Phenylketonuria

ANALOG XPHEN, TYR
ANALOG XPHEN, TYR, MET

Tyrosinaemia

APROTEN GLUTEN-FREE AND LOW-PROTEIN PRODUCTS

See: Gluten-Free and Low-Protein Products.

ARNOTT'S GLUTEN-FREE PRODUCTS

See: Gluten-Free Products

AVEENO CREAM
AVEENO BATH OIL
AVEENO COLLOIDAL (formerly Aveeno Bath Additive Sachets (Oilated))
AVEENO COLLOIDAL BABY

Endogenous and exogenous eczema, xeroderma, ichthyosis and senile pruritus associated with dry skin.

AVEENO BATH ADDITIVE SACHETS (OILATED)

See: Aveeno Colloidal and Aveeno Colloidal Baby.

BAR-KAT GLUTEN-FREE PRODUCTS

See: Gluten-Free products

BATH E45

See: E45 Emollient Bath Oil

BI-AGLUT GLUTEN-FREE PRODUCTS

See: Gluten-Free Products.

XV

CALOGEN

Disease related malnutrition, malabsorption states or other conditions requiring fortification with a high fat supplement.

CALOGEN STRAWBERRY

For use in the dietary management of disease-related malnutrition, malabsorption states, or other conditions requiring fortification with a high fat supplement, with or without fluid and electrolyte restrictions.

LIST A cont

CALOREEN

Disease related malnutrition, malabsorption states or other conditions requiring fortification with a high or readily available carbohydrate supplement.

CALSIP

Disease related malnutrition, malabsorption states or other conditions requiring fortification with a high or readily available carbohydrate supplement.

CAPRILON (formerly CAPRILON FORMULA)

Disorders in which a high intake of MCT is beneficial

CAPRILON FORMULA

See: Caprilon

CASILAN 90

Biochemically proven hypoproteinaemia.

CLARA'S KITCHEN GLUTEN-FREE PRODUCTS

See: Gluten-Free Products.

CLINIFEED 1.0
CLINIFEED 1.5
CLINIFEED FIBRE
CLINIFEED ISO

For use as the sole source of nutrition or as necessary nutritional supplements prescribed on medical grounds for:
Short bowel syndrome, intractable malabsorption, pre-operative preparation of patients who are undernourished, patients with proven inflammatory bowel disease, following total gastrectomy, dysphagia, bowel fistulae, disease-related malnutrition.
Not to be prescribed for any child under one year; use with caution for young children up to five years of age.

CLINUTREN DESSERT (formerly EMELIS)

As a necessary nutritional supplement prescribed on medical grounds for:
Short bowel syndrome, intractable malabsorption, pre-operative preparation of patients who are undernourished, patients with proven inflammatory bowel disease, following total gastrectomy, dysphagia, bowel fistulae, disease-realated malnutrition, continuous ambulatory peritoneal dialysis (CAPD) and haemodialysis. Not to be prescribed for any child under one year; use with caution for young children up to five years of age.

CLINUTREN 1.5
CLINUTREN ISO

As a necessary nutritional supplement prescribed on medical grounds for:
Short bowel syndrome, intractable malabsorption, pre-operative preparation of patients who are undernourished, patients with proven inflammatory bowel disease, following total gastrectomy, dysphagia, bowel fistulae, disease-related malnutrition. Not to be prescribed for any child under one year; use with caution for young children up to five years of age.

COMMINUTED CHICKEN MEAT (SHS)

Carbohydrate intolerance in association with possible or proven intolerance of milk, glucose and galactose intolerance.

LIST A cont

COMPLAN READY-TO-DRINK

For use as the sole source of nutrition or as a necessary nutritional supplement prescribed on medical grounds for:

Short bowel syndrome, intractable malabsorption, pre-operative preparation of patients who are undernourished, patients with proven inflammatory bowel disease, following total gastrectomy, dysphagia, bowel fistulae, disease-related malnutrition. Not to be prescribed for any child under one year; use with caution for young children up to five years of age.

COPPERTONE ULTRASHADE 23

Protection from UV radiation in abnormal cutaneous photosensitivity resulting from genetic disorders or photodermatoses, including vitiligo and those resulting from radiotherapy; chronic or recurrent herpes simplex labialis.

CORN FLOUR AND CORN STARCH

Hypoglycaemia associated with glycogen storage disease.

COVERING CREAMS AND CONCEALMENT OF BIRTH MARKS

Covermark Classic Foundation	Dermacolor Fixing Powder
Covermark Finishing Powder	Keromask Finishing Powder
Dermablend Cover Creme	Keromask Masking Cream
Dermablend Leg and Body Cover	Veil Cover Cream
Dermablend Setting Powder	Veil Finishing Powder
Dermacolor Camouflage Cream	

For post operative scars and other deformities and as adjunctive therapy in the relief of emotional disturbance due to disfiguring skin disease, such as vitiligo.

COVERMARK PRODUCTS

See: Covering Creams

DELPH SUN LOTION SPF15, SPF20, SPF25, SPF30

Protection from UV radiation in abnormal cutaneous photosensitivity resulting from genetic disorders or photodermatoses, including vitiligo and those resulting from radiotherapy, chronic or recurrent herpes simplex labialis.

DERMABLEND

See: Covering Creams

DERMACOLOR CAMOUFLAGE SYSTEM

See: Covering Creams

XV

DEXTROSE

Glycogen storage disease and sucrose/isomaltose intolerance.

DIALAMINE

Oral feeding where essential amino acid supplements are required, for example chronic renal failure, hypoproteinaemia, wound fistula leakage with excessive protein loss, conditions requiring a controlled nitrogen intake and haemodialysis.

LIST A cont

DIETARY SPECIALTIES

See: Gluten-Free Products

DISINFECTANTS (ANTISEPTICS)

May be prescribed on FPIO only when ordered in such quantities and with such directions as are appropriate for the treatment of patients, but not if ordered for general hygienic purposes.

dp LOW-PROTEIN PRODUCTS

See: Low-Protein Products.

DUOBAR

Disease related malnutrition, malabsorption states or other conditions requiring fortification with a fat/carbohydrate supplement.

DUOCAL (LIQUID, MCT POWDER AND SUPER SOLUBLE)

Disease related malnutrition, malabsorption states or other conditions requiring fortification with a fat/carbohydrate supplement.

E45 EMOLLIENT BATH OIL (formerly BATH E45)
E45 EMOLLIENT WASH CREAM (formerly WASH E45)

Endogenous and exogenous eczema, xeroderma, ichthyosis and senile pruritus associated with dry skin.

E45 LOTION

Symptomatic relief of dry skin conditions, such as those associated with atopic eczema and contact dermatitis.

E45 SUN LOTION SPF 15 AND SPF 25 (formerly SUN E45)
E45 SUN 50 SUNBLOCK LOTION (formerly SUN E45)

Protection from UV radiation in abnormal cutaneous photosensitivity resulting from genetic disorders or photodermatoses, including vitiligo and those resulting from radiotherapy; chronic or recurrent herpes simplex labialis.

ELEMENTAL 028 (FLAVOURED AND UNFLAVOURED)
ELEMENTAL 028 EXTRA
ELEMENTAL 028 EXTRA (LIQUID)

For use as the sole source of nutrition or as a necessary nutritional supplement prescribed on medical grounds for: Short bowel syndrome, intractable malabsorption, patients with proven inflammatory bowel disease, bowel fistulae. Not to be prescribed for any child under one year; use with caution for young children up to five years of age.

EMELIS

See: Clinutren Dessert

EMSOGEN (FLAVOURED AND UNFLAVOURED)

For use as the sole source of nutrition or as a necessary nutritional supplement prescribed on medical grounds for: Short bowel syndrome, intractable malabsorption, patients with proven inflammatory bowel disease, bowel fistulae. Not to be prescribed for any child under one year; use with caution for young children up to five years of age.

ENER-G GLUTEN-FREE PRODUCTS

See: Gluten-Free Products

LIST A cont

ENER-G LOW-PROTEIN PRODUCTS

See: Low-Protein Products

ENFAMIL AR

Significant reflux disease. For use not in excess of a 6-month period. Not to be used in conjunction with any other thickener or antacid product.

ENFAMIL LACTOFREE

Proven lactose intolerance

ENLIVE

As a necessary nutritional supplement prescribed on medical grounds for:
Short bowel syndrome, intractable malabsorption, pre-operative prepartion of patients who are undernourished, patients with proven inflammatory bowel disease, following total gastrectomy, dysphagia, bowel fistulae, disease-related malnutrition. Not to be prescribed for any child under one year; use with caution for young children up to five years of age.

ENRICH

For use as the sole source of nutrition or as a necessary nutritional supplement prescribed on medical grounds for:
Short bowel syndrome, intractable malabsorption, pre-operative preparation of patients who are undernourished, patients with proven inflammatory bowel disease, following total gastrectomy, dysphagia, disease-related malnutrition. Not to be prescribed for any child under one year; use with caution for young children up to five years of age.

ENRICH PLUS

For use as a nutritional supplement for patients with disease-related malnutrition, continuous ambulatory peritoneal dialysis (CAPD), and haemodialysis, short bowel syndrome, intractable malasorption, dysphagia, proven inflammatory bowel disease, bowel fistulae, gastrectomy, and for pre-operative preparation of patients who are undernourished. Not to be prescribed for any child under one year; use with caution for young children up to five years of age.

ENSURE, ENSURE POWDER

For use as the sole source of nutrition or as a necessary nutritional supplement prescribed on medical grounds for: Short bowel syndrome, intractable malabsorption, pre-operative preparation of patients who are undernourished, patients with proven inflammatory bowel disease, following total gastrectomy, dysphagia, bowel fistulae, disease-related malnutrition. Not to be prescribed for any child under one year; use with caution for young children up to five years of age.

ENSURE BAR

As a necessary nutritional supplement prescribed on medical grounds for: disease-related malnutrition, intractable malasorption, total gastrectomy, proven inflammatory bowel disease, and pre-operative preparation of patients who are undernourished. Not to be prescribed for any child under two years; use with caution for young children up to five years of age.

ENSURE PLUS

As a necessary nutritional supplement prescribed on medical grounds for:
Short bowel syndrome, intractable malabsorption, pre-operative preparation of patients who are undernourished, patients with proven inflammatory bowel disease, following total gastrectomy, dysphagia, bowel fistulae, disease-related malnutrition, continuous ambulatory peritoneal dialysis (CAPD), and haemodialysis. Not to be prescribed for any child under one year; use with caution for young children up to five years of age.

XV

LIST A cont

ENTERA
ENTERA FIBRE PLUS SIP FEED
ENTERA FIBRE PLUS (NEUTRAL) TUBE FEED

> For use as the sole source of nutrition or as a necessary nutritional supplement prescribed on medical grounds for: Short bowel syndrome, intractable malabsorption, pre-operative preparation of patients who are undernourished, patients with proven inflammatory bowel disease, following total gastrectomy, dysphagia, bowel fistulae, disease-related malnutrition. Not to be prescribed for any child under one year; use with caution for young children up to five years of age.

FARLEY'S SOYA FORMULA

> Proven lactose and associated sucrose intolerance in pre-school children, galactokinase deficiency, galactosaemia and cow's milk protein intolerance.

FATE LOW PROTEIN PRODUCTS

> See: Low-Protein Products

FORMANCE

> As a necessary nutritional supplement prescribed on medical grounds for:
> Short bowel syndrome, intractable malabsorption, pre-operative preparation of patients who are undernourished, patients with proven inflammatory bowel disease, following total gastrectomy, dysphagia, bowel fistulae, disease-related malnutrition, continuous ambulatory peritoneal dialysis (CAPD), and haemodialysis. Not to be prescribed for any child under one year; use with caution for young children up to five years of age.

FORTICREME (formerly Fortipudding)

> As a necessary nutritional supplement prescribed on medical grounds for:
> Short bowel syndrome, intractable malabsorption, pre-operative preparation of patients who are undernourished, patients with proven inflammatory bowel disease, following total gastrectomy, dysphagia, bowel fistulae, disease-related malnutrition, continuous ambulatory peritoneal dialysis (CAPD) and haemodialysis. Not to be prescribed for any child under one year; use with caution for young children up to five years of age.

FORTIFRESH

> For use as the sole source of nutrition or as a necessary nutritional supplement prescribed on medical grounds for:
> Short bowel syndrome, intractable malabsorption, pre-operative preparation of patients who are undernourished, patients with proven inflammatory bowel disease, following total gastrectomy, dysphagia, bowel fistulae, disease-related malnutrition. Not to be prescribed for any child under one year; use with caution for young children up to five years of age.

FORTIJUCE

> As a necessary nutritional supplement prescribed on medical grounds for:
> Short bowel syndrome, intractable malabsorption, pre-operative preparation of patients who are undernourished, patients with proven inflammatory bowel disease, following total gastrectomy, dysphagia, bowel fistulae, disease-related malnutrition. Not to be prescribed for any child under one year; use with caution for young children up to five years of age.

FORTIMEL

> As a necessary nutritional supplement prescribed on medical grounds for:
> Short bowel syndrome, intractable malabsorption, pre-operative preparation of patients who are undernourished, patients with proven inflammatory bowel disease, following total gastrectomy, dysphagia, bowel fistulae, disease-related malnutrition. Not to be prescribed for any child under one year; use with caution for young children up to five years of age.

LIST A cont

FORTIPUDDING

   See: Forticreme

FORTISIP
FORTISIP MULTIFIBRE

   As a necessary nutritional supplement prescribed on medical grounds for:
Short bowel syndrome, intractable malabsorption, pre-operative preparation of patients who are undernourished, patients with proven inflammatory bowel disease, following total gastrectomy, dysphagia, bowel fistulae, disease-related malnutrition. Not to be prescribed for any child under one year; use with caution for young children up to five years of age.

FREBINI

   For use as the sole source of nutrition or as a necessary nutritional supplement prescribed on medical grounds for:
Short bowel syndrome, intractable malabsorption, pre-operative preparation of patients who are undernourished, patients with proven inflammatory bowel disease, following total gastrectomy, dysphagia, bowel fistulae, disease-related malnutrition and/or growth failure. Not to be prescribed for any child under one year of age.

FRESENIUS OPD

   See: Survimed OPD

FRESUBIN ISOFIBRE

   For use as the sole source of nutrition or as a necessary nutritional supplement prescribed on medical grounds for:
Short bowel syndrome, intractable malabsorption, pre-operative preparation of patients who are undernourished, patients with proven inflammatory bowel disease, following total gastrectomy, dysphagia, disease-related malnutrition. Not to be prescribed for any child under two years; use with caution for young children up to five years of age.

FRESUBIN LIQUID AND SIP FEEDS

   For use as the sole source of nutrition or as a necessary nutritional supplement prescribed on medical grounds for:
Short bowel syndrome, intractable malabsorption, pre-operative preparation of patients who are undernourished, patients with proven inflamatory bowel disease, following total gastrectomy, dysphagia, bowel fistulae, disease-related malnutrition and Refsum's Disease. Not to be prescribed for any child under one year; use with caution for young children up to five years of age.

FRESUBIN 750

   See: Fresubin 750 MCT

FRESUBIN 750 MCT (formerly FRESUBIN 750)

   As a necessary nutritional supplement prescribed on medical grounds for:
Short bowel syndrome, intractable malabsorption, pre-operative preparation of patients who are undernourished, patients with proven inflammatory bowel disease, following total gastrectomy, dysphagia, bowel fistulae, disease-related malnutrition continuous ambulatory peritoneal dialysis (CAPD), and haemodialysis. Not to be prescribed for any child under one year; use with caution for young children up to five years of age.

FRUCTOSE

   Proven glucose/galactose intolerance.

LIST A cont

GALACTOMIN 17 (formerly GALACTOMIN 17 (NEW FORMULA))

Proven lactose intolerance in pre-school children, galactosaemia and galactokinase deficiency.

GALACTOMIN 17 (NEW FORMULA)

See: Galactomin 17

GALACTOMIN 19 (FRUCTOSE FORMULA)

Glucose plus galactose intolerance

GENERAID

Patients with chronic liver disease and/or porto-hepatic encephalopathy.

GENERAID PLUS

Children over one year of age with hepatic disorders.

GLANDOSANE

Patients suffering from a dry mouth as a result of having or having undergone radiotherapy or sicca syndrome.

GLUCOSE

Glycogen storage disease and sucrose/isomaltose intolerance.

GLUTAFIN GLUTEN-FREE PRODUCTS

See: Gluten-Free Products.

GLUTANO GLUTEN-FREE PRODUCTS

See: Gluten-Free Products.

GLUTEN-FREE PRODUCTS

(Not necessarily low-protein, lactose or sucrose free).

> Aproten gluten-free flour
> Arnott's gluten-free rice cookies
> Bar-Kat brown rice pizza crust
> Bar-Kat gluten-free bread mix
> Bar-Kat gluten-free brown rice bread
> Bar-Kat gluten-free white rice bread
> Bar-Kat white rice pizza crust
> Bi-Aglut gluten-free biscuits
> Bi-Aglut gluten-free cracker toast
> Bi-Aglut gluten-free crackers
> Bi-Aglut gluten-free pastas (fusilli, lasagne, macaroni, penne, spaghetti)
> Clara's Kitchen gluten-free bread mix
> Clara's Kitchen gluten-free high fibre bread mix
> Dietary Specialties gluten-free (brown bread mix, corn bread mix, fibre mix, pizza bases, white
>   bread mix, white cake mix, white mix)
> Ener-G gluten-free brown rice bread
> Ener-G gluten-free brown rice and maize bread
> Ener-G gluten-free brown rice pasta (lasagne, macaroni, spaghetti)
> Ener-G gluten-free rice loaf
> Ener-G gluten-free rice pasta (cannelloni, lasagna, macaroni, shells, small shells, spaghetti,
>   tagliatelle, vermicelli)
> Ener-G gluten-free tapioca bread

LIST A cont
GLUTEN -FREE PRODUCTS - cont

Ener-G gluten-free white rice bread
Glutafin gluten-free biscuits
Glutafin gluten-free cake mix
Glutafin gluten-free crackers
Glutafin gluten-free digestive biscuits
Glutafin gluten-free fibre loaf (sliced and unsliced)
Glutafin gluten-free fibre mix
Glutafin gluten-free high fibre crackers
Glutafin gluten-free loaf (sliced and unsliced)
Glutafin gluten-free multigrain fibre bread (sliced and unsliced)
Glutafin gluten-free multigrain fibre mix
Glutafin gluten-free multigrain fibre rolls
Glutafin gluten-free multigrain white bread (formerly Glutafin gluten-free
    whitebread loaf (sliced and unsliced))
Glutafin gluten-free multigrain white rolls (formerly Glutafin gluten-free wheat-free bread rolls)
Glutafin gluten-free multigrain white mix
Glutafin gluten-free part-baked fibre loaf
Glutafin gluten-free part-baked fibre rolls
Glutafin gluten-free part-baked rolls
Glutafin gluten-free part-baked white loaf
Glutafin gluten-free pasta (lasagne, long-cut spaghetti, macaroni penne, shells, spirals,
    tagliatelle nests)
Glutafin gluten-free pastry mix
Glutafin gluten-free pizza base
Glutafin gluten-free savoury biscuits
Glutafin gluten-free sweet biscuits (without chocolate or sultanas)
Glutafin gluten-free tea biscuits
Glutafin gluten-free white bread (canned) with added soya bran
Glutafin gluten-free white mix
Glutano gluten-free biscuits
Glutano gluten-free crackers
Glutano gluten-free flour mix
Glutano gluten-free par-baked (baguette, rolls, white sliced bread)
Glutano gluten-free pasta (animal shapes, macaroni, spaghetti, spirals, tagliatelle)
Glutano gluten-free wholemeal bread (sliced)
Glutano gluten-free wholemeal par-baked bread
Gratis gluten-free pasta (alphabets, macaroni, shells, short cut spaghetti, spirals)
Juvela gluten-free bread rolls
Juvela gluten-free crispbread
Juvela gluten-free digestive biscuits
Juvela gluten-free fibre bread rolls
Juvela gluten-free fibre loaf (sliced and unsliced)
Juvela gluten-free fibre mix
Juvela gluten-free Harvest mix
Juvela gluten-free loaf (sliced and unsliced)
Juvela gluten-free mix
Juvela gluten-free part-baked bread rolls
Juvela gluten-free part-baked fibre loaf
Juvela gluten-free part-baked loaf
Juvela gluten-free pizza base
Juvela gluten-free savoury biscuits
Juvela gluten-free sweet biscuits
Juvela gluten-free tea biscuits
Lifestyle gluten-free bread rolls
Lifestyle gluten-free brown bread
Lifestyle gluten-free high fibre bread
Lifestyle gluten-free high fibre bread rolls
Lifestyle gluten-free white bread
Liga gluten-free rusks (Jacob's)
Orgran gluten-free buckwheat spirals pasta
Orgran gluten-free corn lasagne, corn spaghetti, corn spirals pasta
Orgran gluten-free crispbread corn, crispbread rice

XV

LIST A cont

GLUTEN-FREE PRODUCTS - cont

        Orgran gluten-free organic brown rice spirals
        Orgran gluten-free pizza & pastry mix
        Orgran gluten-free rice spaghetti, rice spirals
        Orgran gluten-free rice and millet spirals
        Orgran gluten-free ris o'mais (rice and maize) lasagne, ris o'mais spaghetti,
                ris o'mais spirals
        Orgran gluten-free split pea & soya pasta shells
        Pleniday gluten-free bread (sliced country loaf, petit pain (par-baked), rustic loaf sliced)
        Pleniday gluten-free pasta (penne, rigate)
        Polial gluten-free biscuits
        Rite-Diet gluten-free fibre mix
        Rite-Diet gluten-free fibre rolls
        Rite-Diet gluten-free high fibre bread (sliced and unsliced)
        Rite-Diet gluten-free white bread (sliced and unsliced)
        Rite-Diet gluten-free white mix
        Riet-Diet gluten-free white rolls
        Rite-Diet part-baked fibre loaf
        Rite-Diet part-baked long fibre rolls
        Rite-Diet part-baked gluten-free fibre loaf
        Rite-Diet part-baked gluten-free long fibre rolls
        Schar gluten-free biscuits
        Schar gluten-free bread
        Schar gluten-free bread mix
        Schar gluten-free bread rolls
        Schar gluten-free cake mix
        Schar gluten-free crackers
        Schar gluten-free cracker toast
        Schar gluten-free crispbread
        Schar gluten-free flour mix for cooking
        Schar gluten-free french bread (baguette)
        Schar gluten-free pasta (alphabet pasta, bavette, fusilli, lasagne, macaroni, pasta rings, pasta shells,
        penne, rigati, spaghetti)
        Schar gluten-free pizza base
        Schar gluten-free savoy biscuits
        Schar gluten-free wheat-free bread buns (white)
        Schar gluten-free wheat-free lunch rolls
        Schar gluten-free wholemeal bread
        Schar gluten-free wholemeal flour mix
        Sunnyvale gluten-free mixed grain sourdough bread
        Tinkyada gluten-free brown rice pastas
        Tritamyl gluten-free brown bread mix
        Tritamyl gluten-free flour
        Tritamyl gluten-free white bread mix
        Trufree flour mix no.1 for loaves
        Trufree flour mix no.4 white for loaves and rolls
        Trufree flour mix no.5 brown for loaves and scones
        Trufree flour mix no.6 white for pastry
        Trufree flour mix no.7 white, self-raising
        Ultra gluten-free baguette
        Ultra gluten-free bread
        Ultra gluten-free bread rolls
        Ultra gluten-free cracke;bread
        Ultra gluten-free high fibre bread
        Ultra gluten-free pizza base
        Valpiform gluten-free bread mix
        Valpiform gluten-free country loaf
        Valpiform gluten-free pastry mix
        Valpiform gluten-free petites baguettes

Gluten-sensitive enteropathies including steatorrhoea due to gluten-sensitivity, coeliac disease and
dermatitis herpetiformis.

LIST A cont

GRATIS GLUTEN-FREE PRODUCTS

See: Gluten-Free Products

HARIFEN WHITE CHIP COOKIES

As part of the low protein dietary management of phenylketonuria, and similar amino acid abnormalities, renal and hepatic failure, cirrhosis of the liver.

HYCAL

Disease related malnutrition, malabsorption states or other conditions requiring fortification with a high or readily available carbohydrate supplement.

INFASOY

Proven lactose and associated sucrose intolerance in pre-school children, galactokinase deficiency, glactosaemia and proven whole cows milk sensitivity.

INSTANT CAROBEL

Thickening feeds in the treatment of vomiting.

ISOMIL

Proven lactose intolerance in pre-school children, galactokinase deficiency, galactasaemia and proven whole cows milk sensitivity.

ISOSOURCE ENERGY (formerly Nutrodrip Energy)
ISOSOURCE FIBRE (formerly Nutrodrip Fibre)
ISOSOURCE STANDARD (formerly Nutrodrip Standard)

For use as the sole source of nutrition or as a necessary nutritional supplement prescribed on medical grounds for:

Short bowel syndrome, intractable malabsorption, pre-operative preparation of patients who are undernourished, patients with proven inflammatory bowel disease, following total gastrectomy, dysphagia, bowel fistulae, disease-related malnutrition. Not to be prescribed for any child under one year; use with caution for young children up to fives years of age.

JEVITY

For use as the sole source of nutrition or as a necessary nutritional supplement prescribed on medical grounds for:
Short bowel syndrome, intractable malabsorption, pre-operative preparation of patients who are undernourished, patients with proven inflammatory bowel disease, following total gastrectomy, dysphagia, disease-related malnutrition. Not to be prescribed for any child under one year; use with caution for young children up to five years of age.

JEVITY PLUS

For use as the sole source of nutrition or as a necessary nutritional supplement prescribed on medical grounds for:
Short bowel syndrome, intractable malabsorption, pre-operative preparation of patients who are undernourished, patients with proven inflammatory bowel disease, following total gastrectomy, dysphagia, bowel fistulae, disease-related malnutrition. Not recommended for any child under ten years of age.

JUVELA GLUTEN-FREE PRODUCTS

See: Gluten-Free Products.

XV

LIST A cont

JUVELA LOW-PROTEIN PRODUCTS

See: Low-Protein Products.

KEROMASK

See: Covering creams.

KINDERGEN P.R.O.D.

Complete nutritional support or supplementary feeding for infants and children with chronic renal failure who are receiving peritoneal rapid overnight dialysis.

L-ARGININE SUPPLEMENT FOR UREA CYCLE DISORDERS (S.H.S.)

Urea cycle disorders other than arginase deficiency, such as hyperammonaemia types I and II, citrullaemia, arginossuccinic aciduria, and deficiency of N-acetyl glutamate synthetase.

LEUCINE FREE AMINO ACID MIX

Isovaleric acidaemia

LIFESTYLE GLUTEN-FREE PRODUCTS

See: Gluten-Free Products

LIGA GLUTEN-FREE RUSKS (JACOB'S)

See: Gluten-Free Products.

LIQUIGEN

Steatorrhoea associated with cystic fibrosis of the pancreas, intestinal lymphangiectasia, surgery of the intestine, chronic liver disease, liver cirrhosis, other proven malabsorption syndromes, a ketogenic diet in the management of epilepsy and in type 1 hyperlipoproteinaemia.

LIQUISORBON MCT

See: Nutrison MCT

LOCASOL (formerly LOCASOL NEW FORMULA)

Calcium intolerance

LOCASOL NEW FORMULA

See: Locasol

LOFENALAC

Phenylketonuria.

LOPROFIN LOW-PROTEIN PRODUCTS

See: Low-Protein Products

LOPROFIN PKU DRINK

Phenylketonuria

LIST A cont

LOW-PROTEIN PRODUCTS

> Aglutella low-protein rice
> Aminex low-protein biscuits
> Aminex low-protein cookies
> Aminex low-protein rusks
> Aproten low-protein biscuits
> Aproten low-protein bread mix
> Aproten low-protein cake mix
> Aproten low-protein crispbread
> Aproten low-protein pastas (anellini, ditalini, rigatini, spaghetti, tagliatelle)
> dp low-protein butterscotch and chocolate flavoured chip cookies
> Ener-G low-protein egg replacer
> Ener-G low-protein rice bread
> Fate low-protein cake mix
> Fate low-protein chocolate flavour cake mix
> Fate low-protein flour
> Juvela low-protein chocolate chip, cinnamon and orange flavour cookies
> Juvela low-protein bread rolls
> Juvela low-protein loaf (sliced and unsliced)
> Juvela low-protein mix.
> Loprofin low-protein breakfast cereal
> Loprofin low-protein chocolate flavour cream biscuits
> Loprofin low-protein chocolate, orange and vanilla flavour cream wafers
> Loprofin low-protein cinnamon and chocolate chip cookies
> Loprofin low-protein crackers
> Loprofin low-protein egg replacer
> Loprofin low-protein egg white replacer
> Loprofin low-protein fibre bread (sliced and unsliced)
> Loprofin low-protein loaf (sliced and unsliced)
> Loprofin low-protein mix
> Loprofin low-protein part baked rolls
> Loprofin low-protein pasta (long-cut spaghetti, macaroni penne, spirals vermicelli)
> Loprofin low-protein sweet biscuits
> Loprofin low-protein white bread (canned)
> Loprofin low-protein white bread (canned) with no added salt.
> Loprofin low-protein white bread rolls
> Promin low-protein imitation rice
> Promin low-protein pasta (alphabets, macaroni, shells, short cut spaghetti, spirals)
> Promin low-protein pastameal
> Promin low protein tricolour pasta (alphabets, shells, spirals)
> Rite-Diet low-protein baking mix.
> Rite-Diet low-protein flour mix
> Ultra low-protein canned brown bread
> Ultra low-protein canned white bread
> Ultra PKU biscuits
> Ultra PKU bread
> Ultra PKU cookies
> Ultra PKU flour mix
> Ultra PKU pizza base
> Ultra PKU savoy biscuits
> Valpiform low-protein cookies with chocolate nuggets and hazelnut flavour
> Valpiform low-protein shortbread biscuits

XV

> Inherited metabolic disorders, renal or liver failure requiring a low-protein diet

L-TYROSINE SUPPLEMENT FOR PHENYLKETONURIA

> Maternal Phenylketonurics who have low plasma tyrosine levels

LUBORANT SALIVA REPLACEMENT

> Patients suffering from a dry mouth as a result of having or having undergone radiotherapy or sicca syndrome.

LIST A cont

MAXAMAID
MAXAMUM

See various entries now listed under the appropriate prefix

MAXIJUL LE
MAXIJUL LIQUID
MAXIJUL SUPER SOLUBLE

Disease related malnutrion, malabsorption states or other conditions requiring fortification with a high or readily available carbohydrate supplement.

MAXIPRO SUPER SOLUBLE

Biochemically proven hypoproteinaemia. Not to be prescribed for any child under one year; unsuitable as a sole source of nutrition

MAXISORB

Biochemically proven hypoproteinaemia.

MCT PEPDITE 0-2
MCT PEPDITE 2+

Disorders in which a high intake of MCT is beneficial

MEDIUM-CHAIN TRIGLYCERIDE (MCT) OIL

Steatorrhoea associated with cystic fibrosis of the pancreas, intestinal lymphangiectasia, surgery of the intestine, chronic liver disease, liver cirrhosis, other proven malabsorption syndromes, in a ketogenic diet in the management of epilepsy and in type 1 hyperlipoproteinaemia.

MEGASHAKE NUTRITIONAL SUPPLEMENT

Disease related malnutrition, malabsorption states or other conditions requiring fortification with a fat/carbohydrate supplement

METABOLIC MINERAL MIXTURE

Mineral supplement in synthetic diets.

METHIONINE - FREE AMINO ACID MIX

Homocystinuria or hypermethioninaemia

METHIONINE, THREONINE & VALINE FREE, ISOLEUCINE-LOW AMINO ACID MIX

Methylmalonic acidaemia or propionic acidaemia

MILUPA LOW-PROTEIN DRINK

Inherited disorders of amino acid metabolism in childhood.

MODULEN IBD

For the sole source of nutrition during the active phase of Crohn's disease, and for nutritional support during the remission phase in patients who are malnourished. Not to be prescribed for any child under one year; use with caution for young children up to five years of age.

LIST A cont

MONOGEN

> Long chain acyl-CoA dehydrogenase deficiency (LCAD), carnitine palmitoyl transferase deficiency (CPTD), and primary and secondary lipoprotein lipase deficiency.

MSUD AID III

> Maple syrup urine disease (MSUD) and related conditions when it is necessary to limit the intake of branched chain amino acids

MSUD MAXAMAID
MSUD MAXAMUM

> Maple syrup urine disease

NEOCATE

> Proven whole protein intolerance, short bowel syndrome, intractable malabsorption, and other gastrointestinal disorders where an elemental diet is specifically indicated.

NEOCATE ADVANCE

> Proven whole protein intolerance, short bowel syndrome, intractable malabsorption, and other gastrointestinal disorders where an elemental diet is specifically indicated.

NEPRO

> Patients with chronic renal failure who are on haemodialysis or complete ambulatory peritoneal dialysis (CAPD), or patients with cirrhosis or other conditions requiring a high energy, low fluid, low electrolyte diet.

NESTARGEL

> Thickening of foods in the treatment of vomiting.

NOVASOURCE GI CONTROL (formerly Sandosource GI Control)

> For use as the sole source of nutrition, or as a necessary nutritional supplement prescribed on medical grounds for:
> Short bowel syndrome, intractable malabsorption, pre-operative preparation of patients who are undernourished, patients with proven inflammatary bowel disease, following total gastrectomy, dysphagia, bowel fistulae, disease-related malnutrition. Not to be prescribed for any child under one year, use with caution for young children up to five years of age.

NUTILIS

> Thickening of foods in dysphagia. Not to be prescribed for children under one year old except in cases of failure to thrive.

NUTRAMIGEN

> Disaccharide and/or whole protein intolerance where additional MCT is not indicated

NUTRICIA INFATRINI

> Disease-related malnutrition, malabsorption, and growth failure in infancy.

XV

LIST A cont

NUTRINI (formerly NUTRISON PAEDIATRIC)

For use as the sole source of nutrition or as a necessary nutritional supplement prescribed on medical grounds for:
Short bowel syndrome, intractable malabsorption, pre-operative preparation of patients who are undernourished, dysphagia, bowel fistulae, disease-related malnutrition and/or growth failure. Not to be prescribed for any child under one year.

NUTRINI EXTRA (formerly NUTRISON PAEDIATRIC ENERGY PLUS)

For use as the sole source of nutrition or as a necessary nutritional supplement prescribed on medical grounds for:
Disease-related malnutrition and growth failure.

NUTRINI FIBRE

For use as the sole source of nutrition, or as a necessary nutritional supplement prescribed on medical grounds for:
Short bowel syndrome, intractable malabsorption, pre-operative preparation of patients who are undernourished, patients with proven inflammatory bowel disease, following total gastrectomy, dysphagia, bowel fistulae, disease-related malnutrition. Not to be prescribed for any child under one year.

NUTRISON ENERGY (formerly NUTRISON ENERGY PLUS)

As a necessary nutritional supplement prescribed on medical grounds for:
Short bowel syndrome, intractable malabsorption, pre-operative preparation of patients who are undernourished, patients with proven inflammatory bowel disease, following total gastrectomy, dysphagia, bowel fistulae, disease-related malnutrition. Not to be prescribed for any child under one year; use with caution for young children up to five years of age.

NUTRISON ENERGY PLUS

See: Nutrison Energy

NUTRISON FIBRE

See: Nutrison Multifibre

NUTRISON MCT (formerly LIQUISORBON MCT)

As a necessary nutritional supplement prescribed on medical grounds for:
Short bowel syndrome, intractable malabsorption, pre-operative preparation of patients who are undernourished, patients with proven inflammatory bowel disease, following total gastrectomy, dysphagia, bowel fistulae, disease-related malnutrition. Not to be prescribed for any child under one year; use with caution for young children up to five years of age.

NUTRISON MULTIFIBRE (formerly NUTRISON FIBRE)

For use as the sole source of nutrition or as a necessary nutritional supplement prescribed on medical grounds for:
Short bowel syndrome, intractable malabsorption, pre-operative preparation of patients who are undernourished, patients with proven inflammatory bowel disease, following total gastrectomy, dysphagia, bowel fistulae, disease-related malnutrition. Not to be prescribed for any child under one year; use with caution for young children up to five years of age.

NUTRISON PAEDIATRIC

See: Nutrini

NUTRISON PAEDIATRIC ENERGY PLUS

See: Nutrini Extra

LIST A cont

NUTRISON PEPTI (formerly PEPTI 2000 LF LIQUID AND PEPTI 2000 LF POWDER)

For use as the sole source of nutrition or as a necessary nutritional supplement prescribed on medical grounds for:
Short bowel syndrome, intractable malabsorption, patients with proven inflammatory bowel disease, bowel fistulae. Not to be prescribed for any child under one year; use with caution for young children up to five years of age.

NUTRISON SOYA

For use as the sole source of nutrition or as a necessary nutritional supplement prescribed on medical grounds for:
Short bowel syndrome, intractable malabsorption, pre-operative preparation of patients who are undernourished, patients with proven inflammatory bowel disease, following total gastrectomy, dysphagia, bowel fistulae, disease-related malnutrition, cows milk protein and lactose intolerance. Not to be prescribed for any child under one year; use with caution for young children up to five years of age.

NUTRISON STANDARD

For use as the sole source of nutrition or as a necessary nutritional supplement prescribed on medical grounds for:
Short bowel syndrome, intractable malabsorption, pre-operative preparation of patients who are undernourished, patients with proven inflammatory bowel disease, following total gastrectomy, dysphagia, bowel fistulae, disease-related malnutrition. Not to be prescribed for any child under one year; use with caution for young children up to five years of age.

NUTRODRIP ENERGY
NUTRODRIP FIBRE
NUTRODRIP STANDARD

See: Isosource Energy
          Isosource Fibre
          Isosource Standard

ORALBALANCE DRY MOUTH SALIVA REPLACEMENT GEL

Patients suffering from a dry mouth as a result of having or having undergone radiotherapy or sicca syndrome.

ORGRAN GLUTEN-FREE PRODUCTS

See: Gluten-Free Products

OSMOLITE

For use as the sole source of nutrition or as a necessary nutritional supplement prescribed on medical grounds for:
Short bowel syndrome, intractable malabsorption, pre-operative preparation of patients who are undernourished, patients with proven inflammatory bowel disease, following total gastrectomy, dysphagia, bowel fistulae, disease-related malnutrition. Not to be prescribed for any child under one year; use with caution for young children up to five years of age.

OSMOLITE PLUS

For use as the sole source of nutrition or as a necessary nutritional supplement prescribed on medical grounds for:
Short bowel syndrome, intractable malabsorption, pre-operative preparation of patients who are undernourished, patients with proven inflammatory bowel disease, following total gastrectomy, dysphagia, bowel fistulae, disease-related malnutrition. Not recommended for any child under ten years of age.

XV

LIST A cont

PAEDIASURE

For use as the sole source of nutrition or as a necessary nutritional supplement prescribed on medical grounds for:
Short bowel syndrome, intractable malabsorption, pre-operative preparation of patients who are undernourished, dysphagia, bowel fistulae, disease-related malnutrition and/or growth failure. Not to be prescribed for any child under one year.

PAEDIASURE PLUS

For use as the sole source of nutrition, or as a necessary nutritional supplement prescribed on medical grounds for: short bowel syndrome, intractable malasorption, pre-operative preparation of patients who are undernourished, dysphagia, bowel fistulae, disease-related malnutrition, and/or growth failure. Not to be prescribed for any child under one year.

PAEDIASURE WITH FIBRE

For use as the sole source of nutrition, or as a necessary nutritional supplement prescribed on medical grounds for: short bowel syndrome, intractable malasorption, pre-operative preparation of patients who are undernourished, dysphagia, bowel fistulae, disease-realted malnutrition, and/or growth failure. Not to be precribed for any child under one year.

PAEDIATRIC SERAVIT

Vitamin and mineral supplement in restrictive therapeutic diets in infants and children.

PEPDITE 0-2
PEPDITE 2 +

Disaccharide and/or whole protein intolerance, or where amino acids or peptides are indicated in conjunction with MCT.

PEPTAMEN (FLAVOURED AND UNFLAVOURED)

For use as the sole source of nutrition or as a necessary nutritional supplement prescribed on medical grounds for:
Short bowel syndrome, intractable malabsorption, patients with proven inflammatory bowel disease, bowel fistulae. Not to be prescribed for any child under one year; use with caution for young children up to five years of age.

PEPTAMEN FLAVOUR SACHETS

For use with VANILLA-FLAVOURED PEPTAMEN

PEPTI 2000 LF LIQUID
PEPTI 2000 LF POWDER

See: Nutrison Pepti

PEPTI - JUNIOR

Disaccharide and/or whole protein intolerance, or where amino acids and peptides are indicated in conjunction with MCT.

PERATIVE

As a necessary nutritional supplement prescribed on medical grounds for:
Short bowel syndrome, intractable malabsorption, pre-operative preparation of patients who are undernourished, patients with proven inflammatory bowel disease, following total gastrectomy, bowel fistulae, disease-related malnutrition. Not to be prescribed for any child under five years of age.

LIST A cont

PHENYLALANINE, TYROSINE & METHIONINE-FREE AMINO ACID MIX

See: XPTM Tyrosidon

PHLEXY-10 EXCHANGE SYSTEM (BAR, CAPSULES AND DRINK MIX)

Phenylketonuria

PHLEXYVITS

For use as a vitamin and mineral component of restricted therapeutic diets for older children, from the age of around eleven years, and adults with phenylketonuria and similar amino acid abnormalities.

PIZ BUIN SUN BLOCK LOTION SPF 20

Protection from UV radiation in abnormal cutaneous photosensitivity resulting from genetic disorders or photodermatoses, including vitiligo and those resulting from radiotherapy; chronic or recurrent herpes simplex labialis.

PK AID 4 (formerly PK AID III)

Phenylketonuria.

PKU 2 (MILUPA)

Phenylketonuria

PKU 3 (MILUPA)

Phenylketonuria (not normally to be prescribed for a child below about 8 months old.)

PLENIDAY GLUTEN-FREE PRODUCTS

See: Gluten-Free Products

POLIAL GLUTEN-FREE PRODUCTS

See: Gluten-Free Products.

POLYCAL LIQUID
POLYCAL POWDER

Disease related malnutrition, malabsorption states or other conditions requiring fortification with a high or readily available carbohydrate supplement.

POLYCOSE POWDER

Disease related malnutrition, malabsorption states or other conditions requiring fortification with a high or readily available carbohydrate supplement.

XV

PREGESTIMIL

Disaccharide and/or whole protein intolerance, or where amino acids or peptides are indicated in conjunction with MCT.

PREJOMIN (MILUPA)

Disaccharide and/or whole protein intolerance where additional MCT is not indicated

LIST A cont

PRINTANIA

As a necessary nutritional supplement prescribed on medical grounds for:
Short bowel syndrome, intractable malabsorption, pre-operative preparation of patients who are undernourished, patients with proven inflammatory bowel disease, following total gastrectomy, dysphagia, bowel fistulae, disease-related malnutrition. Not to be prescribed for any child under one year; use with caution for young children up to five years of age.

PRO-CAL

Disease-related malnutrition, malabsorption states or other conditions requiring fortification with a fat/carbohydrate supplement. Not to be prescribed for any child under one year; use with caution for young children up to five years of age.

PROMIN LOW-PROTEIN PRODUCTS

See: Low-Protein Products

PRO-MOD

Biochemically proven hypoproteinaemia.

PROSOBEE LIQUID AND POWDER

Proven lactose and associated sucrose intolerance in pre-school children, glactokinase deficiency, galactosaemia and proven whole cows milk sensitivity.

PROTEIN FORTE

See: Protenplus

PROTENPLUS (formerly PROTEIN FORTE)

As a necessary nutritional supplement prescribed on medical grounds for:
Short bowel syndrome, intractable malabsorption, pre-operative preparation of patients who are undernourished, patients with proven inflammatory bowel disease, following total gastrectomy, dysphagia, bowel fistulae, disease-related malnutrition, continuous ambulatory peritoneal dialysis (CAPD) and haemodialysis. Not to be prescribed for any child under one year; use with caution for young children up to five years of age.

PROTIFAR

Biochemically proven hypoproteinaemia.

PROVIDE XTRA

As a necessary nutritional supplement prescribed on medical grounds for:
Short bowel syndrome, intractable malabsorption, pre-operative preparation of patients who are undernourished, patients with proven inflammatory bowel disease, following total gastrectomy, dysphagia, bowel fistulae, disease-related malnutrition. Not to be prescribed for any child under one year; use with caution for young children up to five years of age.

QUICKCAL

Disease-related malnutrition, malabsorption states or other conditions requiring fortification with a fat/carbohydrate supplement. Not to be prescribed for any child under one year; use with caution for young children up to five years of age.

RECTIFIED SPIRIT

Where the therapeutic qualities of alcohol are required rectified spirit (suitably flavoured and diluted) should be prescribed.

LIST A cont

RENAMIL

Chronic renal failure. Not suitable for infants and young children under one year of age.

RENAPRO

Dialysis and hypoproteinaemia. Not suitable for infants and children under one year of age.

RESOURCE BENEFIBER

As a necessary nutritional supplement prescribed on medical grounds for:
Short bowel syndrome, intractable malabsorption, pre-operative preparation of patients who are undernourished, patients with proven inflammatory bowel disease, following total gastrectomy, bowel fistulae, disease-related malnutrition. Not to be prescribed for any child under five yeas of age.

RESOURCE SHAKE NUTRITIONAL SUPPLEMENT

As a necessary nutritional supplement prescribed on medical grounds for:
Disease-related malnutrition, short bowel syndrome, intractable malabsorption, proven inflammatory bowel disease, bowel fistalae, dysphagia. May also be used for pre-operative preparation of undernourished patients and after total gastrectomy.

RESOURCE THICKENUP WITHOUT VITAMINS AND MINERALS

Thickening of foods in dysphagia. Not to be prescribed for children under three years of age.

RESOURCE THICKENED SQUASH AND RESOURCE READY THICKENED DRINKS

Dyphagia. Not suitable for infants and children under one year of age.

RITE-DIET GLUTEN-FREE AND LOW-PROTEIN PRODUCTS

See: Gluten-Free and Low-Protein Products.

ROC TOTAL SUNBLOCK CREAM SPF 25

Protection from UV radiation in abnormal cutaneous photosensitivity resulting from genetic disorders or photodermatoses, including vitiligo and those resulting from radiotherapy; chronic or recurrent herpes simplex labialis.

RVHB MAXAMAID

See: XMET MAXAMAID

RVHB MAXAMUM

See: XMET MAXAMUM

SALIVA ORTHANA
SALIVACE
SALIVEZE
SALIVIX PASTILLES

XV

Patients suffering from a dry mouth as a result of having or having undergone radiotherapy or sicca syndrome.

SANDOSOURCE GI CONTROL

See: Novasource GI Control

SCANDISHAKE MIX FLAVOURED AND UNFLAVOURED

Disease related malnutrition, malabsorption states or other conditions requiring fortification with a fat/carbohydrate supplement.

LIST A cont

SCHAR GLUTEN-FREE PRODUCTS

  See: Gluten-Free Products

SHS FLAVOUR MODJUL

  For use with any unflavoured product based on peptides or amino acids

SHS FLAVOUR SACHETS

  For use with SHS unflavoured amino acid and peptide based products

SMA HIGH ENERGY

  Disease-related malnutrition, malabsorption and growth failure in infancy.

SMA LF

  Proven lactose intolerance

SNO-PRO DRINK

  Phenylketonuria, chronic renal failure, and other inborn errors of metabolism.

SONDALIS 1.5 LIQUID FEED
SONDALIS FIBRELIQUID FEED
SONDALIS ISO LIQUID FEED

  For use as the sole source of nutrition or as necessary nutritional supplements prescribed on medical grounds
  for:
  Short bowel syndrome, intractable malabsorption, pre-operative preparation of patients who are
  undernourished, patients with proven inflammatory bowel disease, following total gastrectomy, dysphagia,
  bowel fistulae, disease-related malnutrition.
  Not to be prescribed for any child under one year; use with caution for young children up to five years of age.

SONDALIS JUNIOR

For use as the sole source of nutrition, or as a necessary nutritional supplement prescribed on medical grounds
for:
Short bowel syndrome, intractable malabsorption, pre-operative preparation of patients who are undernourished,
patients with proven inflammatory bowel disease, following total gastrectomy, dysphagia, bowel fistulae, disease-
related malnutrition, growth failure in children aged 1-6 years. Not to be prescribed for any child under one year.

SPECTRABAN 25
SPECTRABAN ULTRA

  Protection from UV radiation in abnormal cutaneous photosensitivity resulting from genetic disorders or
  photodermatoses, including vitiligo and those resulting from radiotherapy; chronic or recurrent herpes simplex
  labialis.

SPS ENERGY BAR

  Disease related malnutrition, malabsorption states or other conditions requiring fortification with a
  fat/carbohydrate supplement.

SUN E45 LOTION SPF 15 and SPF 25
SUN E45 50 SUNBLOCK LOTION

  See: E45 Sun Lotion SPF 15 and SPF 25
        E45 Sun 50 Sunblock Lotion

LIST A con

SUNNYVALE PRODUCTS

　　See: Gluten-Free Products

SUPLENA LIQUID NUTRITION

　　Patients with chronic or acute renal failure who are not undergoing dialysis; patients with chronic or acute liver disease with fluid restriction; other conditions requiring a high energy, low protein, low electrolyte, low volume enteral feed.

SURVIMED OPD (formerly FRESENIUS OPD)

　　As a necessary nutritional supplement prescribed on medical grounds for:
　　Short bowel syndrome, intractable malabsorption, pre-operative preparation of patients who are undernourished, patients with proven inflammatory bowel disease, following total gastrectomy, dysphagia, bowel fistulae, disease-related malnutrition and/or growth failure. Not to be prescribed for any child under one year; use with caution for young children up to five years of age.

THICK AND EASY
THIXO-D

　　Thickening of foods in dysphagia. Not to be prescribed for children under one year old except in cases of failure to thrive.

TINKYADA GLUTEN-FREE PRODUCTS

　　See: Gluten-Free Products

TRITAMYL PRODUCTS

　　See: Gluten-Free Products

TRUFREE GLUTEN-FREE PRODUCTS

　　See: Gluten-Free Products.

TYROSINE & PHENYLALANINE - FREE AMINO ACID MIX

　　See: XPT Tyrosidon

ULTRA GLUTEN-FREE AND LOW-PROTEIN PRODUCTS

　　See: Gluten-Free and Low-Protein Products

UVISTAT SUNBLOCK CREAM FACTOR 20
UVISTAT ULTRABLOCK SUNCREAM FACTOR 30

　　Protection from UV radiation in abnormal cutaneous photosensitivity resulting from genetic disorders or photodermatoses, including vitiligo and those resulting from radiotherapy; chronic or recurrent herpes simplex labialis.

XV

VALPIFORM GLUTEN-FREE AND LOW-PROTEIN PRODUCTS

　　See: Gluten-Free and Low-Protein Products

VASELINE DERMACARE CREAM
VASELINE DERMACARE LOTION

　　Endogenous and exogenous eczema, xeroderma, icthyosis and senile pruritis associated with dry skin.

LIST A cont

VEIL COVER CREAM
VEIL FINISHING POWDER

See: Covering Creams

VITAMIN & MINERAL PREPARATIONS

Only in the management of actual or potential vitamin or mineral deficiency; not to be prescribed as dietary supplements or "pick-me-ups".

VITAJOULE

Disease related malnutrition, malabsorption states or other conditions requiring fortification with a high or readily available carbohydrate supplement.

VITAPRO

Biochemically proven hypoproteinaemia.

VITAQUICK

Thickening of foods in dysphagia. Not to be prescribed for children under one year old except in cases of failure to thrive.

VITASAVOURY

Disease-related malnutritition, malabsorption states or other conditions requiring fortification with a fat/carbohydrate supplement. Not to be prescribed for any child under one year; use with caution for young children up to five years of age.

WASH E45

See: E45 Emollient Wash Oil

WYSOY

Proven lactose and associated sucrose intolerance in pre-school children, galactokinase deficiency, galactosaemia and proven whole cows milk sensitivity.

XLEU ANALOG
XLEU MAXAMAID

Isovaleric acidaemia

XLYS MAXAMAID

Hyperlysinaemia

XLYS, TRY LOW ANALOG

Type 1 glutaric aciduria

XLYS LOW TRY MAXAMAID

Glutaric aciduria

XMET MAXAMAID (formerly RVHB MAXAMAID)
XMET MAXAMUM (formerly RVHB MAXAMUM)

Hypermethioninaemia, homocystinuria

LIST A cont

XMET, THRE, VAL, ISOLEU MAXAMAID
XMET, THRE, VAL, ISOLEU MAXAMUM

    Methylmalonic acidaemia and propionic acidaemia

XP MAXAMAID & XP MAXAMAID ORANGE
XP MAXAMAID CONCENTRATE

    Phenylketonuria

XP MAXAMUM (ORANGE AND UNFLAVOURED)

    Phenylketonuria. Not to be prescribed for children under 8 years old

XPHEN, TYR MAXAMAID

    Tyrosinaemia

XPT TYROSIDON (formerly Tyrosine and Phenylalanine-Free Amino Acid Mix)

    Tyrosinaemia where plasma methionine levels are normal

XPTM TYROSIDON (formerly Phenylalanine, Tyrosine and Methionine-Free Amino Acid Mix)

    Tyrosinaemia type 1 where plasma levels are above normal

XV

LIST B

AMINO ACID METABOLIC DISORDERS AND SIMILAR PROTEIN DISORDERS

   Histidinaemia
   Homocystinuria
   Low-Protein Products
   Maple Syrup Urine Disease
   Phenylketonuria
   Synthetic Diets
   Tyrosinaemia

BIRTHMARKS

 See: Disfiguring Skin Lesions

BOWEL FISTULAE

   Clinifeed 1.0
   Clinifeed 1.5
   Clinifeed Fibre
   Clinifeed ISO
   Clinutren Dessert (as a supplement)
   Clinutren 1.5 (as a supplement)
   Clinutren ISO (as a supplement)
   Complan Ready-to-drink
   Elemental 028
   Elemental 028 Extra
   Elemental 028 Extra (Liquid)
   Emsogen
   Enlive (as a supplement)
   Enrich
   Enrich Plus
   Ensure
   Ensure Plus (as a supplement)
   Ensure Powder
   Entera
   Entera Fibre Plus Sip Feed
   Entera Fibre Plus (Neutral) Tube Feed
   Formance (as a supplement)
   Forticreme (as a supplement)
   Fortifresh
   Fortijuce (as a supplement)
   Fortimel (as a supplement)
   Fortisip (as a supplement)
   Fortisip Multifibre (as a supplement)
   Frebini
   Fresubin Liquid and Sip Feeds
   Fresubin 750 MCT (as a supplement)
   Isosource Energy
   Isosource Fibre
   Isosource Standard
   Jevity
   Jevity Plus
   Modulen IBD
   Novasource GI Control
   Nutrini
   Nutrini Fibre

This is a cross index listing clinical conditions and the products which the ACBS has approved for the management of those conditions. It is essential to consult LIST A for more precise guidance.

BOWEL FISTULAE - cont

Nutrison Energy (as a supplement)
Nutrison MCT (as a supplement)
Nutrison Multifibre
Nutrison Pepti
Nutrison Standard
Osmolite
Osmolite Plus
Paediasure
Paediasure Plus
Paediasure with Fibre
Peptamen
Perative (as a supplement)
Printania (as a supplement)
Protenplus (as a supplement)
Provide Xtra (as a supplement)
Resource Benefiber (as a supplement)
Resource Shake Nutritional Supplement
Sondalis 1.5 Liquid Feed
Sondalis Fibre Liquid Feed
Sondalis Iso Liquid Feed
Sondalis Junior
Survimed OPD (as a supplement)

CALCIUM INTOLERANCE

Locasol

CARBOHYDRATE MALABSORPTION for definition of lactose or sucrose intolerance, see page 427

Calogen
Pro-Cal
QuickCal
Vitasavoury
See: Synthetic Diets
Malabsorption States

a)   Disaccharide intolerance (without isomaltose intolerance)

Alfare
Caloreen
Duocal (Liquid and Super Soluble)
Maxijul LE
Maxijul Liquid
Maxijul Super Soluble
Nutramigen
Nutrison Soya
Pepdite 0-2
Pepdite 2 +
Pepti-Junior
Polycal (Liquid & Powder)
Polycose Powder
Pregestimil
Prejomin

XV

This is a cross index listing clinical conditions and the products which the ACBS has approved for the management of those conditions. It is essential to consult LIST A for more precise guidance.

LIST B cont

CARBOHYDRATE MALABSORPTION - cont

         Pro-Cal
         QuickCal
         Vitajoule
         Vitasavoury
See: Lactose intolerance
         Lactose with associated sucrose intolerance

b)   <u>Isomaltose intolerance</u>

         Glucose

c)   <u>Glucose + galactose intolerance</u>

         Comminuted Chicken Meat (SHS)
         Fructose
         Galactomin 19 (Fructose Formula)

d)   <u>Lactose intolerance</u>

         AL110 (Nestle)
         Comminuted Chicken Meat (SHS)
         Enfamil Lacto free
         Farley's Soya Formula
         Galactomin 17
         Infasoy
         Isomil Powder
         Nutramigen
         Nutrison Soya
         Pepdite 0-2
         Pepdite 2 +
         Pregestimil
         Prejomin
         Prosobee liquid and powder
         SMA LF
         Wysoy

e)   <u>Lactose with associated sucrose intolerance</u>

         Comminuted Chicken Meat (SHS)
         Farley's Soya Formula
         Galactomin 17
         Infasoy
         Nutramigen
         Nutrison Soya
         Pepti-Junior
         Pregestimil
         Prejomin
         Prosobee liquid and powder
         Wysoy

This is a cross index listing clinical conditions and the products which the ACBS has approved for the management of those conditions. It is essential to consult LIST A for more precise guidance.

LIST B cont

CARBOHYDRATE MALABSORPTION - cont

f)   <u>Sucrose intolerance</u>

        Glucose (dextrose)
See: Synthetic Diets
        Malabsorption
        Lactose with associated sucrose intolerance

CARNITINE PALMITOYL TRANSFERASE DEFICIENCY (CPTD)

        Monogen

COELIAC DISEASE
See: Gluten-Sensitive Enteropathies

CONTINUOUS AMBULATORY PERITONEAL DIALYSIS (CAPD)
See: Dialysis

CYSTIC FIBROSIS
See: Malabsorption

DERMATITIS

        Aveeno Bath Oil
        Aveeno Colloidal
        Aveeno Colloidal Baby
        Aveeno Cream
        E45 Emollient Bath Oil
        E45 Emollient Wash Cream
        E45 Lotion
        Vaseline Dermacare Cream
        Vaseline Dermacare Lotion

DERMATITIS HERPETIFORMIS

See: Gluten-Sensitive Enteropathies.

DIALYSIS

Nutritional Supplements for Haemodialysis or Continuous Ambulatory Peritoneal Dialysis
(CAPD) patients.

        Clinutren Dessert
        Clinutren 1.5
        Clinutren ISO
        Enrich Plus
        Ensure Plus
        Formance
        Forticreme
        Fresubin 750 MCT
        Kindergen P.R.O.D.
        Nepro
        Protenplus
        Renapro
        Suplena

XV

This is a cross index listing clinical conditions and the products which the ACBS has approved for the management of those conditions. It is essential to consult LIST A for more precise guidance.

LIST B cont

DISACCHARIDE INTOLERANCE

See: Carbohydrate malabsorption

DISFIGURING SKIN LESIONS (BIRTHMARKS, MUTILATING LESIONS, AND SCARS)

Covermark Classic Foundation
Covermark Finishing Powder
Dermablend Cover Creme
Dermablend Leg and Body Cover
Dermablend Setting Powder
Dermacolor Camouflage Cream
Dermacolor Fixing Powder
Keromask Finishing Powder
Keromask Masking Cream
Veil Cover Cream
Veil Finishing Powder

DYSPHAGIA for definition, see page 427
Clinifeed 1.0
Clinifeed 1.5
Clinifeed Fibre
Clinifeed ISO
Clinutren 1.5 (as a supplement)
Clinutren Dessert (as a supplement)
Clinutren ISO (as a supplement)
Complan Ready-to-drink
Enfamil AR
Enlive (as a supplement)
Enrich
Enrich Plus
Ensure
Ensure Plus (as a supplement)
Ensure Powder
Entera
Entera Fibre Plus Sip Feed
Entera Fibre Plus (Neutral) Tube Feed
Formance (as a supplement)
Forticreme (as a supplement)
Fortifresh
Fortijuce (as a supplement)
Fortimel (as a supplement)
Fortisip (as a supplement)
Fortisip Multifibre (as a supplement)
Frebini
Fresubin Isofibre
Fresubin Liquid and Sip Feeds
Fresubin 750 MCT (as a supplement)
Isosource Energy
Isosource Fibre
Isosource Standard
Jevity
Jevity Plus
Modulen IBD
Novasource GI Control
Nutilis (as a thickener)

This is a cross index listing clinical conditions and the products which the ACBS has approved for the management of those conditions. It is essential to consult LIST A for more precise guidance.

LIST B cont

DYSPHAGIA - cont

> Nutrini
> Nutrini Fibre
> Nutrison Energy (as a supplement)
> Nutrison. MCT (as a supplement)
> Nutrison Multifibre
> Nutrison Soya
> Nutrison Standard
> Osmolite
> Osmolite Plus
> Paediasure
> Paediasure Plus
> Paediasure with Fibre
> Printania (as a supplement)
> Protenplus (as a supplement)
> Provide Xtra (as a supplement)
> Resource Benefiber
> Resource Shake Nutritional Supplement
> Resource ThickenUp without Vitamins and Minerals
> Resource Thickened Squash and Resource Ready Thickened Drinks
> Sondalis 1.5 Liquid Feed
> Sondalis Fibre Liquid Feed
> Sondalis ISO Liquid Feed
> Sondalis Junior
> Survimed OPD (as a supplement)
> Thick and Easy (as a thickener)
> Thixo-D (as a thickener)
> Vitaquick (as a thickener)

ECZEMA

See: Dermatitis

EPILEPSY (KETOGENIC DIET IN)

> Alembicol D
> Liquigen
> Medium-chain triglyceride oil (MCT)

FLAVOURING FOR USE WITH ANY UNFLAVOURED PRODUCT BASED ON PEPTIDES
OR AMINO ACIDS

> SHS Flavour Modjul
> SHS Flavour Sachet

GALACTOKINASE DEFICIENCY AND GALACTOSAEMIA

> AL110 (Nestle)
> Farley's Soya Formula
> Galactomin 17
> Infasoy
> Isomil Powder
> Prosobee Liquid and Powder
> Wysoy

XV

This is a cross index listing clinical conditions and the products which the ACBS has approved for the management of those conditions. It is essential to consult LIST A for more precise guidance.

LIST B cont

GASTRECTOMY (TOTAL)

Clinifeed 1.0
Clinifeed 1.5
Clinifeed Fibre
Clinifeed ISO
Clinutren 1.5 (as a supplement)
Clinutren Dessert (as a supplement)
Clinutren ISO (as a supplement)
Complan Ready-to-drink
Enlive (as a supplement)
Enrich
Enrich Plus
Ensure
Ensure Bar
Ensure Plus (as a supplement)
Ensure Powder
Entera
Entera Fibre Plus Sip Feed
Entera Fibre Plus (Neutral) Tube Feed
Formance (as a supplement)
Forticreme (as a supplement)
Fortifresh
Fortijuce (as a supplement)
Fortimel (as a supplement)
Fortisip Multifibre (as a supplement)
Fortisip (as a supplement)
Frebini
Fresubin Isofibre
Fresubin Liquid and Sip Feeds
Fresubin 750 MCT (as a supplement)
Isosource Energy
Isosource Fibre
Isosource Standard
Jevity
Jevity Plus
Modulen IBD
Novasource GI Control
Nutrini Fibre
Nutrison Energy (as a supplement)
Nutrison MCT (as a supplement)
Nutrison Multifibre
Nutrison Soya
Nutrison Standard
Osmolite
Osmolite Plus
Perative (as a supplement)
Printania (as a supplement)
Protenplus (as a supplement)
Provide Xtra (as a supplement)
Resource Benefiber
Resource Shake Nutritional Supplement
Sondalis 1.5 Liquid Feed
Sondalis Fibre Liquid Feed
Sondalis ISO Liquid Feed
Sondalis Junior
Survimed OPD (as a supplement)

This is a cross index listing clinical conditions and the products which the ACBS has approved for the management of those conditions. It is essential to consult LIST A for more precise guidance.

LIST B cont

GLUCOSE/GALACTOSE INTOLERANCE

Comminuted Chicken Meat (SHS)
Galactomin 19 (Fructose Formula)
See: Carbohydrate Malabsorption

GLUTARIC ACIDURIA

XYLS, TRY Low Analog
XYLS LOW TRY Maxamaid

GLUTEN-SENSITIVE ENTEROPATHIES

Aproten gluten-free flour
Arnott's gluten-free rice cookies
Bar-Kat brown rice pizza crust
Bar-Kat gluten-free bread mix
Bar-Kat gluten-free brown rice bread
Bar-Kat gluten-free white rice bread
Bar-Kat white rice pizza crust
Bi-Aglut gluten-free biscuits
Bi-Aglut gluten-free cracker toast
Bi-Aglut gluten-free crackers
Bi-Aglut gluten-free pastas (fusilli, lasagne, macaroni, penne, spaghetti)
Clara's Kitchen gluten-free bread mix
Clara's Kitchen gluten-free high fibre bread mix
Dietary Specialties gluten-free (brown bread mix, corn bread mix, fibre mix, pizza bases, white
     bread mix, white cake mix, white mix)
Ener-G gluten-free brown rice bread
Ener-G gluten free brown rice and maize bread
Ener-G gluten-free brown rice pasta (lasagna, macaroni, spaghetti)
Ener-G gluten-free rice loaf
Ener-G gluten-free rice pasta (cannelloni, lasagna, macaroni, shells, small shells, spaghetti,
     tagliatelle, vermicelli)
Ener-G gluten-free tapioca bread
Ener-G gluten-free white rice bread
Glutafin gluten-free biscuits
Glutafin gluten-free cake mix
Glutafin gluten-free crackers
Glutafin gluten-free digestive biscuits
Glutafin gluten-free fibre loaf (sliced and unsliced)
Glutafin gluten-free fibre mix
Glutafin gluten-free high fibre crackers
Glutafin gluten-free loaf (sliced and unsliced)
Glutafin gluten-free multigrain fibre bread (sliced and unsliced)
Glutafin gluten-free multigrain fibre mix
Glutafin gluten-free multigrain fibre rolls
Glutafin gluten-free multigrain white bread (formerly Glutafin gluten-free
     white bread loaf (sliced and unsliced))
Glutafin gluten-free multigrain white mix
Glutafin gluten-free part-baked fibre loaf
Glutafin gluten-free part-baked fibre rolls
Glutafin gluten-free part-baked rolls
Glutafin gluten-free part-baked white loaf
Glutafin gluten-free pasta (lasagne, long-cut spaghetti, macaroni penne, shells, spirals, tagliatelle
     nests)
Glutafin gluten-free pastry mix

XV

This is a cross index listing clinical conditions and the products which the ACBS has approved for the management
of those conditions. It is essential to consult LIST A for more precise guidance.

LIST B cont

GLUTEN-SENSITIVE ENTEROPATHIES - cont

   Glutafin gluten-free pizza base
   Glutafin gluten-free savoury biscuits
   Glutafin gluten-free sweet biscuits (without chocolate or sultanas)
   Glutafin gluten-free tea biscuits
   Glutafin gluten-free multigrain white rolls (formerly Glutafin gluten-free wheat-free white bread rolls)
   Glutafin gluten-free white bread (canned) with added soya bran
   Glutafin gluten-free white mix
   Glutano gluten-free biscuits
   Glutano gluten-free crackers
   Glutano gluten-free flour mix
   Glutano gluten-free par-baked (baguette, rolls, white sliced bread)
   Glutano gluten-free pasta (animal shapes, macaroni, spaghetti, spirals, tagliatelle)
   Glutano gluten-free wholemeal bread (sliced)
   Glutano gluten-free wholemeal par-baked bread
   Gratis gluten-free pasta (alphabets, macaroni, shells, short cut
      spaghetti, spirals)
   Juvela gluten-free bread rolls
   Juvela gluten-free crispbread
   Juvela gluten-free digestive biscuits
   Juvela gluten-free fibre bread rolls
   Juvela gluten-free fibre loaf (sliced and unsliced)
   Juvela gluten-free fibre mix
   Juvela gluten-free Harvest mix
   Juvela gluten-free loaf (sliced and unsliced)
   Juvela gluten-free mix
   Juvela gluten-free part-baked bread rolls
   Juvela gluten-free part-baked fibre loaf
   Juvela gluten-free part-baked loaf
   Juvela gluten-free pizza base
   Juvela gluten-free savoury biscuits
   Juvela gluten-free sweet biscuits
   Juvela gluten-free tea biscuits
   Lifestyle gluten-free bread rolls
   Lifestyle gluten-free brown bread
   Lifestyle gluten-free high fibre bread
   Lifestyle gluten-free high fibre bread rolls
   Lifestyle gluten-free white bread
   Liga gluten-free rusks (Jacobs)
   Orgran gluten-free buckwheat spirals pasta
   Orgran gluten-free corn lasagne, corn spaghetti, corn spirals pasta
   Orgran gluten-free crispbread corn, crispbread rice
   Orgran gluten-free organic brown rice spirals
   Orgran gluten-free pizza & pastry mix
   Orgran gluten-free rice spaghetti, rice spirals
   Orgran gluten-free rice and millet spirals
   Orgran gluten-free ris o'mais (rice and maize) lasagne, ris o'mais spaghetti, ris o'mais spirals
   Orgran gluten-free split pea & soya pasta shells
   Pleniday gluten-free bread (sliced country loaf, petit pain (par baked), rustic loaf sliced)
   Pleniday gluten-free pasta (penne, rigate)
   Polial gluten-free biscuits
   Rite-Diet gluten-free fibre mix
   Rite-Diet gluten-free fibre rolls
   Rite-Diet gluten-free high fibre bread (sliced and unsliced)
   Rite-Diet gluten-free white bread (sliced and unsliced)
   Rite-Diet gluten-free white mix

This is a cross index listing clinical conditions and the products which the ACBS has approved for the management of those conditions. It is essential to consult LIST A for more precise guidance.

LIST B cont

GLUTEN-SENSITIVE ENTEROPATHIES - cont

Rite-Diet gluten-free white rolls
Rite-Diet part-baked fibre loaf
Rite-Diet part-baked long fibre rolls
Rite-Diet part-baked gluten-free fibre loaf
Rite-Diet part-baked gluten-free long fibre rolls
Schar gluten-free biscuits
Schar gluten-free bread
Schar gluten-free bread mix
Schar gluten-free bread rolls
Schar gluten-free cake mix
Schar gluten-free crackers
Schar gluten-free cracker toast
Schar gluten-free crispbread
Schar gluten-free flour mix for cooking
Schar gluten-free french bread (baguette)
Schar gluten-free pasta (alphabet pasta,bavette, fusilli, lasagne, macaroni, pasta rings, pasta shells
    penne, rigati, spaghetti)
Schar gluten-free pizza base
Schar gluten-free savoy biscuits
Schar gluten-free wheat-free bread buns (white)
Schar gluten-free wheat-free lunch rolls
Schar gluten-free wholemeal bread
Schar gluten-free wholemeal flour mix
Sunnyvale gluten-free mixed grain sourdough bread
Tinkyada gluten-free brown rice pastas
Tritamyl gluten-free brown bread mix
Tritamyl gluten-free flour
Tritamyl gluten-free white bread mix
Trufree flour mix no. 1 for loaves
Trufree flour mix no. 4 white for loaves and rolls
Trufree flour mix no. 5 brown for loaves and scones
Trufree flour mix no. 6 white for pastry
Trufree flour mix no. 7 white, self-raising
Ultra gluten-free baguette
Ultra gluten-free bread
Ultra gluten-free bread rolls
Ultra gluten-free crackerbread
Ultra gluten-free high fibre bread
Ultra gluten-free pizza base
Valpiform gluten-free bread mix
Valpiform gluten-free country loaf
Valpiform gluten-free pastry mix
Valpiform gluten-free petites baguettes

GLYCOGEN STORAGE DISEASE

Caloreen
Corn Flour or Corn Starch
Dextrose
Glucose
Maxijul LE
Maxijul Liquid (Orange flavour only)
Maxijul Super Soluble
Polycal (Liquid & Powder)
Polycose Powder

This is a cross index listing clinical conditions and the products which the ACBS has approved for the management
of those conditions. It is essential to consult LIST A for more precise guidance.

LIST B cont

GLYCOGEN STORAGE DISEASE cont

    Pro-Cal
    QuickCal
    Vitajoule
    Vitasavoury

GROWTH FAILURE (DISEASE RELATED)

    Frebini
    Nutrini
    Nutrini Extra
    Paediasure
    Paediasure Plus
    Paediasure with Fibre
    SMA High Energy
    Sondalis Junior
    Survimed OPD

HISTIDINAEMIA

See: Low-Protein Products
          Synthetic Diets

HAEMODIALYSIS

See: Dialysis

HOMOCYSTINURIA

    Analog RVHB
    Methionine-Free Amino Acid Mix
    XMET Maxamaid
    XMET Maxamum
See: Low-Protein Products
          Synthetic Diets

HYPERLIPOPROTEINAEMIA TYPE 1

    Alembicol-D (MCT Oil)
    Liquigen
    Medium chain triglyceride oil

HYPERLYSINAEMIA

    Analog XLYS
    XLYS Maxamaid

HYPERMETHIONINAEMIA

    Analog RVHB
    Methionine-Free Amino Acid Mix
    XMET Maxamaid
    XMET Maxamum

This is a cross index listing clinical conditions and the products which the ACBS has approved for the management of those conditions. It is essential to consult LIST A for more precise guidance.

LIST B cont

HYPOGLYCAEMIA

    Corn Flour or Corn Starch

  See: Glycogen Storage Disease

HYPOPROTEINAEMIA

    Casilan 90
    Dialamine
    Maxipro Super Soluble
    Maxisorb
    Pro-Mod
    Protifar
    Renapro
    Vitapro

INFLAMMATORY BOWEL DISEASE

    Clinifeed 1.0
    Clinifeed 1.5
    Clinifeed Fibre
    Clinifeed ISO
    Clinutren 1.5 (as a supplement)
    Clinutren Dessert (as a supplement)
    Clinutren ISO (as a supplement)
    Complan Ready-to-drink
    Elemental 028
    Elemental 028 Extra
    Elemental 028 Extra (Liquid)
    Emsogen
    Enlive (as a supplement)
    Enrich
    Enrich Plus
    Ensure
    Ensure Bar
    Ensure Plus (as a supplement)
    Ensure Powder
    Entera
    Entera Fibre Plus Sip Feed
    Entera Fibre Plus (Neutral) Tube Feed
    Formance (as a supplement)
    Forticreme (as a supplement)
    Fortijuce (as a supplement)
    Fortifresh
    Fortimel (as a supplement)
    Fortisip (as a supplement)
    Fortisip Multifibre (as a supplement)
    Frebini
    Fresubin Isofibre
    Fresubin Liquid & Sip Feeds
    Fresubin 750 MCT (as a supplement)
    Isosource Energy
    Isosource Fibre
    Isosource Standard
    Jevity
    Jevity Plus

XV

This is a cross index listing clinical conditions and the products which the ACBS has approved for the management of those conditions. It is essential to consult LIST A for more precise guidance.

LIST B cont

INFLAMMATORY BOWEL DISEASE - cont

> Modulen IBD
> Novasource GI Control
> Nutrini Fibre
> Nutrison Energy (as a supplement)
> Nutrison MCT (as a supplement)
> Nutrison Multifibre
> Nutrison Pepti
> Nutrison Soya
> Nutrison Standard
> Osmolite
> Osmolite Plus
> Peptamen
> Perative (as a supplement)
> Printania (as a supplement)
> Protenplus (as a supplement)
> Provide Xtra (as a supplement)
> Resource Benefiber
> Resource Shake Nutritional Supplement
> Sondalis 1.5 Liquid Feed
> Sondalis Fibre Liquid Feed
> Sondalis ISO Liquid Feed
> Sondalis Junior
> Survimed OPD (as a supplement)

INTESTINAL LYMPHANGIECTASIA
INTESTINAL SURGERY
  See: Malabsorption

ISOMALTOSE INTOLERANCE

  See: Carbohydrate Malabsorption

ISOVALERIC ACIDAEMIA

> Leucine Free Amino Acid Mix
> XLEU Analog
> XLEU Maxamaid

LACTOSE INTOLERANCE

  See: Carbohydrate Malabsorption

LIPOPROTEIN LIPASE DEFICIENCY (PRIMARY AND SECONDARY)

> Monogen

LIVER FAILURE

> Aglutella low-protein rice
> Alembicol D
> Aminex low-protein biscuits
> Aminex low-protein cookies
> Aminex low-protein rusks
> Aproten low-protein biscuits
> Aproten low-protein bread mix

This is a cross index listing clinical conditions and the products which the ACBS has approved for the management of those conditions. It is essential to consult LIST A for more precise guidance.

LIST B cont

LIVER FAILURE - cont

    Aproten low-protein cake mix
    Aproten low-protein crispbread
    Aproten low-protein pasta (anellini, ditalini, rigatini, spaghetti, tagliatelle)
    dp low-protein butterscotch and chocolate flavoured chip cookies
    Ener-G low-protein egg replacer
    Ener-G low-protein rice bread
    Fate low-protein cake mix
    Fate low-protein chocolate flavour cake mix
    Fate low-protein flour
    Generaid
    Generaid Plus
    Harifen white chip cookies
    Juvela low-protein bread rolls
    Juvela low-protein chocolate chip, orange and cinnamon flavour cookies
    Juvela low-protein loaf
    Juvela low-protein mix
    Liquigen
    Loprofin low-protein breakfast cereal
    Loprofin low-protein chocolate flavour cream biscuits
    Loprofin low-protein chocolate, orange and vanilla flavour cream wafers
    Loprofin low-protein cinnamon and chocolate chip cookies
    Loprofin low-protein crackers
    Loprofin low-protein egg replacer
    Loprofin low-protein egg white replacer
    Loprofin low-protein fibre bread (sliced and unsliced)
    Loprofin low-protein loaf (sliced and unsliced)
    Loprofin low-protein mix
    Loprofin low-protein part baked rolls
    Loprofin low-protein pasta (long-cut spaghetti, macaroni penne, spirals, vermicelli)
    Loprofin low-protein sweet biscuits
    Loprofin low-protein white bread (canned)
    Loprofin low-protein white bread (canned) with no added salt
    Loprofin low-protein white rolls
    Medium chain triglyceride (MCT) oil
    Nepro
    Promin low-protein pasta (alphabets, macaroni, shells, short cut spaghetti, spirals)
    Promin low-protein pastameal
    Promin low-protein tricolour pasta (alphabets, shells and spirals)
    Rite-Diet low-protein baking mix
    Rite-Diet low-protein flour mix
    Suplena
    Ultra low-protein canned brown bread
    Ultra low-protein canned white bread
    Ultra PKU biscuits
    Ultra PKU bread
    Ultra PKU cookies
    Ultra PKU flour mix
    Ultra PKU pizza base
    Ultra PKU savoy biscuits
    Valpiform low-protein cookies with chocolate nuggets and hazelnut flavour
    Valpiform low-protein shortbread biscuits

LONG CHAIN ACYL-COA DEHYDROGENASE DEFICIENCY (LCAD)

    Monogen

XV

This is a cross index listing clinical conditions and the products which the ACBS has approved for the management of those conditions. It is essential to consult LIST A for more precise guidance.

LIST B cont

LOW-PROTEIN PRODUCTS

Aglutella low-protein rice
Aminex low-protein biscuits
Aminex low-protein cookies
Aminex low-protein rusks
Aproten low-protein biscuits
Aproten low-protein bread mix
Aproten low-protein cake mix
Aproten low-protein crispbread
Aproten low-protein pasta (anellini, ditalini, rigatini, spaghetti, tagliatelle)
dp low-protein butterscotch and chocolate flavoured chip cookies
Ener-G low-protein egg replacer
Ener-G low-protein rice bread
Fate low-protein cake mix
Fate low-protein chocolate flavour cake mix
Fate low-protein flour
Harifen white chip cookies
Juvela low-protein bread rolls
Juvela low-protein chocolate chip, orange and cinnamon flavour cookies
Juvela low-protein loaf
Juvela low-protein mix
Loprofin low-protein breakfast cereal
Loprofin low-protein chocolate flavour cream biscuits
Loprofin low-protein chocolate, orange and vanilla flavour cream wafers
Loprofin low-protein cinnamon and chocolate chip cookies
Loprofin low-protein crackers
Loprofin low-protein egg replacer
Loprofin low-protein egg white replacer
Loprofin low-protein fibre bread (sliced and unsliced)
Loprofin low-protein loaf (sliced and unsliced)
Loprofin low-protein mix
Loprofin low-protein part baked rolls
Loprofin low-protein pasta (long-cut spaghetti, macaroni penne, spirals, vermicelli)
Loprofin low-protein sweet biscuits
Loprofin low-protein white bread (canned)
Loprofin low-protein white bread (canned) with no added salt
Loprofin low-protein white bread rolls
Milupa low-protein drink
Promin low-protein imitation rice
Promin low-protein pasta (alphabets, macaroni, shells, short cut spaghetti, spirals)
Promin low-protein pastameal
Promin low-protein tricolour pasta (alphabets, shells, spirals)
Rite-Diet low-protein baking mix
Rite-Diet low-protein flour mix
Ultra low-protein canned brown bread
Ultra low-protein canned white bread
Ultra PKU biscuits
Ultra PKU bread
Ultra PKU cookies
Ultra PKU flour mix
Ultra PKU pizza base
Ultra PKU savoy biscuits
Valpiform low-protein cookies with chocolate nuggets and hazelnut flavour
Valpiform low-protein shortbread biscuits

Inherited metabolic disorders, renal or liver failure requiring a low-protein diet.

This is a cross index listing clinical conditions and the products which the ACBS has approved for the management of those conditions. It is essential to consult LIST A for more precise guidance.

LIST B cont

MALABSORPTION STATES

(See also: gluten-sensitive enteropathies, liver failure, carbohydrate malabsorption,
  intestinal lymphangiectasia, milk intolerance and synthetic diets)

(a.)   <u>Protein sources</u>

       Caprilon
       Comminuted Chicken Meat (SHS)
       Duocal (Liquid & Super Soluble)
       Maxipro Super Soluble
       MCT Pepdite 0-2
       MCT Pepdite 2+
       Neocate
       Neocate Advance
       Pepdite 0-2
       Pepdite 2+

(b.)   <u>Fat sources</u>

       Alembicol D
       Calogen
       Calogen Strawberry
       Caprilon
       Liquigen
       MCT Pepdite 0-2
       MCT Pepdite 2+
       Medium chain triglyceride oil
       Pro-Cal
       QuickCal
       Vitasavoury

(c.)   <u>Carbohydrate sources</u>

       Caloreen
       Calsip
       Hycal
       Maxijul LE
       Maxijul Liquid
       Maxijul Super Soluble
       Novasource GI Control
       Nutrini Fibre
       Polycal (Liquid & Powder)
       Polycose Powder
       Pro-Cal
       QuickCal
       Resource Benefiber
       Vitajoule
       Vitasavoury

(d.)   <u>Fat/Carbohydrate sources</u>

       Duobar
       Duocal (Liquid, MCT Powder & Super Soluble)
       Megashake Nutritional Supplement
       Scandishake Mix Flavoured and Unflavoured
       SPS Energy Bar

XV

**This is a cross index listing clinical conditions and the products which the ACBS has approved for the management
of those conditions. It is essential to consult LIST A for more precise guidance.**

LIST B cont

MALABSORPTION STATES - cont

(e.)   <u>Complete Feeds</u>

For use as the sole source of nutrition or as necessary nutritional supplements prescribed on medical grounds

        Caprilon
        Clinifeed 1.0
        Clinifeed 1.5
        Clinifeed Fibre
        Clinifeed ISO
        Complan Ready-to-drink
        Elemental 028
        Elemental 028 Extra
        Elemental 028 Extra (Liquid)
        Emsogen
        Enrich
        Ensure
        Ensure Powder
        Entera
        Entera Fibre Plus Sip Feed
        Entera Fibre Plus (Neutral) Tube Feed
        Fortifresh
        Frebini
        Fresubin Isofibre
        Fresubin Liquid and Sip Feeds
        Isosource Energy
        Isosource Fibre
        Isosource Standard
        Jevity
        Jevity Plus
        MCT Pepdite 0-2
        MCT Pepdite 2 +
        Modulen IBD
        Novasource GI Control
        Nutricia Infatrini
        Nutrini
        Nutrini Fibre
        Nutrison Multifibre
        Nutrison Pepti
        Nutrison Soya
        Nutrison Standard
        Osmolite
        Paediasure
        Paediasure with Fibre
        Paediasure Plus
        Pepdite 0-2
        Pepdite 2 +
        Peptamen
        Pepti - Junior
        Pregestimil
        Reabilan
        SMA High Energy
        Sondalis 1.5 Liquid Feed
        Sondalis Fibre Liquid Feed
        Sondalis ISO Liquid Feed
        Sondalis Junior

This is a cross index listing clinical conditions and the products which the ACBS has approved for the management of those conditions. It is essential to consult LIST A for more precise guidance.

MALABSORPTION STATES - cont

(f.)   Nutritional Supplements

Necessary nutritional supplements prescribed on medical grounds (products should be labelled to
state that they are to be taken under dietetic supervision and that a maximum of x mls containing
80g protein (approximately y cans/packs) may be taken per day)

Clinutren 1.5
Clinutren Dessert
Clinutren ISO
Enlive
Enrich Plus
Ensure Bar
Ensure Plus
Formance
Forticreme
Fortijuce
Fortimel
Fortisip
Fortisip Multifibre
Fresubin 750 MCT
Nutrison Energy
Nutrison MCT
Perative
Printania
Protenplus
Provide Xtra
Resource Benefiber
Resource Shake Nutritional Supplement
Survimed OPD

(g.)   Minerals

Aminogran Mineral Mixture
Metabolic Mineral Mixture

(h.)   Vitamins - as appropriate

See: Synthetic Diets

(i.)   Vitamins and Minerals

Paediatric Seravit

MALNUTRITION (DISEASE RELATED)

Calogen
Calogen Strawberry
Caloreen
Calsip
Clinifeed 1.0
Clinifeed 1.5
Clinifeed Fibre
Clinifeed ISO
Clinutren 1.5 (as a supplement)
Clinutren Dessert (as a supplement)
Clinutren ISO (as a supplement)
Complan Ready-to-drink

XV

**This is a cross index listing clinical conditions and the products which the ACBS has approved for the management
of those conditions. It is essential to consult LIST A for more precise guidance.**

LIST B cont

MALNUTRITION (DISEASE RELATED) - cont

Duobar
Duocal (Liquid, MCT Powder & Super Soluble)
Enlive (as a supplement)
Enrich
Enrich Plus
Ensure
Ensure Bar
Ensure Plus (as a supplement)
Ensure Powder
Entera
Entera Fibre Plus Sip Feed
Entera Fibre Plus (Neutral) Tube Feed
Formance (as a supplement)
Forticreme (as a supplement)
Fortifresh
Fortijuce (as a supplement)
Fortimel (as a supplement)
Fortisip (as a supplement)
Fortisip Multifibre (as a supplement)
Frebini
Fresubin Isofibre
Fresubin Liquid & Sip Feeds
Fresubin 750 MCT (as a supplement)
Hycal
Isosource Energy
Isosource Fibre
Isosource Standard
Jevity
Jevity Plus
Maxijul LE
Maxijul Liquid
Maxijul Super Soluble
Megashake Nutritional Supplement
Modulen IBD
Novasource GI Control
Nutricia Infatrini
Nutrini
Nutrini Fibre
Nutrini Extra
Nutrison Energy (as a supplement)
Nutrison MCT (as a supplement)
Nutrison Multifibre
Nutrison Soya
Nutrison Standard
Osmolite
Osmolite Plus
Paediasure
Paediasure Plus
Paediasure with Fibre
Perative (as a supplement)
Polycal (Liquid & Powder)
Polycose Powder
Printania (as a supplement)
Pro-Cal
Protenplus (as a supplement)
Provide Xtra (as a supplement)

This is a cross index listing clinical conditions and the products which the ACBS has approved for the management of those conditions. It is essential to consult LIST A for more precise guidance.

LIST B cont

MALNUTRITION (DISEASE RELATED) - cont

    QuickCal
    Resource Benefiber
    Resource Shake Nutritional Supplement
    Scandishake Mix Flavoured and Unflavoured
    SMA High Energy
    Sondalis 1.5 Liquid Feed
    Sondalis Fibre Liquid Feed
    Sondalis ISO Liquid Feed
    Sondalis Junior
    SPS Energy Bar
    Survimed OPD (as a supplement)
    Vitajoule
    Vitasavoury

MAPLE SYRUP URINE DISEASE

    Analog MSUD
    MSUD Aid III
    MSUD Maxamaid
    MSUD Maxamum
See: Low-Protein Products
    Synthetic Diets

METHYLMALONIC ACIDAEMIA

    Analog XMET, THRE, VAL, ISOLEU
    Methionine, Threonine & Valine-Free, Isoleucine-Low Amino Acid Mix
    XMET, THRE, VAL, ISOLEU Maxamaid
    XMET, THRE, VAL, ISOLEU Maxamum

MILK PROTEIN SENSITIVITY

    Comminuted Chicken meat (SHS)
    Farley's Soya Formula
    Infasoy
    Isomil Powder
    Nutramigen
    Prosobee Liquid and Powder
    Wysoy
See: Synthetic Diets.

NUTRITIONAL SUPPORT FOR ADULTS (for precise conditions for which these products have been approved see the product listing in List A)

A.   Nutritionally complete feeds

    For use as the sole source of nutrition or as necessary nutritional supplements prescribed on medical grounds

XV

This is a cross index listing clinical conditions and the products which the ACBS has approved for the management of those conditions. It is essential to consult LIST A for more precise guidance.

BORDERLINE SUBSTANCES

LIST B cont

(a) <u>Gluten Free</u>

Clinifeed ISO
Entera
Entera Fibre Plus Sip Feed
Entera Fibre Plus (Neutral) Tube Feed
Fortifresh
Fresubin Liquid and Sip Feeds
Nutrison Multifibre
Nutrison Standard
Paediasure Plus
Sondalis ISO Liquid Feed
Sondalis Junior

(b) <u>Lactose Free</u>

Clinifeed 1.0

(c) <u>Lactose and Gluten Free</u>

Clinifeed 1.5
Enrich
Ensure
Ensure Powder
Fresubin Isofibre
Nutrison Soya
Osmolite
Osmolite Plus
Sondalis 1.5 Liquid Feed

(d) <u>Containing Fibre</u>

Clinifeed Fibre
Enrich
Entera Fibre Plus Sip Feed
Entera Fibre Plus (Neutral) Tube Feed
Fresubin Isofibre
Isosource Fibre
Jevity
Jevity Plus
Novasource GI Control
Nutrini Fibre
Nutrison Multifibre
Paediasure with Fibre
Sondalis Fibre Liquid Feed

(e) <u>Elemental Feeds</u>

Elemental 028
Elemental 028 Extra
Elemental 028 Extra (Liquid)
Emsogen
Nutrison Pepti
Peptamen

This is a cross index listing clinical conditions and the products which the ACBS has approved for the management of those conditions. It is essential to consult LIST A for more precise guidance.

LIST B cont

B.   Nutritional Source Supplements

     See: Synthetic Diets
              Malabsorption States.

     (a)   General Supplements

         Necessary nutritional supplements prescribed on medical grounds for the diseases in List A (products should be labelled to state that they are to be taken under dietetic supervision and that a maximum of xmls containing 80g protein (approximately y cans/packs) may be taken per day)

         Clinutren 1.5
         Clinutren Dessert
         Clinutren ISO
         Enlive
         Enrich Plus
         Ensure Bar
         Ensure Plus
         Formance
         Forticreme
         Fortijuce
         Fortimel
         Fortisip
         Fortisip Multifibre
         Fresubin 750 MCT
         Nutrison Energy
         Nutrison MCT
         Perative
         Printania
         Protenplus
         Provide Xtra
         Survimed OPD

     (b)   Carbohydrates

Caloreen	(Low electrolyte content)
Calsip	(Low electrolyte content)
Hycal	(Low electrolyte content)
Maxijul LE	(Low electrolyte content)
Maxijul Liquid	
Maxijul Super Soluble	
Polycal (Liquid & Powder)	(Low electrolyte content)
Polycose Powder	
Pro-Cal	
QuickCal	
Resource Benefiber	
Vitajoule	
Vitasavoury	

XV

This is a cross index listing clinical conditions and the products which the ACBS has approved for the management of those conditions. It is essential to consult LIST A for more precise guidance.

LIST B cont

(c)   Fat

        Alembicol D
        Calogen
        Calogen Strawberry
        Liquigen
        MCT Oil

(d)   Fat/Carbohydrate sources

        Duobar
        Duocal (Liquid, MCT Powder & Super Soluble)   (Low electrolyte content)
        Megashake Nutritional Supplement
        Scandishake Mix Flavoured and Unflavoured
        SPS Energy Bar

(e)   Nitrogen Sources

        Casilan 90   (Whole protein based, low sodium)
        Maxipro Super Soluble
        Pro-Mod   (Whey protein based, low sodium)

(f)   Minerals

        Aminogran mineral mixture
        Metabolic mineral mixture

PHENYLKETONURIA
        Aglutella low-protein rice
        Aminex low-protein biscuits
        Aminex low-protein cookies
        Aminex low-protein rusks
        Aminogran food supplement
        Aminogran food supplement tablets
        Aminogran mineral mixture
        Analog LCP
        Analog XP
        Aproten low-protein biscuits
        Aproten low-protein bread mix
        Aproten low-protein cake mix
        Aproten low-protein crispbread
        Aproten low-protein pasta (anellini, ditalini, rigatini, spaghetti, tagliatelle)
        dp low-protein butterscotch and chocolate flavoured chip cookies
        Ener-G low-protein egg replacer
        Harifen white chip cookies
        Juvela low-protein bread rolls
        Juvela low-protein chocolate chip; orange and cinnamon flavour cookies
        Juvela low-protein loaf (sliced and unsliced)
        Juvela low-protein mix
        Lofenalac
        Loprofin low-protein breakfast cereal
        Loprofin low-protein chocolate flavour cream biscuits
        Loprofin low-protein chocolate, orange and vanilla flavour cream wafers
        Loprofin low-protein cinnamon and chocolate chip cookies
        Loprofin low-protein crackers
        Loprofin low-protein egg replacer
        Loprofin low-protein fibre bread (sliced and unsliced)
        Loprofin low-protein loaf (sliced and unsliced)

This is a cross index listing clinical conditions and the products which the ACBS has approved for the management of those conditions. It is essential to consult LIST A for more precise guidance.

LIST B cont

PHENYLKETONURIA - cont

         Loprofin low-protein mix
         Loprofin low-protein part baked rolls
         Loprofin low-protein pasta (long-cut spaghetti, macaroni penne, spirals, vermicelli)
         Loprofin low-protein sweet biscuits
         Loprofin low-protein white bread (canned)
         Loprofin low-protein white bread (canned) with no added salt
         Loprofin low-protein white rolls
         Loprofin PKU Drink
         L-Tyrosine Supplement
         Metabolic Mineral Mixture
         Phlexy-10 Exchange System (Bar, Capsules & Drink Mix)
         Phlexyvits
         PK Aid 4 (formerly PK Aid III)
         PKU 2 (Milupa)
         PKU 3 (Milupa)
         Promin low-protein pasta (alphabets, macaroni, shells, short-cut spaghetti, spirals)
         Promin low-protein pastameal
         Promin low-protein tricolour pasta (alphabets, shells, spirals)
         Rite-Diet low-protein baking mix
         Rite-Diet low-protein flour mix
         Sno-Pro Drink
         Ultra low-protein canned white bread
         Ultra PKU biscuits
         Ultra PKU bread
         Ultra PKU cookies
         Ultra PKU flour mix
         Ultra PKU pizza base
         Ultra PKU savoy biscuits
         Valpiform low-protein cookies which chocolate nuggets and hazelnut flavour
         Valpiform low-protein shortbread biscuits
         XP Maxamaid
         XP Maxamaid Concentrate
         XP Maxamaid Orange
         XP Maxamum
See: Low-Protein Products
         Synthetic Diets

PHOTODERMATOSES (SKIN PROTECTION IN)

         Ambre Solaire Total Sunscreen for Sun-sensitive skin SPF 60
         Coppertone Ultrashade 23
         Delph Sun Lotion SPF 15, SPF 20, SPF 25, SPF 30
         E45 Sun Lotion SPF15 and SPF 25
         E45 Sun 50 Sunblock Lotion
         Piz Buin Sun Block Lotion SPF20
         RoC Total Sunblock Cream SPF25
         Spectraban 25
         Spectraban Ultra
         Uvistat Sunblock Cream Factor 20
         Uvistat Ultrablock Suncream Factor 30

XV

This is a cross index listing clinical conditions and the products which the ACBS has approved for the management of those conditions. It is essential to consult LIST A for more precise guidance.

LIST B cont

PROPIONIC ACIDAEMIA

       Analog XMET, THRE, VAL, ISOLEU
       Methionine, Threonine & Valine-Free, Isoleucine-Low Amino Acid Mix
       XMET, THRE, VAL, ISOLEU, Maxamaid
       XMET, THRE, VAL, ISOLEU, Maxamum

PROTEIN INTOLERANCE

   See: Amino Acid Metabolic Disorders
          Low-Protein Products
          Milk Protein Sensitivity
          Synthetic Diets
          Whole Protein Sensitivity

PRURITUS

   See: Dermatitis

PSORIASIS

   See: Scaling of the Scalp

REFSUM'S DISEASE

       Fresubin Liquid and Sip Feeds

RENAL DIALYSIS

   See: Dialysis

RENAL FAILURE

       Aglutella low-protein rice
       Aminex low-protein biscuits
       Aminex low-protein cookies
       Aminex low-protein rusks
       Aproten low-protein biscuits
       Aproten low-protein bread mix
       Aproten low-protein cake mix
       Aproten low-protein crispbread
       Aproten low-protein pasta (anellini, ditalini, rigatini, spaghetti, tagliatelle)
       Dialamine
       dp low-protein butterscotch and chocolate flavoured chip cookies
       Ener-G low-protein egg replacer
       Ener-G low-protein rice bread
       Fate low-protein cake mix
       Fate low-protein chocolate flavour cake mix
       Fate low-protein flour
       Harifen white chip cookies
       Juvela low-protein bread rolls
       Juvela low-protein chocolate chip, orange and cinnamon flavour cookies
       Juvela low-protein loaf
       Juvela low-protein mix
       Kindergen P.R.O.D.
       Loprofin low-protein breakfast cereal
       Loprofin low-protein cinnamon and chocolate chip cookies

---

This is a cross index listing clinical conditions and the products which the ACBS has approved for the management of those conditions. It is essential to consult LIST A for more precise guidance.

LIST B cont

RENAL FAILURE - cont

    Loprofin low-protein chocolate flavour cream biscuits
    Loprofin low-protein chocolate, orange and vanilla flavour cream wafers
    Loprofin low-protein crackers
    Loprofin low-protein egg replacer
    Loprofin low-protein egg white replacer
    Loprofin low-protein fibre bread (sliced and unsliced)
    Loprofin low-protein loaf (sliced and unsliced)
    Loprofin low-protein mix
    Loprofin low-protein part-baked rolls
    Loprofin low-protein pasta (long-cut spaghetti, macaroni penne, spirals, vermicelli)
    Loprofin low-protein sweet biscuits
    Loprofin low-protein white bread (canned)
    Loprofin low-protein white bread (canned) with no added salt
    Loprofin low-protein white rolls
    Nepro
    Promin low-protein pasta (alphabets, macaroni, shells, short-cut spaghetti, spirals)
    Promin low-protein pastameal
    Promin low-protein tricolour pastas (alphabets, shells, spirals)
    Renamil
    Rite-Diet low-protein baking mix
    Rite-Diet low-protein flour mix
    Sno-Pro drink
    Suplena
    Ulltra low-protein canned brown bread
    Ultra low-protein canned white bread
    Ultra PKU biscuits
    Ultra PKU bread
    Ultra PKU cookies
    Ultra PKU flour mix
    Ultra PKU pizza base
    Ultra PKU savoy biscuits
    Valpiform low-protein cookies with chocolate nuggets and hazelnut flavour
    Valpiform low-protein shortbread biscuits

SHORT BOWEL SYNDROME

  See: Malabsorption

SICCA SYNDROME

    Glandosane
    Luborant Saliva Replacement
    Oralbalance Dry Mouth Saliva Replacement Gel
    Saliva Orthana
    Salivace
    Saliveze
    Salivix Pastilles

XV

This is a cross index listing clinical conditions and the products which the ACBS has approved for the management of those conditions. It is essential to consult LIST A for more precise guidance.

LIST B cont

SYNTHETIC DIETS (for precise conditions for which these products have been approved see the product listing in List A)

(a.)   Fat

      Alembicol D
      Calogen
      Calogen Strawberry
      Liquigen
      Medium chain triglyceride oil
      Pro-Cal
      QuickCal
      Vitasavoury

(b.)   Carbohydrate

      Caloreen
      Calsip
      Hycal
      Maxijul LE
      Maxijul Liquid
      Maxijul Super Soluble
      Polycal (Liquid & Powder)
      Polycose Powder
      Pro-Cal
      QuickCal
      Vitasavoury
      Vitajoule

(c.)   Fat/Carbohydrate

      Duobar
      Duocal (Liquid, MCT Powder & Super Soluble)
      Megashake Nutritional Supplement
      Scandishake Mix Flavoured and Unflavoured
      SPS Energy Bar

(d.)   Minerals

      Aminogran Mineral Mixture
      Metabolic Mineral Mixture

(e.)   Protein Sources

  See: Malabsorption states
       Complete feeds

(f.)   Vitamins - as appropriate

  See: Malabsorption States
       Nutritional Support for Adults

(g.)   Vitamins and Minerals

      Paediatric Seravit
      Phlexyvits

This is a cross index listing clinical conditions and the products which the ACBS has approved for the management of those conditions. It is essential to consult LIST A for more precise guidance.

LIST B cont

TYROSINAEMIA

     Analog XPHEN, TYR
     Analog XYPHEN, TYR, MET
     XPHEN, TYR Maxamaid
     XPT Tyrosidon
     XPTM Tyrosidon

UREA CYCLE DISORDERS

     L-Arginine Supplement for urea cycle disorders. (S.H.S.)

VITILIGO

     Covermark Classic Foundation
     Covermark Finishing Powder
     Dermablend Cover Creme
     Dermablend Leg and Body Cover
     Dermablend Setting Powder
     Dermacolor Camouflage Cream
     Dermacolor Fixing Powder
     Keromask Finishing Powder
     Keromask Masking Cream
     Veil Cover Cream
     Veil Finishing Powder

VOMITING IN INFANCY

     Instant Carobel
     Nestargel

WHOLE PROTEIN SENSITIVITY for definition, see page 427

     Alfare
     Caprilon
     MCT Pepdite 2 +
     Neocate
     Neocate Advance
     Nutramigen
     Pepdite 0-2
     Pepdite 2 +
     Pepti - Junior
     Pregestimil
     Prejomin

XEROSTOMIA

     Glandosane
     Luborant Saliva Replacement
     Oralbalance Dry Mouth Saliva Replacement Gel
     Saliva Orthana
     Salivace
     Saliveze
     Salivix Pastilles

XV

This is a cross index listing clinical conditions and the products which the ACBS has approved for the management of those conditions. It is essential to consult LIST A for more precise guidance.

LIST C

The products which have been considered by the ACBS and may not be prescribed on Form FP10, are now included in Part XVIIIA (pages 501-530).

NOTES ON CHARGES FOR DRUGS AND APPLIANCES PAYABLE UNDER REGULATIONS MADE UNDER SECTION 77(1) OF THE NATIONAL HEALTH SERVICE ACT 1977

(N.B: Information is also given on the counting of prescriptions for pricing purposes in para 9 (page 486) with example of the application of the prescription charge arrangements in para 10 (page 487).

1. CHARGES PAYABLE

£6.00 for each prescription item, preparation or type of appliance including each anklet, legging, knee-cap, below-knee, above knee or thigh stocking. No charge is payable for <u>Oxygen concentrators</u> from 1 April 1992.

2. PHARMACY, APPLIANCE AND DRUG STORE CONTRACTORS

Unless a completed declaration of entitlement to exemption or remission (see page 484) is made on the prescription form, a charge is payable for each drug or appliance supplied, including each piece of elastic hosiery. Patients, or their representatives, are required to sign the prescription form to declare that a charge has been paid. The charges are collected and retained by the pharmacy, appliance or drug store contractor, whose remuneration is adjusted accordingly.

In order to secure exemption or remission from prescription charges when presenting a prescription form to a pharmacy, appliance or drug store contractor, the patient, or a person on his behalf, must complete the declaration on the back of the prescription form. The regulations have now been changed to require them to do so.

3. DISPENSING DOCTORS

Unless a completed declaration of entitlement to exemption or remission (see page 484) is made on the prescription form, the charges set out at (1) above are payable in respect of each item supplied by a dispensing doctor. Patients, or their representatives, are required to sign the prescription form to declare that a charge has been paid. Charges collected in respect of prescriptions dispensed in England on and after 1 October 2000 should be retained by the practice and will be deducted from remuneration. Charges collected in respect of prescriptions dispensed in England prior to 1 October 2000 should be paid over to the Health Authority. Charges collected in respect of prescriptions dispensed in Wales continue to be paid over to the Health Authority.

In order to secure exemption or remission from prescription charges when presenting a prescription form to a dispensing doctor, the patient, or a person on his behalf, must complete the declaration on the back of the prescription form. The regulations have now been changed to require them to do so.

When an item dispensed by a dispensing doctor is delivered to a patient outside the surgery, every reasonable effort should be made to obtain a signed declaration from the patient that they have either paid the charge or are exempt.

However, there will be occasions when repeat prescriptions are delivered to points outside the surgery or pharmacy, for example for collection from village shops to rural areas. Where a patient is exempt from charges and it is not practical for the patient to sign the form, a dispensing doctor should mark the reverse of the form as "remote delivery" and sign the form.

XVI

4. PEOPLE ENTITLED TO EXEMPTION

Provided that the appropriate declaration is received, a charge is not payable to the contractor or dispensing doctor for drugs or appliances, including elastic hosiery, supplied for:

Children under 16;
Students aged 16, 17 or 18 in full-time education;
Men and women aged 60 and over.

People holding Health Authority exemption certificates, which are issued to:

Expectant mothers;
Women who have borne a child or women who have given birth to a child registerable as stillborn under the Births and Deaths Registration Act 1953 in the last 12 months;
People suffering from the following specified conditions -

4.1 Permanent fistula (including Caecostomy, Colostomy, Ileostomy or Laryngostomy) requiring continuous surgical dressing or an appliance.

4.2 Forms of hypoadrenalism (including Addison's disease) for which specific substitution therapy is essential.
Diabetes insipidus and other forms of hypopituitarism
Diabetes mellitus except where treatment is by diet alone
Hypoparathyroidism
Myasthenia gravis
Myxoedema (Hypothyroidism) or, in accordance with the application form FP92A, other conditions where supplemental thyroid hormone is necessary.

4.3 Epilepsy requiring continuous anti-convulsive therapy.

4.4 A continuing physical disability which prevents the patient leaving his residence except with the help of another person (this does not mean a temporary disability even if it is likely to last a few months).

War pensioners holding a War Pension exemption certificate for prescriptions needed for treating their accepted disablement;

People who have purchased a prescription prepayment certificate (FP96) from the Health Authority.

5. PEOPLE ENTITLED TO REMISSION

People and their partners receiving Income Support, Income-based Jobseeker's Allowance, full Working Families' Tax Credit (WFTC) or Credit reduced by £70 or less and full Disabled Person's Tax Credit (DPTC) or Credit reduced by £70 or less. The person's WFTC/DPTC award notice will show whether the Credit has been reduced by (or the amount taken off is) £70 or less.

People and their partners who are entitled to full charge remission under the NHS Low Income Scheme (ie those who hold HC2 certificates).

Full details of the exemption and remission arrangements are contained in Leaflet HC11, which can be ordered from: Department of Health, PO Box 777, London, SE1 6XH or by faxing 01623 724524.

6. PREPAYMENT CERTIFICATES (Season Tickets)

Doctors and contractors could greatly assist any patient who makes frequent payments for prescriptions by drawing attention to the availability of prepayment certificates (Season Tickets). These certificates cost £86.20 for one year or £31.40 for four months.

They are worthwhile for anyone requiring more than 14 items on prescription in a year or 5 items in four months. An application form FP95 can be obtained from main Post Offices, Health Authorities or pharmacies.

7. BULK PRESCRIPTION

Charges are not payable in respect of "bulk" prescriptions for schools or institutions supplied in accordance with the Regulations (See Note 6, Part VIII, page 44).

8. CONTRACEPTIVE SERVICES

No charge is payable for contraceptive substances and listed contraceptive appliances for women prescribed on FP10 or any of its variants.

The great majority of family planning prescriptions will be for contraceptive devices (See Part IXA page 117-119) spermicidal gels, creams, films, pessaries and aerosols; or those systemic drugs promoted as contraceptives which are listed below: prescriptions for those products will not be specially marked and a prescription charge should not be levied.

Prescriptions for other drugs - If the prescription is for contraceptive purposes the prescriber may mark the item with the symbol ♀ (or endorse the item in another way which makes it clear that the prescription is for contraceptive purposes) and a prescription charge should not be levied for any items so marked. In the absence of such an endorsement by the prescriber, the normal prescription charge will apply to that item.

Where a dispensing doctor paid on the Drug Tariff basis supplies for contraceptive purposes a drug which is not on the list he should mark the item with the symbol ♀ on the prescription form before it is submitted for pricing.

List of Contraceptive Drugs to be Dispensed Free of Charge:

Progestogen only	50 Micrograms of Oestrogen	Under 50 Micrograms of Oestrogen
Depo-Provera 150mg/ml,	Norinyl-1	Bi Novum
1ml pre-filled syringe	Ovran	Brevinor
Femulen	PC4	Cilest
Implanon		Eugynon 30
Levonelle-2		Femodene
Medroxyprogesterone		Femodene ED
Acetate Injection		Femodette
(Aqueous Suspension)		Loestrin 20
150mg/ml, 1ml		Loestrin 30
pre-filled syringe		Logynon
Micronor		Logynon ED
Microval		Marvelon
Mirena System		Mercilon
Neogest		Microgynon 30
Norgeston		Microgynon 30 ED
Noriday		Minulet
Noristerat Injection		Norimin
		Ovran 30
		Ovranette
		Ovysmen
		Synphase
		Triadene
		Tri-Minulet
		Trinordiol
		Trinovum

XVI

9. NOTES ON CHARGES PAYABLE

9.1 SINGLE PRESCRIPTION CHARGE PAYABLE

Unless the patient claims exemption or the prescription is covered by the provisions at 9.1.5 and 9.1.6 a single prescription charge is payable where:

9.1.1	The same drug or preparation is supplied in more than one container.
9.1.2	Different strengths of the same drug are ordered as separate prescriptions at the same time.
9.1.3	More than one appliance of the same type (other than hosiery*) is supplied.
9.1.4	A set of parts making up a complete appliance is supplied.
9.1.5	Drugs are supplied in powder form with the solvent separate for subsequent admixing.
9.1.6	A drug is supplied with a dropper, throat brush, or vaginal applicator.
9.1.7	Several flavours of the same preparation are supplied.

9.2 MULTIPLE PRESCRIPTION CHARGES PAYABLE

More than one prescription charge is payable where:

9.2.1	Different drugs, types of dressing or appliances are supplied.
9.2.2	Different formulations or presentations of the same drug or preparation are supplied.
9.2.3	Additional parts are supplied together with a complete set of apparatus or additional dressing(s) together with a dressing pack.
9.2.4	More than one piece of elastic hosiery* is supplied.

---

* (Anklet, legging, knee-cap, below-knee, above knee or thigh stocking).

10 EXAMPLES OF APPLICATION OF PRESCRIPTION CHARGE ARRANGEMENTS

"NO CHARGE" ITEM

The number of "no charge" items (ie items which are counted as prescriptions for pricing purposes but which do not carry a prescription charge) should be included on the invoice submitted with the prescription forms to the Pricing Authority.

		Professional Fees	Number of Prescription Charges	No Charge Prescriptons
10.1	**LIQUIDS** - Required by the prescriber to be supplied in more than one container. Certain preparations, if extemporaneously dispensed, may be subject to additional fees, (see Part IIIA page 15).			
	Ammonium Chloride 300ml x 3	1	1	-
	Boric Acid Eye Lotion 100ml x 2	1	1	-
	Chloramphenicol Ear Drops 10ml x 2	1	1	-
	Ferric Chloride Gargle 200ml x 2	1	1	-
	Hydrogen Peroxide Ear Drops 10ml x 3	1	1	-
	Lead Lotion 200ml x 3	1	1	-
	Sulphacetamide Sodium Eye Drops 10ml x 2	1	1	-

10.2 **INJECTIONS**

     10.2.1 **Sets containing graded strength of the same drug**

	Professional Fees	Number of Prescription Charges	No Charge Prescriptons
Migen - set of 6 graded strength unit-dose syringes	1	1	-

     10.2.2 **Same injection, different strength**

	Professional Fees	Number of Prescription Charges	No Charge Prescriptons
Deca-Durabolin 25mg x 3 } Deca-Duralolin 100mg x 3 }	1	1	-

     10.2.3 **Dispensed in powder form with solvent**

	Professional Fees	Number of Prescription Charges	No Charge Prescriptons
Amoxil Inj. Powder 500mg x 1 } Water for Injection 5ml x 1 }	2	1	1
Digoxin Amps 0.5mg x 10 } Normal Saline Amps 5ml x 10 }	2	1	1

     10.2.4 Influenza Vaccine (2 different strains in separate ampoules)

	Professional Fees	Number of Prescription Charges	No Charge Prescriptons
	2	1	1

XVI

10 EXAMPLES OF APPLICATION OF PRESCRIPTION CHARGE ARRANGEMENTS - cont

	Professional Fees	Number of Prescription Charges	No Charge Prescriptons
10.3 TABLETS, CAPSULES, OINTMENTS, etc. - Different strengths of the same drug ordered as separate prescriptions at the same time			
Dithranol ½% in Lassar's Paste ⎫ Dithranol 1% in Lassar's Paste ⎬ Dithranol 1½% in Lassar's Paste ⎭	3	1	2

Phenindione Tabs 50mg/one three ⎫
   times daily, 90   ⎬
Phenindione Tabs 10mg/one three ⎪
   times daily, 90   ⎭
	2	1	1

Phenindione Tabs 50mg/one in the ⎫
   morning, 30   ⎬
Phenindione Tabs 10mg/three at   ⎪
   night, 90   ⎭
	2	1	1

Prednisolone Tabs 5mg/one in the ⎫
   morning, 28   ⎬
Prednisolone Tabs 1mg/one in the ⎪
   morning, 28   ⎭
	2	1	1

Sulphacetamide Eye Drops 10% ⎫ Sulphacetamide Eye Drops 30% ⎭	2	1	1
10.4 TABLETS, CAPSULES, etc.			
10.4.1 Different formulations or presentations of the same drug ordered as separate prescriptions			
Indocid Caps ⎫ Indocid R Caps ⎭	2	2	-
Isordil Tabs ⎫ Isordil Sublingual Tabs ⎭	2	2	-
Achromycin Caps 250mg ⎫ Achromycin Tabs 250mg ⎭	2	2	-
Camcolit 250 Tabs ⎫ Camcolit 400 Tabs sustained ⎬ release ⎭	2	2	-
Bezalip Tabs 200mg ⎫ Bezalip Mono Tabs ⎭	2	2	-
Prednisolone Tabs 1mg ⎫ Prednesol Tabs 5mg (ie ⎬ Prednisolone Sodium Phosphate) ⎭	2	2	-
Prednisolone Tabs 1mg ⎫ Prednisolone Tabs 2.5mg enteric ⎬ coated ⎭	2	2	-
Ronicol Tabs ⎫ Ronicol Timespan Tabs ⎭	2	2	-
Trasicor Tabs ⎫ Slow Trasicor Tabs ⎭	2	2	-

10 EXAMPLES OF APPLICATION OF PRESCRIPTION CHARGE ARRANGEMENTS - cont

	Professional Fees	Number of Prescription Charges	No Charge Prescriptons
10.4.2 **Strength ordered not listed** - must be dispensed and priced by a combination of two different strengths and/or presentations.			
Tolanase Tabs - 350mg x 60			
Contractor endorses 100mg x 60 }			
250mg x 60 }	2	1	1
Prothiaden - 100mg x 100			
Contractor endorses			
Caps 25mg x 100 }			
Tabs 75mg x 100 }	2	1	1
10.5 COMBINATION PACKS			
Adgyn Combi	2	2	-
Canesten Combi	2	2	-
Climagest Tablets	2	2	-
Cyclo-Progynova Tabs 1mg or 2mg	2	2	-
Cyclo-Progynova Tabs 1mg (prescribed }			
Cyclo-Progynova Tabs 2mg together) }	4	3	1
Didronel PMO 90 day Treatment Pack	2	2	-
Dutonin Starter (Treatment) Pack	3	1	2
Ecostatin Twin Pack	2	2	-
Elleste Duet Tablets 1mg or 2mg	2	2	-
Estracombi TTS	2	2	-
Estrapak 50	2	2	-
Estrapak 50 (prescribed }			
Estraderm 100mg together) }	3	2	1
Evorel Pak	2	2	-
Evorel Sequi	2	2	-
Femapak 40 or 80	2	2	-
Femoston Tablets 1/10, 2/10 or 2/20	2	2	-
Femoston Tablets 2/10 (prescribed }			
Femoston Tablets 2/20 together) }	3	2	1
Flagyl Compak	2	2	-
Gyno-Daktarin Combipack	2	2	-
Gyno-Pevaryl 150 Combipack	2	2	-
Gyno-Pevaryl 1 CP Pack	2	2	-
Heliclear Triple Pack	3	3	-
Hypovase BD Starter Pack	2	1	1
Hytrin Starter Pack	2	1	1
Hytrin-BPH Starter Pack	3	1	2
Migraleve Complete Tablets (formerly Duo Pack)	2	2	-
Moraxen Suppositories 35mg, 50mg, 75mg or 100mg (Suppositories and Lubri Gel)	2	2	-
Napratec Combination Pack Tablets	2	2	-
Norprolac Starter Pack	2	1	1
Nuvelle Tablets	2	2	-
Nuvelle TS Patches	2	2	-
Premique Cycle	2	2	-
Prempak-C 0.625	2	2	-
Prempak-C 1.25	2	2	-
Rehidrat Multipack	3	1	2
Seroquel Starter Pack (4 day titration)	3	1	2
Tridestra	3	2	1
Trisequens	3	2	1
Trisequens Forte Combination Pack Tablets	3	2	1

XVI

10 EXAMPLES OF APPLICATION OF PRESCRIPTION CHARGE ARRANGEMENTS - cont

	Professional Fees	Number of Prescription Charges	No Charge Prescriptons
10.6 MULTIPLES OF SAME APPLIANCE OF SAME OR DIFFERING SIZE			
Becotide Rotahaler (prescribed ⎫			
Ventolin Rotahaler together) ⎬	2	2	-
Crepe Bandages 2 x 5cm	1	1	-
Open-Wove Bandages 1 x 2.5cm⎫			
1 x 5cm⎬	1	1	-
1 x 7.5cm⎭			
Polythene Occulusive Dressings ⎫			
Gloves - Polythene 100 gauge ⎬	1	1	-
Arm Sleeve - Polythene 150 gauge ⎫			
Leg Sleeve - Polythene 150 gauge ⎪			
Foot Bag - Polythene 150 gauge ⎬ *	4	1	3
Torso Vest - Polythene 150 gauge ⎭			
Shorts - Polythene 150 guage	1	1	-
Trousers - Polythene 150 guage	1	1	-
10.7 SET OF APPLIANCES OR DRESSINGS			
Atomizer	1	1	-
Douche	1	1	-
Hypodermic Syringe	1	1	-
Multiple Pack Dressing No.1	1	1	-
Multiple Pack Dressing No.2	1	1	-
Portable Urinal	1	1	-
Suprapubic Belt	1	1	-
Higginson's Enema Syringe	1	1	-
10.8 SETS OF APPLIANCES ORDERED WITH EXTRA PARTS			
Hypodermic Syringes ⎫			
Hypodermic Needles ⎬	2	2	-
Multiple Pack Dressing No.2 ⎫			
Absorbent Cotton 25g ⎬	2	2	-
Portable Urinal ⎫			
Spare Sheaths 2 ⎬	1	1	-
10.9 DIFFERENT APPLIANCES			
Lint 25g ⎫			
Absorbent Cotton 25g ⎬	3	3	-
Gauze 90cm x 1m ⎭			

*(Arm Sleeves, leg sleeves, foot bag and torso vest are all regarded as Plastics Sleeves).

10 EXAMPLES OF APPLICATION OF PRESCRIPTION CHARGE ARRANGEMENTS - cont

	Professional Fees	Number of Prescription Charges	No Charge Prescriptons
10.10 DRUGS ORDERED WITH DRUG TARIFF APPLIANCES			
Ametop Gel 4% Dispensing Pack (12 tubes 1.5g Gel and 15 Opsite Flexigrid Dressings)	2	2	-
Becloforte-VM	2	2	-
Broven Inhalant / Broven Inhaler	2	2	-
Clinitest Set and extra / Clinitest Tablets	2	1	1
Intal Spincaps / Spinhaler	2	2	-
Iodine Compd. Paint 25ml / Iodine Brush	2	1	1
Ventolin Tablets / Ventolin Inhaler	2	2	-
10.11 DRUGS PACKED WITH NON DRUG TARIFF APPLIANCES* (including metered aerosols with refills)			
Alupent Inhaler / Alupent Refill(s)	1	1	-
Betadine Vaginal Preparation:-			
Gel (with applicator)	1	1	-
Pessaries (with applicator)	1	1	-
V.C. Kit	1	1	-
Syntaris Nasal Spray	1	1	-
Verrugon Ointment (Composite Pack)	1	1	-

* (These appliances are being allowed because they are packed with drug/preparation).

10.12 ELASTIC HOSIERY			
1 pr Knee-caps - One Way Strech	1	2	-
1 pr Thigh Stockings - Class II	1	2	-
1 pr Spare Suspenders	1	1	-
1 Suspender Belt	1	1	-

XVI

10 **EXAMPLES OF APPLICATION OF PRESCRIPTION CHARGE ARRANGEMENTS** - cont

	Professional Fees	Number of Prescription Charges	No Charge Prescriptons
10.13 MISCELLANEOUS			
10.13.1 Preparation supplied as separate parts for admixing as required for use			
Chlorhexidine 0.2% Aqueous Solution - 400ml)			
Sodium Fluoride 2% Aqueous Solution - 400ml)	2	1	1
10.13.2 Preparation having various flavours			
Dioralyte Plain			
Dioralyte Blackcurrant　　)	2	1	1
Hycal assorted flavours. Mitte 3	3	1	2
Hycal assorted flavours. Mitte 8	4	1	3
(At present 4 flavours available)			
Rite-Diet Gluten Free Biscuits Sweet)			
Rite-Diet Gluten Free Biscuits Savoury)	2	1	1
10.13.3 Different but related preparations			
Aminogran Food Supplement	1	1	-
Aminogran Mineral Mixture	1	1	-
Brasivol-fine, medium and coarse	3	1	2
Parentrovite IM Maintenance	2	2	-
Parentrovite IV High Potency	2	2	-
Parentrovite IM High Potency	2	2	-
Rite-Diet Gluten Free Flour)			
Rite-Diet Gluten Free Bread)	2	2	-
Migraleve Tabs, yellow	1	1	-
Migraleve Tabs, pink	1	1	-
Migraleve Tabs, yellow and pink	2	2	-
Migraleve Duo Pack with additional tablets	2	2	-
(yellow and/or pink)			
Triptafen-M Tabs)			
Triptafen Tabs)	2	2	-
10.13.4 Eye, Ear and Nasal Drops (supplied with dropper bottles, or with a separate dropper where appropriate) (See Part IV.Containers - page 31).	1	1	-
10.13.5 A drug in powder form together with a solvent in the same packs (Treatment Pack) (2 vials of powder and 2 vials of solvent)			
Actinac	2	1	1
10.13.6 Oxygen			
Oxygen Therapy Set with cylinder(s)	1	1	-
Oxygen Cylinders	1	1	-
(See Part X, Domicilary Oxygen Therapy Service, page 393).			

10 EXAMPLES OF APPLICATION OF PRESCRIPTION CHARGE ARRANGEMENTS - cont

	Professional Fees	Number of Prescription Charges	No Charge Prescriptons
10.13 **MISCELLANEOUS** - cont			
10.13.7 Trusses			
Spring Truss Inguinal - Single }	1	1	-
Elastic Band Truss Scrotal-Double }	1	1	-
10.13.8 Vaginal Creams and Applicators* Duracreme Vaginal Applicator - Type 2 }	2	-	2
Ortho Creme Vaginal Applicator - Type 1 }	2	-	2
Sultrin (Triple Sulfa) Cream Vaginal Applicator - Type 1 }	2	1	1
Vaginal Applicator (see page 97) Type 1 (Ortho) Type 2 (Durex)	1 1	- -	1 1

XVI

* (No attempt should be made to determine whether or not the applicator is required for use with a contraceptive)

This Page Is Intentionally Blank

List of Preparations approved by the Secretary of State for Health as respects England and the National Assembly for Wales as respects Wales which may be prescribed on form FP10(D) by Dentists for National Health Service patients

Aciclovir Cream, BP (Syn: Acyclovir Cream)
Aciclovir Oral Suspension,BP 200mg/5ml
  (Syn: Acyclovir Oral Suspension 200mg/5ml)
Aciclovir Tablets BP, 200mg
  (Syn: Acyclovir Tablets 200mg)
Amoxycillin Capsules, BP
Amoxycillin Oral Powder, DPF
Amoxycillin Oral Suspension, BP
  (Syn: Amoxycillin Mixture,
    Amoxycillin Syrup)
  (includes sugar-free formulation)
Amphotericin Lozenges, BP
Amphotericin Oral Suspension, DPF[1]
Ampicillin Capsules, BP
Ampicillin Oral Suspension BP
  (Syn: Ampicillin Mixture
    Ampicillin Syrup)
Artificial Saliva, DPF
Ascorbic Acid Tablets BP
  (Syn: Vitamin C Tablets)
Aspirin Tablets, Dispersible, BP

Ephedrine Nasal Drops, BP
Erythromycin Ethyl Succinate Oral Suspension BP,
  (includes sugar-free formulation)
Erythromycin Ethyl Succinate Tablets, BP
Erythromycin Stearate Tablets, BP
Erythromycin Tablets, BP

Fluconazole Capsules 50mg, DPF
Fluconazole Oral Suspension 50mg/5ml, DPF

Hydrocortisone Cream BP, 1%
Hydrocortisone Lozenges, BPC
Hydrocortisone and Miconazole Cream, DPF
Hydrocortisone and Miconazole Ointment, DPF
Hydrogen Peroxide Solution BP

Benzydamine Mouthwash, BP 0.15%
Benzydamine Oromucosal Spray, BP 0.15%

Ibuprofen Oral Suspension BP, sugar free
Ibuprofen Tablets, BP

Carbamazepine Tablets, BP
Carmellose Gelatin Paste, DPF
Cephalexin Capsules, BP
Cephalexin Oral Suspension BP,
  (Syn: Cephalexin Mixture)
Cephalexin Tablets, BP
Cephradine Capsules, BP
Cephradine Oral Solution, DPF
Chlorhexidine Gluconate 1% Gel, DPF
Chlorhexidine Mouthwash, DPF[1]
Chlorhexidine Oral Spray, DPF
Chlorpheniramine Tablets, BP
Choline Salicylate Dental Gel, BP
Clindamycin Capsules, BP

Lignocaine 5% Ointment, DPF

Menthol and Eucalyptus Inhalation, BP 1980
Metronidazole Oral Suspension, DPF
Metronidazole Tablets, BP
Miconazole Oral Gel, DPF[2]
Mouth-wash Solution - tablets, DPF

Nitrazepam Tablets, BP
Nystatin Ointment, BP
Nystatin Oral Suspension, BP
  (Syns: Nystatin Mixture,
    Nystatin Oral Drops, Nystatin Suspension)
  (includes sugar-free formulation)
Nystatin Pastilles, DPF[1]

Diazepam Oral Solution, BP 2mg/5ml
  (Syn: Diazepam Elixir)
Diazepam Tablets, BP
Diflunisal Tablets, BP
Dihydrocodeine Tablets BP, 30mg
Doxycycline Capsules BP, 100mg

Oxytetracycline Tablets, BP

XVIIA

[1] incorporated into BP 2000 (effective 1 December 2000)
[2] incorporated into BP 2000 (effective 1 December 2000) as Miconazole Oromucosal Gel

List of Preparations approved by the Secretary of State for Health as respects England and the
National Assembly for Wales as respects Wales which may be prescribed on
form FP10(D) by Dentists for National Health Service patients

*   Paracetamol Oral Suspension, BP
        (includes sugar-free formulation)
    Paracetamol Tablets BP
    Paracetamol Tablets, Soluble, BP
    Penciclovir Cream, DPF
    Pethidine Tablets, BP
    Phenoxymethylpenicillin Oral Solution, BP
    Phenoxymethylpenicillin Tablets, BP
        (Syn: Penicillin VK Tablets)
    Povidone-Iodine Mouthwash, BP 1%
    Probenecid Tablets, BP
    Promethazine Hydrochloride Tablets, BP
    Promethazine Oral Solution, BP
        (Syn: Promethazine Elixir)

    Sodium Chloride Mouthwash, Compound, BP
    Sodium Fluoride Oral Drops, BP
    Sodium Fluoride Tablets, BP
    Sodium Fusidate Ointment, BP
    Sodium Perborate Mouthwash, DPF

    Temazepam Oral Solution, BP
    Temazepam Tablets, BP
    Tetracycline Capsules, BP
    Tetracycline Tablets, BP
    Thymol Glycerin, Compound BP 1988
    Triamcinolone Dental Paste, BP

    Vitamin B Tablets, Compound, Strong, BPC

    Zinc Sulphate Mouthwash, DPF

*   The title covers strengths of 120mg/5ml and
    250mg/5ml, it is therefore necessary to specify the
    strength required.

List of Preparations approved by the Secretary of State for Health as respects England and the National Assembly for Wales as respects Wales which may be prescribed on forms FP10(CN) and FP10(PN) by Nurses for National Health Service patients

See Also: Drug Tariff Part I, Clauses 1, 2, 3; Note 7 to Part IXA, B, C and Note 1 to Part IXR

These preparations will only be prescribable as listed

Medicinal Preparations

Almond Oil Ear Drops BP
Arachis Oil Enema NPF
[1]Aspirin Tablets Dispersible 300mg, BP
Bisacodyl Suppositories BP (includes 5mg and
    10mg strengths)
Bisacodyl Tablets BP
Cadexomer-Iodine Ointment NPF
Cadexomer-Iodine Paste NPF
Cadexomer-Iodine Powder NPF
Calamine Cream, Aqueous BP
Calamine Lotion BP
Calamine Lotion, Oily BP 1980
Catheter Maintenance Solution Chlorhexidine NPF
Catheter Maintenance Solution Mandelic Acid NPF
Catheter Maintenance Solution Sodium Chloride NPF
Catheter Maintenance Solution 'Solution G' NPF
Catheter Maintenance Solution 'Solution R' NPF
Clotrimazole Cream 1%, BP
Co-danthramer Capsules NPF
Co-danthramer Capsules Strong NPF
Co-danthramer Oral Suspension NPF
Co-danthramer Oral Suspension Strong NPF
Co-danthrusate Capsules BP
Co-danthrusate Oral Suspension NPF
Crotamiton Cream, BP
Crotamiton Lotion, BP
Dextranomer Beads NPF
Dextranomer Paste NPF
Dimethicone barrier creams containing at least 10%
Docusate Capsules BP
Docusate Enema NPF
Docusate Enema Compound BP
Docusate Oral Solution BP
Docusate Oral Solution Paediatric BP
Econazole Cream 1% BP
Emollients as listed below:
    Alcoderm Cream
    Alcoderm Lotion
    Aqueous Cream, BP
    Arachis Oil, BP
    Dermamist
    Diprobase Cream
    Diprobase Ointment
    E45 Cream
    Emulsifying Ointment, BP
    Epaderm
    Humiderm Cream
    Hydromol Cream
    Hydrous Ointment, BP
    Keri Therapeutic Lotion
    LactiCare Lotion

    Lipobase
    Liquid and White Soft Paraffin Ointment, NPF
    Neutrogena Dermatological Cream
    Oilatum Cream
    Paraffin, White Soft, BP
    Paraffin, Yellow Soft, BP
    Ultrabase
    Unguentum M
Emollient Bath Additives as listed below:
    Alpha Keri Bath Oil
    [2]Balneum
    Dermalo Bath Emollient (Formerly Emmolate
        Bath Oil)
    Diprobath
    Hydromol Emollient
    Oilatum Emollient
    Oilatum Fragrance Free
    Oilatum Gel
Folic Acid 400 microgram/5ml Oral Solution, NPF
Folic Acid Tablets 400 micrograms, BP
Glycerol Suppositories BP
Ispaghula Husk Granules BP
Ispaghula Husk Granules Effervescent BP
Ispaghula Husk Oral Powder BP
Lactitol Powder NPF
Lactulose Powder NPF
Lactulose Solution BP
Lidocaine Gel/Lignocaine Gel, BP
Lidocaine Ointment/Lignocaine Ointment, NPF
Lidocaine and Chlorhexidine Gel/Lignocaine and
    Chlorhexidine Gel, BP
Macrogol Oral Powder, Compound, NPF
Magnesium Hydroxide Mixture BP
Magnesium Sulphate Paste BP
Malathion Alcoholic Lotions (containing at least
    0.5%)
Malathion Aqueous Lotions (containing at least
    0.5%)
Mebendazole Oral Suspension NPF
Mebendazole Tablets NPF
Methylcellulose Tablets, BP
Miconazole Cream 2% BP
Miconazole Oral Gel NPF
Mouthwash Solution-tablets, NPF
Nystatin Oral Suspension BP
Nystatin Pastilles NPF
Olive Oil Ear Drops BP

XVIIB

[1]Only quantities up to 96 in packs of not more than 32
[2]Except pack sizes that are not to be prescribed under the NHS (See Part XVIIIA)

List of Preparations approved by the Secretary of State for Health as respects England and the National Assembly for Wales as respects Wales which may be prescribed on forms FP10(CN) and FP10(PN) by Nurses for National Health Service patients

See Also: Drug Tariff Part I, Clauses 1, 2, 3; Note 7 to Part IXA, B, C and Note 1 to Part IXR

These preparations will only be prescribable as listed

Medicinal Preparations - Cont.

Paracetamol Oral Suspension, BP
    (includes 120mg/5ml and 250mg/5ml strengths
    both of which are available as sugar-free
    formulations)
[1]Paracetamol Tablets, BP
[1]Paracetamol Tablets Soluble BP
Permethrin Cream NPF
Permethrin Cream Rinse NPF
Phenothrin Alcoholic Lotion NPF
Phenothrin Aqueous Lotion, NPF
Phenothrin Foam Application, NPF
Phosphates Enema BP
Piperazine Citrate Elixir BP
Piperazine and Senna Powder NPF
Povidone-Iodine Solution, BP
Senna Granules Standardised BP
Senna Oral Solution NPF
Senna Tablets BP
Senna and Ispaghula Granules NPF
Sodium Bicarbonate Ear Drops, BP
Sodium Chloride Solution Sterile BP
Sodium Citrate Compound Enema NPF
Sodium Picosulfate Elixir NPF
Sterculia Granules NPF
Sterculia and Frangula Granules NPF
Streptokinase and Streptodornase Topical
    Powder NPF
Thymol Glycerin, Compound BP 1988
Titanium Ointment NPF
Zinc and Castor Oil Ointment BP
Zinc Oxide and Dimeticone Spray NPF
Zinc Oxide Impregnated Medicated Stocking NPF

List of Preparations approved by the Secretary of State for Health as respects England and the National Assembly for Wales as respects Wales which may be prescribed on forms FP10(CN) and FP10(PN) by Nurses for National Health Service patients

Appliances and Reagents (Including Wound Management Products)

All Appliances and Reagents included in this list must comply with the description, specifications, sizes, packs and quantities as specified in the relevant entry in Part IX of the Drug Tariff

Chemical Reagents,
- the following as listed in Part IXR
  Detection Tablets for Glycosuria
  Detection Tablets for Ketonuria
  Detection Strips for Glycosuria
  Detection Strips for Ketonuria
  Detection Strips for Proteinuria
  Detection Strips for Blood Glucose

Fertility (Ovulation) Thermometer
  as listed in Part IXA

Film Gloves, Disposable, EMA
  as listed in Part IXA

Elastic Hosiery including accessories
  as listed in Part IXA

Eye Drops Dispensers
  as listed in Part IXA

Hypodermic Equipment,
- the following as listed in Part IXA
  Hypodermic Syringes - U100 Insulin
  Hypodermic Syringe - Single Use Or Single-
  patient Use, U100 Insulin with needle
  Hypodermic Needles - Sterile, Single Use
  Lancets - Sterile, Single Use
  Needle Clipping Device

Incontinence Appliances as listed in Part IXB

Irrigation Fluids as listed in Part IXA

Pessaries, Ring as listed in Part IXA

Stoma Appliances and Associated Products
  as listed in Part IXC

Urethral Catheters as listed in Part IXA

Urine Sugar Analysis Equipment
  as listed in Part IXA

Wound Management and Related Products (including bandages, dressings, gauzes, lint, stockinette, etc),
- the following as listed in Part IXA
  Absorbent Cottons
  Absorbent Cotton Gauzes
  Absorbent Cotton and Viscose Ribbon Gauze, BP 1988
  Absorbent Lint, BPC
  Absorbent Perforated Plastic Film Faced Dressing
  Arm Slings
  Cellulose Wadding, BP 1988
  Cotton Conforming Bandage, BP 1988
  Cotton Crêpe Bandage, BP 1988
  Cotton Crepe Bandage, Hospicrepe 239
  Cotton, Polyamide and Elastane Bandage
  Cotton Stretch Bandage BP 1988
  Crêpe Bandage, BP 1988
  Elastic Adhesive Bandage, BP
  Elastic Web Bandages
  Elastomer and Viscose Bandage, Knitted
  Gauze and Cotton Tissues
  Heavy Cotton and Rubber Elastic Bandage, BP
  High Compression Bandages (Extensible)
  Knitted Polyamide and Cellulose Contour Bandage BP 1988
  Knitted Viscose Primary Dressing, BP, Type 1
  Multi-layer Compression Bandaging
  Multiple Pack Dressing No 1
  Open-wove Bandage, BP 1988, Type 1
  Paraffin Gauze Dressing, BP
  Polyamide and Cellulose Contour Bandage, BP 1988
  Povidone-Iodine Fabric Dressing, Sterile
  Short Stretch Compression Bandage
  Skin Closure Strips, Sterile
  Sterile Dressing Packs
  Stockinettes
  Sub-compression Wadding Bandage
  Surgical Adhesive Tapes
  Suspensory Bandages, Cotton
  Swabs
  Triangular Calico Bandage, BP 1980
  Vapour-permeable Adhesive Film Dressing, BP
  Vapour-permeable Waterproof Plastic Wound Dressing, BP, Sterile
  Wound Management Dressings (including alginate, cavity, hydrocolloid, hydrogel and foam)
  Zinc Paste Bandages (including both plain and with additional ingredients)

All Appliances and Reagents which may **not** be prescribed by Nurses are, for guidance, annotated Ⓝ against the specific entry in the relevant Part of the Drug Tariff.

List of Preparations approved by the Secretary of State for Health as respects England and the National Assembly for Wales as respects Wales which may be prescribed on forms FP10(CN) and FP10(PN) by Nurses for National Health Service patients

This Page Is Intentionally Blank

Part XVIIIA reproduces Schedule 10 to the National Health Service (General Medical Services) Regulations 1992, as amended.

10.10 Cleaning and Disinfecting Solution
10.10 Rinsing and Neutralising Solution
10 Day Slimmer Tablets
10 Hour Capsules
4711 Cologne
Abidec Capsules
Acarosan Foam
Acarosan Moist Powder
Acclaim Flea Control Aerosol Plus
Acnaveen Bar
Acne Aid Bar
Actal Suspension
Actal Tablets
Actifed Compound Linctus
Actifed Cough Relief
Actifed Expectorant
Actifed Linctus with Codeine
Actifed Syrup
Actifed Tablets
Actomite
Actonorm Gel
Actonorm Powder
Actonorm Tablets
Actron Tablets
Adpack Europe Gamolenic Acid (GLA) Capsules
Adreno-Lyph Plus Tablets
Adult Cough Balsam (Cupal)
Adult Meltus Cough & Catarrh Linctus
Adult Tonic Mixture (Thornton & Ross)
Advanced Nutrition Bee Pollen Granules
Advanced Nutrition Bee Propolis Tablets
Advanced Nutrition Chromium Compound Liquid
Advanced Nutrition Ener-B NSL Gel
Advanced Nutrition Herbal Aloe Juice
Advanced Nutrition L-Arginine Capsules
Advanced Nutrition Linseed Oil
Advanced Nutrition Silica-Organic Capsules
Advanced Nutrition Sulphur Capsules
Advanced Nutrition Vitamin E Capsules
Aerocide 2 Spray 400ml
Afrazine Nasal Drops
Afrazine Nasal Spray
Afrazine Paediatric Nasal Drops
Agarol Emulsion
Agiolax Granules
Airbal Breathe Easy Vapour Inhaler
AL Tablets
Alagbin Tablets
Alcin Tablets
Alcon Salette Aerosol Saline Solution
Aletres Cordial (Potters)
Alexitol Sodium Suspension 360 mg/5 ml
Alexitol Sodium Tablets
Algipan Rub
Algipan Tablets
Alka-Donna P Mixture
Alka-Donna P Tablets
Alka-Donna Suspension
Alka-Donna Tablets
Alka Mints

Alka-Seltzer Tablets
Alket Powders
All Clear Shampoo
All Fours Cough Mixture (Harwood)
All Fours Mixture (Glynwed
    Wholesale Chemists)
All Fours Mixture (Roberts Laboratories)
Allbee with C Capsules
Allbee with C Elixir
Aller-eze Plus Tablets
Aller-eze Tablets
Allinson's Wholemeal Flour
Almasilate Tablets 500 mg
Almay Aftersun Soother
Almay Face Powder
Almay Sun Protection Cream SPF 12
Almay Ultra Protection Lotion SPF 12
Almazine Tablets 1mg
Almazine Tablets 2.5 mg
Aloin Tablets 40 mg
Alophen Pills
Alpine Tea
Alprazolam Tablets 0.25mg
Alprazolam Tablets 0.5mg
Alprazolam Tablets 1 mg
Altacaps
Altacite Plus Tablets
Altacite Suspension
Altacite Tablets
Altelave Liquid
Aludrox Gel
Aludrox Liquid
Aludrox M H Suspension
Aludrox S A Suspension
Aludrox Tablets
Aluhyde Tablets
Aluminium Hydroxide & Silicone
    Suspension
Aluminium Phosphate Gel
Aluminium Phosphate Tablets 400 mg
Alupent Expectorant Mixture
Alupent Expectorant Tablets
Aluphos Gel
Aluphos Tablets
Alupram Tablets 2 mg
Alupram Tablets 5 mg
Alupram Tablets 10 mg
Aluzyme Tablets
Alzed Tablets
Ambre Solaire Cream Factor 8
Ambre Solaire Cream Factor 10
Ambre Solaire High Protection Cream SPF10
Ambre Solaire High Protection Milk SPF 12
American Nutrition Strezz B-Vite Tablets
Ami - 10 Rinsing and Storage Solution
Amiclear Contact Lens Cleanser Tablets
Amidose Saline Solution 30 ml
Amin-Aid
Amisyn Tablets

XVIIIA

Ammonium Chloride and Morphine
    Mixture BP
Amplex Mint Capsules
Amplex Mouthwash
Amplex Original Capsules
Anadin Analgesic Capsules Maximum
    Strength
Anadin Analgesic Tablets
Anadin Extra Analgesic Tablets
Anadin Extra Soluble
Anadin Ibuprofen Tablets
Anadin Paracetamol Tablets
Anadin Tablets Soluble
Anaflex Cream
Andrews Answer
Andrews Antacid Tablets
Andrews Liver Salts Effervescent Powder
Andrews Liver Salts (Diabetic Formula)
    Effervescent Powder
Andursil Liquid
Andursil Tablets
Anestan Bronchial Tablets
Anethaine Cream
Aneurone Mixture
Angiers Junior Aspirin Tablets
Angiers Junior Paracetamol Tablets
Anorvit Tablets
Antasil Liquid
Antasil Tablets
Anthisan Cream
Antistin-Privine Nasal Drops
Antistin-Privine Nasal Spray
Antitussive Linctus (Cox)
Antoin Tablets
Antussin Liquid (Sterling Winthrop)
Anxon Capsules 15 mg
Anxon Capsules 30 mg
Anxon Capsules 45 mg
Aperient Tablets (Brome & Schimmer)
Aperient Tablets (Kerbina)
Apodorm Tablets 2.5 mg
Apodorm Tablets 5 mg
APP Stomach Powder
APP Stomach Tablets
Applefords Gluten-Free Rice Cakes
Arnica Lotion
Arocin Capsules
Arret Capsules
Ascorbef Tablets
Ascorbic Acid & Hesperidin Capsules
    (Regent Laboratories)
Asilone Antacid Liquid
Asilone Antacid Tablets
Asilone Orange Tablets
Askit Capsules
Askit Powders
Askit Tablets
Aspergum Chewing Gum Tablets 227 mg
Aspirin Chewing-Gum Tablets 227 mg
Aspirin Tablets, Effervescent Soluble 300 mg
Aspirin Tablets, Effervescent Soluble 500 mg

Aspirin Tablets, Slow
    (Micro-Encapsulated) 648 mg
Aspro Clear Extra Tablets
Aspro Clear Tablets
Aspro Extra Strength Tablets 500 mg
Aspro Junior Tablets
Aspro Microfined Tablets
Aspro Paraclear Junior Tablets
Aspro Paraclear Tablets
Asthma Tablets (Cathay)
Astral Moisturising Cream
Astroplast Analgesic Capsules
Atensine Tablets 2 mg
Atensine Tablets 5 mg
Atensine Tablets 10 mg
Ativan Tablets 1 mg
Ativan Tablets 2.5 mg
Atrixo
Audax Ear Drops
Autan Insect Repellent
Aveeno Baby
Aveeno Bar
Aveeno Bar Oilated
Aveeno Emulave Bar
Aveenobar
Ayrtons Analgesic Balm
Ayrtons Macleans Formula Tablets

B Complex Capsules (Rodale)
B Complex Super Capsules (Rodale)
B Extra Tablets (British
    Chemotherapeutic Products)
Babezone Syrup
Baby Chest Rub Ointment (Cupal)
Babylix Syrup
Babysafe Tablets
Badedas Bath Gelee
Balm of Gilead (Robinsons)
Balm of Gilead Cough Mixture (Wicker
    Herbal Stores)
Balm of Gilead Liquid (Culpeper)
Balm of Gilead Mixture (Potters)
Balneum Bath Treatment 150ml pack
Balneum Plus Bath Treatment 150ml pack
Banfi Hungarian Hair Tonic
Banimax Tablets
Barker's Liquid of Life Solution
Barker's Liquid of Life Tablets
Barkoff Cough Syrup
Barnes - Hind Cleaning and Soaking Solution
Barnes - Hind Intensive Cleaner
Barnes - Hind No 4 Cleaner
Barnes - Hind Wetting and Soaking Solution
Bausch and Lomb Cleaning Tablets
Bausch and Lomb Concentrated Cleaner
    (for Hard Lenses)

Bausch and Lomb Daily Lens Cleaner
Bausch and Lomb Saline Solution
Bausch and Lomb Soaking and Wetting Solution
Bayer Aspirin Tablets 300 mg
BC500 Tablets
BC500 with Iron Tablets
BC500 Vitamin Sachets effervescent
Becosym Forte Tablets
Becosym Syrup
Becosym Tablets
Becotab Tablets
Bee Health Propolis Capsules
Beecham Analgesic Cream
Beechams Catarrh Capsules
Beechams Day Nurse Capsules
Beechams Day Nurse Syrup
Beechams Night Nurse Capsules
Beechams Night Nurse Cold Remedy
Beechams Pills
Beechams Powders
Beechams Powders Capsule Form
Beechams Powders Mentholated
Beechams Powders Tablet Form
Beehive Balsam
Bekovit Tablets
Belladonna and Ephedrine Mixture,
    Paediatric, BPC
Bellocarb Tablets
Bemax Natural Wheatgerm
Benadon Tablets 20 mg
Benadon Tablets 50 mg
Benafed Linctus
Benerva Compound Tablets
Benerva Injection 25 mg/ml
Benerva Injection 100 mg/ml
Benerva Tablets 3 mg
Benerva Tablets 10 mg
Benerva Tablets 25 mg
Benerva Tablets 50 mg
Benerva Tablets 100 mg
Benerva Tablets 300 mg
Bengers Food
Bengue's Balsam
Benylin Chesty Coughs Original
Benylin Children's Coughs
Benylin Children's Cough Linctus
Benylin Cough & Congestion
Benylin Day & Night Tablets
Benylin Day & Night Cold Treatment
Benylin Dry Coughs Original
Benylin Expectorant
Benylin Fortified Linctus
Benylin Mentholated Cough &
    Decongestant Linctus
Benylin Non-Drowsy Cough Linctus
Benylin Paediatric
Benylin with Codeine
Benzedrex Inhaler
Benzoin Inhalation BP
Bepro Cough Syrup
Beres Drops Plus
Bergasol After Sun Soother

Bergasol Ultra Protection Tanning Lotion
Best Royal Jelly Capsules
Beta Carotene Capsules (Nutri Imports & Exports)
Biactol Anti-Bacterial Face Wash
Bile Beans Formula 1 Pill
Bio-Antioxidant Tablets
Biocare Acidophilus Powder
Biocare AD206 (Adreno-Zyme) Capsules
Biocare Allicin Compound Capsules
Biocare Amino-Plex Capsules
Biocare Artemisia Compound Capsules
Biocare ATP Factor Capsules
Biocare Beetroot Concentrate
    (Bioflavour Complex) Capsules
Biocare Beta-Carotene Capsules
Biocare Betaine HCL/Pepsin Capsules
    200/100mg
Biocare BGF Bifidophilus Growth Factor Powder
Biocare Bio Acidophilus Milk Free Capsules
Biocare Bio-A Emulsifying Liquid
Biocare Biogard Capsules
Biocare Bio-Cysteine Capsules
Biocare Bio-Magnesium Capsules 100mg
Biocare Bio-Manganese Capsules
Biocare Bio-Plex Powder
Biocare Butyric Acid Compound Capsules
Biocare Calcidophilus Capsules
Biocare Calcium EAP2 Capsules
Biocare Candistatin Capsules
Biocare Catalase Compound Liquid
Biocare Cervagyn Vaginal Cream
Biocare Cellguard Forte Capsules
Biocare CG233 Capsules
Biocare Children's Multi Vitamin/Mineral Capsules
Biocare Cholesteraze Capsules
Biocare Chromium Polynicotinate Liquid
Biocare Colleginase Capsules
Biocare Colon Care Capsules
Biocare Cystoplex Powder
Biocare Dermasorb Skin Cream
Biocare Digestaid Capsules
Biocare DMSA Capsules
Biocare Efaplex Linseed/GLA Blend Capsules
Biocare Enteroplex Powder
Biocare Eradicin Forte Capsules
Biocare Femforte Capsules
Biocare Garlicin Capsules
Biocare GLA Complex Tablets
Biocare GLA/Co Q10 Catalase Capsules
Biocare Glutenzyme Capsules
Biocare Hep 194 (Hepaguard) Capsules
Biocare HCL Pepsin Capsules
Biocare Histazyme Capsules
Biocare IMU Power Pack
Biocare Int B2 Bifidophilus Bacterium Powder
Biocare Iron EAP2 Capsules
Biocare Kalmar Capsules
Biocare Lactase Enzyme Liquid
Biocare Ligazyme Capsules
Biocare Linseed Oil Emulsifying Capsules
Biocare Lipazyme Capsules
Biocare Lipo-Plex Capsules

XVIIIA

Biocare Lipo-Plex Co-Q10 EPA/DHA Capsules
Biocare Magnesium Calcium 2:1 Capsules
Biocare Magnesium EAP2 Capsules
Biocare Mega GLA Complex Capsules 163mg
Biocare Molybdenum Liquid
Biocare Multi-Mineral Complex Capsules
Biocare Multivitamin Mineral Capsules
Biocare Mycopryl 250 Junior Strength
   Capsules
Biocare Mycopryl 400 Capsules
Biocare Mycopryl 680 Capsules
Biocare N-Acetyl Glucosamine Capsules
Biocare NT 188 (Neurotone) Capsules
Biocare Organic Selenium Capsules 100mcg
Biocare Oxy-B15 Complex Capsules
Biocare Oxyplex Tablets
Biocare Oxy Pro Liquid
Biocare Pancrogest Capsules
Biocare Paracidin (Citricidal) Oral Drops
Biocare Permatrol Capsules
Biocare Pit-Enzyme Capsules
Biocare Polyzyme Capsules
Biocare Polyzyme Forte & Acidophilus Capsules
Biocare Polyzyme Forte Capsules
Biocare Potassium Ascorbate Capsules
Biocare Prolactazyme Capsules
Biocare Prolactazyme Tablets
Biocare Reduced Glutathione Capsules
Biocare Replete Sachets
Biocare Sea Plasma Capsules 500mg
Biocare Selenium Complex Tablets 50mcg
Biocare Selenium Liquid
Biocare Shiitake Mushroom Extract Capsules
Biocare Spectrumzyme Capsules
Biocare TH207 (Thyro-Zyme) Capsules
Biocare Thioproline Capsules
Biocare Uritol Capsules
Biocare Vegi-Dophilus Capsules
Biocare Vitamin B6 Capsules
Biocare Vitamin B Compound Capsules
Biocare Vitamin B12 Timed Release
   Capsules
Biocare Vitamin C Capsules
Biocare Vitamin C Magnesium Ascorbate
   Powder
Biocare Vitamin E Emulsifying Capsules
Biocare Vyta Mins Capsules
Biocare Zinc Tablets
Bio-Carotene Softgel Capsules
Bioflav Complex Tablets
Bioflav Complex + C Tablets
Bioflavonoid C Capsules
Bio-Glandin 25 Capsules
Bio Harmony Sachets
Bio-Health Buffered C500 Capsules
Bio-Health Extra Calcium Capsules
Bio-Health Zinc Gluconate Capsules
Bio-Light Slimming Food Supplement
Bio-Quinone Q10 Softgel Capsules
Bio-Quinone Q10 Super Softgel Capsules
Bioscal Hair Formula
Bio Science Basic Health AM Capsules

Bio Science Basic Health PM Capsules
Bio Science Bio-C Powder
Bio Science Cal-Mag Alkaline Capsules
Bio Science Chelated Cal-Mag Compound Capsules
Bio Science Chelated Zinc Capsules
Bio Science Full Spectrum Aminos Powder
Bio Science Lipid Enzyme Capsules
Bio Science Lo-pH Complete Spectrum
   Digestive Enzyme Capsules
Bio Science Lo-pH Digestive Enzyme Capsules
Bio Science MSM Organic Sulphur Capsules
Bio Science Non-Acidic Sustained
   Release Vitamin C Tablets
Bio Science Organic Iron Capsules
Bio Science Pro Enzyme Capsules
Bio Science Pyroxidal 5 Phosphates Capsules
Bio Science Selenium Plus Capsules
Bio Science Timed Release Vitamin
   C Tablets
Bio Science Vitamin B1 Capsules
Bio Science Vitamin B3 Nicotinamide Capsules
Bio Science Vitamin B5 Calcium
   Pantothenate Capsules
Bio Science Vitamin B6 Capsules
Bio Science Vitamin E Capsules
Bio-Selenium + Zinc Tablets
Bio-Strath Drops
Bio-Strath Elixir
Biovital Tablets
Biovital Vitamin Tonic
Birley's Antacid Powder
Bis-Mag Lozenge
Bis-Peps Tablets
Bisma-Calna Cream
Bisma-Rex Powder
Bisma-Rex Tablets
Bismag Antacid Powder
Bismag Tablets
Bismuth Compound Lozenges BPC
Bismuth Dyspepsia Lozenges
Bismuth Pepsin and Pancreatin Tablets
Bismuth, Soda and Pepsin Mixture
Bisodol Antacid Powder
Bisodol Extra Tablets
Bisodol Tablets
Bisolvomycin Capsules
Bisolvon Elixir
Bisolvon Tablets
Blackcurrant Cough Elixir
   (Thornton & Ross)
Blackcurrant Seed Oil Capsules
Blackcurrant Syrup Compound (Beben)
Blackmore's Acidophilus & Pectin Tablets
Blackmore's Bio C Tablets
Blackmore's Celloid CS36 Calcium
   Sulphate Tablets
Blackmore's Celloid IP82 Iron pH Tablets
Blackmore's Celloid SS69 Sodium
   Sulphate Tablets
Blackmore's Citrus C & Acerola Tablets
Blackmore's Duocelloid PP/MP Tablets
Blackmore's Duocelloid PS/MP Tablets

Blackmore's Duocelloid S/CF Tablets
Blackmore's Duocelloid SP/S Tablets
Blackmore's Echinacea ACE + Zinc Tablets
Blackmore's Hypericum Tablets
Blackmore's Sodical Plus Tablets
Blandax Suspension
Blavig Tablets
Blood Tonic Mixture (Thompsons)
Boldolaxine Tablets
Bonemeal Calfos, Vit A Ester, Vit D
   Tablets
Bonomint Chewing Gum
Bonomint Tablets
Booth's Cough & Catarrh Elixir
Boots Aromatherapy Massage Oil
Boots Baby Oil
Boots Cold Relief Powder for Solution
Boots Compound Laxative Syrup of Figs
Boots Cough Relief for Adults
Boots Glycerin & Blackcurrant Soothing
   Cough Relief
Boots Hard Lens Soaking Solution
Boots Hard Lens Wetting Solution
Boots Health Salts
Boots Indigestion Plus Mixture
Boots Indigestion Powder
Boots Lip Salve
Boots Menthol & Wintergreen Embrocation
Boots Nasal Spray
Boots No 7 Vitamin E Skin Cream
Boots Orange Drink
Boots Soft Lens Cleaning Solution
Boots Soft Lens Comfort Solution
Boots Soft Lens Soaking Solution
Boots Soya Milk
Boots Vapour Rub Ointment
Boston Lens Cleaning Solution
Boston Lens Wetting and Soaking Solution
Box's Balm of Gilead Cough Mixture
Bravit Capsules
Bravit Tablets
Breoprin Tablets 648 mg
Brewers Yeast Super B Tablets (Rodale)
Brewers Yeast Tablets (3M Health Care)
Brewers Yeast Tablets (Phillips Yeast
   Products)
Bricanyl Compound Tablets
Bricanyl Expectorant
Brogans Cough Mixture
Brogans Cough Syrup
Bromazepam Tablets 1.5 mg
Bromazepam Tablets 3 mg
Bromazepam Tablets 6 mg
Bromhexine Hydrochloride Elixir 4 mg/5 ml
Bromhexine Hydrochloride Tablets 8 mg
Bronalin Decongestant
Bronalin Dry Cough Linctus
Bronalin Expectorant
Bronalin Paediatric Cough Syrup
Bronchial & Cough Mixture
   (Worthington Walter)
Bronchial Balsam (Cox)

Bronchial Catarrh Syrup (Rusco)
Bronchial Cough Mixture (Evans Medical)
Bronchial Emulsion (Three Flasks)
   (Thornton & Ross)
Bronchial Emulsion AS Extra Strong
   (Ayrton Saunders)
Bronchial Mixture (Rusco)
Bronchial Mixture Extra Strong (Cox)
Bronchial Mixture Sure Shield Brand
Bronchial Tablets (Leoren)
Bronchialis Mist Liquid (Industrial
   Pharmaceutical Services)
Bronchialis Mist Nig Double Strength
   (Phillip Harris Medical)
Bronchisan Childrens Cough Syrup
Bronchisan Cough Syrup
Broncholia Mixture
Bronchotone Solution
Bronkure Cough & Bronchitis Mixture
   (Jacksons)
Brontus Syrup
Brontus Syrup for Children
Brontussin Cough Suppressant Mixture
Brooklax Tablets
Brotizolam Tablets 0.125 mg
Brotizolam Tablets 0.25 mg
Bufferin Tablets
Build-Up (Nestle Health Care)
Buttercup Baby Cough Linctus
Buttercup Syrup
Buttercup Syrup Honey and Lemon

Cabdrivers Adult Linctus
Cabdrivers Diabetic Linctus
Cabdrivers Junior Linctus
Cabdrivers Nasal Decongestant Tablets
Cadbury's Coffee Compliment
Cafadol Tablets
Caffeine & Dextrose Tablets
Cal-A-Cool Aftersun Moisturising Cream
Caladryl Cream
Caladryl Lotion
Calamage
Calcia Calcium Supplement Tablets
Calcimax Syrup
Calcinate Tablets
Calcium Syrup (Berk Pharmaceuticals)
Calendolon Ointment
California Syrup of Figs
Calpol Extra Tablets
Calpol Infant Suspension
Calpol Six Plus Suspension
Calpol Tablets
Calsalettes Sugar Coated Tablets
Calsalettes Uncoated Tablets
Camfortix Linctus P1

XVIIIA

Camphor Spirit
Candacurb Capsules
Candacurb-E Capsules
Canderel Intense Sweetener Spoonful
Candermyl Liposome Cream
Cantaflour
Cantamac Tablets
Cantamega 1000 Tablets
Cantamega 2000 Divided Dose Tablets ¼ Size
Cantamega 2000 Naturtab Tablets
Cantassium Amino M.S. Tablets
Cantassium Discs
Cantassium Fructose
Cantassium Multivitamin Tablets
Capramin Tablets
Caprystatin Capsules
Carbellon Tablets
Carbo-Cort Cream
Carisoma Compound Tablets
Carnation Coffeemate
Carnation Slender Meal Replacement
    (All Flavours)
Carrzone Powder
Carters Little Pills
Carylderm Shampoo
Cascara Evacuant Liquid Mixture
Cascara Tablets BP
Castellan No 10 Cough Mixture
Catarrh & Bronchial Syrup (Thornton & Ross)
Catarrh Cough Syrup (Boots)
Catarrh Mixture (Herbal Laboratories)
Catarrh Syrup for Children (Boots)
Catarrh Tablets (Cathay)
Catarrh-Ex Tablets
Ce-Cobalin Syrup
Ceeyees Tablets
Celaton Rejuvenation Tablets
Celaton CH3 Strong & Calm Tablets
Celaton CH3 Triplus Tablets
Celaton CH3 + Ease & Vitality Tablets
Celaton Whole Wheat Germ Capsules
Celavit 1 Powder
Celavit 2 Powder
Celavit 3 Powder
Celevac Granules
Centrax Tablets 10 mg
Cephos Powders
Cephos Tablets
Cetaphil Lotion
Charabs Tablets
Charvita Tablets
Cheroline Cough Linctus
Cherry Bark Cough Syrup Childrens
    (Loveridge)
Cherry Bark Linctus Adults (Loveridge)
Cherry Cough Balsam (Herbal
    Laboratories)
Cherry Cough Linctus (Savoury & Moore)
Cherry Cough Mixture (Rusco)
Cherry Flavoured Extract of Malt
    (Distillers)

Chest & Cough Tablets (Brome &
    Schimmer)
Chest & Cough Tablets (Kerbina)
Chest & Throat Tablets No 8,000
    (English Grains)
Chest Pills (Brome & Schimmer)
Chest Tablets (Kerbina)
Chesty Cough Syrup (Scott & Browne)
Chickweed Ointment
Chilblain Tablets (Boots)
Child's Cherry Flavoured Linctus (Cupal)
Children's Blackcurrant Cough Syrup
    (Rusco)
Children's Cherry Cough Syrup
    (Thornton & Ross)
Children's Cough Linctus (Ransoms)
Children's Cough Mixture (Beecham)
Children's Cough Mixture (Loveridge)
Children's Cough Syrup (Ayrton
    Saunders)
Children's Cough Syrup (Cox)
Children's Cough Syrup (Evans Medical)
Children's Cough Syrup (Thornbers)
Children's Medicine Liquid (Hall's)
Children's Phensic Tablets
Children's Wild Cherry Cough Linctus
    (Evans Medical)
Chilvax Tablets
Chlorasol Sachets
Chocolate Laxative Tablets (Isola)
Chocovite Tablets
Christy's Rich Lanolin
Christy's Skin Emulsion
Cidal
Cidex Longlife
Cidex Sterilising Solution
Cinnamon Essence Medicinal Mixture (Langdale)
Cinnamon Tablets Medicinal (Langdale)
Cinota Drops
Citrosan Powder
Claradin Effervescent Tablets
Clara's Kitchen Gluten-Free Porridge
Clarityn Allergy
Clarkes Blood Mixture
Clean and Soak
Cleansing Herb Dried (Potters)
Cleansing Herbs (Brome & Schimmer)
Cleansing Herbs Powder (Dorwest)
Clen-Zym Tablets
Clerz Lubricating and Rewetting Eye Drops
Clerz Lubricating Cleaning and
    Comfort Sachets
Clinique Clarifying Lotion
Clinique Continuous Coverage
Clinique Crystal Clear Cleaning Oil
Clinique Dramatically Different
    Moisturising Lotion
Clinique Facial Mild Soap
Clinisan Skin Cleansing Foam
Clinisan Skin Cleansing Foam Aerosol 500ml
Clorazepate Dipotassium Capsules 7.5 mg

Clorazepate Dipotassium Capsules
15 mg
Clorazepate Dipotassium Tablets 15 mg
Co-op Aspirin Tablets BP 300 mg
Co-op Bronchial Mixture
Co-op Halibut Liver Oil Capsules BP
Co-op Paracetamol Tablets BP 500 mg
Co-op Soluble Aspirin Tablets BP 300 mg
Cobalin H Injection 250 mcg/ml
Cobalin H Injection 1000 mcg/ml
Cobalin Injection 100 mcg/ml
Cobalin Injection 250 mcg/ml
Cobalin Injection 500 mcg/ml
Cobalin Injection 1000 mcg/ml
Coda - Med Tablets
Cod Liver Oil & Creosote Capsules
(5 Oval) (R P Scherer)
Cod Liver Oil & Creosote Capsules
(10 Oval) (R P Scherer)
Cod Liver Oil Caps 10 Minims
(Woodward)
Cod Liver Oil High Potency Capsules
(R P Scherer)
Cod Liver Oil with Malt Extract &
Hypophosphite Syrup (Distillers)
Cod Liver Oil 0.3 ml Capsules
(R P Scherer)
Cod Liver Oil 0.6 ml Capsules
(R P Scherer)
Codalax
Codalax Forte
Codanin Analgesic Tablets
Codis Soluble Tablets
Codural Tablets
Cojene Tablets
Cold & Influenza Capsules (Regent
Laboratories)
Cold & Influenza Mixture (Boots)
Cold & Influenza Mixture (Davidson)
Cold & Influenza Mixture (Rusco)
Cold & Influenza Mixture (Thornton &
Ross)
Cold Relief (Blackcurrant Flavour)
Granular Powder (Boots)
Cold Relief Capsules (Scott & Bowne)
Cold Relief Tablets (Boots)
Cold Tablets (Roberts)
Coldrex Powder
Coldrex Tablets
Colgard Emergency Essence (Lane
Health Products)
Colgate Dental Cream with MFP Fluoride
Colgate Disclosing Tablets
Collins Elixir
Colocynth & Jalap Tablets Compound
BPC 1963
Colocynth Compound Pills BPC 1963
Cologel Liquid
Communion Wafers
Complan
Comploment Continus Tablets
Compound Fig Elixir BP

Compound Rhubarb Oral Powder BP
Compound Rhubarb Tincture BP
Compound Syrup of Glycerophosphates
BPC 1963
Compound Syrup of Hypophosphites
BPC 1963
Comtrex Capsules
Comtrex Liquid
Comtrex Tablets
Concavit Capsules
Concavit Drops
Concavit Injection
Concavit Syrup
Confiance Dietary Supplement Tablets
Congreves Balsamic Elixir
Constipation Herb Dried (Potters)
Constipation Herbs (Hall's)
Constipation Herbs (Mixed Herbs)
(Brome & Schimmer)
Constipation Mixture No 105 (Potters)
Contac 400 Capsules
Contac Coughcaps
Contactaclean Cleaning Solution
Contactasoak Disinfecting and Soaking Solution
Contactasol O2 Care Solution
Contactasol Complete Care All-In-One Solution
Contactasol Solar Saline Spray
Contactasol Wetting Solution
Copholco Cough Syrup
Copholcoids
Coppertone Apres Plage Aftersun Milk
Coppertone Children's Cream SPF25
Coppertone Children's Lotion SPF15
Coppertone Dark Tanning Lotion SPF4
Coppertone Sun Tanning Lotion SPF6
Coppertone Water Resistant Tanning
Cream SPF8
Co-QIO Tablets
Core Level Adrenal Tablets
Core Level Auto Sym Tablets
Core Level C Timed Release Tablets
Core Level Health Reserve Tablets
Core Level Ilioduodenal Tablets
Core Level Magnesium Tablets
Core Level Zinc Tablets
Corrective Tablets (Ayrton Saunders)
Correctol Tablets
Cosalgesic Tablets
Cosylan Syrup
Coterpin Syrup
Cough & Bronchitis Mixture (Davidson)
Cough & Cold Mixture (Beecham)
Cough Balsam (Abernethy's)
Cough Balsam (Thornbers)
Cough Expectorant Elixir (Regent
Laboratories)
Cough Linctus (Sanderson's)
Cough Linctus Alcoholic (Thomas Guest)
Cough Linctus for Children (Boots)
Cough Medicine for Infants & Children
Solution (Boots)
Cough Mixture (Tingles)

XVIIIA

Cough Mixture Adults (Thornton & Ross)
Cough Mixture Adults (Wicker Herbal Stores)
Cough Syrup Best (Diopharm)
Cough Tablets (Kerbina)
Country Basket Rice Cakes
Covermark Removing Cream
Covonia Bronchial Balsam Linctus
Cow & Gate Babymeals Stage One
Cow & Gate Baby Milk Plus
Cow & Gate Follow-On Babymilk Step Up
Cow & Gate Junior Meal
Cow & Gate Nutriprem 2
Cow & Gate Olvarit Stage Two Main Course
Cow & Gate Premium Baby Food
Cox Pain Tablets
Crampex Tablets
Cranberry Juice
Cream of Magnesia Tablets 300 mg
Cremaffin Emulsion
Cremalgin Balm
Creosote Bronchial Mixture (Loveridge)
Crookes One-a-Day Multivitamins with Iron
Crookes One-a-Day Multivitamins without Iron
Crookes Wheat Germ Oil Capsules
Croupline Cough Syrup (Roberts)
Crusha Milk Shake Syrup
Cullen's Headache Powders
Culpepper Healing Ointment
Culpepper Rheumatic Cream
Cupal Health Salts
Cupal Nail Bite Lotion
Cuprofen Soluble Tablets
Cuprofen Tablets
Cuticura Medicated Foam Bath
Cuticura Talcum Powder
Cyanocobalamin Solution (any strength)
Cytacon Liquid
Cytacon Tablets
Cytamen 250 Injection
Cytamen 1000 Injection
Cytoplan Acidophilus Capsules (Milk Free)
Cytoplan Acidophilus/Bifidophilus 50%/50% Capsules
Cytoplan Aloe Vera Concentrate
Cytoplan Betaine & Pepsin Capsules 345mg/10mg
Cytoplan Bifidophilus Extra Tablets
Cytoplan Biotin Capsules 100mcg
Cytoplan Children's Chewable Mineral/Vitamin Tablets
Cytoplan Choline/Inositol Capsules 250mg/250mg
Cytoplan Co-Factor Compound Plus Capsules
Cytoplan Cytocleanse Formula Capsules
Cytoplan Cytomin Mineral/Vitamin Tablets
Cytoplan Cytoplex Tablets
Cytoplan Cytophilus Milk Free Capsules
Cytoplan De-Toxifying Compound Capsules
Cytoplan Dolomite Magnesium Carbon Calcium Carbon Tablets

Cytoplan EPA Capsules
Cytoplan Iron Extra Tablets
Cytoplan Lecithin Capsules
Cytoplan Magnesium Ascorbic Capsules

Cytoplan Magnesium/Calcium Capsules 250mg/250mg
Cytoplan Magnesium Citric Capsules
Cytoplan Magnesium Complex Capsules
Cytoplan Manganese Complex Capsules
Cytoplan Multex Multivitamin and Mineral Formulation
Cytoplan Pantothenic Acid Tablets
Cytoplan Potassium Pantothenate Capsules
Cytoplan Pryoxidal-5-pH Complex Capsules
Cytoplan Selenium Capsules
Cytoplan Supermag-Plus Capsules
Cytoplan Vitamin A Capsules
Cytoplan Vitamin C 1000mg + Bioflavour 50mg Capsules
Cytoplan Vitamin C Powder
Cytoplan Vitamin E Capsules
Cytoplan Zinc Lozenge Wafers

Dakin's Golden Vitamin Malt Syrup
Daktarin Cream 15g
Daktarin Powder
Daktarin Twin Pack
Dalivit Capsules
Dalivit Syrup
Dalmane Capsules 15 mg
Dalmane Capsules 30 mg
Dansac Skin Lotion
Davenol Linctus
Daxaids Tablets
Day-Vits Multivitamin & Mineral Tablets
Dayovite
De Witt's Analagesic Pills
De Witt's Antacid Powder
De Witt's Antacid Tablets
De Witt's Baby Cough Syrup
De Witt's Cough Syrup
De Witt's PL Pills
Dead Sea Natural Mineral Soap
Deakin & Hughes Cough & Cold Healer Mixture
Deakin's Fever & Inflammation Remedy Mixture
Delax Emulsion
Delial Lotion SPF2
Delial Lotion SPF6 Water Resistant
Delimon
Deltasoralen Bath Lotion
Dencyl Spansules
Dentakit Toothache First Aid Kit
Dentu-Hold Liquid

Derbac C Shampoo
Derbac Soap
Derl Dermatological Soap
Dermablend Chromatone Fade Creme Plus
Dermablend Cleanser/Remover
Dermablend Maximum Moisturiser
Dermablend Quick Fix Concealment Stick
Dermacolor Body Cover
Dermacolor Cleansing Cream
Dermacolor Cleansing Lotion
Dermacolor Cleansing Milk
Dermacolor 6 Colour Palette
Dermacolor Creme Effective No.2
Dermacolor Fixier Spray
Dermacolor Skin Plastic
Dermacort Cream
Dermalex Skin Lotion
Dermidex Dermatological Cream
Dermo-Care Soapless Soap
Desiccated Liver Tablets
Desiccated Liver USNF Tablets
Detox Tablets (Hursdrex)
Dettox Antibacterial Cleanser
Dextro Energy Glucose Tablets
Dextrogesic Tablets
Dextromethorphan Hydrobromide
    Solution 3.75 mg/5 ml
Dextromethorphan Hydrobromide
    Solution 7.5 mg/5 ml
Dextromethorphan Hydrobromide
    Syrup 6.6 mg/5 ml
Dextromethorphan Hydrobromide
    Syrup 13.5 mg/5 ml
Dextropropoxyphene & Paracetamol
    Dispersible Tablets
Dextropropoxyphene & Paracetamol
    Soluble Tablets
DF 118 Elixir
DF 118 Tablets
DGL 1 Suspension
DGL 2 Suspension
DGT 1 Tablets
DGT 2 Tablets
DHL Rheumatic Massage Cream
Diabetic Bronal Syrup
Dialar Forte Syrup 5 mg/5 ml
Dialar Syrup 2 mg/5 ml
Dialume Capsules 500 mg
Diazepam Capsules, Slow 10 mg
Diazepam Elixir 5 mg/5 ml
Diazepam Oral Solution 5mg/5ml
Diazepam Oral Suspension 5mg/5ml
Dietade Diabetic Jam
Dietade Diabetic Marmalade
Dietade Diabetic Squash
Dietade Dietary Foods Fruit Sugar
Dietade Fruit Sugar
Dietade Jelly Crystals
Digesprin Antacid Tablets
Digestells Lozenges
Dihydroxyaluminium Sodium Carbonate
    Tablets

Dijex Liquid
Dijex Tablets
Dimotane Expectorant
Dimotane Expectorant DC
Dimotane with Codeine Elixir
Dimotane with Codeine Paediatric Elixir
Dimotapp Elixir
Dimotapp Elixir Paediatric
Dimotapp LA Tablets
Dimotapp P Tablets
Dimyril Linctus
Dinnefords Gripe Mixture
Diocalm Ultra Capsules
Dioctyl Ear Drops
Disprin Direct Tablets
Disprin Extra Tablets
Disprin Solmin Tablets
Disprin Tablets
Disprinex Tablets
Disprol Infant Suspension
Disprol Junior Tablets Soluble
Distalgesic Soluble Tablets
Distalgesic Tablets
Ditemic Spansules
Do-Do Linctus
Do-Do Tablets
Dolasan Tablets
Doloxene Capsules
Doloxene Compound Pulvules
Dolvan Tablets
Dorbanex Capsules
Dorbanex Liquid
Dorbanex Liquid Forte
Dormonoct Tablets 1 mg
Dove Cleansing Bar
Dr Brandreth's Pills
Dr D E Jongh's Cod Liver Oil with Malt
    Extract & Vitamins Fortified Syrup
Dr William's Pink Pills
Dragon Balm
Drastin Tablets
Dristan Decongestant Tablets with
    Antihistamine
Dristan Nasal Spray
Droxalin Tablets
Dry Cough Linctus (Scott & Bowne)
Dual-Lax Extra Strong Tablets
Dual-Lax Tablets
Dubam Cream
Dubam Spray Relief
Dulca Tablets
Dulcodos Tablets
Dulco-Lax Suppositories
Dulco-Lax Tablets
Duo-Gastritis Mixture (Baldwin's)
Duphalac Syrup
Duralin Capsules Extra Strength
Duralin Tablets
Dusk Insect Repellent Cream
Duttons Cough Mixture
Dynese Aqueous Suspension
Dynese Tablets

XVIIIA

D001 Capsules
D002 Capsules
D004 Capsules
D006 Capsules
D007 Capsules
D009 Capsules
D010 Capsules
D011 Capsules
D012 Capsules
D013 Capsules
D014 Capsules
D017 Capsules
D018 Capsules
D019 Capsules
D020 Capsules
D021 Capsules
D024 Capsules
D029 Capsules
D030 Capsules
D031 Capsules
D032 Capsules
D033 Capsules
D034 Capsules
D036 Capsules

Elizabeth Arden Sunscience Superblock
    Cream spf 34
Elkamol Tablets
Ellimans Universal Embrocation
Elsan Blue Liquid
Emuwash
Endet Powders
Ener-G Gluten-free and Soya-free Macaroon Cookies
Ener-G Gluten-free Rice and Peanut-Butter Cookies
Ener-G Gluten-free Rice Walnut Cookies
Energen Starch Reduced Crispbread
Enfamil Human Milk Fortifier
English Grains Mixed Gland Compound Tablets
English Grains Red Kooga Multivitamins & Minerals
Engran HP Tablets
Engran Tablets
Eno Fruit Salts
Enzyme Process Achol Tablets
Enzyme Process Enzastatin Tablets
Enzyme Process Liver Tablets
Enzyme Process Pancreas 523 Tablets
Enzyme Process Pro-T-Compound Tablets
Enzyme Process Vitamin B12 + Liver Tablets
EP Tablets
EPOC Capsules
Equagesic Tablets
Equisorb High Fibre Guar Bread Rolls
Eskamel Cream
Eskornade Spansule Capsules
Eskornade Syrup
Eso-Col Cold Treatment Tablets

Earex Ear Drops
Earthdust Aged Garlic Tablets
Earthdust Capricin Forte Capsules
Earthdust Formula 1 Capsules
Earthdust Pro-Biotic New Complex Powder
Earthdust Super-Pro-Bifidus Powder
Earthdust Super-Pro-Dophilus Powder
Earthlore Vitamin B Compound Tablets
Ecologic 315 Granules
Ecdilyn Syrup
Educol Tablets
Efamol
Efamol Capsules
Efamol Marine Capsules
Efamol Oil
Efamol Plus Capsules
Efamol Plus Evening Primrose Oil & Coenzyme Q10
    Capsules
Efamol PMP
Efamolia Enriched Moisture Cream
Efamolia Moisture Cream
Efamolia Night Cream
Efavite Tablets
Efavite Vitamin & Zinc Supplement Tablets
Effer-C Tablets
Effico Syrup
Elagen
Eldermint Cough Mixture (Herbal Laboratories)
Elgydium Toothpaste
Elizabeth Arden Flawless Finish
Elizabeth Arden Sunblock Cream Factor 15

Esoterica Fortified Cream
Essentia Special E Cream
Ester-C Powder
Ester-C Tablets
Euhypnos Capsules 10 mg
Euhypnos Elixir 10 mg/5 ml
Euhypnos Forte Capsules 20 mg
Evacalm Tablets 2 mg
Evacalm Tablets 5 mg
Evans Cough Balsam
Evening Primrose Oil
Evening Primrose Oil Capsules
Evian Mineral Water
Evident Disclosing Cream
Ex-Lax Chocolate Laxative Tablets
Ex-Lax Pills
Expectorant Cough Mixtures (Beecham)
Expulin Cough Linctus
Expulin Decongestant Linctus for Babies & Children
Expulin Paediatric Cough Linctus
Extil Compound Linctus
Extravite Tablets
Extren Tablets
Exyphen Elixir
E001 Capsules
E015 Capsules
E018 Capsules
E021 Capsules
E031 Capsules
E032 Capsules

Fabrol Granules
Fade Out Skin Lightening Cream
Fairy Household Liquid
Falcodyl Linctus
Falkamin
Fam Lax Tablets
Famel Expectorant
Famel Linctus
Famel Original Linctus
Family Cherry Flavoured Linctus (Cupal)
Family Health Multivitamin Tablets
Family Herbal Pills
Fanalgic Syrup
Fanalgic Tablets
Farex Fingers
Farley's Farex Weaning Food
Farley's First Milk
Farley's Follow-On Milk
Farley's Premcare
Farley's Premcare Ready-to-Feed
Farleys Rusks
Farley's Tea Timer
Father Pierre's Monastery Herbs
Fe-Cap C Capsules
Feac Tablets
Feen-a-Mint Tablets
Fefol Spansule Capsules
Fefol-Vit Spansules
Fefol Z Spansule Capsules
Femafen Capsules
Femerital Tablets
Femeron Cream
Feminax Tablets
Fendamin Tablets
Fennings Adult Cooling Powders
Fennings Children's Cooling Powders
Fennings Little Healers Pills
Fennings Mixture
Fennings Soluble Junior Aspirin Tablets
Fenox Nasal Drops
Fenox Nasal Spray
Feospan Spansule Capsules
Ferfolic SV Tablets
Ferfolic Tablets
Fergluvite Tablets
Fergon Tablets
Ferraplex B Tablets
Ferrlecit Tablets/Dragees
Ferrocap Capsules
Ferrocap F-350 Capsules
Ferroglobin B12 Vitamin/Mineral Compound
Ferrograd C Tablets
Ferrol
Ferrol Compound Mixture
Ferromyn B Elixir
Ferromyn B Tablets
Ferrous Gluconate Compound Tablets
Ferrous Sulphate Compound Tablets BP
Fesovit Spansules
Fesovit Z Spansules
Fibre Biscuits
Fibrosine Analgesic Balm

Fiery Jack Cream
Fiery Jack Ointment
Filetti Sensitive Skin Soap
Finasteride 1mg Tablets
Fine Fare Aspirin Tablets 300 mg
Fine Fare Hot Lemon Powders
Fink Linusit Gold Pure Golden Linseeds
Flar Capsules
Flavelix Syrup
Flexcare Soft Lens Solution
Flexsol Solution
Flora Margarine
Floradix Formula Liquid
Floradix Tablets
Floral Arbour Tablets (Cathay)
Flucaps
Fluimucil Granules
Flunitrazepam Tablets 1 mg
Fluralar Capsules 15 mg
Fluralar Capsules 30 mg
Flurazepam Capsules 15 mg
Flurazepam Capsules 30 mg
Flurazepam Hydrochloride Capsules 15 mg
Flurazepam Hydrochloride Capsules 30 mg
Flu-Rex Tablets
Flurex Bedtime Cold Remedy
Flurex Capsules
Flurex Decongestant Inhalant Capsules
Flurex Hot Lemon Concentrate
Flurex Tablets
Folex-350 Tablets
Folicin Tablets
Folped
Foresight Tablets Mineral Formula
Foresight Tablets Vitamin
  (Multivitamins)
Formula M.E. (Multiple Elevator)
  No 1 Capsules
Formula M.E. (Multiple Elevator)
  No 2 Capsules
Formula M.E. (Multiple Elevator)
  No 3 Capsules
Formule B Spot Treatment Roll On
Formulix
Forprin Tablets
Fortagesic Tablets
Fortespan Spansules
Fort-E-Vite Capsules
Fort-E-Vite 1000 Capsules
Fort-E-Vite Cream
Fort-E-Vite Plus Capsules
Fort-E-Vite Super Plus Capsules
Fortison Low Sodium
Fortral Capsules 50 mg
Fortral Injection
Fortral Suppositories
Fortral Tablets 25 mg
Fortral Tablets 50 mg
Fortris Solution
Fosfor Syrup
Franol Expectorant
Franolyn Sed Liquid

XVIIIA

Frisium Capsules 5 mg
Frisium Capsules 10 mg
Frisium Capsules 20 mg
FSC Betaine HCL Capsules
FSC Beta Plus Capsules
FSC Evening Primrose Oil + Vitamin E Cream
FSC Lactobacillus Acidophilus Capsules
FSC Multivitamin Addlife For Over 50s
   Capsules
FSC Natural Vitamin E Capsules
FSC Organic Linseed Oil Capsules
FSC Super B-Supreme High-Potency
   Tablets
FSC Super Calcium 200mg + Vitamin
   A & D Tablets
FSC Vitamin B6 Tablets
FSC Vitamin D 400u
Fybranta Tablets
Fynnon Calcium Aspirin Tablets
Fynnon Salt

G Brand Linctus
Galake Tablets
Gale's Honey
Galfer-Vit Capsules
Galloway's Baby Cough Linctus
Galloway's Bronchial Cough Care
Galloway's Bronchial Expectorant
Galloway's Cough Syrup
Gammolin Capsules
Gamophase Gamolenic Acid Capsules
Gamophen
Gastalar Tablets
Gastric Ulcer Tablets No 1001
Gastrils Pastilles
Gastritabs
Gastrovite Tablets
Gatinar Syrup
Gaviscon Granules
Gaviscon 250 Tablets
Gelusil Lac Powder
Gelusil Tablets
Genasprin Tablets
Genatosan
Gentian Acid Mixture with Nux Vomica
Gentian Alkaline Mixture with Nux Vomica
Gentian & Rhubarb Mixture BPC
Georges Vapour Rub Ointment
Gericaps Capsules
Gericare Multivitamin & Mineral Capsules
Gerimax Original Korean Panax Ginseng with
   Vitamins, Minerals and Amino Acid.
Geriplex Capsules
Germolene Ointment
Gevral Capsules
Gevral Tablets

Ginkgo Biloba Extract Capsules 40mg
Ginkgo Biloba Liquid
Givitol Capsules
Gladlax Tablets
Glemony Balsam (Baldwin's)
Glenco Elixir
Gluca-Seltzer Effervescent Powder
Glucodin
Glutafin Gluten-Free Chocolate Chip Cookies
Glutafin Gluten-Free Custard Cream Biscuits
Glutafin Gluten-Free Gingernut Cookies
Glutafin Gluten-Free Milk Chocolate Biscuits
Glutafin Gluten-Free Milk Chocolate Digestive Biscuits
Glutafin Gluten-Free Shortcake Biscuits
Glutano Gluten-Free Chocolate Hazelnut Wafer Bar
Glutano Gluten-Free Muesli
Glutano Gluten-Free Pretzel
Glutano Gluten-Free Wafer
Glutano Gluten-Free Wafer, Cream Filled
Glycerin Honey & Lemon Cough
   Mixture (Isola)
Glycerin Honey & Lemon Linctus (Boots)
Glycerin Honey & Lemon Linctus with
   Ipecacuanha (Boots)
Glycerin Lemon & Honey and
   Ipecacuanha (Thomas Guest)
Glycerin Lemon & Honey Linctus (Rusco)
Glycerin Lemon & Honey Syrup (Cupal)
Glycerin Lemon & Honey Syrup (Thomas
   Guest)
Glycerin Lemon & Honey Syrup
   (Waterhouse)
Glycerin Lemon & Ipecacuanha Cough
   Mixture (Isola)
Glykola Infants Elixir
Glykola Tonic
Glymiel Hand Care
Goat's Milk Spray Dried Powder
Goddard's White Oils Embrocation
Golden Age Vitamin & Mineral Capsules
Golden Health Feverfew Tablets
Golden Health Super Sea Kelp Tablets
Golden Health Tablets (Kerbina)
Golden Health Tablets (Brome &
   Schimmer)
Gon Tablets
Gonfalcon Tablets
Grangewood Insomnia Tablets
Granogen
Granose Liquid Soya Milk
Granose Soya Yogert
Granoton Emulsion
Gratis Gluten-Free Tricolour Pasta
Gregovite C Tablets
GS Tablets
Guaiphenesin Syrup (any strength)
Guanor Expectorant
Gynovite Plus Nutritional Supplement
   Tablets

H-Pantoten Tablets
Hactos Chest & Cough Mixture
  (Thomas Hubert)
Halaurant Syrup
Halcion Tablets 0.125 mg
Halcion Tablets 0.25 mg
Haliborange Syrup
Haliborange Tablets
Halibut Liver Oil A & D Capsules
  (Rodale)
Halibut Oil A & D Capsules (GR Lane
  Health Products)
Halin Tablets
Halocaps Inhalant Capsules
Halycitrol Emulsion
Harvestime Malt Extract with Cod Liver
  Oil and Butterscotch
Hayphryn Nasal Spray
HC45 Cream
Head and Shoulders Shampoo
Health Aid Children's Multivitamin
  + Mineral Tablets
Health Aid DL-Phenylalanine Tablets 500mg
Health Aid Dolomite Tablets
Health Aid Eczema Oil
Health Aid EPO Forte Capsules 1000mg
Health Aid Halibut Liver Oil Capsules
Health Aid Magnesium & Calcium Tablets
Health Aid Multivitamins & Minerals Tablets
Health Aid Super Cod Liver Oil Capsules
Health Aid Super Lecithin Capsules
Health Aid Vitamin A Capsules
Health Aid Vitamin A + D Capsules
Health Aid Vitamin B6 Tablets Prolonged Release
Health Aid Vitamin B Complex Supreme Tablets
Health Aid Vitamin C Tablets
Health Aid Vitamin E Capsules
Health Aid Vitamin E Cream
Health Aid Vitamin E Hand and
  Body Lotion
Health Aid Vitamin E Natural Capsules
Health Aid Vitamin E Oil
Health Aid Zinc Sulphate Tablets 200mg
Health Aid Zinc Tablets 10mg
Healthcrafts Aminochel Calcium Tablets
Healthcrafts Aminochel Chelated Magnesium
  Tablets
Healthcrafts Aminochel Zinc Tablets 1.3mg
Healthcrafts Aminochel Zinc Tablets 5mg
Healthcrafts Arteroil Tablets
Healthcrafts Betacarotene Capsules
Healthcrafts Brewers Yeast Tablets
Healthcrafts Calcium + Vitamin D Chewable
  Tablets
Healthcrafts Calcium Chewable Tablets
Healthcrafts Calcium Pantothenate Super
  Tablets
Healthcrafts Cod Liver Oil Capsules
Healthcrafts Cod Liver Oil Compleat Tablets
Healthcrafts Dolomite Tablets 500mg
Healthcrafts EPA Forte Capsules
Healthcrafts High Strength Starflower Oil

Healthcrafts Kelp Tablets
Healthcrafts Lecithin Capsules
Healthcrafts Multivitamin Chewable Tablets
Healthcrafts Multivitamin + Iron &
  Calcium Tablets
Healthcrafts Natural Vitamin C 1g
  Tablets (High Potency)
Healthcrafts Prolonged Release Nutrition
  Mega-B6 Tablets
Healthcrafts Prolonged Release Nutrition
  Mega B-Complex Tablets
Healthcrafts Prolonged Release Nutrition
  Mega C 1500 Tablets
Healthcrafts Prolonged Release
  Nutrition Mega Multis Tablets
Healthcrafts Vitamin E Capsules
Healthcrafts Vitamin E Capsules
  High-Potency
Healthcrafts Vitamin E Capsules Mega
Healthcrafts Vitamin E Capsules Super
Healthcrafts Vitamin E Natural Oil
Healthcrafts Vitamin E One-A-Day
  Capsules
Healthcrafts Zinc One-A-Day Capsules
Healtheries Rice Crispbread
Healthilife Dolomite Tablets 60mg
Healthilife Halibut Oil Capsules
Healthilife Rutin Tablets 60mg
Healthilife Sunflower Seed Oil Capsules 500 mg
Healthilife Vitamin A Capsules
Healthilife Vitamin E Soya Free Capsules
Healthilife Wild Sea Kelp Tablets 300mg
Healthlink High Zinc + Manganese Formula 1
  Capsules
Healthlink Loosemore Herbal Capsules
Healthlink Magnesium Acetate Capsules
Healthlink Psyllium Husks
Health Perception Glucosamine Tablets
Health + Plus Absorb Plus Capsules
Health + Plus Absorb Plus Tablets
Health + Plus Chromium GTF & B3 Tablets
Health + Plus Complex B Tablets
Health + Plus Co-Q Plus Tablets
Health + Plus Dolomite + D Tablets
Health + Plus E500 Tablets
Health + Plus Immunade Tablets
Health + Plus Multiminerals Tablets
Health + Plus Multivite Tablets
Health + Plus Nutrient Pack, Metabolic Pack
Health + Plus Pregnancy Pack
Health + Plus Selenium Tablets 50mcg
Health + Plus Super B6 + Zinc Tablets
Health + Plus Super C1000 Tablets +
  Bioflavour
Health + Plus Supercholine Tablets
Health + Plus Vitamin E Capsules
  High-Potency
Health + Plus VV Pack
Health + Plus Ziman Plus
  (Manganese & Zinc) Tablets
Health Salts (Wicker Herbal Stores)
Health Tonic Mixture (Hall's)

XVIIIA

Healthwise Halibut Oil Capsules
Healthwise Vitamin E Capsules
Heart Shape Indigestion Tablets
Heath & Heather Feverfew Tablets
Heath & Heather Garlic Perles
  (Odourless)
Hedamol Capsules
Hedex Extra Caplets
Hedex Plus Capsules
Hedex Seltzer Granules
Hedex Soluble Granules
Hedex Tablets
Heinz Weight Watcher Baked Beans
Hemingways Catarrh Syrup
Hemoplex Injection
Hepacon B12 Injection
Hepacon B-Forte Injection
Hepacon Liver Extract Injection
Hepacon-Plex
Hepanorm Tablets
Herbal Aperient Tablets (Cathay)
Herbal Aperient Tablets (Kerbina)
Herbal Bronchial Cough Tablets (English
  Grains)
Herbal Laboratories Feverfew Tablets
Herbal Laxative Naturtabs
Herbal Pile Tablets
Herbal Quiet Nite Sleep Naturtabs
Herbal Syrup (Baldwin's)
Herbalene Herbs
Hermesetas (blue)
Hermesetas Gold
Hermesetas Light
Hermesetas Liquid Sweetener
Hermesetas Sprinkle Sweet
Hexidin Solution
Hi-g-ah Tea
Higher Nature Paraclear Capsules
Hi-pro Liver Tablets
Hill's Adult Balsam
Hill's Balsam Children's Mixture for Chesty
  Coughs
Hip C Rose Hip Syrup
Hismanal Tablets 10-tablet pack
Histalix Expectorant
Hofels Cardiomax Garlic Pearles
Hofels Garlic Pearles
Hofels One-A-Day Garlic Pearles
Hofels One-A-Day Neo Garlic Pearles
Honey & Molasses Cough Mixture (Lane
  Health Products)
Hot Blackcurrant Cold Remedy (Beechams)
Hot Lemon Cold Remedy (Beechams)
Hot Lemon Cold Treatment (Scott &
  Bowne)
Hot Measure Solution (Reckitt & Colman)
Hydrex Hand Rub
Hydrocare Boiling/Rinsing Solution
Hydrocare Cleaning and Soaking Solution
Hydrocare Preserved Saline Solution
Hydrocare Protein Remover Tablets
Hydroclean Solution

Hydron Europe Cleaning Solution
Hydron Europe Comfort Soaking Solution
Hydron Europe Solusal
Hydron Europe Solution Comfort
Hydrosoak Disinfecting and Soaking Solution
Hydrosol Comfort Solution
Hymosa Vitamin E Cream
Hypomultiple Capsules
Hypon Tablets

Iberet 500 Tablets
Iberol Tablets
Ibrufhalal Tablets
ICC Analgesic Tablets
Idoloba Tablets
Iliadin Mini Nasal Drops
Iliadin Mini Paediatric Nasal Drops
Imarale Agba Suspension
Imarale Omode Suspension
Imedeen Skin Regenerating Tablets
Imedeen Tablets
Imodium Capsules Pharmacy Packs 8 and 12
  Capsules
Importal
Imuderm Body Wash
Imuderm Hand & Face Wash
Imuderm Shower Gel
Inabrin Tablets 200 mg
Indian Brandy Solution
Indigestion Mixture (Boots)
Indigestion Mixture (Thornton & Ross)
Indigestion Mixture (William Ransom)
Indigo Indigestion Lozenges
Infa-Care Baby Bath
Infaderm Baby Bath
Infaderm Baby Cream
Infaderm Baby Hair Wash
Infaderm Baby Lotion
Influenza and Cold Mixture 2315
  (Wright Layman & Umney)
Inhalit Liquid Inhalation
Innoxa Concealing Cream
Innoxa Creme Satin Foundation
Innoxa Finishing Touch Loose Powder
Innoxa Foundation
Innoxa Moisturised Liquid Make-up
Innoxa Sensitive/Dry Range: Enriched
  Moisture Cream
Innoxa Sensitive/Normal Range:
  Creamy Moisturiser
Innoxa Young Solution Spot Gel
Inoven Caplets
Iodinated Glycerol Elixir 60 mg/ 5 ml
Iodised Vitamin Capsules
Iodo-Ephedrine Mixture

Ionax Scrub
Ipecacuanha Pills 20 mg
Ipecacuanha & Morphine Mixture BP
Ipecacuanha & Squill Linctus
   Paediatric BPC
Ipsel Hygienic Babysalve
Irofol C
Iron & Brewers Yeast Tablets
   (3M Health Care)
Iron & Vitamin Tablets (Davidson)
Iron Formula Tablets (Rodale)
Iron Jelloids Tablets
Iron Tonic Tablets (Boots)
Ironorm Capsules
Ironorm Tonic
Ironplan Capsules
Isoaminile Linctus
Isocal
Ivy Tablets (Ayrton Saunders)

Jaap's Health Salts
Jacksons All Fours Cough Mixture
Jacksons Febrifuge
Jambomins Tablets
Jenners Suspension
Jenners Tablets
Jochem Hormone Hair Preparation
Johnson & Johnson Baby Bath
Johnson & Johnson Baby Cream
Johnson & Johnson Baby Lotion
Johnson & Johnson Baby Oil
Johnson & Johnson Baby Powder
Johnson & Johnson Baby Shampoo
Johnson & Johnson Baby Sunblock Stick
Johnson & Johnson Prickly Heat Powder
Jolen Creme Bleach
Jordans Crunchy Bar
Junamac
Jung Junipah Tablets
Jungle Formula Insect Repellent Gel
Jungle Formula Insect Repellent Pump Spray
Junior Cabdrivers Linctus
Junior Disprin Tablets
Junior Disprol Tablets
Junior Ex-Lax Chocolate Tablets
Junior Lemsip Powder
Junior Meltus Cough & Catarrh Linctus
Junior Mucron Liquid
Junior Paraclear Tablets
Junior Tablets (Rodale)
Juno-Junipah Mineral Salts
Juvel Elixir
Juvel Tablets
Juvela Gluten-Free Mince Pies
Juvela Gluten-Free Sage & Onion Stuffing Mix
Juvela Low-Protein Savoury Snack

Kamillosan Baby Cleansing Bar
K'An Herbal Preparations
Kaodene Suspension
Kaopectate
Karvol Capsules
Kelsoak 2 Solution
Kelvinol 2 Wetting Solution
Kenco Instant Decaffeinated Coffee
Kendales Adult Cough Syrup
Kendales Cherry Linctus
Kentogam Gamolenic Acid Capsules
Kest Tablets
Ketazolam Capsules 15 mg
Ketazolam Capsules 30 mg
Ketazolam Capsules 45 mg
Keybells Linctus of Glycerine, Lemon &
   Ipecacuanha
Kingo Cough Syrup
Koladex Tablets
Kolanticon Tablets
Kolanticon Wafers
Kolantyl Gel
Kolorex Capsules
Kolynos Denture Fixative
Krauses Cough Linctus
Kruschen Salts
Kuralax Herbs
Kwai Garlic Tablets
Kylie Skin Guard

Labiton Kola Tonic
Laboprin Tablets
Lac Bismuth Mixture
Lactaid Lactase enzyme for milk drops
Lactaid Lactase enzyme tablets
Lactaid Lactose reduced, skimmed and whole
   milk UHT
Lacto Calamine
Ladycare No 2 (Menopausal) Tablets
Laevoral
Lamberts Acidophilus Extra Capsules
Lamberts Bee Propolis Tablets
Lamberts Beta Carotene Capsules
Lamberts Betaine HCL/Pepsin Tablets
Lamberts Betasec Tablets
Lamberts Betasec Timed Release Antioxidant Tablets
Lamberts Calcium Extra Tablets
Lamberts Calcium/Magnesium Balance Capsules
Lamberts Calcium & Magnesium Chelates Tablets
Lamberts Calcium 500/Magnesium 250 Amino
   Acid Chelated Tablets

XVIIIA

Lamberts Calcium/Magnesium/Zinc Orotates
  Capsules
Lamberts Caprylic Acid Tablets
Lamberts Chelating Mega Mineral Complex Tablets
Lamberts Co-Enzyme Q10 Capsules
Lamberts DLPA Complex + Vitamin B & C
  Capsules
Lamberts Dolomite Tablets
Lamberts Enzygest Capsules
Lamberts EPA Marine Lipid Concentrate Capsules
Lamberts Evening Primrose Oil 250 mg Capsules
Lamberts Evening Primrose Oil 500 mg Capsules
Lamberts Evening Primrose Oil 1000 mg Capsules
Lamberts Gentle Vitamin C Tablets
Lamberts Ginkgo Biloba Extract Tablets
Lamberts GTF Chromium Capsules
Lamberts Health Insurance Plus Tablets
Lamberts High Potency EPA Capsules
Lamberts L-Carnitine Capsules
Lamberts L-Carnitine Tablets
Lamberts L-Glutamic Acid Powder
Lamberts L-Glutamine Capsules
Lamberts L-Glutathione Complex Capsules
Lamberts L-Histidine HCL Capsules
Lamberts L-Isoleucine Capsules
Lamberts L-Leucine Capsules
Lamberts L-Threonine 500mg Capsules
Lamberts Magnesium Amino Acid Chelated Tablets
Lamberts Magnesium Orotate Capsules
Lamberts Magnesium Sustained Release Tablets
Lamberts Magnesium Sustained Release
  Timed Release Tablets
Lamberts Mega Mineral Compound Tablets
Lamberts Mega 3 Vitamins/Minerals Tablets
Lamberts Multi-Max Tablets
Lamberts Natural Vitamin E Capsules
Lamberts One Daily Vitamin/Mineral Tablets
Lamberts Playfair Tablets
Lamberts PMT Supplement Optivite Tablets
Lamberts Protein Deficiency Formula Capsules
Lamberts Protein Deficiency Formula Powder
Lamberts Pycnogenol Capsules
Lamberts Pyridoxal-5-Phosphate Capsules
Lamberts Pyridoxal-5-Phosphate Plus Capsules
Lamberts Selenium Capsules
Lamberts Selenium Tablets
Lamberts Senior Capsules
Lamberts Super Acidophilus Plus Capsules
Lamberts Taurine Capsules
Lamberts Ultra Detoxifying Capsules
Lamberts Vitamin B-50 Complex Capsules
Lamberts Vitamin B-50 Complex Tablets
Lamberts Vitamin B-100 Complex Tablets
Lamberts Vitamin C Ascorbic Acid &
  Calcium Ascorbate Crystals
Lamberts Vitamin C Ascorbic Acid Powder
Lamberts Vitamin C & Bioflav Tablets
Lamberts Vitamin C Calcium Ascorbate Crystals
Lamberts Vitamin C-Time Bioflav
  Timed-Release Tablets
Lamberts Vitamin E 200 D-Alpha Tablets

Lamberts Vitamin E 200 D-Alpha/Selenium Tablets
Lamberts Vitamin E 400 D-Alpha/Selenium Tablets
Lamberts Vitamin/Mineral Compound Tablets
Lamberts Zinc Citrus Capsules
Lamberts Zinc Gluconate Tablets
Lamberts Zinc Tablets
Lanacane Cream
Lanacort Cream
Lanacort Ointment
Lance B & C Tablets
Lancome Nutrix Cream
Lane's Cut-a-Cough
Lane's Laxative Herb Tablets
Lane's Sage and Garlic Catarrh Remedy
Lanes Glanolin Capsules 250/500
Lanes Lecigran Granules
Lantigen B
Larkhall Acidophilus 500 Tablets
Larkhall B13 Zinc Tablets
Larkhall Beta Carotene Capsules
Larkhall Calcimega 500 Tablets
Larkhall DLPA 375 Tablets
Larkhall Dolomite Tablets
Larkhall Folic Acid Tablets 100mcg
Larkhall Folic Acid Tablets 500mcg
Larkhall L-Carnitine Capsules
Larkhall Magnesium Orotate B13 Tablets
Larkhall Selenium Supplement Tablets
Larkhall Vitamin C Naturtabs 1000mg Buffered
Lavender Bath
Laxaliver Pills
Laxatabs Leoren
Laxipurg Tablets
Laxoberal Elixir
LC 65 Cleaning Solution
Lecithin Capsules
Ledercort Cream
Lederplex Capsules
Lederplex Liquid
Lejfibre Biscuit
Lemeze Cough Syrup
Lemon Eno Powder
Lemon Flu-Cold Concentrated Syrup
Lemon Glycerine & Honey Cough Syrup
  Compound (Carter Bond)
Lemon Glycerine & Honey Lung
  Mixture (Whitehall Laboratories)
Lemon Glycerine & Ipecac Cough Syrup
  Compound (Carter Bond)
Lemon Juice, Glycerine & Honey A S
  Syrup (Ayrton Saunders)
Lemon Linctus 1-472
Lem-Plus Capsules
Lem-Plus Hot Lemon Drink
Lemsip Expectorant
Lemsip Flu Strength
Lemsip Lemcaps Cold Relief Capsules
Lemsip Linctus
Lemsip Flu Strength Night Time Formula
Lemsip Powder
Lendormin Tablets 0.125 mg

Lendormin Tablets 0.25 mg
Lensept Solution
Lensine 5 All in One Solution
Lensplus Sterile Saline Spray
Lensrins Solution
Leoren Tonic Tablets
Lexotan Tablets 1.5 mg
Lexotan Tablets 3 mg
Lexotan Tablets 6 mg
Libraxin Tablets
Librium Capsules 5 mg
Librium Capsules 10 mg
Librium Tablets 5 mg
Librium Tablets 10 mg
Librium Tablets 25 mg
Librofem Tablets
Lifeplan Acidophilus Capsules
Lifeplan Boron 3 Tablets
Lifeplan Cod Liver Oil One-A-Day Capsules
Lifeplan DL-Phenylalanine (DLPA) Tablets 500
Lifeplan Dolomite Tablets 500mg
Lifeplan Dolomite Tablets 800mg
Lifeplan Dolomite (Natural) Tablets
Lifeplan Super Galanol Starflower Capsules
Lifeplan Vitamin B6 Tablets
Lightning Cough Remedy Solution (Potters)
Limbitrol Capsules "5"
Limbitrol Capsules "10"
Linctifed Expectorant
Linctifed Expectorant Paediatric
Linctoid C
Linituss
Linoleic Acid
Linus Vitamin C Powder
Lipoflavonoid Capsules
Lipotriad Capsules
Lipotriad Liquid
Liqufruta Blackcurrant Cough Medicine
Liqufruta Honey & Lemon Cough
    Medicine
Liqufruta Medica
Liqufruta Medica Garlic Flavoured
    Cough Medicine
Liquid Formula (Food Concentrate)
    (Rodale)
Liquid Paraffin & Phenolphthalein
    Emulsion BP
Liquid Paraffin Emulsion with Cascara
    BPC
Liquifilm Wetting Solution
Listerine Antiseptic Mouthwash
Listermint Mouthwash
Liver Herbs (Hall's)
Livibron Mixture
Lloyds Cream (Odour Free)
Lloyds Heat Spray
Loasid Tablets
Lobak Tablets
Lofthouse's Original Fisherman's Friend
    Honey Cough Syrup
Logado
London Herb and Spice Herbal Tea Bags

Loramet Capsules 1 mg
Loramet Tablets 0.5 mg
Loramet Tablets 1 mg
Lotil Facial Cream
Lotussin Cough Syrup
L-Threonine Capsules
L-Threonine Tablets
Lucozade
Luma Bath Salts
Lung Balsam (Rusco)
Lyons Ground Coffee Beans
Lypsyl Lemon
Lypsyl Mint
Lypsyl Original
Lysaldin

M & B Children's Cough Linctus
MA4 Herbal Fruit Concentrate Paste
MA572 Tablets
Maalox Concentrate Suspension
Maalox Plus Tablets
Mackenzies Smelling Salts
Maclean Indigestion Powder
Maclean Indigestion Tablets
Macleans Toothpaste
Magaldrate Tablets
Magnesium Citrus Tru-Fil Capsules
Magnesium Glycerophos Tablets
Magnesium OK Tablets
Mainstay Pure Cod Liver Oil
Male Gland Double Strength Supplement
    Tablets
Male Sex Hormone Tablets (Diopharm)
Malinal Plus Tablets
Malinal Suspension 500 mg/5 ml
Malinal Tablets 500 mg
Malt Extract with Cod Liver Oil &
    Chemical Food (Distillers)
Malt Extract with Cod Liver Oil BPC &
    Hypophosphites (Distillers)
Malt Extract with Cod Liver Oil BPC
    Soft Extract (Jeffreys Miller)
Malt Extract with Haemoglobin &
    Vitamins Syrup (Distillers)
Malt Extract with Halibut Liver-Oil
    Syrup (Distillers)
Malvern Water
Mandarin Tablets
Manna Herbal Rheumapainaway Tablets
Marly Skin
Marvel
Matthew Cough Mixture
Maturaplus Tablets
Maws Sterilising Tablets
Max Factor Face Powder
Max Factor Pan-Stik

XVIIIA

Maxivits Tablets
Medathlon Aspirin Tablets 300 mg
Medazepam Capsules 5 mg
Medazepam Capsules 10 mg
Medex Elixir
Mediclean Soft Lens Solutions
Medilax Tablets
Medinol Over 6 Paracetamol Oral Suspension
Medinol Under 6 Paracetamol Junior Suspension
Medipain Tablets
Medised Suspension
Medised Tablets
Medisoak Soft Lens Solution
Meditus Syrup
Medocodene Tablets
Meggeson Dyspepsia Tablets
Melissin Syrup
Melo Brand Glycerin Lemon & Honey
   with Ipecac
Meloids Lozenges
Meltus Adult Dry Cough Elixir
Meltus Adult Expectorant
Meltus Baby Cough Linctus
Meltus Honey and Lemon Cough Linctus
Meltus Junior Expectorant
Memo Boost Capsules
Menopace Capsules
Menthacol Liquid
Menthells Pellet/Pill
Menthol & Benzoin Inhalation BP
Menthol & Eucalyptus (M in P) Pastilles
   (Thomas Guest)
Menthol Inhalation
Mentholated Balsam (Loveridge)
Mentholated Balsam (Savory & Moore)
Mentholated Balsam (Wright Laymen & Umney)
Mentholated Balsam Mixture (Pilsworth
   Manufacturing)
Mentholatum Balm
Mentholatum Deep Freeze Spray
Mentholatum Deep Heat Massage Liniment
Mentholatum Deep Heat Maximum Strength Rub
Mentholatum Deep Heat Rub
Mentholatum Nasal Inhaler
Mercurochrome Solution
Metatone
Methylcisteine Tablets 100 mg
Micaveen
Midro-Tea Powder
Migrafen Tablets
Mijex Cream
Milgard Baby Cleansing Milk
Milk of Magnesia Tablets
Mil-Par Suspension
Milton Sterilising Tablets
Milumil Baby Milk
Milupa 7 Cereal Breakfast
Milupa Aptamil Baby Milk
Milupa Braised Steak & Vegetable Infant Food
Milupa Camomile Infant Drink
Milupa Cauliflower Cheese Special Infant
   Food

Milupa Country Chicken & Vegetable Casserole
Milupa Fennel Variety Infant Drink
Milupa Forward Follow-On Milk
Milupa Harvest Muesli Breakfast
Milupa Infant Dessert, Banana & Apple Yoghurt
Milupa Infant Dessert, Caribbean Fruit
Milupa Infant Dessert, Semolina & Honey
Milupa Infant Tea-Time, Cheese & Tomato
Milupa Modified Yoghurt
Milupa Special Formula HN25
Milupa Sunshine Orange Breakfast
Milupa Vegetable Hotpot Infant Food
Minadex Chewable Vitamin Tablets
Minadex Syrup
Minamino Syrup
Minivits Tablets
Minoxidil Cream
Minoxidil Lotion
Minoxidil Ointment
Minoxidil Solution (for external use)
Mira Flow Cleaning Solution
Mira Flow Soft Lens Solution
Mira Soak Lens Soaking Solution
Mira Sol Soft Lens Solution
Mitchell's Wool Fat Soap
Modifast Nutritionally Complete
   Supplemented Fasting Formula
Mogadon Capsules 5 mg
Mogadon Tablets 5 mg
Moorland Indigestion Tablets
Morning Glory Tablets
Morny Lavender Talc
Mosquito Milk Mosquito Repellent Tropical
   Formula
Mrs Cullen's Lemsoothe Powder
Mrs Cullen's Powders
Mucodyne Capsules
Mucodyne Forte Syrup
Mucodyne Forte Tablets
Mucodyne Paediatric Syrup
Mucodyne Syrup
Mucofalk Sachets
Mucolex Syrup
Mucolex Tablets
Mu-Cron Junior Syrup
Mu-Cron Tablets
Mucron Liquid
Muflin Linctus
Multi-Vitamin Tablets (English Grains)
Multivitamin Capsules (Regent
   Laboratories)
Multivitamin Tablets
   (Approved Prescription Services)
Multivitamin Tablets (Chemipharm)
Multivitamin Tablets (Evans Medical)
Multivitamin Tablets (UAC
   International)
Multivitamin with Mineral Capsules
   (Potters)
Multivitamin with Minerals Tablets
   (Chemipharm)
Multivite Pellets

Multone Tablets
My Baby Cough Syrup
Mycocidin Perles
Mycolactine Tablets
Mylanta Liquid
Mylanta Tablets
Myolgin Tablets

N Tonic Syrup (Cupal)
N-300 Capsules
Nair Depilatory Cream
Nanny Goat's Milk Infant Formula
Napca Skin Lotion
Napisan Nappy Treatment
Napoloids Tablets
Napsalgesic Tablets
Nasal Drops for Children (Boots)
Natex 12A Tablets
Natural Bran
Natural Flow Acidophilus Capsules
Natural Flow Amino Acid Complex Capsules
Natural Flow Animal Fun Children's
   Chewable Tablets
Natural Flow Boron + Calcium & Silica
   Tablets
Natural Flow Calcium Ascorbate Tablets
Natural Flow Calcium & Magnesium Chelated
   Tablets
Natural Flow Candiforte Capsules
Natural Flow Digestive Enzyme Compound
   Tablets
Natural Flow Dolomite + A & D Tablets
Natural Flow Mega B Complex Tablets
Natural Flow Mega Multi Tablets
Natural Flow Multimineral Tablets
Natural Flow Organic Germanium Capsules
Natural Flow Primedophilus Powder
Natural Flow Probion Bifidus Powder
Natural Flow Probion Tablets
Natural Flow Psyllium Husks
Natural Flow Psyllium Husk Capsules
Natural Flow Selenium Chelated Tablets
Natural Flow Selenium Tablets
Natural Flow Super Vitamin C Complex Tablets
Natural Flow Super Vitamin C Tablets
Natural Flow Tangerine C Chewable Tablets
Natural Flow Thiamin Tablets (Vitamin B1)
Natural Flow Vega Mins Tablets
Natural Flow Vitamin A Tablets
Natural Flow Vitamin C Powder
Natural Flow Zinc Chelated Tablets
Natural Herb Laxative Tablets (Brome &
   Schimmer)
Natural Herb Laxative Tablets (Kerbina)
Natural Herb Tablets (Dorwest)
Natural Herb Tablets (Kerbina)

Natural Herb Tablets (Lane)
Naturavite Tablets
Nature's Aid Co-Enzyme Q-10 Capsules
Nature's Own Acidophilus Plus Capsules (Supreme)
Nature's Own Betacarotene Capsules
Nature's Own Beta Carotene tablets
Nature's Own Calcium Orotate Tablets
Nature's Own Dolomite Tablets
Nature's Own Dolomite-Calcium Carbonate
   Magnesium Carbonate Tablets
Nature's Own Food State Beta Carotene Tablets
Nature's Own Food State Calcium Tablets
Nature's Own Food State "Euro Formula" Vitamin
   B Complex + Vitamin C & MagnesiumTablets
Nature's Own Food State Magnesium Tablets
Nature's Own Food State Selenium Tablets
Nature's Own Food State Vitamin B6
   (Pyridox) Tablets
Nature's Own Food State Vitamin C Tablets
Nature's Own Food State Vitamin E 300 Tablets
Nature's Own Food State Zinc/Copper Tablets
Nature's Own Multi-Vitamin Tablets
Nature's Own Vitamin B Complex Plus Tablets
   High Potency
Nature's Own Vitamin B6 (Pyridox) Tablets
Nature's Own Vitamin C Ascorbic Acid Powder
Nature's Own Vitamin C as Calcium
   Ascorbate Tablets
Nature's Own Vitamin C (as Sodium Ascorbate)
   Tablets
Nature's Own Vitamin C with Bioflavonoids
Nature's Own Vitamin E 100 Capsules
Nature's Own Vitamin E 100 Emulsifying Capsules
Nature's Own Vitamin E 200 Capsules
Nature's Own Zinc Orotates
Nature's Plus Calcium/Magnesium Tablets
Nature's Plus Green Magma Powder
Nature's Plus Liquid B Complex & Iron
Nature's Plus Mega C Tablets
Nature's Plus Rutin Tablets 500mg
Nature's Plus Super B50 Capsules
Naturtabs Choline
Naturtabs Nicotinamide
Naturtabs Nicotinic Acid
Naturtabs Paba
Natusan Baby Ointment
Naudicelle
Nella Red Oil Liniment
Neo-Cytamen Injection 250 mcg/ml
Neo-Cytamen Injection 1000 mcg/ml
Neoklenz Powder
Neophryn Nasal Drops
Neophryn Nasal Spray
Nescafe Instant Coffee
Nestle Nativa HA
Nethaprin Expectorant
Neuro Phosphates
Neurodyne Capsules
Neutradol Concentrated Air Deodoriser
Neutradonna Powder
Neutradonna Sed Powder
Neutradonna Sed Tablets

XVIIIA

Neutradonna Tablets
Neutrogena Body Oil
  (Scented and Unscented)
Neutrogena Conditioner
Neutrogena Hand Cream
Neutrogena Lip Care
Neutrogena Liquid
Neutrogena Moisture
Neutrogena Norwegian Formula
  Body Emulsion
Neutrogena Rainbath Shower and
  Bath Gel
Neutrogena Shampoo
Neutrogena Soap
Neutrogena Sun Care Lotion SPF 14
Neutrolactis Tablets
New Formula Beechams Powders
  Capsules
New Life Herbs
New Life Tablets
Newton's Children's Cough Treatment
Newton's Cough Mixture for Adults
Nezcaam Syrup
Nezeril Nose Drops (single dose pipette)
Nicabate Nicotine Transdermal Patch
Nico Patch
Nicobrevin
Nicodex Patch
Niconil Transdermal Patch
Nicorette
Nicorette Nasal Spray
Nicorette Patch
Nicorette Plus
Nicostop Patch
Nicotine Patch (QHR Limited)
Nicotinell Gum
Nicotinell TTS Patches
Niferex 150 Capsules
Nilbite
Nirolex Expectorant Linctus
Nitrados Tablets 5 mg
Nitrazepam Capsules 5 mg
Nivea
No 177 Tablets (Leoren)
Nobacter Medicated Shaving Foam
Nobrium Capsules 5 mg
Nobrium Capsules 10 mg
Nocold Tablets
Noctamid Tablets 0.5 mg
Noctamid Tablets 1 mg
Noctesed Tablets 5 mg
Noradran Bronchial Syrup
Norgesic Tablets
Normax Capsules
Normison Capsules 10 mg
Normison Capsules 20 mg
Norvits Syrup
Noscapine Linctus BP
Nourkrin Tablets
Novaprin Tablets
Novasil Antacid Tablets
Novasil Antacid Viscous Suspension

Noxzema Medicated Skin Cream
Nucross Coconut Oil
Nulacin Tablets
Numark Multivitamin Tablets
Nurodol Tablets
Nurofen Soluble Tablets
Nurofen Tablets 200 mg
Nurse Sykes Bronchial Balsam
Nurse Sykes Powders
Nu-Soft Baby Oil
Nutricare Beta Carotene Capsules
Nutricare Capricin Capsules
Nutricare Selenium Tablets
Nutricare Vitamin C Tablets
Nutricare Zinc Orotate Tablets
NutriTec Vitamin Mineral Complex Food
  Supplement
Nutrition Associates Beta Carotene Capsules
Nutrition Associates Reduced Glutathione Capsules
Nux Vomica Acid Mixture
Nux Vomica Alkaline Mixture
Nux Vomica Elixir BPC
Nylax Tablets
Nytol Tablets

Octovit Tablets
Ocuvite Multivitamin & Mineral Tablets
Oilatum Bar
Oilatum Soap
Olbas Oil
Omeiri Iron Tonic Tablets
Omilcaf Suspension
Onadox 118 Tablets
One Gram C Capsule
Opas Powder
Opas Tablets
Opobly Bailly Pills
Optivite Tablets
Oral B Plaque Check Disclosing Tablets
Orange & Halibut Vitamins (Kirby
  Warrick Pharmaceuticals)
Organidin Elixir
Organidin Solution
Organidin Tablets
Original Indigestion Tablets (Boots)
Orovite 7
Orovite Elixir
Orovite Tablets
Orthoxicol Syrup
Osteocare Calcium & Magnesium Tablets
Ostermilk Complete Formula
Ostermilk Two Milk Powder
Osterprem
Otrivine Nasal Drops 0.05%
Otrivine Nasal Drops 0.1%
Otrivine Nasal Spray 0.1%

Otrivine-Antistin Nasal Drops
Otrivine-Antistin Nasal Spray
Overnight Bedtime Cold Medicine
Owbridge's Cough Mixture
Oxanid Tablets 10 mg
Oxanid Tablets 15 mg
Oxanid Tablets 30 mg
Oxy 5 Acne Lotion
Oxy 10 Acne Lotion
Oxy Clean Facial Wash Gel
Oxy Clean Medicated Cleanser
Oxymetazoline Hydrochloride Nasal
    Drops 0.025%
Oxymetazoline Hydrochloride Nasal
    Drops 0.05%
Oxymetazoline Hydrochloride Nasal
    Spray 0.05%
Oxysept 1 Disinfecting Solution
Oxysept 2 Rinsing, Neutralising and
    Storing Solution
Ozium 500 Air Sanitizer
Ozium 1500 Air Sanitizer
Ozium Air Sanitizer
Ozium 3000

Pacidal Tablets
Pacifene Tablets
Paedo-Sed Syrup
Pain Relief Tablets (Cox)
Pain Relief Tablets (Davidson)
Paldesic Elixir
Pameton Tablets
Panacron Nasal Spray
Panacron Tablets
Panadeine Co Tablets
Panadeine Forte Tablets
Panadeine Soluble Effervescent Tablets
Panadeine Tablets
Panadol Baby & Infant Suspension
Panadol Caplets
Panadol Extra Soluble Tablets
Panadol Extra Tablets
Panadol Junior Sachets
Panadol Soluble Tablets
Panadol Tablets
Panaleve Junior
Panaleve Six Plus Suspension
Panasorb Tablets
Panax 600 Ginseng Tablets
Panerel Tablets
Panets Tablets
Pango Pain Paracetamol Codeine Tablets
    (Cupal)
Pantene Hair Tonic
Papain Compound Tablets
Paprika Tablets (Kerbina)

Para-Seltzer Effervescent Tablets
Paracetamol & Caffeine Capsules
Paracetamol & Caffeine Tablets
Paracetamol DC Tablets
Paracetamol Tablets Soluble (Boots)
Paracetamol Tablets, Sorbitol Basis
    500 mg
Paracets Tablets 500 mg
Paraclear Tablets
Paracodol Capsules
Paracodol Tablets
Paradeine R Tablets
Paragesic Effervescent Tablets
Parahypon Tablets
Parake Tablets
Paralgin Tablets
Paramin Capsules
Paramol Tablets
Paranorm Cough Syrup
Pardale Tablets
Parenamps Intramuscular Injection
Pastilaids Pastilles
Pavacol Cough Syrup
Paxadon Tablets
Paxalgesic Tablets
Paxidal Tablets
Paynocil Tablets
PEM Linctus
Penetrol Inhalant
Pentazocine-Aspirin Compound Tablets
Peplax Peppermint Flavoured Laxative
    Tablets
Peppermint Indigestion Tablets (Boots)
Pepto-Bismol Suspension
Perform 1 Disinfecting Solution
Perform 2 Rinsing and Neutralising Solution
Pernivit Tablets
Perrier Mineral Water
Persomnia Tablets
Pestroy Flea and Insect Powder
Petrolagar Emulsion Plain
Petrolagar Emulsion with
    Phenolphthalein
PF Plus Tablets
Pharmacin Capsules
Pharmacin Effervescent Plus C Tablets
Pharmacin Effervescent Tablets 325 mg
Pharmaton Capsules
Pharmidone Tablets
Phenergan Compound Expectorant
    Linctus
Phenolphthalein Compound Pills BPC
Phenolphthalein Compound Tablets BPC
    1963
Phenolphthalein Tablets BP
Phensedyl Cough Linctus
Phensic Tablets
Phensic 2 Tablets
Phenylephrine Hydrochloride Nasal
    Drops 0.25%
Phenylephrine Hydrochloride Nasal
    Spray 0.5%

XVIIIA

Phillips Brewers Yeast Tablets
Phillips Iron Tonic Tablets
Phillips Tonic Yeast Tablets
Phillips' Toothpaste
Phisoderm
Phisohex System Medicated Face Wash
pHiso-Med Solution
Pholcolix Syrup
Pholcomed D Linctus
Pholcomed Diabetic Forte Linctus
Pholcomed Expectorant
Pholcomed Forte Linctus
Pholcomed Linctus
Pholcomed Pastilles
Pholtex Syrup
Pholtussa Mixture
Phor Pain
Phor Pain Double Strength
Phosferine Liquid
Phosferine Multi-Vitamin Liquid
Phosferine Tablets
Phygeine Liquid
Phyllosan Tablets
Physeptone Linctus
Pickles Nail Bite Lotion
PIL Food Capsules
Pile Mixture (Ayrton Saunders)
Pile Tablets (Ayrton Saunders)
Pine Bath Milk
Pine Catarrh Drops Lozenges
Piriton Allergy
Piz Buin After Sun Lotion
Piz Buin After Sun Shower Gel
Piz Buin Children's Balm SPF 8
Piz Buin Cream Factor 12
Piz Buin Creme factor 6
Piz Buin Creme factor 8
Piz Buin Factor 4 Cold Air Protection Cream
Piz Buin Glacier Cream SPF 15
Piz Buin Lip Protection Stick SPF 8
Piz Buin Sun Allergy Lotion SPF 12
Piz Buin Sun Protection Lotion SPF 12
Piz Buin SPF 6 Lotion
Piz Buin SPF 8 Lotion
Plax Anti-Plaque Pre-Brushing Rinse
Plenamin Super
Plenivite with Iron Tablets
Pliagel Soft Lens Solution
Plurivite M Tablets
Plurivite Tablets
Poli-grip Denture Fixative Cream
Pollen-Eze Tablets
Polyalk Gel
Polyalk Tablets
Polyvite Capsules
Porosis D Calcium Supplement Tablets
Potaba + 6 Capsules
Potaba + 6 Tablets
Potassium Bromide & Nux Vomica
    Mixture BPC 1963

Potters Household Liniment
Potters Nine Rubbing Oils
Powdered Bran Tablets 2 g
Power Cranberry Juice Capsules
Power Cranberry Juice Concentrated Powder
Power Dolomite Tablets
Power Dophilus Capsules
Power Feverfew Capsules
Power GLA 65 (Borage Oil) Capsules
Power Halibut Liver Oil Capsules
Power Kelp Tablets 500mg
Power Nature Vitamin E Cream
Power Nutrimental 24 Tablets
Power Plus Super Multivitamin and
    Mineral Capsules
Powerin Tablets
PP Tablets
PR Freeze Spray
PR Heat Spray
PR Tablets
Prazepam Tablets 10 mg
PRD 200 Tablets 600 mg
Preflex Solution
Pregaine Shampoo
Pregnacare Capsules
Pregnadon Tablets
Pregnavite Forte Tablets
Pregnavite Forte F Tablets
Prematil with Milupan
Premence-28 Capsules
Premit Tablets 20 mg
Prenatal Dri-Kaps Capsules
Prenatol Anti Stretch Mark Cream
Pre-Nutrison
Primes Premiums Tablets
Prioderm Cream Shampoo
Priory Cleansing Herbs Powder
Probase 3 Cream
Pro-Bifidus Powder (Dairy Free)
Procol Capsules
Proctofibre Tablets
Prodexin Tablets
Pro-Dophilus Powder (Dairy Free)
Proflex Capsules
Proflex Tablets 200 mg
Progress Powder
Propain Tablets
Propecia
Pro-Plus He-Vite Elixir
Proteolised Liver Tablets
Protexin B Powder
Protexin Natural Care Powder
Protexin Natural Care Tablets
Pro-Vitamin A Capsules (Rodale)
Pru Sen Tablet Bar
Prymecare Tablets for Soft and
    and Gas Permeable Lenses
Prymeclean Cleaning Solution for
    Soft Lenses
Prymesoak Soaking Solution for
    Soft Lenses

Pulmo Bailly Liquid
Purgoids Tablets
Pyridoxine Tablets, Slow 100 mg

Quest Balanced Ratio Cal-Mag Tablets
Quest Beta Carotene Tablets
Quest Folic Acid with Vitamin B Capsules
Quest Gamma EPA Capsules 1000mg
Quest Herbal Range Feverfew Formula Capsules
Quest Improved Once-A-Day Tablets
Quest Kyolic 350 Tablets
Quest Mega B50 Tablets
Quest Mega B-100 Timed Release Tablets
Quest Mega B Complex Plus 1000mg C Tablets
Quest Multi B Complex Plus 500mg C Tablets
Quest Multi C Complex Tablets
Quest Non-Dairy Acidophilus Plus Capsules
Quest Once-A-Day Tablets
Quest Super Mega B-50 Timed Release Tablets
Quest Super Mega B + C Tablets
Quest Super Once-A-Day Tablets
Quest Super Once-A-Day Divided Dose Tablets
Quest Synergistic Boron Tablets
Quest Synergistic Iron Capsules
Quest Synergistic Magnesium Tablets
Quest Synergistic Selenium Capsules
Quest Synergistic Zinc Capsules
Quest Vitamin C Tablets
Quest Vitamin C Tablets Sustained Release
Quest Vitamin E Capsules
Quick Action Cough Cure (Brian C Spencer)
Quiet Life Tablets

Rabenhorst Tomato Juice
Radian-B Mineral Bath Liquid
Radian-B Mineral Bath Salts
Radian-B Muscle Lotion
Radian-B Muscle Rub
Ralgex Cream
Ralgex Stick
Rappell Head Louse Repellent Pump Spray
Raspberry Tablets No B039
Rayglo Chest Rub Ointment
Rayglo Laxative Tablets
Reach Mouthwash
Reactivan Tablets
Red Catarrh Pastilles (Baldwin)
Redelan Effervescent Tablets
Redoxon Adult Multivitamin Tablets
Redoxon C Effervescent Tablets 1 g

Redoxon C Tablets 25 mg
Redoxon C Tablets 50 mg
Redoxon C Tablets 200 mg
Redoxon C Tablets 250 mg
Redoxon C Tablets 500 mg
Redoxon Childrens Multivitamins Tablets
Redoxon Effervescent Tablets 1 g
Regaine
Regina Royal Jelly Capsules
Reg-U-Lett Tablets
Relanium Tablets 2 mg
Relanium Tablets 5 mg
Relanium Tablets 10 mg
Relcofen Tablets
Relcol Tablets
Remegel Tablets
Remnos Tablets 5 mg
Remnos Tablets 10 mg
Rennie Tablets
Rennie Gold Tablets
Rennie Plus Tablets
Rennie Rap-Eze Tablets
Replens Vaginal Moisturiser
Resolve Granules
Respaton
Retinova
Revlon Nurtrasome Shampoo
Revlon ZP11 Medicated Shampoo
Rheumavit Tablets
Rhuaka Herbal Syrup
Rhuaka Tablets
Rhubarb & Soda Mixture Ammoniated BP
Rhubarb Compound Mixture BPC
Rhubarb Mixture Compound Paediatric BPC
Ribena
Riddovydrin Liquid
Rinurel Linctus
Rinurel Tablets
Rite-Diet Egg White Replacer
Rite-Diet Gluten-Free Baking Powder
Rite-Diet Gluten-Free Banana Cake
Rite-Diet Gluten-Free Bourbon Biscuits
Rite-Diet Gluten-Free Christmas Pudding
Rite-Diet Gluten-Free Half Covered Chocolate
     Digestive Biscuits
Rite-Diet Gluten-Free Coconut Cookies
Rite-Diet Gluten-Free Date and Walnut Cake
Rite-Diet Gluten-Free Gingernut Cookies
Rite-Diet Gluten-Free Muesli Cookies
Rite-Diet Gluten-Free Lemon Madeira Cake
Rite-Diet Gluten-Free Rich Fruit Cake
Rite-Diet Gluten-Free Wheat-Free Mince Pies
Rite-Diet Hot Breakfast Cereal
Robaxisal Forte Tablets
Roberts Aspirin & Caffeine Tablets
Robinsons Baby Rice
Robinsons Instant Baby Foods Baby Breakfast
Robinsons Instant Baby Foods Baby Dessert
Robitussin AC Liquid
Robitussin Cough Soother
Robitussin Cough Soother
     Junior Formula

XVIIIA

Robitussin Expectorant
Robitussin Expectorant Plus
Robitussin Liquid
Robitussin Plus Liquid
Robitussin Syrup
RoC Amino Moisturising Cream
RoC Compact Cleanser
RoC Eye Make-up Remover Lotion
RoC Face Powder Loose
RoC Foundation Cream
RoC High Protection Sun Cream SPF 7/9
RoC Hydra and Body Cream
RoC Hydra Plus
RoC Intensive Hand Cream
RoC Lipo Moisturising Treatment
RoC Lipo Vitamin Treatment
RoC Pre-Tanning Lotion
RoC Soap for Delicate Skin
RoC Soothing After Sun Lotion
RoC Soothing Eye Gel
RoC Treatment Lipstick
RoC Vitamin Cream
Roche Starflower Oil Capsules 500mg
Roche Starflower Oil (GLA) Capsules 250mg
Rock Salmon Cough Mixture
Rohypnol Tablets 1 mg
Roscorbic Effervescent Tablets
Roscorbic Tablets 25 mg
Roscorbic Tablets 50 mg
Roscorbic Tablets 200 mg
Roscorbic Tablets 500 mg
Rose Hip C-100 Capsules
Rose Hip C-200 Capsules
Rose Hip Tablets (English Grains)
Rose Hip Tablets (Potters)
Rose Hip Tablets (Roberts)
Rosemary Bath
Roskens Ultracare 3
Rosmax Syrup
Roter Tablets
Rovigon
RRC1 Cream
Rubelix Syrup
Rubraton B Elixir
Ruby Tonic Tablets (Jacksons)
Rum Cough Elixir
Ruthmol
Rutin Plus Tablets (Gerard)

Safapryn Tablets
Safapryn-Co Tablets
Safflower Seed Oil
Sainsbury's Aspirin Tablets 300mg
Sainsbury's Cold Powders with
   Blackcurrant
Sainsbury's Hot Lemon Powders

Sainsbury's Indigestion Tablets
Sainsbury's Junior Soluble Aspirin
   Tablets
Sainsbury's Paracetmaol Tablets 500 mg
Sainsbury's Soluble Aspirin Tablets
St. Clements Fruit Juice Concentrate
Salonair Spray
Salzone Syrup
Salzone Tablets 500 mg
Sanatogen Childrens Vitamins Plus Minerals
Sanatogen Cod Liver Oil Capsules
Sanatogen Garlic Oil Perle One-A-Day
Sanatogen Junior Vitamins Tablets
Sanatogen Multivitamin Plus Iron
   (Formula One) Tablets
Sanatogen Multivitamins Tablets
Sanatogen Multivitamins & Calcium Tablets
Sanatogen Nerve Tonic Powder
Sanatogen Selected Multivitamins Plus
   Iron (Formula Two) Tablets
Sanatogen Tonic
Sanatogen Vitamin B6 Capsules
Sanatogen Vitamin E Capsules
Sancos Compound Linctus
Sancos Syrup
Savant Tablets
Savlon Dry Skin Cream
Saxin
SBL Junior Cough Linctus
SBL Soothing Bonchial Linctus
Schar Gluten Free Sponge Cake
Scholl Foot Refresher Spray
Scott's Cod Liver Oil Capsules
Scott's Emulsion
Scott's Husky Biscuits
Seatone Capsules
Seatone Super Strength Capsules
Seaweed Vitamin A Ester BP & Vitamin
   D BP Capsules (Regent Laboratories)
Seba-Med Cleansing Bar
Seba-Med Cream
Seba-Med Facial Wash
Seba-Med Lotion
Seba-Med Shampoo
Sebbix Shampoo
Secaderm Salve
Seclodin Capsules
Sedazin Tablets 1 mg
Sedazin Tablets 2.5 mg
Seldane Tablets
Selenium ACE Tablets
Selora Sodium-free Salt Substitute
Selsun Soft Conditioner
Senlax Tablets
Senna Laxative Tablets (Boots)
Senna Tablets (Potters)
Senokot Tablets
Senotabs Tablets
Senselle Natural Feminine Moisture
Sensodyne Toothpaste
Serenid D Tablets 10 mg
Serenid D Tablets 15 mg

Serenid Forte Capsules 30 mg
Sergeant's Dust Mite Patrol Powder
Sertin Tablets
Setamol Soluble Tablets
Setlers Extra Strength Tablets
Setlers Liquid
Setlers Tablets
Seven Seas Antioxidant Beta Carotene Capsules
Seven Seas Antioxidant Vitamin E Capsules
Seven Seas Beta Carotene Capsules
Seven Seas Calcium Chewables (Chewable Caps)
Seven Seas Cod Liver Oil
Seven Seas Evening Primrose Oil Capsules
Seven Seas Folic Acid & Vitamin B12 One-A-Day
    Tablets
Seven Seas Formula 70 Multivitamin-
    Multimineral Capsules
Seven Seas Garlic Oil Perles
Seven Seas Iron Chewables (Chewable Caps)
Seven Seas Korean Ginseng Capsules
Seven Seas Lecithin Capsules
Seven Seas Magnesium Berries
Seven Seas Malt and Cod Liver Oil
Seven Seas Multivitamin & Mineral Capsules
Seven Seas Natural Vitamin E in Wheatgerm
    Capsules
Seven Seas Orange Syrup & Cod Liver
    Oil
Seven Seas Pulse Capsules
Seven Seas Pure Cod Liver Oil Capsules
Seven Seas Pure Starflower Oil
Seven Seas Selenium E & Cod Liver Oil
    Capsules
Seven Seas Start Right Cod Liver Oil for
    Babies
Seven Seas Vitamin and Mineral Tonic
Seven Seas Wheatgerm Oil Capsules
Seven Seas Zinc Chewables (Chewable Caps)
Sidros Tablets
Silk-Lax Tablets
Siloxyl Suspension
Siloxyl Tablets
Simeco Suspension
Simeco Tablets
Simple Hair Conditioner
Simple Moisturising Lotion
Simple Night Cream
Simple Protective Moisture Cream
Simple Refreshing Shower Gel
Simple Shampoo
Simple Soap
Simple Sun Block
Simple Talcum Powder
Sine-Off Tablets
Sinitol Capsules
Sinutab Tablets
Sionon Sweetner
Skin Glow Capsules
Slim-Fast Meal Replacement
SMA Gold Cap Powder and Ready-to-
    Feed
SMA Powder and Concentrated Liquid

Snufflebabe Vapour Rub
Soaclens Solution
Soframycin Ointment
Softab Soft Lens Care Tablets
Solgar Cartilade Capsules
Solgar Ester-C Tablets
Solgar Evening Primrose Oil
Solgar Maxi Coenzyme Q10 Capsules
Solgar Maxi L-Carnitine Tablets
Solgar Provatene Softgel Capules
Solis Capsules 2 mg
Solis Capsules 5 mg
Solis Capsules 10 mg
Solmin Tablets
Solpadeine Capsules
Solpadeine Forte Tablets
Solpadeine Tablets
Solpadeine Tablets Effervescent
Solprin Tablets
Soluble Aspirin Tablets for Children (Boots)
Soluble Phensic Tablets
Solusol Solution
Sominex Tablets
Somnite Suspension 2.5 mg/5 ml
Somnite Tablets 5 mg
Soquette Soaking Solution
Sovol Liquid
Sovol Tablets
Soya Powder & Nicotinamide Tablets
SP Cold Relief Capsules
Special E Moisture Cream
Special Stomach Powder (Halls)
Spectraban 4 Lotion
SPHP Tablets
SPS Low-Protein Drink
Squill Linctus Opiate BP (Gee's Linctus)
Squill Linctus Opiate, Paediatric, BP
Squire's Soonax Tablets
SR2310 Expectorant
SR Toothpaste (Gibbs)
Staffords Mild Aperient Tablets
Staffords Strong Aperient Tablets
Steradent Mouthwash
Steri-Clens Solution
Steri-Solve Soft Lens Solution
Sterling Health Salts Effervescent
Sterling Indigestion Tablets
Sterling Paracetamol Tablets
Sterogyl Alcoholic Solution
Stomach Aids Tablets
Stomach Mixture (Herbal Laboratories)
Stomach Mixture H138 (Southon
    Laboratories)
Stomach Powder (Diopharm)
Stomach Tablets (Ulter)
Stop 'N' Grow Nail Biting Deterrent
Street's Cough Mixture
Strengthening Mixture (Hall's)
Stress B Supplement Tablets
Strychnine & Iron Mixture BPC 1963
Strychnine Mixture BPC 1963
Stute Diabetic Blackcurrant Jam

XVIIIA

Stute Diabetic Marmalade	Tablets No B070
Sudafed Co Tablets	Tablets No 268A (Potters)
Sudafed Expectorant	Tablets to Formula A10
Sudafed Linctus	Tablets to Formula A11
Sudafed Nasal Spray	Tablets to Formula A18
Sudocrem Baby Lotion	Tablets to Formula A19
Suleo C Shampoo	Tablets to Formula A20
Sun E45 Lotion SPF8	Tablets to Formula A22
Sunerven Tablets	Tablets to Formula A23
Sunnyvale Gluten-Free Rich Plum Pudding	Tablets to Formula A31
Sun Yums Gluten Free & Dairy Free Almond &	Tablets to Formula A32
Coconut Cake	Tablets to Formula A33
Sun Yums Gluten Free & Dairy Free Banana &	Tablets to Formula A45
Sesame Seed Cake	Tablets to Formula A51
Sun Yums Gluten Free & Dairy Free Carob &	Tablets to Formula A63
Mint Cake	Tablets to Formula A67
Sun Yums Gluten Free & Dairy Free Ginger &	Tablets to Formula A68
Pecan Nut Cake	Tablets to Formula A69
Sun Yums Gluten Free & Dairy Free Jaffa Spice	Tablets to Formula A70
Cake	Tablets to Formula A71
Super Plenamins Tablets	Tablets to Formula A105
Super Yeast + C Tablets	Tablets to Formula A111
Superdophilus Powder	Tablets to Formula A114
Superdrug Health Salts	Tablets to Formula A120
Superdrug Heat Spray	Tablets to Formula A147
Supradyn Capsules	Tablets to Formula A157
Supradyn Effervescent Tablets	Tablets to Formula A158
Supradyn Tablets for Children	Tablets to Formula A161
Surbex-T Tablets	Tablets to Formula A162
Surem Capsules 5 mg	Tablets to Formula A164
Surem Capsules 10 mg	Tablets to Formula A165
Surelax Laxative Tablets	Tablets to Formula A166
Sweetex	Tablets to Formula A167
Sylopal Suspension	Tablets to Formula A169
Sylphen Tablets	Tablets to Formula A175
Syn-Ergel	Tablets to Formula A183
Syndol Tablets	Tablets to Formula A184
Syrtussar Cough Syrup	Tablets to Formula A190
	Tablets to Formula A195
	Tablets to Formula A202
	Tablets to Formula A203
	Tablets to Formula A213
	Tablets to Formula A221
	Tablets to Formula A244
	Tablets to Formula A245
T-Zone Decongestant Tablets	Tablets to Formula A246
Tabasan Tablets	Tablets to Formula A247
Tablets No B006	Tablets to Formula A248
Tablets No B011	Tablets to Formula A249
Tablets No B015	Tablets to Formula A250
Tablets No B024	Tablets to Formula A264
Tablets No B025	Tablets to Formula A266
Tablets No B029	Tablets to Formula A270
Tablets No B034	Tablets to Formula A271
Tablets No B035	Tablets to Formula A272
Tablets No B036	Tablets to Formula A273
Tablets No B037	Tablets to Formula A274
Tablets No B038	Tablets to Formula A275
Tablets No B040	Tablets to Formula A276
Tablets No B041	Tablets to Formula A277
Tablets No B045	Tablets to Formula A298
Tablets No B048	Tablets to Formula A301

Tablets to Formula A316
Tablets to Formula BA6
Tablets to Formula B10
Tablets to Formula B15
Tablets to Formula B18
Tablets to Formula B19
Tablets to Formula B20
Tablets to Formula B21
Tablets to Formula B22
Tablets to Formula B25
Tablets to Formula B26
Tablets to Formula B29
Tablets to Formula B41
Tablets to Formula B48
Tablets to Formula B51
Tablets to Formula B56
Tablets to Formula B58
Tablets to Formula B64
Tablets to Formula B65
Tablets to Formula B66
Tablets to Formula B67
Tablets to Formula B68
Tablets to Formula B70
Tablets to Formula B71
Tablets to Formula B72
Tablets to Formula B73
Tablets to Formula B74
Tablets to Formula B75
Tablets to Formula B76
Tablets to Formula B77
Tablets to Formula B78
Tablets to Formula B79
Tablets to Formula B80
Tablets to Formula B81
Tablets to Formula B82
Tablets to Formula B83
Tablets to Formula B85
Tablets to Formula B86
Tablets to Formula B87
Tablets to Formula B90
Tablets to Formula B91
Tablets to Formula B93
Tablets to Formula B94
Tablets to Formula B96
Tablets to Formula B98
Tablets to Formula B100
Tablets to Formula B102
Tablets to Formula B104
Tablets to Formula B117
Tablets to Formula B118
Tablets to Formula B120
Tablets to Formula B122
Tablets to Formula B124
Tablets to Formula B128
Tablets to Formula B141
Tablets to Formula B143
Tablets to Formula B145
Tablets to Formula B148
Tablets to Formula B156
Tablets to Formula B157
Tablets to Formula B158

Tablets to Formula B160
Tablets to Formula B163
Tablets to Formula B169
Tablets to Formula B178
Tablets to Formula B180
Tablets to Formula B181
Tablets to Formula B182
Tablets to Formula B190
Tablets to Formula B193
Tablets to Formula B207
Tablets to Formula B209
Tablets to Formula B210
Tablets to Formula B211
Tablets to Formula B212
Tablets to Formula B213
Tablets to Formula B214
Tablets to Formula B215
Tablets to Formula B216
Tablets to Formula B217
Tablets to Formula B218
Tablets to Formula B222
Tablets to Formula B223
Tablets to Formula B224
Tablets to Formula B225
Tablets to Formula B227
Tablets to Formula B228
Tablets to Formula B231
Tablets to Formula B234
Tablets to Formula B235
Tablets to Formula B236
Tablets to Formula B243
Tablets to Formula B248
Tablets to Formula B250
Tablets to Formula B251
Tablets to Formula B252
Tabmint Anti-Smoking Chewing Gum Tablets
Tanacet Feverfew 125
Tancolin Childrens Cough Linctus
Tedral Expectorant
Temazepam Gelthix Capsules
Temazepam Planpak
Temazepam Soft Gelatin Gel-Filled Capsules
Tenaset Wash Cream
Tenaset Wash Cream (Unperfumed)
Tensium Tablets 2 mg
Tensium Tablets 5 mg
Tensium Tablets 10 mg
Tercoda Elixir
Tercolix Elixir
Terpalin Elixir
Terperoin Elixir
Terpoin Antitussive
Terrabron
T-Gel Conditioner
Thermogene Medicated Rub
Thixo-D Thickened Drink Mixes
Three Noughts Cough Syrup
Tidmans Bath Sea Salt
Tidman's Sea Salt Coarse
Tiger Balm Liquid
Tiger Balm Red

XVIIIA

Tiger Balm White
Timotei Herbal Shampoo
Tinaderm Cream
Titan Hard Cleanser
Tixylix Cough and Cold Linctus
Tixylix Cough Linctus
Tixylix Day-Time Cough Linctus
Tixylix Decongestant Inhalant Capsules
Tolu Compound Linctus Paediatric BP
Tolu Solution BP
Tolu Syrup BP
Tonatexa Mixture
Tonic Tablets (Thomas Guest)
Tonic Wines
Tonivitan A & D Syrup
Tonivitan B Syrup
Tonivitan Capsules
Top C Tablets
Topfit Amino Acid Powder
Topfit L Threonine + Vitamin B6 Capsules
        500/12.5mg
Toptabs
Total All Purpose Solution
Total Nutrient Liquid
Totavit D R Capsules
Totolin Paediatric Cough Syrup
Tramil Capsules
Trancoprin Tablets
Transclean Cleaning Solution
Transdrop
Transoak Solution
Transol Solution
Tranxene Capsules 7.5 mg
Tranxene Capsules 15 mg
Tranxene Tablets 15 mg
Triludan Forte Tablets 7-tablet pack
Triludan Tablets 10-tablet pack
Triocos Linctus
Triogesic Elixir
Triogesic Tablets
Triominic Syrup
Triominic Tablets
Triopaed Linctus
Triotussic Suspension
Triovit Tablets
Triple Action Cold Relief Tablets
Tropium Capsules 5 mg
Tropium Capsules 10 mg
Tropium Tablets 5 mg
Tropium Tablets 10 mg
Tropium Tablets 25 mg
Trufree Crispbran
Trufree Tandem IQ Tablets
Trufree Vitamin & Minerals Tablets
Tudor Rose Bay Rhum
Tums Tablets
Tusana Linctus
Tussifans Syrup
Tussimed Liquid
Two-A-Day Iron Jelloids Tablets
Tymasil
Tysons Catarrh Syrup

Ucerax Tablets
Udenum Gastric Vitamin Powder
Ultracach Analgesic Capsules
Ultradal Antacid Stomach Tablets
Ultralief Tablets
Uncoated Tablets to Formula A323
Uncoated Tablets to Formula A325
Undecyn Capsules
Unguentum Merck Cream 60g
Unicap M Tablets
Unicap T Tablets
Unichem Baby Oil
Unichem Chesty Cough Linctus
Unichem Children's Dry Cough Linctus
Unichem Cod Liver Oil Capsules
Unichem Cold Relief Capsules
Unichem Cold Relief Day-Time Liquid
Unichem Cold Relief Night-Time Liquid
Unichem Cold Relief Powders
Unichem Dry Cough Linctus
Unichem Extract of Malt with Cod Liver Oil
Unichem Multivitamins + Iron Tablets
Unichem Multivitamins & Minerals One-A-Day
        Capsules
Uniflu Tablets
Unigesic Capsules
Unigest Tablets
Unisomnia Tablets 5 mg
United Skin Care Programme
(Uni-Derm; Uni-Salve; Uni-Wash)
Uvistat Aftersun Lotion
Uvistat Baby Sun Cream SPF 12
Uvistat Cream SPF 4
Uvistat Facial Cream SPF 8
Uvistat Facial Cream SPF 22
Uvistat Lipscreen SPF 5 Lipstick
Uvistat SPF 8 Suncream
Uvistat SPF 10 Suncream
Uvistat Sun Lotion SPF 6
Uvistat Sun Lotion SPF 8

Vadarex Wintergreen Heat Rub
Vagisil Feminine Powder
Valium Capsules 2 mg
Valium Capsules 5 mg
Valium Syrup 2 mg/5 ml
Valium Tablets 2 mg

Valium Tablets 5 mg
Valium Tablets 10 mg
Valonorm Tonic Solution
Valrelease Capsules
Vanamil Tablets
Vantage Baby Shampoo
Vantage Garlic One-A-Day Capsules
Vantage Halibut Fish Oil One-A-Day Capsules
Vantage Sterilising Fluid
Vapex Inhalent
Vaseline Intensive Care Lotion
Vaseline Intensive Care Lotion Herbal and Aloe
Veganin Tablets
Veno's Adult Formula Cough Mixture
Veno's Cough Mixture
Veno's Honey & Lemon Cough Mixture
Veracolate Tablets
Verdiviton Elixir
Vervain Compound Tablets
Vichy Total Sunscreen
Vicks Coldcare Capsules
Vicks Cremacoat Syrup
Vicks Cremacoat Syrup with Doxylamine
  Succinate
Vicks Cremacoat Syrup with Guaiphenesin
Vicks Cremacoat Syrup with Paracetamol
  & Dextromethorphan
Vicks Daymed
Vicks Formula 44 Cough Mixture
Vicks Inhaler
Vicks Medinite
Vicks Pectorex Solution
Vicks Sinex Nasal Spray
Vicks Vapo-Lem Powder Sachets
Vicks Vaposyrup Children's Dry Cough
Vicks Vaposyrup for Chesty Coughs
Vicks Vaposyrup for Chesty Coughs and Nasal
  Congestion
Vicks Vaposyrup for Dry Coughs
Vicks Vaposyrup for Dry Coughs and Nasal
  Congestion
Vicks Vapour Rub
Vi-Daylin Syrup
Videnal Tablets
Vigour Aids Tablets
Vigranon B Complex Tablets
Vigranon B Syrup
Vikelp Coated Tablets
Vikonon Tablets
Villescon Liquid
Villescon Tablets
Viobin Octacosanol Tablets 50,000mcg
Viobin Pancreatin Tablets 325mg
Vipro Vegetable Protein
Virvina Elixir
Visclair Tablets
Vitabrit Beta Carotene Capsules
Vita Diem Multi Vitamin Drops
Vita-E 200 (D-Alpha Tocopherol) Capsules
Vita-E Cream
Vita-E Ointment
Vital Dophilus Powder

Vitalia Calcium Formula A + D Tablets
Vitalia Lecithin Capsules High Potency
Vitalia Multivitamins & Minerals Children's
  Chewable Sugar-Free Tablets
Vitalia Multivitamin & Minerals with Iron
  Tablets
Vitalia Multivitamin & Minerals Tablets
  without Iron
Vitalia Natural E Capsules
Vitalia Vitamin A Tablets
Vitalia Vitamin B Complex Super Tablets
Vitalia Vitamin B6 Tablets
Vitalia Vitamin C Chewable Tablets
Vitalia Vitamin E Tablets
Vitalia Zinc Amino Acid Chelated Tablets 15mg
Vitalia Zinc Chelated Tablets
Vitalife Vital E Capsules
Vitalife Vitamin B6 Capsules
Vitalife Vitamin B Complex Tablets
Vitalin Tablets
Vitalzymes Capsules
Vitamin & Iron Tonic (Epitone) Solution
Vitamin A & D Capsules BPC 1968
  (Regent Laboratories)
Vitamin A Ester & Vitamin D2 Capsules
  (Regent Laboratories)
Vitamin A Ester Capsules
  (Regent Laboratories)
Vitamin A Ester Conc, Alpha Tocopherol
  Acetate Nat Capsules
  (Regent Laboratories)
Vitamin A 4500 Units & Vitamin D2
  Capsules (Regent Laboratories)
Vitamin A 6000 Units & Vitamin D2
  Capsules (Regent Laboratories)
Vitamin A, C & D Tablets (Approved
  Prescription Services)
Vitamin A, D & C Tablets
  (Regent Laboratories)
Vitamin B Complex Tablets (English Grains)
Vitamin B Complex with Brewer's Yeast
  Tablets (English Grains)
Vitamin B1 Dried Yeast Powder (Distillers)
Vitamin B1 Yeast Tablets (Distillers)
Vitamin B12 Tablets 0.01 mg
Vitamin B12 Tablets 0.025 mg
Vitamin B12 Tablets 0.05 mg
Vitamin B12 Tablets 0.10 mg
Vitamin B12 Tablets 0.25 mg
Vitamin B12 Tablets 0.5 mg
Vitamin B12 Tablets 1 mg
Vitamin C Tablets (G & G Food Supplies)
Vitamin C Tablets Effervescent 1g
Vitamin Capsules (Regent Laboratories)
Vitamin Malt Extract with Orange Juice
  (Distillers)
Vitamin Mineral Capsules
  (Regent Laboratories)
Vitamin Tablets No B077
Vitamin Tablets No B081
Vitamin Tablets No B084

Vitaminised Iron & Yeast Tablets
   (Kirby Warrick Pharmaceuticals)
Vita Natura Evening Primrose Oil +
   Vitamin E Tablets
Vitanorm Malt Extract
Vitanorm Malt Extract Syrup
Vitapointe Conditioner
Vitasafe's CF Kaps Tablets
Vitasafe's WCF Kaps Tablets
Vita-Six Capsules
Vitathone Chilblain Tablets
Vitatrop Tablets
Vitavel Powder for Syrup
Vitavel Solution
Vitepron Tablets
Vitorange Tablets
Vitrite Multi-Vitamin Syrup
Vykamin Fortified Capsules

Zactirin Tablets
Zam Buk Ointment
Zefringe Sachets
Zemaphyte Chinese Herbal Eczema Remedy
Zendium Toothpaste
Zenoxone Cream
Zirtek 7
Zubes Expectorant Cough Syrup
Zubes Original Cough Mixture
Zyriton Expectorant Linctus

W L Tablets
Wallachol Syrup
Wallachol Tablets
Wate-on Emulsion
Wate-on Emulsion Super
Wate-on Tablets
Wate-on Tablets Super
Wate-on Tonic
Waterhouses All Fours
Wines
Woodwards Nursery Cream
Wrights Glucose with Vitamin D Powder
Wrights Vaporizing Fluid

Xanax Tablets 0.25 mg
Xanax Tablets 0.5 mg
Xanax Tablets 1.0 mg

Yeast & B12 Tablets (English Grains)
Yeast Plus Tablets (Thomas Guest)
Yeast-Vite Tablets
Yellow Phenolphthalein Tablets
   (any strength)
Yestamin Vitamin B5 Tablets

Part XVIIIB reproduces Schedule 11 to the National Health Service (General Medical Services) Regulations 1992, as amended.

Drugs in Column 1 of this part may be prescribed for persons mentioned in Column 2, only for the treatment of the purpose specified in Column 3. The Doctor must endorse the prescription with the reference "SLS".

Drug	Patient	Purpose
Acetylcysteine Granules	Any Patient	Abdominal complications associated with cystic fibrosis.
Carbocisteine	A patient under the age of 18 who has undergone a tracheostomy.	Any condition which, through damage or disease, affects the air ways and has required a tracheostomy.
Clobazam	Any Patient	Epilepsy
Cyanocobalamin Tablets	A patient who is a vegan or who has a proven vitamin B12 deficiency of dietary origin.	Treatment or prevention of vitamin B12 deficiency.
Locabiotal Aerosol	Any Patient	Treatment of infections and inflammation of the oropharynx.
Niferex Elixir 30ml Paediatric Dropper Bottle	Infants born prematurely	Prophylaxis in treatment of iron deficiency
Nizoral Cream	Any patient	Treatment of seborrhoeic dermatitis and pityriasis versicolor

The following drugs for the treatment of erectile dysfunction -
 	
Alprostadil
  (Caverject), (MUSE),
  (Viridal)
Moxisylyte Hydrochloride
  (Erecnos)
Thymoxamine Hydrochloride
  (Erecnos)
Sildenafil (Viagra)
	(a) a man with erectile dysfunction who on 14 September 1998 was receiving a course of treatment under the Act, the National Health Service (Scotland) Act 1978(a) or the Health and Personal Social Services (Northern Ireland) Order 1972(b) for this condition with any of the following drugs -
	  Alprostadil (Caverject),
	  (MUSE), (Viridal)
	  Moxisylyte Hydrochloride
	  (Erecnos)
	  Thymoxamine Hydrochloride
	  (Erecnos)
	  Sildenafil (Viagra); or
		Treatment of erectile dysfunction.

(a) 1978 c.29
(b) SI 1972/1265 (NI 14)

The following drugs for the treatment of erectile dysfunction -

Alprostadil
    (Caverject, (MUSE),
    (Viridal)
Moxisylyte Hydrochloride
    (Erecnos)
Thymoxamine Hydrochloride
    (Erecnos)
Sildenafil (Viagra)

(b) a man who is a national of an EEA State who is entitled to treatment by virtue of Article 7(2) of Council Regulation 1612/68(c) as extended by the EEA Agreement or by virtue of any other enforceable Community right who has erectile dysfunction and was on 14th September 1998 receiving a course of treatment under a national health insurance system of an EEA State for this condition with any of the drugs listed in sub-paragraph (a); or

(c) a man who is not a national of an EEA State but who is the member of the family of such a national who has an enforceable Community right to be treated no less favourably than the national in the provision of medical treatment and has erectile dysfunction and was being treated for that condition on 14th September 1998 with any of the drugs listed in sub-paragraph (a); or

(d) a man who is suffering from any of the following -
    diabetes
    multiple sclerosis
    Parkinson's disease
    poliomyelitis
    prostate cancer
    severe pelvic injury
    single gene neurological
      disease
    spina bifida
    spinal cord injury; or

(e) a man who is receiving treatment for renal failure by dialysis; or

(f) a man who has had the following surgery -
    prostatectomy
    radical pelvic surgery
    renal failure treated by
      transplant.

Treatment of erectile dysfunction - cont.

(c) OJ No.L257, 19.10.68, p.22 (OJ/SE 1968(II) p.475)

Criteria notified to the European Commission under Article 7 of the Council Directive relating to the transparency of measures regulating the pricing of medicinal products for human use and their inclusion in the scope of national heatlh insurance schemes (89/105/EEC)

The following six criteria have been separately notified by the UK Government to the European Commission since 1989 to comply with Article 7 of the Transparency Directive.

First, under the Selected List Scheme, medicinal products in seventeen therapeutic categories which are excluded from prescription on the grounds that, on expert advice, they had no clinical or therapeutic advantage over other, cheaper, drugs in the following categories:-

mild to moderate painkillers
indigestion remedies
laxatives
cough and cold remedies
vitamins
tonics
benzodiazepine sedatives and tranquillisers
anti-diarrhoeal drugs
drugs for allergic disorders
hypnotics and anxiolytics
appetite suppressants
drugs for vaginal and vulval conditions
contraceptives
drugs used in anaemia
topical anti-rheumatics
drugs acting on the ear and nose
drugs acting on the skin

Second, products may be considered as "borderline substances" which are not truly medicinal products with clinical or therapeutic value and are excluded from NHS prescription on that ground.

Third, as well as being freely available on sale over the counter to the general public the cost to the NHS if the product(s) were to be supplied on prescription could not be justified at any price likely to be economic to the manufacturer and that the supply of the product is not considered a priority for the use of the limited resources available to the NHS.

Fourth, that products which nonetheless may meet a legitimate clinical or therapeutic need when properly prescribed, are subject to misuse by drug misusers, and such misuse, or the manner in which the product is administered by drug misusers, gives rise to the risk of physical or mental morbidity and alternative products are available to meet all legitimate clinical or therapeutic needs.

Fifth, a medicinal product or a category of medicinal products may be excluded entirely from supply on NHS prescription. It may alternatively be excluded except in specified circumstances, or except in relation to specified conditions or categories of condition, or specified categories of patient. A medicinal product or a category of them may be so excluded where the forecast aggregate cost to the NHS of allowing the product (or category of products) to be supplied on NHS prescription, or to be supplied more widely than the permitted exceptions, could not be justified having regard to all the relevant circumstances including in particular: the Secretary of State's duties pursuant to the NHS Act 1977 and the priorities for expenditure of NHS resources.

Sixth, products which comprise an injection device prefilled with a drug may be excluded from supply on NHS prescription if the same drug is available and can be used more economically in a container which may be used in conjunction with a refillable injection device.

This Page Is Intentionally Blank

Page   Page

A

AAA-Flex 102
Above-Knee Stockings Elastic 137
 Dispensing Fee, Appliance
  Contractors 29
 Prescription Charge 483
 Professional Fee, Pharmacy
  Contractors 15-18
Absorbent Cellulose
 Dressing with Fluid Repellent Backing 120
Absorbent Cottons 97,499
Absorbent Dressing (Perforated) 120
Absorbent Gauze 140, 499
 Ribbon 140, 499
 Tissue 142
Absorbent Lint 148, 499
Absorbent, Perforated Dressing
 with Adhesive Border 121
Absorbent Perforated Plastic Film
 Faced, Dressing 120, 499
Acacia Powder 45
Acarbose Tablets 45
Acebutolol
 Capsules 45
 Tablets 45
Aceclofenac Tablets 45
Acemetacin Capsules 45
Acetazolamide
 Capsules 45
 Tablets 45
Acetest Tablets 383
Acetic Acid 45
Acetone 45
Acetylcysteine Granules 531
Acetylsalic Acid 48
 Mixture 45
 Tablets 48
Aciclovir (Acyclovir)
 Cream 45, 495
 Eye Ointment 45
 Oral Suspension 45, 495
 Tablets 45, 495
 Tablets Dispersible 45
Acids (See Under Separate Names)
Acriflavine Emulsion 45
Acrivastine Capsules 45
Actiban Bandage 104
Actico (Cohesive) Bandage 104
Actisorb Silver 220 126
Activated Charcoal Dressing 126
Activated Dimethicone & Hydrotalcite
 Suspension 59
 Tablets 59
Additional Pharmacist Access Services 413
Additional Professional Fees,
 Pharmacy Contractors 15-18
Adhesive Bandages Elastic 100
Adhesive Elastic Wound Dressing 120
Adhesive Felt 116
Adhesive Latex Foam 148
Adhesive Tapes 158-159

Adhesives
 Incontinence 167
 Stoma 223
Advice to Care Homes 421
Adrenaline Injection 45
Adrenaline Tartrate Injection 45
Aerosol Inhalations (See Under
 Separate Names)
 Chamber Devices 98
Albufilm Surgical Tape 159
Albupore Surgical Tape 159
Albustix 384
Alcoderm
 Cream 497
 Lotion 497
Alcohol 45, 63
 Customs & Excise Duty
  Rebate, Unclaimed 43
 Supply Or Use of Industrial
  Methylated Spirit 43
Alendronic Acid Tablets 45
Alfacalcidol Capsules 45
Alfuzosin Hydrochloride Tablets 46
Alginate Dressings 126
 Algisite M 126
 Algosteril 126
 Comfeel Seasorb 126
 Kaltogel 126
 Kaltostat 126
 Melgisorb 126
 Sorbsan 126
 Tegagen 126
 Algisite M 126
 Algisite M-Rope 127
 Algosteril 126
 Algosteril Rope 127
Alkaline Eye Drops 69
Alkaline Ipecacuanha Mixture 46
Allevyn 133
 Allevyn Adhesive 132
 Allevyn Cavity 127
 Allevyn LM 133
Allopurinol Tablets 46
Almond Oil 46
 Ear Drops 497
Alpha Keri Bath Oil 497
Alprostadil Injection 46
Alum Granules 46
Aluminium Hydroxide
 and Magnesium Trisilicate Tablets 74
Aluminium Potassium Sulphate 46
Alverine Citrate Capsules 46
Amantadine
 Capsules 46
 Oral Solution 46
Amaranth Solution 46
Amiloride and Frusemide Tablets 56
Amiloride and Hydrochlorthiazide
 Tablets 56
Amiloride Tablets 46
Aminoglutethimide Tablets 46

INDEX

Aminophylline
  Injection   46
Amiodarone Tablets   46
Amitriptyline Tablets   46
Amitriptyline Hydrochloride
  Capsules   46
  Oral Solution   46
Amlodipine Besylate Tablets   46
Ammonia Aromatic Solution   46
Ammonia and Ipecacuanha
  Mixture   46
  Oral Solution   46
Ammonia Solution, Strong   383
Ammonium Acetate Solution, Strong   46
Ammonium Bicarbonate   46
Ammonium Chloride   46
  Mixture   47
  Oral Solution   47
Ammonium Ichthosulphonate   69
Amorolfine
  Cream   47
  Nail Laquer   47
Amoxycillin
  Capsules   47, 495
  Injection   47
  Mixture/Syrup   47, 495
  Mixture/Syrup (Paediatric)   47, 495
  Oral Powder   47, 495
  Oral Suspension   47, 495
  Oral Suspension (Paediatric)   47, 495
  Sachets   47
Amoxycillin and Potassium Clavulanate
  Injection
  Suspension
  Tablets
  Tablets Disp
  See:- Co-amoxiclav
Amphotericin
  Lozenges   47, 495
  Oral Suspension   47, 495
  Tablets   47
Ampicillin
  Capsules   47, 495
  Mixture   47, 495
  Oral Suspension   47, 495
  Syrup   47, 495
Anal Plugs   167
Analysis Set, Urine Sugar   166
Anastrozole Tablets   47
Anhydrous Lanoline   91
Animal Wool (Chiropody)   116
Anionic Emulsifying Wax   63
Anise
  Oil   47
  Water, Concentrated   47
Aniseed Oil   47
Anklets, Elastic   139
  Dispensing Fee, Appliance Contractors   29
  Prescription Charge   483
  Professional Fee, Pharmacy
    Contractors   16
Antitoxins (See Under Separate Names)

Anusol Suppositories   41
Apothecaries System - Requirement
  To Convert to Metric System   8
Appliance Contractors - Provision
  For Payments for Prescriptions
  Dispensed Each Month   6
Appliances
  Approved List - Notes   93
  Approved List   97-166
  Bandages, Interpretation   99
  Chiropody   116
  Definition   93
  Dispensing Fees, Appliance Contractors   29
  Incontinence Appliances   167
  Invoice Price - Definition   93
  Limitation on Supply   3
  Meaning of Basic Price   7
  Out of Pocket Expenses   9
  Prescription Charges   483-493
  Professional Fees - Pharmacy
    Contractors   15-18
  Provision for Determination
    Of Basic Price   7
  Sealed Packets, Quantity to Supply   93
  Stoma Appliances   223
  Technical Specifications   93
    List of   95-96
  Weights-Net   93
Applications (See Under Separate Names)
Applicator, Vaginal   97
Aquacel   130
Aquacel Ribbon   127
Aquaform Hydrogel   131
Aqueous Cream   47, 497
Arachis Oil   48, 497
Arachis Oil Enema   48, 497
Arch Support   117
Arm Sleeve, Polythene,
  Disposable   151
Arm Sling   97, 499
Artificial
  Saliva   495
  Tears   69
Ascorbic Acid   48
  Tablets   48, 495
Askina
  Biofilm   129
  Derm   123
  Jet Saline   147
  Spray   147
  Transorbent   133
Aspirin   48
Aspirin Tablets   48
  Dispersible   48, 495, 497
  With Codeine, Dispersible   58
Aspirin Soluble Tablets
  See:- Aspirin Dispersible.
Atenolol
  Oral Solution   48
  Tablets   48
Atenolol and Chlorthalidone Tablets   59
Atomizers   98

Page   Page

Atorvastatin Tablets	48	Belts		
Atropine		Incontinence	167	
Eye Drops	48	Stoma	223	
Eye Ointment	48	Suprapubic	155	
Injection	48	Suspender	136-138	
Tablets	48	Benadryl Allergy Relief Capsules	41	
Auranofin Tablets	48	Bendrofluazide Tablets	49	
Autopen	145	Benorylate		
Azapropazone		Mixture	49	
Capsules	48	Oral Suspension	49	
Tablets	48	Tablets	49	
Azathioprine Tablets	41, 48	Benserazide Hydrochloride		
Azelastine Hydrochloride Nasal Spray	48	And Levodopa		
Azithromycin		Capsules		
Capsules	48	Tablets, Dispersible		
Oral Suspension	48	See :- Co-beneldopa		
Tablets	48	Benzhexol Tablets	49	
		Benzoic Acid Ointment, Compound	49	
B		Benzoin		
		Tincture	49	
Baclofen		Tincture, Compound	49	
Oral Solution	49	Benztropine Tablets	49	
Tablets	49	Benzydamine Hydrochloride		
Bactigras - See:- Chlorhexidine Gauze Dressing		Cream	49	
Bags		Mouthwash	49, 495	
Closing Clip (Stoma)	223	Oral Spray	49, 495	
Covers (Stoma)	223	Benzyl Benzoate	49	
Drainage	167	Application	49	
Foot	153	Benzylpenicillin Injection	49	
Leg (Portable Urinal)	167	Betahistine Dihydrochloride Tablets	41, 50	
Night Drainable	167	Betamethasone Eye Drops	50	
Plastics (Stoma) Drainable	223	Betamethasone Sodium Phosphate		
Plastics (Stoma) Disposable	223	Ear Drops	50	
Rubber (Stoma)	223	Nasal Drops	50	
Balneum	497	Betamethasone Valerate		
Bambuterol Hydrochloride Tablets	49	Cream/Ointment	50	
Bandaging - Multi-Layer	102	Scalp Application	50	
Bandages	99-104	Betaxolol Hydrochloride		
Basic Price	10	Eye Drops	50	
Meaning for Approved Appliances	3, 91	Bezafibrate Tablets	50	
Meaning for Chemical Reagents	3	Biatain	132, 133	
Bath Eye	139	Bicalutamide Tablets	50	
BD Ultra Pen	145	Biloptin Capsules	383	
Beclomethasone		Bioclusive Dressing	124	
Nasal Spray	49	Biosensor Strips	387-388	
Pressurised Inhalations	49	Bisacodyl		
Beclomethasone Dipropionate		Suppositories	50, 497	
Dry Powder Capsules for Inhalation	49	Tablets	50, 497	
Becotide Rotahaler	147	Bisgaard Leg Bandage See:-		
Beeswax	49	Elastic Web with Foot Loop Bandages		
Belladonna		Bismuth Carbonate	50	
Plaster	153	Bismuth Subcarbonate	50	
Tincture	49	Bisoprolol Fumarate Tablets	50	
Below-Knee Stockings Elastic	136-138	Black Currant Syrup	50	
Dispensing Fee, Appliance Contractors	29	"Black List"	501-530	
Prescription Charge	483	Bladder/Irrigating Syringe	160	
Professional Fee, Pharmacy Contractors	18	Blenderm Surgical Tape	156	
		Blood Glucose Strips	385-389	
		Appendix	391	

INDEX

Page | Page

Blue Line Bandages 102
Bm-Accutest Strips 388
Bm-Test 385
Boil Dressing Pack 121
Borderline Substances
  List A 426
  List B 451
  List C 480
Boric Acid 50
  Lint 148
Breast Reliever 106
Breast Shields 106
Broken Bulk - Provisions For Payment 9
Bromocriptine
  Capsules 50
  Tablets 50
Brompheniramine Maleate
  Elixir 50
  Tablets 50
Brompheniramine Tablets 50
Brovon Midget Inhaler 98
Brufen Tablets 41
Brushes
  Iodine 106
  Tracheostomy 163
Buchanan
  Deltanex Protector 164
  Larynectomy Protector 164
Budesonide
  Dry Powder Inhaler 50
  Nasal Spray 50
Buffered Cream 51
Bulk Prescriptions -
  Additional Professional Fees -
  Pharmacy Contractors 16
  Definition 44
  Exemption From Container
  Allowance Payment 31
  Exemption From Prescription Charges 484
Bumetanide
  Oral Solution 51
  Tablets 51
Bumetanide and Amiloride
  Hydrochloride Tablets 51
Bumetanide and Slow Potassium Tablets 51
Bunion Rings 116
Buprenorphine Tablets 51
Buspirone Hydrochloride Tablets 51

C

Cabergoline Tablets 51
Cade Oil 51
Cadexomer-Iodine
  Ointment 497
  Paste 497
  Powder 497
Calaband 105

Calamine 51
  Aqueous Cream 51, 497
  Compound Application 51
  Lotion 51, 497
  Lotion Oily 51, 497
Calciferol
  Injection 51
  Tablets 51
Calcipotriol
  Cream 51
  Ointment 51
  Scalp Solution 51
Calcium Carbonate 51
  Mixture, Compound Paediatric 51
  Tablets Chewable 52
Calcium Gluconate
  Tablets Effervescent 52
Calcium Lactate Tablets 52
Calcium Sulphate
  Dried 52
  Exsiccated 52
Calcium and Ergocalciferol
  Tablets 51
Calcium with Vitamin D Tablets 51
Calendar Packs 11
Calico Bandage Triangular 104
Camel Hair Brush 105
Camphor 52
  Water, Concentrated 52
Camphorated-Opium Tincture 52
Capoten Tablets 41
Capsicum
  Ointment 52
  Tincture 52
Capsules *(See Under Separate Names)*
Captopril Tablets 52
Carbamazepine
  Liquid 52
  Tablets 51, 495
Carbaryl
  Lotion Alcoholic 52
  Lotion Aqueous 52
Carbidopa and Levodopa Tablets
  See :- *Co-careldopa Tablets*
Carbimazole Tablets 52
Carbocisteine 531
  Capsules 52
  Syrup 52
Carboflex 125
Carbopad VC 125
Cardamom Tinctures
  Aromatic 53
  Compound 53
Care Homes, Advice to 421
Carmellose Gelatin Paste 53, 495
Carteolol Eye Drops 53
Castor Oil 53
Categories 43
Catgut Sutures 160

Page   Page

Catheters
  Accessories   106
  External   172
  Maintenance Solutions   106, 497
  Suprapubic   158
  Urethral   107-115, 499
  Valves   167
Catheter Maintenance Solution
  Chlorhexidine   497
  Mandelic Acid   497
  Sodium Chloride   497
  Solution 'G'   497
  Solution 'R'   497
Caustic Pencil   53
Cavi-Care   127
Cavity Dressing   127, 499
Cefaclor
  Capsules   53
  Suspension   53
  Tablets   53
Cefadroxil
  Capsules   53
  Suspension   53
Cefixime
  Oral Suspension   53
  Tablets   53
Cefpodoxime Proxetil Tablets   53
Cefuroxime Axetil Tablets   53
Celiprolol Hydrochloride Tablets   53
Cellona   103, 104
Cellulose
  Wadding   116, 499
Cephalexin
  Capsules   53, 495
  Mixture   53, 495
  Oral Suspension   53, 495
  Tablets   53, 495
Cephradine
  Capsules   53, 495
  Oral Solution   53, 495
Ceporex
  Capsules   41
  Tablets   41
Cetirizine Dihydrochloride Tablets   53
Cetomacrogol Cream   53
Chalk Powder   54
Charcoal Dressing   125
Chemical Reagents (See Also
  Under Separate Names)
  Approved List   383-389
  Limitation on Supply   3
Chiropody Appliances   116
Chloral
  Mixture   54
  Oral Solution   54
  Syrup   54
Chloral Betaine Tablets   54
Chloral Hydrate   54
  Mixture   54

Chloramphenicol
  Capsules   54
  Ear Drops   54
  Eye Drops   54
  Eye Oint   54
Chlordiazepoxide Capsules   54
Chlordiazepoxide Hydrochloride
  Tablets   54
Chlorhexidine
  Dental Gel   53, 495
  Gauze Dressing   140
  Gluconate Gel   54, 495
Chlorhexidine
  Gluconate Mouthwash   54, 495
  Gluconate Oral Spray   54, 495
  Mouthwash   54, 495
  Oral Spray   495
Chlormethiazole
  Capsules   54
  Oral Solution   54
Chlorodyne   54
Chloroform
  Spirit   54
  Water, Concentrated   54
  And Morphine Tincture   54
Chloroquine Phosphate Tablets   54
Chloroquine Sulphate Tablets   54
Chlorpheniramine
  Elixir   54
  Oral Solution   54
  Tablets   54, 495
Chlorpromazine
  Elixir   54
  Oral Solution   54
  Tablets   54
Chlorthalidone Tablets   54
Cholecystographic Examination   383
Cholestyramine Powders   54
Choline Salicylate Dental Gel   55, 495
Choline Salicylate Dental Paste
  See:- Choline Salicylate Dental Gel
Chromic Catgut Suture   160
Cica-Care   134
Cimetidine
  Oral Solution   55
  Oral Suspension   55
  Tablets   55
Cinnarizine Tablets   55
Ciprofibrate Tablets   55
Ciprofloxacin Tablets   55
Cisapride
  Suspension   55
  Tablets   55
Citalopram Tablets   55
Citric Acid Monohydrate Powder   55
Clarithromycin
  Suspension   55
  Tablets   55
Clemastine
  Oral Solution   55
  Tablets   55
Clement Clarke   149-151

	Page		Page
Clindamycin		Codeine Linctus	58
Capsules	55, 495	Diabetic	58
Lotion	55	Paediatric	58
Oral Suspension Paediatric	55	Codeine Phosphate	58
Topical Solution	55	Oral Solution	58
Clindamycin Phosphate Cream	55	Syrup	58
Clinisorb	125	Tablets	41, 58
Clinistix	384	Codeine Phosphate and Paracetamol	
Clinitest (Set and Spares)	166	See:- Co-codamol	
Tablets	383	Co-dergocrine Tablets	58
Clobazam	531	Co-dydramol Tablets	41, 58
Tablets	55, 531	Co-fluampicil	
Clobetasol		Capsules	59
Cream	56	Syrup	59
Ointment	56	Co-Flumactone Tablets	59
Clobetasone		Cohfast Bandage	102
Cream	56	Colchicine Tablets	59
Ointment	56	Collodions (See Under Separate Names)	
Clomiphene Tablets	56	Colostomy Appliances	223
Clomipramine Capsules	56	Professional Fees, Pharmacy Contractors	16
Clomipramine Hydrochloride		CombiDERM	130
Capsules	56	CombiDERM-N	130
Tablets	56	Comfeel	128
Clonazepam Tablets	56	Comfeel Plus	127, 128
Clonidine Hydrochloride Tablets	56	Comfeel Plus Contour	127
Clonidine Tablets	56	Comfeel Seasorb	126
Clotrimazole		Common Pack List	41-42
Cream	56, 497	Compound Aneurine Tablets	91
Pessaries	56	Compound Magnesium Trisilicate	
Clotrimazole and Hydrochloride		Mixture	73
Cream	56	Tablets Strong	74
Clove Oil	56	Compound Macrogol Oral Powder	497
Coal Tar		Compound Sodium Chloride Mouth-Wash	496
Solution	56	Compound Thiamine Tablets	91
Solution Strong	56	Compound Thymol Glycerin	496
Co-amilofruse Tablets	56	Compression Bandages High	
Co-amilozide Tablets	41, 56	P.e.c.	101
Co-amoxiclav		Peche	101
Suspension	57	Setopress	101
Tablets	57	Surepress	101
Tablets Disp	57	Tensopress	101
Coban Bandage	102	V.e.c	101
Co-beneldopa		Veche	101
Capsules	57	Compression Hosiery - See	
Tablets, Dispersible	57	Elastic Hosiery	136-139
Cocaine Hydrochloride	57	Comprilan Bandage	104
Co-careldopa Tablets	57	Conforming Foam Cavity	
Co-codamol		Wound Dressing	127, 499
Capsules	58	Connector (Suprapubic Glass/Plastics)	155
Tablets	41, 58	Container - Allowance and	
Tablets Effervescent	58	Suitability	5, 31
Co-codaprin Tablets Dispersible	58	Contraceptive Devices	117-119
Coconut Oil	58	Services - Notes on	
Fractionated	58	Prescription Charges	483
Co-danthramer		Controlled Drugs - Additional	
Capsules	58, 497	Professional Fees, Pharmacy	
Capsules Strong	58, 497	Contractors	16
Oral Suspension	58, 497	Co-Plus Bandage	103
Oral Suspension Strong	58, 497	Copper Solution Reagent Tablets	383
Co-danthrusate		Copper Sulphate	59
Capsules	58, 497		
Oral Suspension	58, 497		

Page   Page

Copper Sulphate Pentahydrate   59
Co-prenozide Tablets   59   **D**
Co-proxamol Tablets   59
Corn Plasters   116   Danazol Capsules   60
  Rings   116   Danthron and Docusate Sodium Capsules
Cortisone Tablets   59   *See :- Co-danthrusate*
Co-simalcite Suspension   59   Danthron and Poloxamer
Cosmopor E   121   Suspension
Co-tenidone Tablets   59   Suspension, Strong
Co-triamterzide Tablets   59   *See :- Co-danthramer*
Co-trimoxazole   Dantrolene Sodium Capsules   60
  Mixture   59   Dapsone Tablets   60
Cotton Absorbent   97, 499   Deltacortril Tablets   41
Cotton Bandages   Deduction Scale   33-35
  Conforming   99, 499   Deltanex Protector   164
  Crepe   99, 499   Dental Gel   495
  Elastic, Heavy   99, 499   Dental Practitioners - Approved
  Stretch   99, 499   List of Prescribable Preparations 495-496
  Suspensory   103   Deodorants (Stoma)   223
Cotton Gauze   De-Pezzer Suprapubic Catheter   158
  Absorbent   140, 499   Dermabond   160
  And Viscose   140, 499   Dermalo Bath Emollient   497
Cotton and Gauze Pads *See:-*   Dermamist   496
  Filmated Gauze Swabs   161   Desmopressin
Cotton, Polyamide and Elastane Bandage 99   Intranasal Solution   60
Cotton Stockinette   154   Nasal Spray   60
Cotton Wools   97   Detection Strips   384-389, 499
Counting of Prescriptions for   Detection Tablets   383, 499
  Pricing Purposes - Examples   483-493   Dexamethasone Tablets   41, 60
Cow and Gate Foods *(See Under*   Dexamethasone and Hypromellose
  Separate Names)*   Eye Drops   60
Cream of Magnesia   73   Dexamphetamine Sulphate Tablets   60
Creams *(See Under Separate Names)*   Dexomon SR Tablets   41
Crepe Bandages   99, 499   Dextranomer
Crinx Bandage   99   Beads   497
Criteria notified under the   Paste   497
  Transparency Directive   533   Dextropropoxyphene Capsules   60
Crotamiton Cream   59, 497   Dextropropoxyphene Hydrochloride
Crotamiton Lotion   497   And Paracetamol Tablets
Cutifilm   123   *See :- Co-Proxamol Tablets*
Cutilin Dressing   120   Dextrose Strong Injection   60
Cutinova Cavity   127   Diabur Test 5000   384
Cutinova Foam   128   Diachylon Bandages   100
Cutinova Hydro   128   Diamorphine Hydrochloride Tablets   60
Cyanocobalamin   Diamorphine Injection   60
  Injection   59   Diaphragm
  Tablets   59, 531   Pessary   152
Cyclizine   Vaginal Contraceptive   119
  Injection   59   Diastix   384
  Lactate Injection   59   Diazepam
  Tablets   59   Elixir   495
Cyclopenthiazide Tablets   59   Oral Solution   495
Cyclopenthiazide and Amiloride   Solution Rectal Tube   61
  Hydrochloride Tablets   59   Syrup   61
Cyclopentolate Eye Drops   60   Tablets   61, 495
Cyclophosphamide Tablets   60   Diclofenac Diethylammonium Salt Gel 61
Cyclosporin Capsules   60   Diclofenac Sodium
Cyclosporin Oral Solution   60   Capsules   61
Cyproterone Acetate Tablets   60   Suppositories   61
                                             Suppositories Paediatric   61
                                             Tablets   41, 61
                                             Tablets Dispersible   61
                                           Diclofenac and Misoprostol Tablets 61

INDEX

Page | Page

Dicyclomine		Domperidone	
Elixir	61	Suppositories	62
Oral Solution	61	Suspension	62
Solution Rectal Tube	61	Tablets	62
Syrup	61	Dorzolamide Ophthalmic Solution	62
Tablets	61	Dothiepin	
Dienoestrol Cream	61	Capsules	62
Diethylamine Salicylate Cream	61	Tablets	62
Diflunisal Tablets	61, 495	Douches	
Digitoxin Tablets	61	Plastics	119
Digoxin		Professional Fees, Pharmacy	
Elixir Paediatric	61	Contractors	15
Oral Solution	61	Spare Plastics Tubing	119
Tablets	61	Dowse's Suprapubic Catheter	158
Dihydrocodeine		Doxazosin Tablets	62
Elixir	61	Doxepin Capsules	62
Injection	61	Doxycycline Capsules	62, 495
Oral Solution	61	Drainable Bags	
Tablets	41, 61, 495	Plastics (Incontinence)	167
Dihydrocodeine Tartrate Tablets	61	Plastics (Stoma)	225
Dihydrocodeine and Paracetamol Tablets	58	Drainable Dribbling Appliances	167
Dilators, Rectal	154	Drainage Bags	
Dill Water Concentrated	62	Night (Incontinence)	167
Diltiazem Hydrochloride		Plastics, Suprapubic Belt	157
Capsules	62	Urinal, Portable	167
Tablets	62	Dressings	120-132
Dimethicone Cream	62, 497	Boil	121
Dipivefrine Hydrochloride Eye Drops	62	Gauze (Impregnated)	141-142
Diprobase		Knitted Viscose	121
Cream	497	Multiple Packs	122
Ointment	497	Perforated Film Absorbent Sterile	122
Diprobath	497	Povidone Iodine Fabric	122
Dipyridamole Tablets	41, 62	Standard	122
Disc (Stoma)	223	Sterile Pack	123
Discount		With Non-Woven Pads	123
Provision	5	Vapour-Permeable Adhesive Film	124
Scale Pharmacy Contractors	33-37	Vapour-Permeable Waterproof	
Disodium Etidronate Tablets	62	Plastic Wound	124
Disopyramide		Wound Management Dressings	124-132
Capsules	62	Absorbent Cellulose	120
Tablets	62	Alginate	125
Dispensing Fees - Appliance Contractors	29	Cavity	127
Provision for Payment	6	Hydrocolloid	127, 128
Scale of Fees	29	Hydrocolloid Thin	129
Dispos-A-Gloves	153	Hydrogel	130
Disposable Bags		Polyurethane Foam	130
Incontinence, Plastics	167	Polyurethane Foam Film	130
Stoma, Plastics	225	Soft Silicone	132
Disposable Protectives	153	Dribbling Appliances	167
Disulfiram Tablets	62	Droperidol Tablets	62
Dithranol	62	Droppers Glass	
Diumide-K Tablets	41	For Eye, Ear and Nasal Drops	31, 135
Capsules	62, 497	Drugs - Categories	43
Enema	497	Prescription Charges	483
Docusate		Dumas Cap	118
Enema, Compound	497	Duoderm	129
Oral Solution	62, 497	Durex Vaginal Applicator	97
Oral Solution, Paediatric	62, 497	Dusting Powders (*See Under Separate Names*)	
		Dydrogesterone Tablets	62

Page | | Page

E

E45 Cream	497
Ear Drops *(See Under Separate Names)*	
Ear Syringe	162
Easifix Bandage	103
easiGRIP	155
Econazole Cream	497
Eesiban Ribbed Stockinette	157
Elantan Tablets	41
Elastic Adhesive Tape	158
Elasticated Stockinette	154-157
Cotton and Viscose	157
Foam Padded	155
Net	155
Tubular	155-157
Viscose	156
Elastic Bandages	
Adhesive	100, 499
Diachylon	100
Heavy Cotton and Rubber	100
Web, Without Foot Loop	100, 499
Web, Blue Line	100, 499
Web, with Foot Loop	100, 499
Elastic Band Trusses	163
Dispensing Fees, Appliance Contractors	29
Professional Fees, Pharmacy Contractors	15
Elastic Hosiery	134-137
Circular Knit	134-137
Descriptions and Diagrams	134-137
Dispensing Fees, Appliance Contractors	29
Flatbed Knit	136-137
Lightweight Elastic Net	136
One Way Stretch	136-137
Nurse Prescribable	497
Prescription Charge	483-493
Elastomer and Viscose Bandage Knitted	100
Elastoplast Airstrip Wound Dressing	125
Elastoweb *(See Heavy Cotton and Rubber Elastic Bandage)*	
Elixirs *(See Under Separate Names)*	
Elset	100, 102
Elset S	100
Ema Film Gloves	153
Emollients *(See Under Separate Names)*	
Emulsifying Ointment	63, 497
Emulsifying Wax	63
Emulsions *(See Under Separate Names)*	
Endorsement Requirements	7
Enalapril Maleate Tablets	63
Enemas *(See Under Separate Names)*	
Enema Syringe (Higginson's)	162
Enprin Tablets	41
Epaderm	497
Ephedrine	
Elixir	63
Nasal Drops	63, 495
Oral Solution	63

Ephedrine Hydrochloride Tablets	63
EpiVIEW	124
Epsom Salts	73
Dried	73
Erythrocin 250 Tablets	41
Erythromycin	
Capsules	63
Tablets	63, 495
Topical Solution	63
Erythromycin Ethyl Succinate	
Oral Suspension	63, 495
Oral Suspension, Paediatric	63, 495
Tablets	63, 495
Erythromycin Stearate Tablets	63, 495
Erythromycin and Zinc	
Acetate Lotion	63
Essential Small Pharmacies Scheme	417-419
Ests	155
Estropipate Tablets	63
Ethamsylate Tablets	63
Ethanol	63
Customs & Excise Duty Rebate	43
Supply Or Use of Industrial Methylated Spirit	43
Ethanolamine Oleate Injection	63
Ether Solvent	63
Ethinyloestradiol Tablets	63
Ethosuximide	
Capsules	63
Elixir	63
Oral Solution	63
Eucalyptus Oil	63
Exactech Strips	387
Exemptions From Prescription Charges	484
Extemporaneously Prepared Preparations Professional Fees	15
Extracts *(See Under Separate Names)*	
Eye Bath	140
Eye Drop Dispensers	140
Eye Drops *(See Under Separate Names)*	
Eye Lotions *(See Under Separate Names)*	
Eye Ointments *(See Under Separate Names)*	
Eye Pad with Bandage	122
Eye Shade	140

F

Faecal Collectors (Incontinence)	167
Famciclovir Tablets	64
Famotidine Tablets	64
Fees for Prescriptions Dispensed -	
Provision for Payment	5
Appliance Contractors	6, 29
Examples of	487-493
Pharmacy Contractors	5, 15-18

Page

Page

Felbinac
  Foam Aerosol 64
  Gel 64
Felodipine Tablets 64
Felt, Adhesive 116
Felt Wool, Surgical 117
Fenbufen
  Capsules 64
  Tablets 64
Fenofibrate Capsules 64
Fenoterol Hydrobromide
  Aerosol Inhalation 64
Fenoterol Hydrobromide and
  Ipratropium Bromide Aerosol Inhalation 64
Fermathron 160
Ferraris 149-151
Ferric Chloride Solution 64, 383
Ferrous Fumerate
  Oral Solution 64
  Tablets 64
Ferrous Gluconate Tablets 64
Ferrous Sulphate Tablets 64
Fertility Thermometer 117, 499
Filmated Swabs
  Gauze 161
  Non-Woven Fabric 161
Finger Cots 140
Finger Stalls 140
Fisonair - See:- Aerosol Inhalation
  Chamber Devices 98
Fixing Strips (Incontinence) 167
Flange (Stoma) 223
Flaps (Suprapubic Belt) Rubber 157
Flavine Cream 82
Flavoxate Tablets 64
Flecainide Acetate Tablets 64
Flexi T-300 117
Flexi-Ban Bandage 104
Flexible Collodion 64
Flexipore 133
Flucloxacillin
  Capsules 64
  Elixir 64
  Mixture 64
  Oral Solution 64
  Oral Suspension 64
  Syrup 64
Flucloxacillin Magnesium &
  Ampicillin - See Co-fluampicil
Flucloxacillin Sodium &
  Ampicillin - See Co-fluampicil
Fluconazole
  Capsules 65, 495
  Oral Suspension 65, 495
Fludrocortisone Tablets 65
Fluid Ring Pessary 152
Flunisolide Nasal Spray 65
Fluoxetine Liquid 65
Fluoxetine Hydrochloride Capsules 65
Flupenthixol Tablets 65
Flurbiprofen
  Capsules 65
  Tablets 65

Flutamide Tablets 65
Fluticasone Propionate
  Aerosol Inhalation 65
  Aqueous Nasal Spray 65
  Cream 65
Fluvastatin Capsules 65
Fluvoxamine Maleate Tablets 65
Folic Acid
  Oral Solution 497
  Syrup 65
  Tablets 65, 497
Foot Bag, Polythene, Disposables 153
Formaldehyde
  Solution 65
Formalin 65
Fosinopril Sodium Tablets 65
Framycetin Sulphate Gauze Dressing 141
Fraudulent Prescription Forms
  Reward Scheme 427-428
Friars Balsam 49
Frusemide Tablets 41, 65
Fucidin Intertulle Dressing 142
Fusidic Acid
  Cream 66
  Gel 66
  Viscose Eye Drops 66
Fusidic Acid and
  Betamethasone Valerate Cream 66
  Hydrocortisone Cream 66
Fybogel Orange Sachets 41

G

Ga 386
Gabapentin Capsules 66
Galpseud
  Linctus 41
  Tablets 41
Gargles (See Under Separate Names)
Gauzes 138
Gauze Dressings (Impregnated) 141-142
  Chlorhexidine 141
  Framycetin 141
  Paraffin 141, 499
  Povidone Iodine Fabric 142, 499
  Sodium Fusidate 142
Gauze Pads 161
Gauze Swab
  Filmated 161
  Non-Sterile 161
  Sterile 161
Gauze Tissue 142
Gauze Tissues 142
  Cotton 142, 499
Gaviscon Liquid 41
Gels (See Under Separate Names)
Gemfibrozil
  Capsules 66
  Tablets 66

Page | Page

H

Gentamicin Ear/Eye Drops 66
Gentamicin and Hydrocortisone
  Acetate Ear Drops 66
Gentian
  Acid Mixture 66
  Acid Oral Solution 66
  Alkaline Mixture 66
  Alkaline Oral Solution 66
  Alkaline with Phenobarbitone Mixture 66
Gentian Compound Infusion (Concentrated) 66
Gerhardt's Reagent 383
Ginger
  Essence 66
  Syrup 66
  Tincture Strong 66
Glass Droppers 31
Glibenclamide Tablets 41, 66
Gliclazide Tablets 66
Glipizide Tablets 66
Gloves
  E.m.a. Disposable 153, 499
  Polythene, Disposables 153
GlucoMen Sensors 387
Glucose for Oral Use 66
Glucose Intravenous Infusion 66
Glucose Liquid 66
Glucostix 385
Glucotide 389
Glucotrend 389
Glucotrend Plus 389
Glucometer Esprit 388
Glucose VT 386
Glycerin 66
  Suppositories 67
Glycerins (See Under Separate Names)
Glycerol 66
Glycerol Suppositories 67, 497
Glyceryl Trinitrate
  Spray 67
  Tablets 67
Glycosuria Detection Strips 384
Glycosuria Detection Tablets 383
Goserelin Implant 67
Grade of Drug Or Preparation
  General Requirements 3
Graduated Compression Hosiery
  See Elastic Hosiery 136-139
Granuflex 127, 128
Granugel Hydrocolloid Gel 131
Granules (See Under Separate Names)
Griseofulvin Tablets 67
Ground Nut Oil 48
GyneFix IN 117
GyneFix PT 117
Gyne-T380S 117
Gypsona Bandage 103

Halibut-Liver Oil Capsules 67
Haloperidol
  Capsules 67
  Oral Drops 67
  Oral Solution 67
  Solution 67
  Tablets 41, 67
Hamamelis Water 67
Hexopal Tablets 41
Higginson's Enema Syringe 162
High Compression Bandages
  Nurse Prescribable 499
  P.e.c. 101
  Pecche 101
  Setopress 101
  Surepress 101
  Tensopress 101
  V.e.c. 101
  Vecche 101
Hirst Laryngectomy Protector 164
Hodges Pessaries 152
Holders (tapeless)
  Dressing 162
  IV 162
  Tracheostomy Tube 163
Homatropine Eye Drops 67
Hosiery, Elastic 136-139
  Dispensing Fees, Appliance
    Contractors 29
  Prescription Charges 483-493
  Professional Fees, Pharmacy
    Contractors 15
Hospicrepe 233 99
Hospicrepe 239 99, 102, 499
Hospi Four 102
Hospital Cotton Wool 97
Humiderm Cream 497
Hydralazine Tablets 67
Hydrochloric Acid, Dilute 67
Hydrochlorothiazide Tablets 67
Hydrocoll Dressings 127-129
Hydrocolloid Wound Dressing 127-130
  Aquacel 130
  Combiderm 129
  Comfeel 128
  Comfeel Plus 127, 128
  Cutinova Foam 128
  Duoderm 129
  Granuflex 127, 128
  Hydrocoll Basic 128
  Hydrocoll Border (Bevelled Edge) 127
  Hydrocoll Thin Film 129
  Tegasorb 127, 129
Hydrocortisone 68
  Cream 68, 495
  Eye Ointment 68
  Lozenges 495
  Ointment 68
  Tablets 68

Page | Page

Hydrocortisone and Butyrate
Cream 68
Ointment 68
Hydrocortisone and Miconazole
Cream 68, 495
Ointment 68, 495
Hydrocortisone Sodium Succinate
Injection 68
Hydrofilm 124
Hydroflumethiazide and Spironolactone
Tablets See:- Co-flumactone
Hydrogel Wound Dressing 130
Aquaform 130
Granugel 130
IntraSite 130
IntraSite Conformable 130
Novogel 130
Nu-Gel 130
Purilon 130
Sterigel 130
Hydrogen Peroxide
Ear Drops 68
Mouth-Wash 495
Solution 68
Hydromol
Cream 497
Emollient 497
Hydrotalcite Suspension 68
Hydrous Ointment 68, 497
Wool Fat Ointment 68
Hydroxocobalamin Injection 68
Hydroxychloroquine Tablets 68
Hydroxyurea Capsules 68
Hydroxyzine Hydrochloride Tablets 68
Hylan G-F20 162
Hyoscine Injection 68
Hyoscine Butylbromide Tablets 68
Hyoscine Hydrobromide Injection 68
Hyoscyamus Tincture 68
Hypodermic Equipment Non-Sterile
Needles 143
Needle Clipping Device 146, 499
Syringe 143
Insulin 143, 499
Ordinary Purpose 143
Hypodermic Equipment Sterile
Insulin Syringe U100 144, 499
Needles 144, 499
Lancets 145, 499
Hypromellose Eye Drops 69
Hypoguard Supreme Strips
Supreme Strips 386
Supreme Spectrum Strips 386

I

Ibuprofen
Cream 69
Gel 69
Granules Effervescent 69
Oral Suspension 69, 495
Syrup 69
Tablets 69, 495
Ichthammol 69
Glycerin 69
Ointment 69
Ichthopaste 105
Icthaband 105
Ileostomy Appliances 223
Professional Fees, Pharmacy Contractors 16
Imipramine Hydrochloride Syrup 69
Imipramine Tablets 69
Imodium Capsules 42
Imodium Plus Tablets 42
Imperial System - Requirement to
Convert to Metric System 11
Impermeable Plastic Adhesive Tape 158
Plastic Synthetic Adhesive Tape 158
Ims 69
Inadine Dressing 120
Incontinence Appliances
List of Contents 167
Nurse Prescribable 499
Professional-Fee Pharmacy Contractors 16
Urinal, Portable 166
Indapamide Tablets 69
Indermil 160
Indomethacin
Capsules 69
Suppositories 69
Indoramin Tablets 69
Industrial Methylated Spirit 69
Supply Or Use 43
Infusions (See Under Separate Names)
Inhalations (See Under Separate Names)
Inhaler (Spare Top) 146
Injectable Preparations (See Under
Separate Names)
Insufflations (See Under Separate Names)
Insufflators (Plastics for Fine Powders) 147
Insulin Syringe 143
Intal Spinhaler 147
Intersurgical Mask 396-398
Constant Performance 395-396
Illustrations 397
Variable Performance 396
IntraSite Conformable 131
IntraSite Gel 131
Intrauterine Contraceptive Devices 117-118
Introducers (For Self Retaining
Catheters) 158
Iodine 69
Brush 104
Iodine Solutions
Aqueous 69
Aqueous Oral Solution 69
Strong 69

Page

Ipecacuanha
  Alkaline Mixture 46
  And Ammonia Mixture, Paediatric 70
  Mixture Paediatric 70
  Opiate Mixture, Paediatric 70
  Tincture 70
Ipratropium Bromide
  Aerosol Inhalation 70
  Nasal Spray 70
Irriclens 147
Irrigating/Bladder Syringe 162
Irrigation Equipment (Stoma) 223
Irrigation Fluids 147
Irrigation, Sheath, Drain Bag (Stoma) 223
Irrigation, Wash-Out Appliance (Stoma) 223
Isoniazid Tablets 70
Isosorbide Dinitrate Tablets 70
Isosorbide Mononitrate
  Capsules 70
  Tablets 70
Ispaghula Husk
  Granules 70, 497
  Powder 70, 497
Itraconazole Capsules 70
Iucd 117-118

J

Jelonet 141

K

Kaltogel 124
Kaltostat 124
Kaltostat Cavity 126
Kaolin Light 70
Kaolin
  Mixture 70
  Mixture, Paediatric 70
  Oral Suspension 70
  And Morphine
    Mixture 70
    Oral Suspension 70
Kaolin Poultice 70
K-Band 103
Keflex Pulvules 42
  Tablets 42
Keri Therapeutic Lotion 497
Ketoconazole
  Cream 71
  Shampoo 71
Ketonuria Detection Strips 384
Ketonuria Detection Tablets 383
Ketoprofen
  Capsules 71
  Gel 71
Ketostix 384
Ketotifen Elixir 71
Ketur Test Strips 384

Page

K-Flex 102
K-Four 102
Kling Conforming Bandage 99
K-Lite Bandage 100, 102
K-Plus Bandage 100, 102
Knee-Caps, Elastic 137
Dispensing Fees,
  Appliance Contractors 29
  Prescription Charges 483-493
  Professional Fees, Pharmacy
    Contractors 16
Knitted Elastomer and
  Viscose Bandage 100
Knitted Polyamide and 102, 499
  Cellulose Contour Bandage
Knitted Viscose Dressing Sterile 121
Knitted Viscose Primary Dressing 121, 499
Kolanticon Gel 42
K-Soft 102,104

L

Labetalol Hydrochloride Tablets 71
Labetalol Tablets 71
Lacidipine Tablets 71
Lactic Acid 71
Lacticare Lotion 497
Lactitol Oral Powder 71, 497
Lactose 71
Lactose Monohydrate 71
Lactulose
  Powder 497
  Solution 71, 497
Lamotrigine
  Dispersible Tablets 71
  Tablets 71
Lancets 145-146, 497
Lanolin (Hydrous) 91
Lanolin Anhydrous 91
Lansoprazole
  Capsules 71
  Granules 71
  Sachets 71
Laryngectomy Protectors 164
Laryngofoam, Laryngectomy
  Protector 164
Lassar's Paste 92
Lasix Tablets 42
Latanoprost Eye Drops 71
Latex Foam, Adhesive 148
L-Dopa Tablets 72
Leg Bags (Incontinence) 167
Leg Sleeve, Polythene (Disposable) 153
Lemon Spirit 72
Lestreflex, Elastic Bandage 100
Leukopor Surgical Tape 158
Leukosilk Surgical Tape 157
Leukostrip 160
Levobunolol Eye Drops 72

INDEX

Page

Levodopa and Carbidopa Tablets
 See :- Co-careldopa Tablets
Levodopa Tablets 72
Lidocaine/Lignocaine
 Gel 497
 Ointment 497
 and Chlorhexidine Gel 497
Lignocaine
 Gel 72
 Injection 72
 Ointment 72, 495
Lignocaine Hydrochloride
 Gel 72
 Injection 72
Linctuses (See Under Separate Names)
Liniments (See Under Separate Names)
Linseed Oil 72
Lints
 Absorbent 148
 Boric Acid 148
Liothyronine Tablets 72
Lipobase 497
Liquefied Phenol 72
Liquid Paraffin
 Emulsion 72
 Oral Emulsion 72
 and Magnesium Hydroxide
  Emulsion 72
  Oral Emulsion 72
 and Soft White Paraffin 497
Liquorice Liquid Extract 72
Lisinopril Tablets 72
Litepress Bandage 103
Litetex Bandage 100
Litetex Plus Bandage 100,102
Lithium Carbonate Tablets 73
Lodoxamide Eye Drops 73
Lofepramine Tablets 73
Loperamide Hydrochloride
 Capsules 73
 Syrup 73
Loprazolam Tablets 73
Loratadine
 Syrup 73
 Tablets 73
Lorazepam Tablets 73
Lormetazepam Tablets 42, 73
Losartan Potassium Tablets 73
Lotions (See Under Separate Names)
Lozenges (See Under Separate Names)
L-Thyroxine Sodium Tablets 89
L Tri-Iodothyronine Sodium Tablets 72
Lubricating Jelly 148
Lugols Solution 69
Lyofoam 131
Lyofoam C 124
Lyofoam Extra 133
Lyofoam Extra Adhesive 132

Page

M
Magnesium Carbonate, Heavy 73
Magnesium Carbonate, Light 73
Magnesium Carbonate
 Mixture 73
 Aromatic, Mixture 73
 Aromatic Oral Suspension 73
Magnesium Hydroxide
 Mixture 73, 497
 Oral Suspension 73
Magnesium Sulphate 73
 Dried 73
 Injection 73
 Mixture 73
 Oral Suspension 73
 Paste 73, 497
Magnesium Trisilicate 73
 Mixture 73
 Oral Powder 73
 Oral Powder Compound 74
 Oral Suspension 73
 Powder 73
 Powder Compound 74
 And Belladonna Mixture 74
Malathion
 Lotion Alcoholic 74, 497
 Lotion Aqueous 74, 497
 Shampoo 74, 497
Malecots Suprapubic Catheter 158
Masks, Oxygen 395-398
Measuring Spoons 31
Mebendazole
 Oral Suspension 74, 497
 Tablets 74, 497
Mebeverine Tablets 74
Medic-Aid Personal Best 149-151
Medicine Measure Oral 31
Medisense "G2" Strips 387
Medisense Optium Strips 387
Meditest Glucose 384
Medi-Test Glycaemie C 387
Medi-Test Protein 2 384
Medroxyprogesterone Acetate
 Injection 74
 Tablets 74
Mefanamic Acid
 Capsules 74
 Tablets 74
Mefilm Dressing 124
Mefix 158
Megestrol Tablets 74
Melgisorb 126
Melgisorb Cavity 127
Melleril Tablets 42
Melolin Dressing 120
Meloxicam SuppositoriesTablets 74
Menthol And Eucalyptus Inhalation 74, 495
Mepitel 135
Mepilex 135

Page | Page

Mepore Dressing	121
Mepore Ultra	124
Meptazinol Tablets	74
Mesalazine Tablets	74
Mesorb	119
Metalline	161
Metatarsal	
Arch Supports	116
Pads	116
Meter, Peak Flow	149-151
Metformin Tablets	42, 74
Methadone	
Injection	74
Linctus	74
Mixture	75
Oral Solution	75
Tablets	75
Methadone Hydrochloride	75
Methionine Tablets	75
Methocarbamol Tablets	75
Methotrexate Tablets	75
Methylated Spirit - Supply Or Use of	
Industrial Methylated Spirit	43
Methylcellulose '20'	75
Methylcellulose Tablets	75, 497
Methyldopa Tablets	75
Methylphenidate HydrochlorideTablets	75
Methyl Salicylate	75
Liniment	75
Ointment	75
Ointment Strong	75
Metoclopramide Tablets	75
Metolazone Tablets	75
Metoprolol Tartrate Tablets	42, 75
Metric Doses - Measuring Spoon	31
Metronidazole	
Oral Suspensions	75, 495
Tablets	75, 495
Mianserin Tablets	75
Miconazole	
Cream	75, 497
Oral Gel	75, 497
Miconazole Nitrate Cream	75
Micropore Surgical Tape	159
Mini-Wright - See:- Clement Clarke	
Minocin Tablets	42
Minocycline Hydrochloride Capsules	76
Minocycline Tablets	76
Misoprostol Tablets	76
Mixtures (See Under Separate Names)	
Moclobemide Tablets	76
Mometasone Furoate	
Cream	76
Ointment	76
Morison's Paste	73
Morphine and Cocaine Elixir	76
Morphine Hydrochloride	76
Morphine Sulphate	76
Injection	76
Suppositories	76
Tablets	76

Mouth Bath (See Under Separate Names)	
Mouth Wash (See Under Separate Names)	
Mouthwash Solution-Tablets	76, 495, 497
Multi-Layer Compression	
Bandaging	102, 103, 499
Multiload Cu 250	117
Multiload Cu 250 Short	118
Multiload Cu 375	118
Multiple Pack Dressing	122, 499
Multiple Prescription Charges	486
Mupirocin	
Nasal Ointment	76
Ointment	76
Myrrh Tincture	76

N

Na Dressing	122
Na Ultra Dressing	122
Nabumeton	
Oral Suspension	76
Tablets	76
Naftidrofuryl Capsules	76
Naproxen	
Suppositories	76
Tablets	76
Naproxen Sodium Tablets	76
Naratriptan Tablets	76
Nasal Drops (See Under Separate Names)	
Natrilix Tablets	42
Nebuhaler - See:- Aerosol	
Inhalation Chamber Devices	98
Nebulizers	98
Nedocromil Sodium	
Aqueous Eye Drops	76
Needle Clipping Device	146, 500
Needles for Pre-filled and Reusable	
Pen Injectors	145
Needles, Hypodermic	143-145, 499
Nefazodone Hydrochloride Tablets	76
Nefopam Hydrochloride Tablets	76
Neomycin	
Cream	77
Eye Ointment	77
Neomycin Sulphate Eye Ointment	77
Neo-Naze	162
Netelast Tubular Stockinette	156
Neutrogena	
Dermatological Cream	497
Nicardipine Hydrochloride Capsules	77
Nicef Capsules	42
Nicorandil Tablets	77
Nifedipine	
Capsules	42, 77
Tablets	77
Niferex Elixir	531
Night Drainage Bags	167
Nipple Shields	149

Page | Page

Nitrazepam
  Mixture 77
  Oral Suspension 77
  Tablets 77, 495
Nitrofurantoin
  Capsules 77
  Tablets 77
Nitroglycerin Tablets 67
Nitroprusside Reagent Tablets 383
Nizatidine Capsules 77
"No Charge" Items (Prescription
  Charges) 487
Nizoral Cream 531
Non Prescribable Products 500-530
Norethisterone Tablets 77
Norfloxacin Tablets 77
Normasol 147
Normasol Twist 147
Nortriptyline Tablets 77
Nova T 118
Novogel 131
Novonorm Tablets 42
NovoPen 3 Classic, Demi, Fun 145
Nu-Gel Dressing 131
Nurse Prescribable - Approved List
  Of Prescribable Preparations 497-499
Nylon & Viscose Stretch Bandage 103
Nylon Sutures See:- Polyamide Sutures 160
Nystatin
  Cream 77
  Mixture 77, 495
  Ointment 77, 495
  Oral Drops 77
  Oral Suspension 77, 495
  Pastilles 77, 495, 497
  Pessaries 77
  Suspension 77, 495, 497
Nystatin Tablets 77
Nystatin Vaginal Cream 77

O

Occlusives Disposable 153
Oestradiol Implant 78
Oestrogens, Conjugated Tablets 78
Ofloxacin Tablets 78
Oilatum
  Cream 497
  Emollient 497
  Fragrance Free 497
  Gel 497
Oils (See Under Separate Names)
Oily Cream 68
Ointments (See Under Separate Names)
Olanzapine Tablets 78
Oleic Acid 78
Olive Oil 78
  Ear Drops 497
Olsalazine Sodium Capsules 78

Omeprazole Capsules 78
On-Cost - Appliance Contractors 39
One Touch Strips 388
Open-Wove Bandage 103, 498
OptiFlo G 106
OptiFlo R 106
OptiFlo S 106
Opium Tincture 78
OpSite Flexigrid 124
OpSite Plus 124
OpSite Post-Op 124
Opticare 140
Opticare Arthro 5 140
Opticare Arthro 10 140
Oral Contraceptive Drugs 485
  Prescription Charges 485
  Professional Fee 15
Oral Medicine Measure 31
Oral Powders (See Under Separate Names)
Oral Syringe 31
Orange
  Syrup 78
  Tincture 78
Orciprenaline
  Elixir 78
  Oral Solution 78
Ordinary Purpose Syringe 143
Orphenadrine Hydrochloride
  Tablets 78
Ortho-Band Plus 102,104
Ortho Vaginal Applicator 97
Orthovisc 162
Out of Pocket Expenses
  Provision for Payment 9
Oxazepam Tablets 78
Oxerutins Capsules 78
Oxitropium Bromide Inhaler 78
Oxpentifylline Tablets 78
Oxprenolol Tablets 78
Oxprenolol Hcl &
  Cyclopenthiazide Tablets 59
Oxybutynin Hydrochloride
  Oral Solution 78
  Tablets 42, 78
Oxygen
  Concentrator Services -
    Description 406
    Prescribable Equipment 408
    Claims for Payment 408
    List of Suppliers 409-411
    Guidelines for Prescribing 404
    Prescribing Arrangements 407
    Under Use of 407
    Transfer of Patients From
      Cylinders 408
    Withdrawal of Emergency
      Back-Up Supply of Cylinders 408

Page

Oxygen Cylinder Services
  Arrangement of Service 393
  Basic Price of 398
  Equipment 395-396
  Procedure for Loaning of
    Equipment That May Be
    Provided 394-395
  Compensation for Financial
    Loss of 398
  Termination of Continued
    Use of 394
  Guidance on Prescribing 393
  Illustrations 397, 400-403
  Masks 394, 396
  Sets 395
  Specifications 399
  Stands 394
  "Use" 393-406
Oxymel of Squill 87
Oxytetracycline Tablets 495

P

Pack Dressings
  Multiple 122
  Sterile 123
Pads
  Eye, with Bandage 122
  Gauze 161
  Metatarsal 117
Paints (See Under Separate Names)
Pantoprazole Tablets 79
Paracetamol
  Elixir, Paediatric 79
  Oral Solution Paediatric 79
  Oral Suspension 79, 496, 498
  Suppositories 79
  Suppositories Paediatric 79
  Tablets Soluble 79, 497
  Tablets 79, 497
Paracetamol and Metoclopramide
  Hydrochloride Tablets 79
Paraffin
  Gauze Dressings 141-142, 499
  Hard 79
  Liquid 79
  Liquid, Light 79
  Soft White 79, 497
  Soft Yellow 79, 497
Paranet 141
Paratex 102, 122
Paratulle 141
Paregoric 52
Paroxetine Tablets 79
Pastes (See Under Separate Names)
Patient Medication Records 423

Page

Payment for Prescriptions Dispensed 5
Payment for Additional Professional
  Services 37
Provision - Pharmacy Contractors 5
  Appliance Contractors 6
  Oxygen Contractors 398
Scale of Professional Fees
  Pharmacy Contractors 15
Scale of Dispensing Fees
  Appliance Contractors 29
Scale of on-Cost
  Appliance Contractors 39
  Container Allowance - Pharmacy
    Contractors 31
  Rota Service - Pharmacy
    Contractors 413
  Essential Small Pharmacies-
    Pharmacy Contractors 415
Payments - Monthly Provision
  Pharmacy Contractors 5
  Appliance Contractors 6
  Drug Store Contractors 6
Peak Flow Meters 149-151
Peanut Oil 48
P.e.c. High Compression Bandage 101,498
Pecche Bandage 101
Penbritin Capsules 42
Penciclovir Cream 79
Penicillamine Tablets 79
Penicillin-V
Penicillin-Vk) See:-
  Phenoxymethylpenicillin 80, 496
Pentazocine
  Capsules 79
  Injection 79
  Suppositories 79
  Tablets 79
Pentazocine Lactate Injection 79
Peppermint
  Emulsion, Concentrated 79
  Oil 79
  Oil Capsules 79
  Water, Concentrated 79
Pergolide Tablets 80
Perindopril Tert-Butylamine
  Tablets 80
Permeable Adhesive Tape
  Woven 158
  Non-Woven 159
  Aperatured Non-woven 159
Permethrin
  Cream 80, 497
  Cream Rinse 80, 497
Pessaries
  Hodges 150
  Polythene 150
  Pvc 150
  Ring 150, 499
  Rubber Diaphragm 150
  Watch Spring 150

INDEX

Page

Page

Pethidine	
Injection	80
Tablets	80, 496
PFA Dressing	122
Phenelzine Tablets	11, 80
Phenobarbitone	
Elixir	80
Oral Solution	80
Tablets	80
Phenobarbitone Sodium	80
Phenol	
Liquified	72
Crystals	80
Phenothrin Alcoholic Lotion	80
Aqueous Lotion	497
Foam Application	497
Phenoxymethylpenicillin	
Oral Solution	80, 496
Tablets	80, 496
Phenothrin Alcoholic Lotion	497
Phenylephrine Eye Drops	80
Phenytoin	
Capsules	80
Oral Suspension	80
Tablets	80
Pholcodine	
Linctus	80
Linctus Paediatric	80
Linctus Strong	80
Phosphates Enema	80, 497
Phytomenadione	
Injection	80
Tablets	80
Pills (See Under Separate Names)	
Pilocarpine Eye Drops	81
Pilocarpine Hydrochloride Eye Drops	81
Pimozide Tablets	81
Piperazine Citrate Elixir	497
Piperazine and Senna Powder	81, 497
Piroxicam	
Capsules	81
Gel	81
Tablets Dispersible	81
Pizotifen	
Elixir	81
Tablets	81
Place(s) of Business in Respect of Prescription Payments	
Pharmacy Contractors	5
Appliance Contractors	6
Plaster of Paris	52
Bandage	103
Plasters	
Belladonna	151
Corn	116
Salicylic Acid	116
Spool	158-159
Plastics	
Connector (Suprapubic Belt)	157
Tubing for Douches	119
Pocket Riddopag Inhaler	98
Pocket Scan Strips	387
Podophyllin	81
Paint	81
Paint, Compound	81
Podophyllum Resin	81
Polyamide and Cellulose	
Contour Bandage	103, 499
Contour Bandage Knitted	103, 499
Polyamide, Elastane and Cotton Compression Bandage	102
Polyamide Sutures	
Braided	160
Monofilament	160
Polythene	
Finger Stalls	139
Ring Pessary	152
Polythene Occlusives Disposable	
Arm Sleeve	153
Foot Bag	153
Gloves	153
Leg Sleeve	153
Torso Vests	153
Trousers	153
Polyurethane Foam Dressing	131
Lyofoam	131
Polyurethane Foam Film Dressing	132-134
Allevyn	133
Allevyn Adhesive	132
Flexipore	133
Lyofoam Extra	132
Lyofoam Extra Adhesive	132
Spyrosorb	134
Tielle	132
Tielle Lite	132
Tielle Sacrum	132
Portable Urinals	157
Potash Alum	46
Potassium Bromide	81
Mixture	81
Potassium Chlorate	81
Potassium Chloride	81
Potassium Chloride Tablets	
Effervescent	81
Slow	81
Potassium Citrate	81
Mixture	81
Mixture Concentrated	81
Oral Solution	81
And Hyoscyamus Mixture	81
Potassium Effervescent Tablets	81
Potassium Iodide	81
and Ammonia Mixture	81
Mixture Ammoniated	81
Potassium Nitrate	81
Potassium Permanganate	81
Solution	81
Poviderm	122
Povidone - Iodine	
Solution	497
Dry Powder Spray	82
Mouth-Wash	82, 496
Fabric Dressing	119, 498
Powdered Tragacanth	89
Compound	89

Page — Page

Powders (*See Under Separate Names*)
Pravastatin Sodium Tablets — 82
Praxilene Capsules — 42
Prazosin Tablets — 82
Prednisolone Tablets — 82
  Enteric-Coated — 42, 82
  Gastro-Resistant — 42, 82
Prednisolone Acetate Eye Drops — 82
Prednisolone Sodium Phosphate
  Ear Drops — 82
  Eye Drops — 82
  Tablets — 82
Prentif Cap — 116
Preparations - Prescription Charges — 483
Pre-Registration Trainees - Payments — 419
Prescription Charges Arrangements
  Pharmacy Contractors — 483
  Appliance and Drug Store Contractors — 483
  Bulk Prescriptions — 485
  Dispensing Doctors — 483
  Charges Payable — 483
  - Notes on — 486
  Contraceptive Services — 485
  Exemptions — 484
  Number of Charges Applicable — 486
  - General Guidance
  Examples of:
  A Drug in Powder Form
    Together with A Solvent
    In the Same Pack
    (Treatment Packs) — 492
  Combination Packs — 489
  Different Appliances — 490
  Different But Related Preparations — 492
  Drug Ordered with Drug
    Tariff Appliances — 491
  Drugs Packed with Non
    Drug Tariff Appliances — 491
  Eye, Ear and Nasal Drops — 492
  Elastic Hosiery — 491
  Injections - Various Situations
  Liquids - Extempraneously
    Dispensed and Required
    By the Prescriber to Be
    Supplied in More Than
    One Container — 487
  Multiples of Same Appliances
    Of Same Or Differing Size — 490
  Oxygen Cylinder Service — 492
  Preparations Having Various Flavours — 492
  Preparations Supplied As
    Separate Parts for
    Admixing As Required for Use — 492
  Remission — 484
  Set of Appliances Or Dressings — 490
  Sets of Appliances Ordered
    With Extra Parts — 490
  Tablets, Capsules, Etc
  - Different Strengths of
    The Same Drug Ordered As
    Separate Prescriptions At
    The Same Time — 488

Prescription Charges Arrangements - Cont
  - Different Formulations
    Of the Same Drug Ordered
    As Separate Prescriptions — 488
    Combination of Strengths
      Providing Unlisted Strengths — 489
    Trusses — 493
    Vaginal Creams & Applicators — 493
Prescription Forms Submission of — 5, 483
Prepayment Certificates — 484
Pressure Plate (Stoma) — 223
Prices for Drugs, Preparations and
  Approved Appliances
    Provision — 6
    Revision — 7
Primapore Dressing — 121
Primodone Tablets — 82
Probenecid Tablets — 495
Prochlorperazine
  Oral Solution — 82
  Tablets — 82
Prochlorperazine Maleate
  Suppositories — 82
Prochlorperazine Mesylate Granules — 82
Procyclidine Hydrochloride Syrup — 82
Procyclidine Tablets — 82
Professional Fees Pharmacy — 15
Professional Fees for Prescriptions
  Dispensed: Provision for Payment
  - Pharmacy Contractors — 5
  - Oxygen Contractors — 398
  Scale - Pharmacy Contractors — 15-18
  Related to Threshold Quantity — 17
  Examples of — 487-493
Proflavine
  Cream — 42,82
  Emulsion — 82
  Solution — 82
Proflavine Hemisulphate — 82
Profore Bandage — 103
Proguanil Tablets — 83
Promazine Hydrochloride
  Suspension — 83
Promazine Tablets — 83
Promethazine Hydrochloride
  Elixir — 496
  Tablets — 83, 496
Promethazine
  Elixir — 83, 496
  Oral Solution — 83, 496
Propafenone Hydrochloride Tablets — 83
Propranolol Tablets — 83
Proprietary Preparations
  Basic Price Meaning — 6
  Broken Bulk — 9
  Commonly Used Pack Sizes — 41-43
  Out of Pocket Expenses — 9
  Provision for Determination
    Of Basic Price — 6
    Provision for Prices — 6
Propylene Glycol — 83
Propylthiouracil Tablets — 83

Page   Page

Protectives	153	Replicare Ultra		127
Protector, Laryngectomy	147	Residential Homes, Advice to		421
Tracheostomy	163	Reusable Pens		145
Proteinuria Detection Strips	384	Reward Scheme - Fraudulent		
Prothiaden Capsules/Tablets	42	Prescription Forms		425-426
Provera Tablets	42	Ribbed Cotton and Viscose		
Provox Stomafiller	163	Stockinette		157
Pseudoephedrine Hydrochloride		Ribbon Gauze (Absorbent)		139
Elixir	83	Riddell Minor Inhaler		98
Linctus	83	Riddopag Pocket Inhaler		98
Pseudoephedrine Tablets	83	Rifampicin Capsules		84
Purified Talc	83	Ring Pessaries		152
Purified Water	83	Diaphragm		152
Conditions of Payment	44	Fluid		152
Purilon Gel	131	Polythene		152
PVC Ring Pessary	152	Pvc		152
Pyridostigmine Tablets	83	Watch Spring		152
Pyridoxine Tablets	83	Rings		
		Bunion		116
		Corn		117
Q		Risperidone Tablets		84
		Rosidal K Bandage		104
		Rotahaler		146
Quality of Drug Or Preparation		Rota Service		413
General Requirements	3	Rothera's Tablets		383
Quantity to Be Supplied -		Rubber		
Payment Thereof	8	Bags (Stoma)		223
Quinaband	105	Flaps (Suprapubic Belt)		157
Quinapril Tablets	83	Leg Bag (Incontinence)		167
Quinine Acid Sulphate Tablets	83	Shields (Suprapubic Belt)		157
Quinine Bisulphate Tablets	83	Understraps (Suprapubic Belt)		157
Quinine Sulphate Tablets	83	Urethral Catheter	107-115,	499
		Urinal (Suprapubic Belt)		157
		Rybar Standard Inhaler		98
R				
Ramipril Capsules	84	**S**		
Ranitidine				
Effervescent Tablets	84	Saccharin		
Tablets	84	Sodium		84
Oral Solution	84	Soluble		84
Raspberry Syrup	84	Sal Volatile Solution		46
Rat-Tail Syringe *See:- Ear Syringe*	162	Salbutamol		
Rectal Dilators	154	Aerosol Inhalation		84
Rectified Spirit	63, 84	Dry Powder Capsules		84
Customs and Excise Duty		Nebuliser Solution		84
Rebate Unclaimed	43	Pressurised Inhalation		84
Supply Or Use of Industrial		Syrup		84
Methylated Spirit	43	Tablets		84
Red Line Bandage	100	Salicylic Acid		
Rediform	155	Lotion		85
Redoxon Slow Release		Ointment		85
Vit C Capsules	42	And Sulphur Ointment		85
Refined Sugar	87	Plasters		116
Reflexions Flat Spring Diaphragm	119	Salicylic Acid Powder		85
Regal Swabs	161	Saline Irrigation Fluids		147
Release Dressing	120	Saliva Stimulating Tablets		154
Reliever, Breast	104	Salmeterol Aerosol		
Repairs to Trusses		Inhalation		85
Dispensing Fee, Appliance		Scalp Cleansers and Shampoos		
Contractors	29	(*See Under Separate Products*)		
Professional Fee, Pharmacy		Scanpor Surgical Tape		159
Contractors	15-18	Scott Curwen		100

Page

SeaSorb 126
SeaSorb Filler 127
Selegiline Hydrochloride Tablets 85
Senna
  Granules 85, 497
  Oral Solution 85, 497
  Tablets 85, 497
Senna and Ispaghula Granules 497
Senokot Syrup 42
Serotulle See:- Chlorhexidine
  Gauze Dressing 141
Sertraline Tablets 85
Setocrepe 99, 103
Seton Ribbed Stockinette 157
Setopress 101
Setoprime 102, 122
Shade Eye 140
Sheaths (Incontinence) 167
Shields
  Breast 105
  Nipple 147
  Rubber 155
Short Stretch
  Compression Bandage 104
Sigma ETB 155
Silgel 135
Silicone Gel Sheet 134
Silicone Topical Cream 135
Silk Sutures Braided 160
Silver Nitrate, Toughened See:- Caustic Pencil
Simple Eye Oint 85
Simple Linctus 85
  Paediatric 85
Simple Ointment (White) 85
Simulated Leather
  Finger Stalls 140
Simvastatin Tablets 85
Skin Adhesives
  Incontinence 167
  Sterile 160
  Stoma 223
Skin Care Products (See Under
  Separate Names)
Skin Cleansers (See Under Separate Names)
Skin Closure Strips 160, 499
Skin Gel (Stoma) 223
Skin Protectives (Stoma) 223
Skintact Dressing 120
Sleeve
  Arm 153
  Leg 153
Sling, Arm 97
Slinky Bandage 103
Slo-Phyllin Capsules 42
Soap
  Liniment, Methylated 85
  Spirit, Methylated 85
Soda Mint Tablets 85
Sodium Acid Phosphate 86
Sodium Benzoate 85

Page

Sodium Bicarbonate 85
  Capsules 85
  Ear Drops 85, 498
  Injection 85
  Intravenous Infusion 85
  Mixture, Paediatric 85
  Tablets 85
  Tablets, Compound 85
Sodium Chloride 85
  Eye Drops 85
  Injection 85, 86
  Intravenous Infusion 85, 86
  Mixture, Compound 86
  Mouth-Wash, Compound 86, 496
  Solution 86
  Solution Sterile 497
Sodium Citrate 86
  Enema, Compound 497
Sodium Cromoglycate
  Aerosol Inhalation 86
  Aqueous Eye Drops 86
  Aqueous Nasal Spray 86
Sodium Dihydrogen Phosphate
  Dihydrate 86
Sodium Disulphite 86
Sodium Fluoride
  Oral Drops 86, 496
  Paediatric Drops 86
  Tablets 86, 496
Sodium Fusidate
  Gauze Dressing 141
  Ointment 86, 496
Sodium Iopodate Capsules 383
Sodium Ironedetate Elixir 86
Sodium Metabisulphite 86
Sodium Perborate 86
  Mouth-Wash 86, 496
Sodium Phosphates Enema 80
Sodium Picosulphate Elixir 86, 498
Sodium Pyrosulphite 86
Sodium Salicylate 86
Sodium Valproate
  Enteric-Coated Tablets 87
  Oral Solution 87
  Syrup 87
  Tablets 87
Soffban Natural Bandage 103, 104
Soffcrepe Bandage 99, 103
Sofra Tulle 140
Softclix II 146
Softexe 102, 104
Soft Silicone Wound Contact Dressing 135
Sohfast Bandage 102, 104
Solutions (See Under Separate Names)
Solution Tablets (See Under
  Separate Names)
Solvaline N 120
Sorbalgon 126
Sorbalgon T 127
Sorbide Nitrate Tablets 70
Sorbitol Solution 87
Sorbsan 126
Sorbsan Packing 127

	Page
Sorbsan Plus	126
Sorbsan Ribbon	127
Sotalol Tablets	87
Special Container	8
List of	13-14
Specification of Appliances	
General Requirements	3
Spirits (See Under Separate Names)	
Spironolactone Tablets	87
Spool Plasters	158-159
Spoons Measuring	31
Spray (See Under Separate Names)	
Spring Trusses	165
Dispensing Fees, Appliance	
Contractors	29
Spyrosorb	134
Squill Oxymel	87
Squill Tincture	87
SST	154
Standard Dressings	122
Standard Drugs and Preparations	
Basic Price, Meaning	7
Broken Bulk	9
List of Standard Drugs and	
Preparations - Part VIII	43-92
Out of Pocket Expenses	9
Provision for Determination	
Of Basic Price	7
Provision for Prices	7
Revision of Prices	8
Starch Maize (Powder)	87
Stayform Bandage	103
Stearic Acid	87
Sterculia Granules	498
Sterculia and Frangula Granules	498
Sterifix	121
Sterigel	130
Sterile	
Dressing Pack	123, 499
Eye Pad	122
Steripaste Bandage	105
Steripod	147
Steri-Strip	160
Sterile Knitted	
Viscose Dressing	121
Stilboestrol Tablets	87
Stockinettes	154-157, 499
Stockings, Elastic	
Below-Knee	136-139
Thigh	136-139
Dispensing Fees, Appliance	
Contractors	29
Prescription Charges	486
Professional Fees, Pharmacy	
Contractors	16
Stoma Appliances	
List of Contents	223
Nurse Prescribable	499
Stoma Cap	225
Stretch Bandage	
Nylon & Viscose	103
Streptokinase and Streptodornase	
Topical Powder	498

	Page
Stugeron Tablets	42
Sub-compression	
Wadding Bandage	104, 499
Submission of Prescription Forms	
To Processing Divisions	5
Sucralfate Tablets	87
Sucrose	87
Sudafed Elixir	42
Tablets	42
Sulindac Tablets	87
Sulphasalazine Tablets	87
Sulphur	
Precipitated	85
Sublimed	85
Sulphuric Acid Dilute	85
Sulpiride Tablets	85
Sumatriptan Tablets	85
Supartz	162
Suppositories (See Under Separate Names)	
Suprapubic Belts	
Catheters	158
Professional Fees, Pharmacy	
Contractors	16
Replacement Parts for	157
Supreme	386
Surepress Bandage	101, 102, 104
Surgical Adhesive Tapes	158-159, 499
Surgical Spirit	87
Surgical Suture	160
Surgical Tapes	158-159
Suspender Belts	137-138
Suspenders, Mens	137-138
Suspensory Bandages, Cotton	105, 499
Suspensory Systems	167
Sutherland Lubricating Jelly	148
Synovial Fluid	162
Sutures	
Absorbable	160
Non-Absorbable	160
Swabs Gauze	
Non-Woven Fabric, Non Sterile	161, 499
Non-Woven Fabric, Sterile	161, 499
Non-Woven Fabric, Filmated	161, 499
Gauze Non Sterile	161, 499
Sterile	161, 499
Filmated	161, 499
Synvisc	162
Synovial Fluid	162
Syringes	
Bladder/Irrigating	162
Ear	162
Enema (Higginsons)	162
Spare Vaginal Pipes	162
Hypodermic Equipment	
Ordinary Purpose	143
Insulin	143-144, 499
Pre-Set	143
U.100	143, 499
Sterile U100	144, 499
Medicine (Oral)	31

	Page
Syrup	87
Syrup (Unpreserved)	87
Syrups (See Under Separate Names)	
System 4 Bandages	102

T

	Page
Tablets (See Under Separate Names)	
Tacrolimus Capsules	87
Tamoxifen Tablets	87
Tamsulosin Hydrochloride Capsules	87
Tapes	
Surgical Adhesive	158-159
Synthetic Adhesive	158-159
Tartaric Acid	87
Technical Specifications List of	95-96
Tegaderm Dressing	124
Tegagen	125, 127
Tegasorb	128
Tegasorb Thin	130
Temazepam	
Elixir	88, 496
Oral Solution	88, 496
Tablets	88, 496
Tenoxicam Tablets	88
Tensolan K Bandage	104
Tensopress	101, 103
Terbinafine Hydrochloride Cream	88
Terbinafine Tablets	88
Terbutaline Sulphate	
Aerosol Inhalation	88
Powder for Inhalation	88
Terbutaline Tablets	88
Terfenadine	
Suspension	88
Tablets	88
Test Tubes	163
Testosterone Undecanoate	
Capsules	11, 88
Tetrabenazine Tablets	88
Tetracycline	
Capsules	88, 496
Tablets	88, 496
Texband	103
Textube	155
Theophylline	
Capsules	42, 88
Tablets	88
Thermometer, Fertility	117, 499
Thiamine Compound Tablets,	91
Strong	91
Thiamine Tablets	88
Thigh Stockings, Elastic	136-139
Dispensing Fees, Appliance	
Contractors	29
Prescription Charge	483
Professional Fees, Pharmacy	
Contractors	16
Thioridazine	
Oral Solution	88
Oral Suspension	88

	Page
Threshold Quantity	
List of Preparations	18-27
Thymol	88
Compound Glycerin	88, 495, 498
Thyroxine Tablets	89
Tiaprofenic Acid Capsules	89
Tibolone Tablets	89
Tielle	132
Tielle Lite	134
Tielle Plus	134
Tielle Plus Borderless	134
Tielle Sacrum	132
Timolol	
Eye Drops	89
Tablets	89
Timolol Maleate	
Eye Drops	89
Tablets	89
Tinctures (See Under Separate Names)	
Tinidazole Tablets	89
Tioconazole Nail Solution	89
Tissue Gauze	142
Titanium Ointment	498
Tocopheryl Acetate Tablets	89
Tolbutamide Tablets	89
Torso Vest Polythene, Disposable	153
Toughened Silver Nitrate	
See:- Caustic Pencil	
Tracheo Brush	163
Tracheostomy	
Breathing Aids	163
Brushes	163
Dressings	163
Protectors	164
Trachi-Dress Dressings	163
Trachi-Naze Nasal Restoration	163
Tragacanth	
Mucilage	89
Powder	89
Powder, Compound	89
Tramadol Hydrochloride	
Capsules	89
Tablets	89
Trandate Tablets	42
Tranexamic Acid Tablets	89
Transparency Directive	533
Tranylcypromine Tablets	89
Trazodone Hydrochloride	
Capsules	89
Tablets	89
Triamcinolone Dental Paste	89, 496
Triamterene Capsules	89
Triamterene and Frusemide Tablets	89
Triamterene and	
Hydrochlorothiazide Tablets	59
Triangular Bandage, Calico	105, 499
Triclofos	
Elixir	89
Oral Solution	89
Tricotex	122
Trifluoperazine	
Capsules	89
Tablets	89

Page

Trimeprazine
 Elixir Paediatric 90
  Paediatric Strong 90
 Oral Solution Paediatric 90
  Paediatric Strong 90
 Tablets 90
Trimethoprim
 Suspension 90
 Tablets 90
Trimethoprim and Sulphamethoxazole
 Mixture 59
 Oral Suspension 59
Trimipramine
 Capsules 90
 Tablets 90
Trinitrin Tablets 67
Trisodium Citrate 86
Trousers, Polythene, Disposable 153
Trusses 165-166
 Elastic Band 166
 Spring 165
 Umbilical "Belts" Infants 166
 Understrap, Replacement and
  Repairs 165
 Dispensing Fees, Appliance Contractor 29
 Professional Fees, Pharmacy Contractors 16
Tubifast 156
Tubigrip 155
Tubing
 Incontinence 167
 Plastics 119
 Stoma 223
Tubipad 156
Tubular Bandage 105
Tulle Dressings 141-142
Tulle Gras Dressing 140
Turpentine
 Liniment 90
 Oil 90

U

Ultra Four Bandages 102
Ultrabase 497
Understraps, Rubber (Suprapubic Belts) 157
Unguentum Merck 497
Unmedicated Gauze 139
Urethral Catheters 107-115, 499
Urgent Dispensing
 Professional Fees, Pharmacy Contractors 17
Urinals
 Portable, See Incontinence Systems 167
 Rubber (Suprapubic) 157
Urine Sugar Analysis Set 166
 Droppers 165
 Nurse Prescribable 499
 Professional Fees, Pharmacy
  Contractors 16
 Solution Tablets 383
 Test Tubes 163

Page

Urostomy Appliances 223
 Professional Fees, Pharmacy
  Contractors 16
Ursodeoxycholic Acid
 Capsules 90
 Tablets 90

V

Vaginal Applicator
 Durex 97
 Ortho 97
Vaginal Contraceptive
 Applicators 97
 Caps 118
 Diaphragm 119
Vaginal Pipe Spare, for Enema Syringe 162
Valaciclovir Tablets 90
Valerian Simple Tincture 90
Vapour-Permeable
 Adhesive Film Dressing 123-124, 499
 Waterproof Plastic
  Wound Dressing 126, 499
Varex Short Stretch Bandage 104
Varico Leg Bandage (See Elastic
 Web Bandage with Foot Loop) 100
V.e.c. High Compression Bandage 101, 499
Vecche Bandage 101, 499
Velband Bandage 102, 104
Velosef Capsules 42
Venlafaxine Tablets 90
Venticaire Mask 396-398
Ventide Rotahaler 149
Ventimask 396-398
Ventolin Rotahaler 149
Verapamil Tablets 90
Verapamil Hydrochloride
 Capsules 90
 Tablets 90
Vernaid Dressing Pack 123
Vest, Polythene, Disposable 153
Vigabatrin
 Oral Powder Sachets 91
 Tablets 91
Vimule Cap 118
Viscopaste PB7 105
Viscose and Elastomer Knitted Bandage 100
Viscose & Nylon Stretch Bandage 103
Viscose, Elastane and Cotton
 Compression Bandage 101
Viscose Dressing Sterile Knitted 121
Viscose Gauze 140
Vitalograph 149-151
Vitamin Capsules 91
Vitamin A and D Capsules 91
Vitamin B Tablets Compound 91
Vitamin B Tablets Compound Strong 91, 496
Vitamin B and C Injections 91
Vitamin B1 Tablets 88
Vitamin B12 Tablets 59
Vitamin C 48
 Tablets 48, 495

Page

Page

Vitamin E Tablets 89
Vitamin K1
Injection 79
Tablets 80
Vitrellae *(See Under Separate Names)*
Volumatic *See:- Aerosol*
Inhalation Chamber Devices 98

W

Wadding Cellulose 116
Warfarin Tablets 91
Watch Spring Pessary 152
Water for Injections 91
Water
Purified 44, 83
Potable 44
Waters *(See Under Separate Names)*
Weights and Measures (Equivalents
For Dealing with Drugs)
Regulations 1970 - Requirement
Regarding Dispensing in the
Metric System 8
White Embrocation 91
White Liniment 91
White Petroleum Jelly 79
Whitfield's Ointment 49
Wild Cherry Syrup 91
Wool Alcohols Ointment 91
Wool Fat 91
Wool Fat Hydrous 91
Wool Felt, Surgical 116
Wound Dressings
Elastic Adhesive 122
Plastic 124
Wound Management Dressings 126-134
Nurse Prescribable 499
Absorbent Cellulose 120
Activated Charcoal Dressing 126, 499
Alginate Dressings 126, 499
Cavity 126, 499
Hydrocolloid Dressings 127-129, 499
Hydrogel Dressing 130, 499
Polyurethane Foam Dressing 130, 499
Polyurethane Foam Film Dressing 132, 499
Soft Silicone 132
Wow Bandages 103

X

Xipamide Tablets 91
Xylometazoline
Nasal Drops 91
Nasal Spray 91

Y

Yellow Petroleum Jelly 79

Z

"Zero Deduction" 10-12
Zinc
Ointment 92
And Castor Oil Cream 92
And Castor Oil Ointment 92, 498
And Ichthammol Cream 92
And Salicylic Acid Paste 92
Zinc Oxide 92
And Dimethicone Spray 92
Adhesive Tapes 498
Elastic Adhesive Bandage 100
Impregnated Medicated Stocking 498
Zinc Oxide and Dimethicone Spray 498
Zinc Paste Compound 92
Zinc Paste Bandages 105, 499
Calamine and Clioquinol 105
And Calamine 105
And Coal Tar 105
And Ichthammol 105
Zinc Sulphate 92
Eye Drops 92
Lotion 92
Mouth-Wash 92, 496
Zincaband 105
Zolpidem Tartrate Tablets 92
Zopiclone Tablets 92
Zuclopenthixol
Acetate Injection 92
Decanoate Injection 92
Tablets 92

NOTES

NOTES

NOTES

NOTES

NOTES

NOTES

Printed in the United Kingdom for The Stationery Office
011782027/X C280 11/00 (3840)